CURRENT CONTROVERSIES IN BREAST CANCER

The University of Texas
M. D. Anderson Hospital and Tumor Institute at Houston
26th Annual Clinical Conference on Cancer

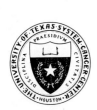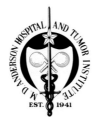

Published for
The University of Texas
M. D. Anderson Hospital and Tumor Institute at Houston
Houston, Texas, by the University of Texas Press, Austin

The University of Texas
M. D. Anderson Hospital and Tumor Institute at Houston
26th Annual Clinical Conference on Cancer

Current Controversies in Breast Cancer

Edited by

Frederick C. Ames, M.D.
Department of General Surgery
The University of Texas
M. D. Anderson Hospital and
Tumor Institute at Houston
Houston, Texas

George R. Blumenschein, M.D.
Department of Internal Medicine
The University of Texas
M. D. Anderson Hospital and
Tumor Institute at Houston
Houston, Texas

Eleanor D. Montague, M.D.
Department of Radiotherapy
The University of Texas
M. D. Anderson Hospital and
Tumor Institute at Houston
Houston, Texas

University of Texas Press, Austin

This volume is a compilation of the proceedings of The University of Texas M.D. Anderson Hospital and Tumor Institute at Houston's 26th Annual Clinical Conference on Cancer, held November 3–5, 1982, in Houston, Texas.

The material contained in this volume was submitted as previously unpublished material, except in instances in which credit has been given to the source from which some of the illustrative material was derived.

Great care has been taken to maintain the accuracy of the information contained in the volume. However, the Editorial Staff, the University of Texas, and the University of Texas Press cannot be held responsible for errors or for any consequences arising from the use of the information contained herein.

Library of Congress Cataloging in Publication Data
Clinical Conference on Cancer (26th : 1982 : M. D.
   Anderson Hospital and Tumor Institute)
   Current controversies in breast cancer.
   Conference held Nov. 3–5, 1982, in Houston, Tex.
   Includes bibliographical references and index.
   1. Breast—Cancer—Congresses.   I. Ames, Frederick C.
II. Montague, Eleanor D.   III. Blumenschein, George R.
IV. M. D. Anderson Hospital and Tumor Institute.
V. Title.
RC280.B8C58   1982   616.99′449   83-23320
ISBN 0-292-71093-3

Preface

Today's physician is presented with a confusing array of data regarding the management of breast cancer. Some questions are now being argued that concern: (1) the efficacy of lesser surgery, (2) the use of pre- or postoperative irradiation, (3) the use of chemotherapy combinations with or without hormonal therapy, (4) the role of dietary supplements to prevent a screening technique, and (5) the use of appropriate laboratory tests, serological markers, nuclear scans, and radiographs to follow the patients with diagnoses of breast cancer. These are but a few of the many dilemmas facing the physician.

The following chapters discuss the multiple phases of the management of breast cancer and shed some light, wherever possible, on the current state of the art at each stage of the decision-making process for the management of this disease.

We are privileged in having acknowledged experts in the fields of epidemiology, diagnostic radiology, radiation therapy, nuclear medicine, laboratory medicine, pathology, surgery, and medical oncology to discuss these multiple aspects of breast cancer. One of the leaders in breast cancer research has been appropriately chosen for the Heath Award; Dr. Bernard Fisher's elegant discussion on the biological observations of breast cancer is one of the outstanding features of this text. Dr. Bonadonna's discussion of the principles of adjuvant chemotherapy appears as the final chapter. This is a most appropriate and significant chapter in honor of one of the outstanding clinical investigators in medical oncology, Jeffrey Gottlieb.

Acknowledgments

We would like to extend our appreciation to all who made the 26th Annual Clinical Conference on Cancer and the publication of this monograph possible. Our special thanks go to the American Cancer Society, Texas Division, Inc., for cosponsoring the conference and to the Texas Society of Pathologists for cosponsoring the 15th Annual Special Pathology Program, held in conjunction with the 26th Annual Clinical Conference on Cancer. For additional support, we would like to thank the following contributors: American Cyanamid Company; Lederle Laboratories, American Cyanamid Company; Bristol Laboratories, Inc., Bristol-Myers Company; Stuart Pharmaceuticals, ICI Americas Inc.; Mead Johnson Pharmaceutical Division, Mead Johnson & Company; and Miles Pharmaceuticals, Miles Laboratories, Inc. We are grateful for support provided for annual clinical and pathology awards and lectureships, including the Heath Memorial Award, established by former University of Texas Board of Regents Chairman William W. Heath and Mavis B. Heath in honor of the former Chairman's brothers, and the William O. Russell lectureship, endowed by Joanne Vandenberge Hill.

For planning and preparation of the conference, we wish to thank members of the Program Committee: Herbert A. Fritsche, Ph.D., Department of Laboratory Medicine, H. Stephen Gallager, M.D., Department of Pathology, and Herman I. Libshitz, M.D., Department of Diagnostic Radiology, all of The University of Texas M.D. Anderson Hospital and Tumor Institute at Houston. We also wish to thank the following representatives of various UT M.D. Anderson Hospital departments who participated in the preparation of the conference: Frances Goff, Coordinator Emeritus for Conference Services; Jeff Rasco, Coordinator for Conference Services/Accreditation and Documentation; E.R. Gilley, Vice President for Administration and Finance; C. Stratton Hill, M.D., Department of Internal Medicine; Glenn R. Knotts, Ph.D., Executive Editor of *The Cancer Bulletin*; Joseph T. Painter, Vice President for Planning and Extramural Programs; and Stephen C. Stuyck, Director of Public Information and Education and Assistant to the President.

For compiling and editing this volume, we are again grateful to the Department of Scientific Publications, UT M.D. Anderson Hospital. We especially wish to thank Dorothy Beane, Department Head, and Margaret Small, Editor, who was assisted by Douglas Rowlett, Editor, and Sally Hartline, Editorial Assistant.

Contents

Adjunctive Therapy

Imaging and Tumor Markers

Stage IV Disease

Newer Surgical Aspects of Breast Oncology

Radiation Oncology and Breast Cancer

New Staging and Prognostic Factors in Breast Cancer

Systemic Therapeutic Trials for Stages II and IV Breast Cancer

The Jeffrey A. Gottlieb Memorial Lecture

HEATH MEMORIAL AWARD LECTURE

Current Controversies in Breast Cancer, edited
by F. C. Ames, G. R. Blumenschein, and E. D. Montague.
University of Texas Press, Austin © 1984.

The Role of Science in the Evolution of Breast Cancer Management

Bernard Fisher, M.D.

Department of Surgery, University of Pittsburgh, Pittsburgh, Pennsylvania

A concept of how a particular pathway of science has developed when obtained from a textbook or journal, which is used by each generation to learn its vocation, is likely to be as inaccurate as is the image of a national culture gleaned from a tourist brochure. Science is usually documented in textbooks as a collection of facts, methods, and currently accepted theories. There is little or no description of scientific development that relates to the incremental process by which information has been added or to the obstacles that have retarded its accumulation. A portrayal of the developmental pathways of the physical sciences would describe the transitions from paradigm to paradigm occurring as the result of scientific revolutions. That approach is equally appropriate to depict the development of components of the biological sciences. The purpose of this presentation is to provide an overview of the developmental pathway associated with the therapy of breast cancer and to examine whether it too has evolved and continues to progress as the result of paradigmatic changes—revolutions that are the products of scientific investigation—or whether it is a consequence of conjuries of observations carried out in random or near random fashion. Despite the constraint of time and the limited perspective of a single individual, it is hoped that this overview will place into focus the dynamics of a process that has led to the present state of affairs relative to breast cancer management and that it will provide an insight into the subject that cannot be gleaned from conventional sources. No detailed data review that can serve as a source for therapeutic recipes will be presented.

THE HALSTEDIAN HYPOTHESIS

Development

The first true paradigm for primary breast cancer therapy came from the fertile mind of William S. Halsted, who 92 years ago synthesized the "Halstedian" hypothesis for cancer management. The hypothesis did not originate because it seemed a better theory than another, unless considered a replacement for the concept of Galen who, in the second century A.D., depicted cancer as a systemic dis-

ease related to excess black bile and beyond cure by operation. Prior to its inception, there was some conceptualization of the nature of the disease based upon
anecdotal information (Fisher 1977). Valsalva (1704) discarded Galenic teaching
and espoused the belief that cancer spread by lymphatics to regional nodes and that
it tended to recur. Le Dran (1757) and Morgagni (1769) assumed that cancer was a
local disease, curable if found sufficiently early. Fact gathering occurred as a random activity during the decade or so prior to Halsted. The findings from those
efforts led him to formulate the anatomical and mechanistic principles recognized
as Halstedian. They provided the basis for both cancer surgery and postoperative
radiation. In effect, around 1880 Halsted wittingly or unwittingly gathered together
a diverse group of findings obtained by others and formulated an hypothesis that had
its expression in the radical mastectomy.

Of particular importance were the findings of Goldman and Schmidt (as cited by
Handley 1922) that cancer cells in blood excited thrombosis. They were of the opinion that the thrombosis destroyed or rendered cancer cells harmless. The report of
Handley (1907) that tumor cells spread along lymphatic pathways by direct extension rather than by embolization had a seminal effect on Halsted's thinking. Finally,
the investigations of Virchow (1863) indicating that regional lymph nodes were
effective filters influenced the evolution of Halstedian concepts.

While I will indicate how the Halstedian hypothesis has been supplanted, it is
important to stress that it was synthesized from principles that were "scientific."
Theories that have been replaced are not in principle unscientific. If one assigns the
term "nonscientific" or "error" to outdated concepts, then scientific knowledge of
today is apt to be judged in the future as nonscience and error as well.

There were surgeons of stature prior to and during Halsted's era who were presenting anecdotal reports of various operative procedures for breast cancer. The
contributions of Gross (1880), Volkmann (1894), Küster (1883), Heidenhain (1889)
and others had little enduring impact because they contained no special concept or
scientific principal that could be the subject for further testing and future investigation. Their contributions were each nothing more than a cul de sac!

Perpetuation

That the Halstedian hypothesis should have resulted in a paradigm for breast cancer management that endured for nearly three quarters of a century seems remarkable. Careful consideration indicates that there was indeed no reason for anything
but a prolonged tenure. (The study of paradigms is what prepares a student for
membership into the particular professional community in which he will practice.)
The Halstedian paradigm became rapidly and universally accepted because of lack
of competition. Indoctrination of others was carried out by ardent and dedicated
proponents. The subsequent practice of the novice was among those who shared the
same rules and standards—the same paradigm—for practice. With such a consensus, it would be unlikely that there would have occurred disagreement over funda-

mentals. Thus, the theory remained essentially unchallenged. Moreover, the paradigm remained intact because there were few substantive challenges to it arising from the results of laboratory and clinical investigation. Findings from studies that were carried out could not be unified to produce a competing hypothesis.

Clinical Challenge

During the 1950s and 1960s and even shortly before, the efficacy of radical mastectomy to fulfill the tenets of the Halstedian hypothesis began to be challenged, at first by a few dissidents and gradually over time by an increasing number. The challenge did not concern the principles upon which the hypothesis was based but rather the question of whether or not the radical mastectomy adequately embodied those principles. If the removal of the entire lymphatic drainage area was of paramount importance, then the radical operation for breast cancer was inadequate, since lymph nodes other than those in the axilla were frequently involved with tumor. A flurry of anecdotal reports by such leaders in surgery as Wangensteen (1952), Margottini (1949), Urban (1952), Dahl-Iverson (Andreassen et al. 1954), Lacour (1967), Veronesi (1967), Caceres (1967), and others (Sugarbaker 1964) appeared; these reports narrated their personal experiences with extended radical mastectomy. In 1970, after an extensive evaluation of the reports, I concluded that the material presented had not demonstrated that the extended radical procedure was more efficacious than the conventional radical mastectomy (Fisher 1970). Despite the large number of patients in many of the studies, the evaluations were inadequate to test the worth of the super-radical operation. Nothing came from those reports that could provide a basis for challenging Halstedian principles. Nothing arose from them that added to comprehension of the disease. There was no research component in those efforts.

At the same time that more encompassing operations were being carried out, others were reporting their experience with operations less extensive than the radical mastectomy. The deviation from radical mastectomy was not because the Halstedian hypothesis was being displaced by new facts or concepts. The change was primarily due to dissatisfaction with the results of the operation. The considerations of McWhirter (1948), who reported his results with simple mastectomy combined with postoperative radiotherapy, best exemplify that attitude. He adopted his "new" therapeutic regimen because of concern that radical operations were not radical enough. They failed to get rid of all tumor tissue in the operative area and that "at the time of operation tissues actually invaded by tumor must often be divided." It was his opinion that, as a result of this trauma, malignant cells would have an increased tendency to disseminate to other sites. Although he appreciated the possibility that such cells could still be liberated from the area of operation when a simple mastectomy was performed, he was of the opinion that they would be trapped by the intact barrier of the axilla. Moreover, since wound healing was likely to take place more rapidly after simple than after radical mastectomy, radiotherapy could be applied with less delay, thus reducing the interval during which cells could be disseminated to distant sites. Those views were in keeping with the mechanistic approach toward both tumor dissemination and eradication. They were not challenging the prevailing paradigm.

Following McWhirter's tampering with tradition, surgeons the world over made known their opinions. Some saw no merit in his findings. Others, seeing an opportunity to break with tradition, uncritically accepted them as proved and adopted simple mastectomy and radiation as their treatment for breast cancer. The great majority maintained a "wait and see" attitude. The 20 years following McWhirter's publication may be characterized as an era best known for its "personal experience" reporting. There were those who used their data to demonstrate that radical mastectomy was still the preferable operation, while others claimed superiority for simple mastectomy.

Again, as with super-radical mastectomy, aside from a demonstration of personal conviction, the plethora of data was nondefinitive. It failed to demonstrate unequivocally whether simple mastectomy was a procedure that should or should not supplant the radical operation. The clinical tests were, almost without exception, "no contests." Only Crile (1961) proposed a new concept that was based on biological considerations. Influenced by the findings of Billingham et al. (1954) and of Mitchison (1955), which indicated the importance of regional lymph nodes in the immunologic response of a host to a transplant, Crile postulated that there might be value in leaving axillary lymph nodes unremoved in breast cancer patients.

While the majority of clinicians were debating the relative merits of radical, super-radical, and simple mastectomy, a few were reporting their experiences with modified radical mastectomy or local excision and radiation. The most ardent supporter (and one of the very few) of the modified radical mastectomy (Patey operation) was Handley (1965). His rationale for that operation was based on his conviction that since the radical mastectomy left behind internal mammary nodes it was not adequate. The use of radiation following modified radical mastectomy would be more rational since the internal mammary nodes would be treated.

The results of local excision of breast tumors followed by breast radiation reported by Mustakallio (1954), and by Porritt (1964), Peters (1967), and Crile (1965), while failing to clearly determine the relative merits of that regimen, did demonstrate that patients could survive for many years free of disease following such treatment. The more recent reports by Calle (1978), Hellman (1980), Prosnitz (1977), Montague (1979), and others (Pierquin et al. 1980) continue to attest to the fact. It is difficult for me to determine the rationale that was employed by the early advocates of the procedure. What seems most certain is that there was no clear biological principal that directed their approach. In many instances, as noted by Mustakallio, the procedure was initially performed for the reason that patients refused to have a recommended radical mastectomy. In a sense, those patients may claim responsibility for the immortality of those pioneers!

Despite the fact that clinical efforts between 1950 and 1970 failed to determine with certainty the relative merits of the various methods for the local-regional treatment of breast cancer, failed to evolve new biological principles, and failed to test the Halstedian hypothesis allowing it to remain the paradigm for breast cancer management, operations of lesser extent were becoming accepted in clinical practice and in some places were considered "standard." As I have said, the retreat from radical mastectomy was more the result of frustration with its inability to fulfill the tenets of the hypothesis than because there were new principles attracting attention.

LABORATORY AND CLINICAL RESEARCH IN THE 1960s

During the time that the anecdotal clinical information was accumulating, we were carrying out a series of laboratory and clinical investigations. Our efforts were directed toward obtaining a better comprehension of the biological process of metastasis. At that time, about 1956, controversy regarding metastatic mechanisms concerned the question of whether anatomical or mechanical factors were responsible for the occurrence of metastases or whether metabolic and biological properties of tissues were responsible. Stimulated by the paucity of investigation and concern regarding the significance of circulating tumor cells disseminated at operation (Fisher and Turnbull 1955), we began to study metastases. No convictions or hypotheses compelled us to embark upon those studies or directed our efforts. We were entirely involved with experiment, driven research, fact finding.

The following highlights findings from a few of the studies carried out by us prior to 1968. The prevailing idea was that lymph-borne tumor cells have one destination—the lymph nodes; that tumor cells in the blood vascular system lodge in the first capillary bed they encounter; and that there is an orderly pattern of tumor cell dissemination based upon temporal and mechanical considerations. Observations indicated otherwise. They revealed that since the blood and the lymphatic vascular systems are so interrelated, it is impractical to consider them as independent routes of tumor cell dissemination (Fisher and Fisher 1966). We found that within minutes, viable tumor cells gaining access to the liver via the portal vein could be identified in lymph coming from the liver. At the same time, using labeled cells, we observed that the residence of a vast majority of tumor cells gaining access to an organ via the bloodstream was transient (B. Fisher and E. Fisher 1967). The findings led us to conclude that patterns of tumor spread are not solely dictated by anatomical considerations but are influenced by intrinsic factors in tumor cells and in the organs to which they gain access. We accepted the thesis that there is no orderly pattern of tumor cell dissemination.

Experiments beginning in 1965 revealed for the first time that regional lymph-nodes (RLN) are not the effective barrier to tumor cell dissemination as proposed by Virchow (1863). Lymph nodes trap red blood cells (RBC) but tumor cells pass through nodes into efferent lymph (E. Fisher and B. Fisher 1966) . They also gain access to the blood vascular system by lymphaticovenous communications in nodes. Additional findings revealed the importance of RLN in the initiation of tumor immunity (Fisher and Fisher 1971) and demonstrated that those nodes may play a role in the maintenance of immunity when tumors of "low" antigenicity are present (Fisher and Fisher 1972). We also demonstrated that RLN cells are capable of destroying tumor cells. This concept indicated that the presence of negative nodes may be the result of such a circumstance, as well as the result of tumor cells traversing nodes; the nodes are not necessarily negative because the tumor is removed prior to its dissemination (Fisher et al. 1974a). In investigations of nodes from women having had radical mastectomies (Fisher et al. 1972, Fisher et al. 1974b), we ascertained that they continued to possess immunological capabilities despite the presence of growing tumors; those capabilities varied in nodes within a patient and between patients, and low-lying nodes differed biologically from those high in the axilla. All these findings indicate that there are biological rather than anatomical reasons why certain nodes contain metastases while others do not. More recently, we obtained evidence to indicate that RLN cells are instigators of a cascade of events giving rise to cytotoxic effector cells of both the lymphoid and myeloid series (Fisher et al. 1977).

Evidence thus indicates that RLN are of biological rather than anatomical importance in cancer. To consider them merely as mechanical receptacles for tumor cells and way stations for further dissemination is an anachronism.

Our studies undertaken in 1958 demonstrated that host factors are important in the development of metastases and that a tumor is not autonomous as was popularly believed (E. Fisher and B. Fisher 1967). We also showed that there are dormant tumor cells and suggested that "cancer cells alive to begin with may be enduringly capable of growth if conditions are favorable" (Fisher and Fisher 1959). Perturbation of the host by a variety of means could produce lethal metastases from dormant cells (Fisher and Fisher 1959, Fisher et al. 1969b). In 1963 we observed that when normal tissue was injected at a site remote from a tumor, growth of tumor at the site of tissue inoculation occurred (Fisher and Fisher 1963). We commented that " . . . there is an almost immediate wide dissemination of tumor cells. These cells may, under ordinary circumstances, fail to grow, but when coming into contact with dead or dying normal cells, a proper microenvironment is supplied for their stimulation and growth." It was considered that local recurrences following an operation were apt to be the result of systemically disseminated cells lodging and growing at a site of trauma rather than of inadequate surgical technique (Fisher et al. 1967). We proposed that a tumor is a systemic disease, probably from its inception. That premise never implied that all patients will develop overt metastases in their lifetime. Conversely, it does not imply that only those with metastases represent the population with disseminated disease. Some tumor cells lodge and develop overt metastases; some lodge and remain dormant never forming tumor microfoci; some form micrometastases that are of no clinical significance; and others are destroyed by the host. The statement that cancer is a systemic disease also signifies that tumors evoke host responses that are systemic in nature.

In the 1960s we adopted the thesis that the RLN is an indicator of host-tumor relations and that negative nodes reflect conditions that, in addition to preventing nodal growth of tumor, also inhibit the occurrence of metastases elsewhere. The lymph node that contains tumor cells is important because it reflects an interrelationship between host and tumor that permits the development of metastases, not because it instigates distant disease.

Concurrently, a series of clinical trials provided new information that raised questions regarding concepts upon which treatment was based. Recurrence and survival was found to be independent of the number of axillary nodes removed and examined (Fisher and Slack 1970), and tumor location failed to influence prognosis (Fisher et al. 1969a).

FORMULATION, TESTING, AND CONFIRMATION OF AN ALTERNATIVE HYPOTHESIS

Results from all of these studies led us to conclude that they were anomalous in that they failed to coincide with the principles of the Halstedian hypothesis. They provided a matrix upon which an alternative hypothesis of breast cancer management could be formulated. That hypothesis, synthesized in 1968, is biological in concept rather than anatomic and mechanistic. Its components are completely antithetical to those in the Halstedian hypothesis (Table 1). While the Halstedian hypothesis, contrary to usual scientific practice, was readily accepted without test of its validity, it was realized that a competitive theory would of necessity require the attainment of credibility before it would attract most of the next generation of practitioners. The opportunity to test the principles upon which the hypothesis was based became available. In August, 1971, a clinical trial was begun to confirm or deny the Halstedian principles of cancer surgery. It was simultaneously testing the validity of the alternative hypothesis. The results of that trial indicated that in patients without clinical evidence of nodal involvement (40% of whom had histologically positive nodes), three distinctly different treatment regimens, —radical mastectomy, total (simple) mastectomy with local-regional radiation, or total mastectomy and removal of nodes that later became clinically positive—yielded no significant difference in overall treatment failure, distant metastasis, or survival after a mean follow-up time of 112 months (8–10 years) (Fisher et al. 1980). There was no significant difference between the two groups of patients with clinical evidence of nodal involvement, including those treated by radical mastectomy and those treated by total mastectomy and local-regional radiation.

The similarity in findings in patients with clinically negative nodes was remarkable, considering that approximately 40% of women subjected to total mastectomy alone had positive nodes unremoved and untreated. Those nodes could have been expected to serve as a source of further tumor dissemination resulting in an increase in distant treatment failure. Just as leaving nodes unremoved was not deleterious, their removal did not adversely affect prognosis, refuting the concept by Crile that leaving behind regional nodes may be beneficial. Once again we observed that tumor location does not influence prognosis. The multiple findings from this study validated the various components of the alternative hypothesis.

During the 1970s, other trials were unwittingly putting the alternative hypothesis

Table 1. *Two Divergent Hypotheses of Tumor Biology*

Halstedian	Alternative
Tumors spread in an orderly defined manner based upon mechanical considerations.	There is no orderly pattern of tumor cell dissemination.
Tumor cells traverse lymphatics to lymph nodes by direct extension supporting en bloc dissection.	Tumor cells traverse lymphatics by embolization challenging the merit of en bloc dissection.
The positive lymph node is an indicator of tumor spread and is the instigator of disease.	The positive lymph nodes are an indicator of a host-tumor relationship that permits development of metastases rather than the instigator of distant disease.
Regional lymph nodes (RLN) are barriers to the passage of tumor cells.	RLN are ineffective as barriers to tumor cell spread.
RLN are of anatomic importance.	RLN are of biological importance.
The blood stream is of little significance as a route of tumor dissemination.	The blood stream is of considerable importance in tumor dissemination.
A tumor is autonomous of its host.	Complex host-tumor interrelationships affect every facet of the disease.
Operable breast cancer is a local regional disease.	Operable breast cancer is a systemic disease.
The extent and nuances of operation are the dominant factors influencing patient outcome.	Variations in local-regional therapy are unlikely to substantially affect survival.
No consideration was given to tumor multicentricity.	Multicentric foci of tumor are not of necessity a precursor of clinically overt cancer.

to further test. A major trial in the United Kingdom employed women with clinical stage I or stage II carcinoma of the breast (Cancer Research Campaign Working Party 1980). A simple mastectomy was performed in all patients without surgical attention to the axillary nodes. Patients either received a course of regional radiotherapy or no further primary treatment, the "watch policy" group. Ten years later no differences have been found between the two groups, findings which lend support to the alternative hypothesis.

A few studies may at first glance be considered nonsupportive since their findings suggest that local-regional treatment of internal mammary nodes affects survival, i.e., that these nodes are instigators of distant disease. Host and Brennhovd (1977) reported that survival of patients with stage II medially located tumors was enhanced as a result of ^{60}CO radiation. The few patients in the study and the questionable comparability of the groups prevents assessment of the findings. Similar problems exist with the observations of Lacour et al. (1976), who noted an improved survival of patients with T_1 and T_2 cancers of the inner or medial quadrants following extended mastectomy. These studies are considered here for the purpose of determining whether their findings lend support to or refute the alternative hypothesis. Two other investigations must be similarly evaluated. The findings by Wallgren (1980) that preoperative radiation results in a better survival of patients with tumors in the inner half of the breast, while of considerable interest, cannot at present be put into proper perspective. It may be that this trial does indeed confirm the alternative hypothesis since the findings may be related to modified host responses resulting from the tumor radiation. Findings from the Guy's Hospital trial are equally uncertain in interpretation (Atkins et al. 1972). The survival rates of patients with clinically uninvolved nodes randomized to receive radical mastectomy or local excision were similar despite a higher incidence of local recurrence in those having tumor excision. These observations seem compatible with the alternative hypothesis. Patients with clinically positive nodes and with wide local excision suffered a poorer survival than did patients receiving radical mastectomy. Since inadequate radiation was employed in the study and local disease, particularly in the axilla, was poorly controlled, the clinical or biological implications of the findings are ambiguous.

It seems that in all of the clinical trials of that period involving radiation therapy the results were sufficiently diverse to preclude formulation of a unifying biological theme that could challenge the alternative hypothesis or that could result in the development of a new concept.

A review of all of the information obtained in the 1970s led to the conclusion that, while there was evidence to confirm the alternative hypothesis, no substantive challenges to it were apparent. It was, therefore, appropriate to set aside the paradigm that was the offspring of the Halstedian hypothesis and accept a new one that was in keeping with the tenets of the alternative hypothesis. There has taken place a transition from one paradigm to another via scientific revolution, just as in the usual developmental pattern of mature science. The current paradigm will be replaced by another in due time if progress is made.

BREAST CONSERVATION

The biological principles embodied in the alternative hypothesis allow for a consideration of breast-conserving operations. The phenomenon of tumor multicentricity, however, remains a limiting factor. As a result of anecdotal clinical information, as well as laboratory and clinical research, there is sound justification to extend the alternative hypothesis so that it includes the premise that multicentric foci of tumor are not necessarily a precursor of clinically overt cancer, which would preclude operations that preserve the breast. The clinical trial being conducted by the National Surgical Adjuvant Breast Project (NSABP) is the only study evaluating the biological importance of multicentricity. Simultaneously, it is retesting the validity of the entire alternative hypothesis.

The objective of trials evaluating segmental mastectomy should not only be to determine whether patients should or should not have that operation. That in itself is a pedestrian objective with little scientific or practical virtue. The challenge is to identify tumor and host characteristics associated with successful use of the operation. We are concerned that if an overall difference between the treatment groups should be found, the less favorable treatment regimen will be completely rejected. Should there be a 10% greater disease-free survival in patients treated by mastectomy, surgeons will be apt to conclude that segmental mastectomy is unjustified in all patients. Similarly, should the group having local excision and radiation demonstrate an overall 10% lower incidence of recurrence in the operated breast than the group treated by local excision alone, radiation therapists will advocate the use of radiation therapy for all patients.

It is important to consider the report from the National Cancer Institute of Milan within the framework of this discussion (Veronesi et al. 1981). Patients with tumors less than 2 cm in diameter and with no palpable axillary nodes were treated between 1973 and 1980 by a Halsted radical mastectomy or a "quadrantectomy" with axillary dissection and radiotherapy to the ipsilateral residual breast tissue. Actuarial curves showed no difference between the two groups. These findings, derived from one subgroup of breast cancer patients, may be interpreted as lending confirmation to the alternative hypothesis. They corroborate the tenet that breast cancer is a systemic disease and that variations of local-regional therapy are unlikely to substantially affect survival. The study fails, however, to provide insight into the problem of multicentricity. Careful examination resulted in uncertainty regarding the rationale for the use of the less radical procedure when it began to be used in 1973. It is unlikely that the Halstedian paradigm had been abandoned. The fact that the Halsted radical mastectomy was the standard against which the new operation was tested and that it was employed unchanged until 1978, when the extent of surgery was slightly reduced with preservation of a large portion of the major pectoral muscle, suggests this. The fact that the quadrantectomy also continued to embody Halstedian principles may be construed as evidence that Halstedian concepts still held sway; they were being modified but not abandoned. The removal in that operation of a large amount of skin and breast tissue, the pectoral fascia, and the pectoralis minor muscle and the performance of en bloc dissection in about 75% of the patients, together with the security contributed by the use of radiation, attests to this. While the results of this study provide a more credible transition bridge from the Halstedian paradigm to the one based on biological principles than do anecdotal reports of experiences with lumpectomy, one cannot extrapolate from it and conclude what the outcome might be if Halstedian principles were truly set aside.

Recent information regarding tumor heterogeneity, receptor content of tumors, and other biological considerations must be taken into account when considering local excision of breast tumors. Increasing evidence indicates that tumor estrogen-receptor (ER) and perhaps progesterone-receptor (PR) content, number of axillary nodes, patient age, pathologic characteristics of tumor, and other variables influence the outcome of breast cancer patients (Knight et al. 1977, Fisher et al. 1981, Fisher et al. 1983b). It would be important to know if patients with ER-positive tumors are better candidates for lumpectomy without radiation than are those with ER-negative tumors. Perhaps radiation is highly efficacious only in the ER-negative group. Treatment with tamoxifen after segmentectomy in ER-positive patients may preclude the need for radiation in this patient subset. These and other questions having biological and clinical importance remain to be answered.

Such findings may never be known if clinical practice is decided by considerations such as the following. "Only a few hundred patients entered into earlier modified radical mastectomy series eased our surgical colleagues into accepting this less mutilating procedure for their patients. How many thousands of cured and non-maimed patients must the radiation therapists of the world accumulate before tylectomy and radiation therapy takes its place as an acceptable method of treatment for early carcinoma of the breast?" Equally inhibitory to the obtaining of knowledge that may be of benefit to humanity is the legislation recently enacted in California and Massachusetts indicating that patients be informed of their options of therapy. There is no dichotomy between preservation of human rights and freedom of inquiry. There must be vigilance to ensure that no conflict occurs between the two.

From a clinical point of view, I believe that the results with local excision of breast tumors are in all probability equivalent to results with mastectomy in certain subsets of patients. In other subsets the results will not be similar; in some subsets, radiation will be of benefit, and in others it will be superfluous. Results from successive clinical trials will determine the correctness of this thesis. In the meantime, however, a variety of factors that have little basis in fact may result in the adoption of local excision and radiation as "standard" therapy.

HYPOTHESIS FOR THE USE OF ADJUVANT CHEMOTHERAPY

Another developmental pathway associated with the therapy of breast cancer is that related to the use of systemic chemotherapy. It originated from an awareness that only by distant disease control could there be an improvement in the outcome of breast cancer patients. That consideration, the observations in the middle 1950s indicating that cancer cells could be found in the circulating blood during surgical removal of tumors, and the findings that chemotherapeutic agents had a favorable effect on disseminated tumor cells in experimental animals (Shapiro and Fugmann 1957) provided the reasons for hypothesizing that the use of adjuvant chemotherapy would lower recurrence and improve the survival of breast cancer patients.

Early Testing

That concept was tested by means of a clinical trial begun in 1958 by the NSABP. It was based on the premise that chemotherapy administered at the time of and for a short period after the operation would destroy tumor cells disseminated as a result of the surgery. The results of that study demonstrated both a decrease in recurrence and improvement in survival in one subgroup of patients (Fisher et al. 1968). The observation in retrospect is of historic importance in that it was the first demonstration that the natural history of breast cancer could be perturbed by the use of adjuvant chemotherapy. It also indicated that there was a difference in patient subset response to a therapy, a prediction of future findings. Disappointment with the overall results, however, led to the conclusion that the hypothesis had not been confirmed. Subsequent events revealed that the hypothesis was still valid, but that the premise upon which the first testing was based was inappropriate. It became appreciated that the killing of surgically disseminated tumor cells was probably less important than was the response of existing micrometastases to cytotoxic agents.

In general, the 1960s were nonproductive. They produced virtually no substantive clinical information that demonstrated that adjuvant chemotherapy was or was not of benefit for adult solid tumors. Advanced disease was the arena for the use of chemotherapy. It was in that forum that evidence accumulated indicating that the use of multiple agents produced greater remission rates than did single drugs. From that information, a rationale evolved that was to influence future trials of adjuvant chemotherapy. At the same time, there was considerable research activity that was also to have significant consequences.

Origins of New Premises

Mendelsohn (1960), and, subsequently, Skipper (1971a) and Skipper and Schabel (1973), defined the concept of a growth fraction in tumor cell populations. During the next few years, Skipper (1971b) provided additional principles that served as a new basis for the use of adjuvant chemotherapy. He (a) quantitated the effects of chemotherapy on cancer cells, (b) demonstrated that cell kill by chemotherapeutic agents follows first-order kinetics, (c) postulated the influence of body tumor burden on the outcome of treatment, and (d) estimated the number of cells remaining in breast cancer patients following operation. Some of the considerations that led us to adopt our clinical trial strategy have been summarized (Table 2). We were in accord with Skipper (1971b) that "it would be foolhardy to expect to hit upon the best drug(s) and best regimens in the first, second, or third clinical trials designed and carried out. Hopefully, such trials could be planned in a manner so that we learn and improve design and end-results in a stepwise fashion." While the prevailing concept at the time was that increasing numbers of chemotherapeutic agents would directly increase therapeutic response, our premise was that since the residual tumor burden would be variable, and it had been suggested by Skipper that tumor cell populations

Table 2. *Kinetic Concepts for Adjuvant Chemotherapy (c. 1970)*

1. Growth fractions and doubling times of primary tumors may differ from those in micrometastases. Consequently, responsiveness to chemotherapy may differ.
2. The magnitude of response of a primary tumor in the plateau of Gompertzian growth need not reflect the response of micrometastases in exponential growth.
3. First-order kinetics relative to cell kill by cytocidal agents apply to those cells with constant growth fractions in exponential growth, i.e., micrometastases of $\leq 10^6$ cells.
4. The degree of synchronization of cell-cycle times of a primary tumor and its micrometastases may differ. On this basis, they may respond to cyclical chemotherapy differently.
5. Ablation of a primary tumor with a resultant decrease in total tumor cell burden may alter the growth characteristics of residual micrometastases. A decrease in tumor doubling time, an increase in growth fraction, and an improved synchronization of cell-cycle times may result. Such changes may enhance the sensitivity of micrometastases to chemotherapy.
6. Micrometastases approaching exponential growth kinetics could be sensitive to single-agent chemotherapy. Consequently, there exists the rationale for first evaluating the effect of single agents as adjuvants.

between 10^6 and 10^7 cells could be amenable to single-agent chemotherapy, it was possible that subsets of patients could be as responsive to single agents as to combinations of drugs. An awakening awareness of the phenomenon of tumor "heterogeneity" also suggested to us the possibility that there might be a variable response to a therapeutic regimen by different patient subsets. There then arose new premises for the use of adjuvant chemotherapy.

Testing During the 1970s

The next decade saw the vigorous testing of the adjuvant chemotherapy hypothesis by means of numerous clinical trials (Fisher et al. 1983a). The results of those studies have been under constant scrutiny and review and have been the subject of continuous comparison. Even prior to the establishment of its worth, adjuvant chemotherapy became the paradigm for the treatment of micrometastatic disease. It is now appropriate to decide whether evidence has accumulated that lends support to the hypothesis that adjuvant chemotherapy is of value and whether new data have arisen that would modify the prevailing hypothesis or establish new premises for future testing. It is also appropriate to consider whether there is evidence that a new paradigm for the treatment of systemic disease is in the making.

Provisional Conclusions

Information from all the major trials indicates that the natural history of breast cancer has been altered. There is justification to conclude that the original hypothesis has been confirmed, but only partially so. The results from a clinical point of view may be disappointing since no "penicillin effect" has been observed. When one considers the empiricism employed in those trials, however, the finding of any positive result seems remarkable. In none was there a preliminary determination of optimal drug dose. The scheduling, length of administration, and decisions concerning drug dose reduction and escalation were arbitrary. Consequently, the results obtained may reflect the application of less than optimal methodology.

Some of the findings in the plethora of data appear to have particular biological importance. It is clearly apparent that there is a heterogeneous response to a particular chemotherapeutic regimen. Some subsets of patients benefit more or less than others. This disparate therapeutic response is concordant with evidence characterizing the biological heterogeneity between and within tumors (Fisher 1980). Results from our own trial indicating that postmenopausal patients with four or more positive nodes are more responsive to chemotherapy than are those who have one to three nodes are inconsistent with the concept that increasing numbers of positive nodes reflect a greater tumor burden and that chemotherapeutic effectiveness is inversely related to tumor burden. As a consequence of these clinical findings, one or the other of those accepted premises must be incorrect. The findings are also discordant when considered in light of the hypothesis relating cell kill to first-order kinetics. In that context, it would have been anticipated that those with one to three positive nodes would have demonstrated better results than those with four or more positive nodes. No available hypothesis (tumor burden, cell kill, drug resistance, etc.) could have been used to predict a priori the unexpected findings.

A major premise upon which the trials of the 1970s were based was that increasing the number of agents in combination would increase the effectiveness of the therapy. It is our opinion that this thesis has not been entirely borne out by the findings. In some subsets of patients, one or two drugs have been as effective as three or five (Figure 1). In others, two, three, or five agents have produced similar results (Figure 2), and in others any number used in combination have failed to demonstrate an effect (Figure 3).

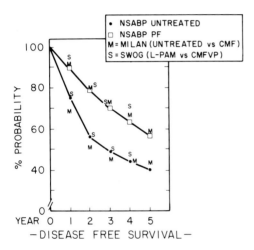

FIG. 1. Comparison of National Surgical Adjuvant Breast and Bowel Project PF with other adjuvant combinations; patients ≤ 49 years. (PF = 1-phenylalanine mustard and 5-fluorouracil; CMF = cyclophosphamide, methotrexate, and 5-fluorouracil; L-PAM = 1-phenylalanine mustard; CMFVP = CMF plus vincristrine and prednisone)

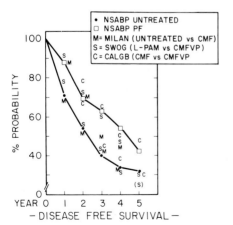

FIG. 2. Comparison of National Surgical Adjuvant Breast and Bowel Project PF with other adjuvant combinations; patients ≥ 50 years with ≥ 4 positive nodes. (PF = 1-phenylalanine mustard and 5-fluorouracil; CMF = cyclophosphamide, methotrexate, and 5-fluorouracil; L-PAM = 1-phenylalanine mustard; CMFVP = CMF plus vincristine and prednisone)

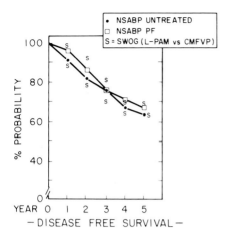

FIG. 3. Comparison of NSABP PF with other adjuvant combinations; patients ≥ 50 years with 1–3 positive nodes. (PF = 1-phenylalanine mustard and 5-fluorouracil; CMFVP = cyclophosphamide, methotrexate, and 5-fluorouracil, vincristine and prednisone; L-PAM = 1-phenylalanine mustard)

To dwell further on those trials and distill from them an overall therapeutic recipe, as I have previously stated, is not the purpose of this report. It is more appropriate to consider them as scientific investigations rather than mechanisms for formulating dicta for a standard breast cancer therapy.

Recent Considerations

Trials carried out in the last decade are almost passé. While they were being conducted, new laboratory and clinical research provided information that modified old premises and gave rise to new ones.

Findings relative to the ER and PR content of tumors have added a new dimension to breast cancer biology. Receptor values are of prognostic importance not only in untreated patients but in patients receiving adjuvant therapy as well. Our own studies indicate that the heterogeneity of response to adjuvant therapy is not only related to the number of positive nodes, age, and tumor characteristics but is also influenced by tumor ER and PR (Fisher 1983b).

A recent concept having important implications is that of Goldie and Coldman (1979). They proposed that the chance of having multiple drug-resistant lines and increasing numbers of drug-resistant cells increases directly with tumor size as a result of the mutation rate of tumor cell populations. That hypothesis provides an explanation unrelated to tumor growth kinetics for the inverse relationship between drug curability and cell number. It, together with the demonstration of kinetic changes in metastases that occur following primary tumor removal (Gunduz et al. 1979), provides a biological hypothesis for the use of adjuvant chemotherapy at an earlier time than is currently employed.

Findings from trials have shown that a population of breast cancer patients is composed of subgroups having different host and tumor characteristics. When a chemotherapeutic regimen is administered, subsets of patients respond to a variable degree or not at all. The therapy serves as a probe that points out differences in subsets utilizing patient response as the marker. Unfortunately, the greater the number of subsets and prognostic variables that are identified, the more difficult becomes evaluation of the outcome of therapy. Sophisticated statistical approaches are required for this purpose. Current methodology may be inadequate, and more complex statistical techniques will require development. It will become increasingly difficult for statisticians to provide data analyses that may be understood and assessed by clinicians responsible for the use of the therapy.

These few examples indicate that the clinical trials employed during the rest of this decade and into the 1990s for chemotherapy hypothesis testing must be based on new and modified premises. Short of an unexpected "breakthrough," which would make this entire discussion academic, those trials will produce results that will require further hypothesis modification, and the cycle of testing will continue. It must be strongly emphasized that in this orderly process we must not become victims of arbitrariness, such as existed in the Halstedian era. We must not be forced into conceptual boxes that preclude speculation and suppress new findings, because they are subversive to an existing paradigm. There must be flexibility that permits retreat and retracing of parts of the past. The use of untreated control groups when indicated and the ability to rapidly adjust to unexpected findings in ongoing studies must take place. It is unfortunate that with accomplishment such flexibility becomes more difficult. The greater the hold a paradigm has on its advocates, the less likely are they to be receptive to change.

At the moment, it seems that despite enthusiasm that has been generated regarding biological response modifiers (interferon) and monoclonal antibodies, investigational findings do not yet allow for the synthesis of a new hypothesis based on those agents that could supplant or modify the one currently in use. It is not unreasonable to predict that in the future the existing chemotherapy paradigm will become displaced by one arising from an hypothesis having a new set of biological principles.

COMMENTS

It is evident that since Halsted there has been an "ebb and flow of the therapeutic tide." Competing forces have continuously played a role in determining the management of breast cancer. For 70 years the Halstedian hypothesis, unproven but nonetheless based on scientific information of the time, provided the paradigm for treatment. The radical mastectomy embodied its concepts. Gradually, during the next 25 years as the flow of less extensive operations increased, the radical mastectomy ebbed in prominence so that by the middle to late 1970s it was the minority operation. This turn of events was primarily the result of anecdotal clinical information that described experiences with unproven operations and was not conceived from new biological information that challenged the credibility of the prevailing hypothesis. By the time a new hypothesis based on biological principles was adequately tested, operations retreating from radical mastectomy had been accepted as "standard" therapy despite their unproven status. As a result of proof of the alternative hypothesis, those previously unproven procedures fortuitously achieved scientific credibility. Once again, clinical practice was in keeping with proven biological concepts, but not for long! Within a short time, anecdotal information, this time supported by populism, began to dictate the use of breast-conserving procedures. Treatment based on a paradigm derived from a scientifically tested hypothesis has again begun to ebb!

The same circumstance has prevailed with the use of chemotherapy. Anecdotal information has influenced practice. The term anecdotalism now has an expanded connotation. It not only signifies acceptance of results from personal experiences, as was the case in the past, but it encompassses findings from ongoing clinical trials that have not reached conclusive endpoints and from poorly designed and implemented trials. Indication that findings have arisen from a clinical trial gives them no more credibility than does the presence of a P value.

There may be argument regarding the relative contribution of science and anecdotalism to the progress that has been made in breast cancer management. That disagreement is of no importance. Our concern must be to define the course necessary for progress to be made in the future. Prior to the inception of clinical trials two decades ago, anecdotalism was the only mechanism available that could lead to therapeutic decision making. It was an acceptable process for evolving breast cancer therapy. It was the "science" of the time. Moreover, comprehension of the disease was so simplistic and narrow in concept that it was not in conflict with science. The consequences of anecdotalism are different today than they were at that time. In its various forms, anecdotalism is now in conflict with properly conceived trials having biological endpoints. While there must always remain the opportunity for reporting clinical observations that suggest new concepts and therapies for proper evaluation, it must be appreciated that those anecdotes, except under rare circumstances, cannot provide proof of the efficacy of a therapy, nor are they able to confirm or reject biological hypotheses. Enhanced laboratory research and clinical investigation employing rigidly controlled scientific principles provide the best course for future progress relative to breast cancer management. The rapidity of the progress depends upon our readiness to accept the discipline imposed by devotion to science. To quote from Lewis Thomas (1977): "From here on, as far ahead as one can see, medicine must be building as a central part of its scientific base, a solid underpinning of statistical knowledge. Hunches and intuitive impressions are essential for getting the work started, but it is only through the quality of the numbers at the end that the truth can be told."

REFERENCES

Andreassen, M., E. Dahl-Iverson, and B. Sorensen. 1954. Extended exeresis of regional lymph nodes at operation for carcinoma of the breast and result of 5-year follow-up of first 98 cases with removal of axillary as well as supraclavicular gland. Acta. Chir. Scand. 107:206–213.

Atkins, H., J. L. Hayward, D. J. Klugman, and A. B. Wayte. 1972. Treatment of early breast cancer: A report after ten years of clinical trial. Br. Med. J. 2:423–429.

Billingham, R. E., L. Brent, and P. B. Medawar. 1954. Quantitative studies on tissue transplantation immunity: Origin, strength and duration of actively and adoptively acquired immunity. Proc. R. Soc. Lond. (Biol.) 143:58–80.

Caceres, E. 1967. An evaluation of radical mastectomy and extended radical mastectomy for cancer of the breast. Surg. Gynecol. Obstet. 125:337–341.

Calle, R., J. P. Pilleron, P. Schleinger, and J. R. Vilcoq. 1978. Conservative management of operable breast cancer: Ten years experience at the Foundation Curie. Cancer 42:2045–2053.

Cancer Research Campaign Working Party. 1980. Cancer research campaign (King's/Cambridge) trial for early breast cancer. Lancet 1:55–60.

Coman, D. R. 1953. Mechanisms responsible for the origin and distribution of blood-borne tumor metastases: A review. Cancer Res. 13:397–404.

Crile, G., Jr. 1961. Simplified treatment of cancer of the breast: Early results of a clinical study. Ann. Surg. 153:745–761.

Crile, G., Jr. 1965. Treatment of breast cancer by local excision. Am. J. Surg. 109:400–403.

Fisher, B. 1970. The surgical dilemma in the primary therapy of invasive breast cancer: A critical appraisal. Curr. Probl. Surg. 7:1–53.

Fisher, B. 1977. The changing role of surgery in the treatment of cancer, *in* Cancer: A Comprehensive Treatise, vol. 6., F. F. Becker, ed. Plenum Publishing Corporation, New York, pp. 401–421.

Fisher, B. 1980. Laboratory and clinical research in breast cancer: A personal adventure. The David A. Karnofsky Memorial Lecture. Cancer Res. 40:3863–3874.

Fisher, B., and E. R. Fisher. 1959a. Experimental evidence in support of the dormant tumor cell. Science 130:918–919.

Fisher, B., and E. R. Fisher, 1959b. Experimental studies of factors influencing hepatic metastases III. Effect of surgical trauma with special reference to liver injury. Ann. Surg. 150:731–744.

Fisher, B., and E. R. Fisher. 1963. Local factors affecting tumor growth I. Effect of tissue homogenates. Cancer Res. 23:1651–1657.

Fisher, B., and E. R. Fisher. 1966. The interrelationship of hematogenous and lymphatic tumor cell dissemination. Surg. Gynecol. Obstet. 122:791–798.

Fisher, B., and E. R. Fisher. 1967. The organ distribution of disseminated ^{51}Cr-labeled tumor cells. Cancer Res. 27:412–420.

Fisher, B., and E. R. Fisher. 1971. Studies concerning the regional lymph node in cancer I. Initiation of immunity. Cancer 27:1001–1004.

Fisher, B., and E. R. Fisher. 1972. Studies concerning the regional lymph node in cancer II. Maintenance of immunity. Cancer 29:1496–1501.

Fisher, B., E. R. Fisher, and N. Feduska. 1967. Trauma and the localization of tumor cells. Cancer 20:23–30.

Fisher, B., J. Hanlon, J. Linta, and E. A. Saffer (with the technical assistance of J. Coyle and C. Ruddock). 1977. Tumor specificity, serum inhibition, and influence of regional lymph nodes on cytotoxic macrophages from cultured bone marrow. Cancer Res. 37:3628–3633.

Fisher, B., R. G. Ravdin, R. K. Ausman, N. H. Slack, G. E. Moore, and R. J. Noer. 1968. Surgical adjuvant chemotherapy in cancer of the breast: Results of a decade of cooperative investigation. Ann. Surg. 168:337–356.

Fisher, B., C. Redmond, N. Abramson, D. Bowman, T. Campbell, R. Desser, N. Dimitrov, R. Frelick, P. Geggie, A. Glass, D. Plotkin, D. Prager, L. Stolbach, J. Wolter, and other NSABP investigators. 1983a. Topics in oncology: Advances in adjuvant chemotherapy of breast cancer, *in* Current Hematology II, Virgil F. Fairbanks, ed. John Wiley & Sons, Inc., New York, pp. 415–446.

Fisher, B., C. Redmond, A. Brown, D. L. Wickerham, N. Wolmark, J. Allegra, G. Escher, M. Lippman, E. Savlov, J. Wittliff, and E. R. Fisher, with the contributions of D. Plotkin, D. Bowman, J. Wolter, R. Bornstein, R. Desser, R. Frelock, and other NSABP investigators. 1983b. The influence of tumor estrogen and progesterone receptor levels on the response to tamoxifen and chemotherapy in primary breast cancer. J. Clin. Oncol. 1:227, 241.

Fisher, B., C. Redmond, A. Brown, N. Wolmark, J. Wittliff, E. R. Fisher, D. Plotkin, D. Bowman, S. Sachs, J. Wolter, R. Frelick, R. Desser, N. LiCalzi, P. Geggie, T. Campbell, E. G. Elias, D. Prager, P. Koontz, H. Volk, N. Dimitrov, B. Gardner, H. Lerner, H. Shibata, and other NSABP investigators. 1981. Treatment of primary breast cancer with chemotherapy and tamoxifen. N. Engl. J. Med. 305:1–6.

Fisher, B., C. Redmond, E. R. Fisher, and Participating NSABP Investigators. 1980. The contribution of recent NSABP clinical trials of primary breast cancer therapy to an understanding of tumor biology: An overview of findings. Cancer 46:1009–1025.

Fisher, B., E. A. Saffer, and E. R. Fisher. 1972. Studies concerning the regional lymph node in cancer III. Response of regional lymph node cells from breast and colon cancer patients to PHA stimulation. Cancer 30:1202–1215.

Fisher, B., E. Saffer, and E. R. Fisher. 1974a. Studies concerning the regional lymph nodes in cancer IV. Tumor inhibition by regional lymph node cells. Cancer 33:631–636.

Fisher, B., E. A. Saffer, and E. R. Fisher. 1974. Studies concerning the regional lymph node in cancer VII. Thymidine uptake by cells from nodes of breast cancer patients relative to axillary location and histopathologic discriminants. Cancer 33:271–279.

Fisher, B., and N. H. Slack. 1970. Number of lymph nodes examined and the prognosis of breast carcinoma. Surg. Gynecol. Obstet. 131:79–88.

Fisher, B., N. H. Slack, R. K. Ausman, and I. D. J. Bross. 1969a. Location of breast carcinoma and prognosis. Surg. Gynecol. Obstet. 129:705–716.

Fisher, B., O. Soliman, and E. R. Fisher. 1969b. Effect of antilymphocyte serum on parameters of tumor growth in a syngeneic tumor-host system. Proc. Soc. Exp. Biol. Med. 131:16–18.

Fisher, E. E., and B. Fisher. 1966. Transmigration of lymph nodes by tumor cells. Science 152:412–420.

Fisher, E. R., and B. Fisher. 1967. Host-tumor relationship in the development and growth of hepatic metastases, *in* Endogenous Factors Influencing Host-Tumor Balance (International Symposium Argonne Cancer Research Hospital, University of Chicago, 1966), R. W. Wissler, T. L. Dao, and S. W. Wood, Jr., eds. University of Chicago Press, Chicago, pp. 149–166.

Fisher, E. R., and R. B. Turnbull, Jr. 1955. Cytologic demonstration and significance of tumor cells in the mesenteric venous blood in patients with colorectal carcinoma. Surg. Gynecol. Obstet. 100:102–108.

Goldie, J. H., and A. J. Coldman. 1979. A mathematic model for relating the drug sensitivity of tumors to the spontaneous mutation rate. Cancer Treat. Rep. 63:1727–1733.

Gross, S. W. 1880. A Practical Treatment of Tumors of the Mammary Gland Embracing Their Histology, Pathology, Diagnosis, and Treatment. D. Appleton & Co., New York, pp. 222–227.

Gunduz, N., B. Fisher, and E. A. Saffer. 1979. Effect of surgical removal on the growth and kinetics of residual tumor. Cancer Res. 39:3861–3865.

Halsted, W. S. 1907. The results of radical operations for the cure of carcinoma of the breast. Ann. Surg. 46:1–19.

Handley, R. S. 1965. The technique and results of conservative radical mastectomy (Patey's operation). Prog. Clin. Cancer 1:462–470.

Handley, W. S. 1922. The inadequacy of the embolic theory, *in* Cancer of the Breast and Its Operative Treatment, A. Murray, ed. P. B. Horber, New York, p. 2.

Heidenhain, L. 1889. On the causes of the local relapses after amputation of the breast. Ann. Surg. 10:383.

Hellman, S., J. R. Harris, and M. B. Levene. 1980. Radiation therapy of early carcinoma of the breast without mastectomy. Cancer 46:988–994.

Host, H., and I. O. Breenhovd. 1977. The effect of postoperative radiotherapy in breast cancer. Int. J. Radiat. Oncol. Biol. Phys. 2:1061–1067.

Knight, W. A., III, R. B. Livingston, E. J. Gregory, and W. L. McGuire. 1977. Estrogen receptor as an independent prognostic factor for early recurrence in breast cancer. Cancer Res. 37:4669–4671.

Küster, E. 1883. Zur behandlung des brustkrebsen. Arch. Klin. Chir. 29:723.

Lacour, J. 1967. The place of the Halsted operation in treatment of breast cancer. Int. Surg. 47:282–287.

Lacour, J., P. Bucalossi, E. Cacers, G. Jacobelli, T. Koszarowski, M. Le, C. Rumeau-Rouquette, and U. Veronesi. 1976. Radical mastectomy versus radical mastectomy plus internal mammary dissection. Five-year results of an international cooperative study. Cancer 37:206–214.

Margottini, M., and P. Bucalossi. 1949. El metastasi lymphoghiandolari mammario interne nel cancro delia mammella. Boll. Oncol. 23:2.

McWhirter, R. 1948. The value of simple mastectomy and radiotherapy in the treatment of cancer of the breast. Br. J. Radiol. 21:599–610.

Mendelsohn, M. L. 1960. The growth fraction: A new concept applied to tumors. Science 132:1496.

Mitchison, N. A. 1955. Studies on immunological response to foreign tumor transplants in mouse: Role of lymph node cells in coferring immunity by adoptive transfer. J. Exp. Med. 102:157–177.

Montague, E. D., A. E. Gutierrez, J. L. Barker, N. D. Tapley, and G. H. Fletcher. 1979. Conservative surgery and irradiation for the treatment of favorable breast cancer. Cancer 43:1058–1061.

Mustakallio, S. 1954. Treatment of breast cancer by tumour extirpation and roentgen therapy instead of radical operation. J. Fac. Radiology 6:23–26.

Peters, M. V. 1967. Wedge resection and irradiation, an effective treatment in early breast cancer. JAMA 200:134–135.

Pierquin, B., R. Owen, C. Maylin, Y. Otmezguine, M. Raynal, W. Mueller, and S. Hannoun. 1980. Radical radiation therapy of breast cancer. Int. J. Radiat. Oncol. Biol. Phys. 6:17–24.

Porritt, A. 1964. Early carcinoma of the breast. Br. J. Surg. 51:214–216.

Prosnitz, E. R., I. S. Goldenberg, R. A. Packard, M. B. Levene, J. Harris, S. Hellman, P. E. Wallner, L. W. Brady, C. M. Mansfield, and S. Kramer. 1977. Radiation therapy as initial treatment for early stage cancer of the breast without mastectomy. Cancer 39:917–923.

Shapiro, D. M., and R. A. Fugmann. 1957. A role for chemotherapy as an adjunct to surgery. Cancer Res. 17:1098–1101.

Skipper, H. E. 1971a. Kinetics of mammary tumor cell growth and implications for therapy. Cancer 28:1479–1499.

Skipper, H. E. 1971b. Some thoughts on surgery-chemotherapy trials against breast cancer, *in* Southern Research Institute Monograph #1, Southern Research Institute, Birmingham, Alabama.

Skipper, H. E., and F. M. Schabel, Jr. 1973. Quantitative and cytokinetic studies in experimental tumor models, *in* Cancer Medicine, J. F. Holland and E. Frei, III, eds. Lea and Febiger, New York, pp. 629–650.

Sugarbaker, E. D. 1964. Extended radical mastectomy: Its superiority in the treatment of breast cancer. JAMA 187:96–99.

Thomas, L. 1977. Biostatistics in medicine. Science 198:676.

Urban, J. A. 1952. Discussion on radical mastectomy in breast cancer with supraclavicular and/or internal mammary node dissection. Proc. Natl. Cancer Conf. 2:243–246.

Veronesi, U., R. Saccozzi, M. DelVecchio, A. Banfi, C. Clemente, M. De Lena, G. Gallus, M. Greco, A. Luini, E. Marubini, G. Muscolino, F. Rilke, B. Salvadori, A. Zecchini, and R. Zucali. 1981. Comparing radical mastectomy with quadrantectomy, axillary dissection, and radiotherapy in patients with small cancers of the breast. N. Engl. J. Med. 305:6–11.

Veronsi, U., and L. Zingo. 1967. Extended mastectomy for cancer of the breast. Cancer 20:677–680.

Virchow, R. 1863. Cellular Pathology (Translated by Frank Chance). J. B. Lippincott Co., Philadelphia.

Volkmann, R. 1894. The results of operations for the cure of cancer of the breast performed at the Johns Hopkins Hospital from June, 1899, to January, 1894. Ann. Surg. 20:497.

Wallgren, A., O. Arner, J. Bergstrom, B. Blomstedt, P. O. Granberg, L. Karnstrom, L. Raf, and C. Silfversward. 1980. The value of preoperative radiotherapy in operable mammary carcinoma. Int. J. Radiat. Oncol. Biol. Phys. 6:287–290.

Wangensteen, O. H. 1952. Super-radical operation for breast cancer in the patient with lymph node involvement. Proc. Natl. Cancer Conf. 2:230–242.

EPIDEMIOLOGY AND SCREENING

Current Controversies in Breast Cancer, edited
by F. C. Ames, G. R. Blumenschein, and E. D. Montague.
University of Texas Press, Austin © 1984.

The Epidemiology of Breast Cancer

Anthony Bernard Miller, M.B., F.R.C.P.(C.)

NCIC Epidemiology Unit, University of Toronto, Toronto, Ontario

"Breast cancer is hormonally mediated and estrogens are the prime agents in tumor expression. . . ." This was the main conclusion of the first of four meetings held by the International Union Against Cancer Multidisciplinary Project on Breast Cancer (Miller and Bulbrook 1980). The role of certain risk factors for breast cancer that are hormonally mediated, e.g. age at menarche, late age at menopause, the protective effect of artificial menopause, the effect of nulliparity and parity, and the effect of age at first pregnancy, is well recognized (MacMahon et al. 1973). However, two aspects of the epidemiology of breast cancer discussed in the 1980 report are still controversial, though further data are now available; these are the role of exogenous estrogens and the role of diet. In this presentation, I shall review both these areas and attempt some resolution, which may aid in the knowledge of breast cancer prevention.

EXOGENOUS ESTROGENS

Oral Contraceptives

In 1980 we concluded that "concern over breast cancer is not a reason for restriction of the use of oral contraceptives" (Miller and Bulbrook 1980). We also warned that findings from all studies of the effects of oral contraceptives will have to be interpreted with caution because of the substantial changes that have occurred in the formulation of oral contraceptives over the years. In addition, we commented that increased risk reported in certain subgroups in some studies of oral contraceptives has not been consistently found after detailed analyses within strata. These caveats still apply. Although the long-term follow-up of some established cohorts continues to show no evidence of increased risk of breast cancer overall (Royal College of General Practitioners 1981, Vessey et al. 1981), subgroups that may have increased risk continue to be reported. These subgroups include nulliparous women (Trapido 1981) and those who use oral contraceptives before first full-term pregnancy (Pike et al. 1981). The elevated risk for the latter subgroup was significant and was possibly mirrored by a nonsignificant elevated risk ratio for women under 35 years old in one of the follow-up studies (Royal College of General Practitioners 1981) and by the finding of increased risk in nulliparous women of Trapido (1981). However, this effect was not confirmed in a special analysis of a case-control study in Britain, where the frequency of women using oral contraceptives before first pregnancy is lower than in California (Vessey et al. 1982).

One of the high-risk subgroups, as suggested by earlier studies, consisted of women who took oral contraceptives and who had previously had benign breast disease. The study of Fasal and Paffenbarger (1975) suggested excess risk of six- to 11-fold for such women if they were long-term (6 or more years) users of oral contraceptives. Lees et al. (1978) largely confirmed this. They found a fivefold increase in risk for recent users with a previous benign biopsy for breast disease, while in such women taking oral contraceptives for 5 years or more, the risk was increased ninefold. Although this issue has not been specifically addressed in the follow-up of the British cohorts (Royal College of General Practitioners 1981, Vessey et al. 1981), in a case-control study of 332 women, aged 45–74 years, with breast cancer and 1,353 controls, Kelsey et al. (1981) did not find such an effect, and, in fact, found no increase in risk for use of oral contraceptives overall. Similarly, in an ongoing case-control study of the Center for Disease Control, in which cases have been identified in eight U.S. locations and population controls sought by random digit dialing, no increased risk for oral contraceptive use overall or in any subgroup has been seen. So far, findings have been reported in 689 patients within the age range of 20–54 years (Layde et al. 1982). In all studies, benign breast disease has been found less often in present or past users of oral contraceptives than expected. However, it is still possible that some who develop benign breast disease and continue taking oral contraceptives are at higher risk of developing breast cancer. Caution over continuing use of oral contraceptives in these circumstances is therefore desirable.

The possibility that a completely different subgroup of women may be at particular risk by continuing use of oral contraceptives was raised by a study of Jick et al. (1980a). They determined the incidence of breast cancer among members of a group health cooperative that maintains computer files of diagnosis and out-patient drug use. Although the incidence of breast cancer was found to be nearly identical in users and nonusers of oral contraceptives age 45 or younger, there was a positive association between current oral contraceptive use and breast cancer in women over 45 years of age. The risk seemed particularly high among current users aged 51–55, in whom, the authors suggest, continuing use of oral contraceptives may have masked the fact that women were no longer premenopausal.

Hence, continuing caution is justified by the possibility that certain subgroups of women may be at increased risk of developing breast cancer if they maintain use of oral contraceptives: Those with benign breast disease and those 45 years of age and older (and perhaps particularly older than 50 years of age). Furthermore, as has been repeatedly stated, the cohorts of women who became users of oral contraceptives have not yet reached the age of maximum incidence of breast cancer.

Noncontraceptive Estrogens

In 1980, we commented that there was cause for concern that the use of non-contraceptive estrogens increases the incidence of breast cancer (Miller and Bulbrook 1980). Only one study in the previous decade had suggested a risk in such use (Hoover et al. 1976), whereas three had found no association (Boston Collaborative Drug Surveillance Program 1974, Casagrande et al. 1976, Sartwell et al. 1977). However, the study of Hoover et al. (1976) showed evidence of a doubling of risk after 15 years of follow-up of a well-identified group of women in one clinic. Since then, four studies have reported a similar association (Jick et al. 1980b, Ross et al. 1980, Brinton et al. 1981, Hoover et al. 1981). All suggest a twofold increase in risk following use of estrogens for menopausal symptoms after a 10- to 15-year latent period. The study of Jick et al. (1980b) also suggests a strong effect for current estrogen use in women aged 45–54 who had had a natural menopause but no increase in risk for estrogen use in women with a previous hysterectomy. Thus, it seems likely that replacement estrogen use does not increase the risk of breast cancer. This suggestion was reinforced by the case-control study of Ross et al. (1980) who found a significant effect of postmenopausal estrogen use in heavy users (relative risk, 2.5) with intact ovaries and no effect in women having had oophorectomy. They also found an interaction in women with intact ovaries with a history of surgically confirmed benign breast disease, who, if they had a high cumulative dose of estrogen, had a risk of 5.7 relative to nonusers with normal breasts. Nevertheless, Brinton et al. (1981) found high risks among women who had received oophorectomy and who used hormones in the presence of other risk factors for breast cancer, including nulliparity, family history (also suggested as increasing the risk of breast cancer in women who take oral contraceptives by Black et al. 1980), and benign breast disease.

Although the relationship of exogenous estrogens and breast cancer is undoubtedly complex, there now seems little justification in questioning the association, in spite of some opinions to the contrary (Meier and Landau 1980). Thus, as we concluded in 1980, prolonged use of these agents, especially at high doses, should be avoided (Miller and Bulbrook 1980). We also suggested that the possible advantages of exogenous estrogens (such as a reduction in senile osteoporosis) should be evaluated in the light of an increase in the risk of breast cancer. Breast cancer is such a common disease that a doubling of risk could have a substantial effect, even in women age 70 or more.

DIET AND NUTRITION

Several lines of evidence now support the importance of dietary factors in association with breast cancer. The first derives from animal experimental studies, which have demonstrated that in the presence as well as in the absence of mammary carcinogens, the incidence of mammary tumors in rats increases substantially with high-fat diets, providing the diet contains a small amount of unsaturated fat (Carroll and Hopkins 1979).

The second type of evidence comes from studies of incidence and mortality (Bjarnason et al. 1974, Hirayama 1977) that suggest that changing environmental factors in a country have increased the incidence of breast cancer. Studies of migrants (Buell 1974, Dunn 1977) suggest that acculturation results in a slow change in incidence over several generations. In Japanese migrants to California, the incidence of breast cancer in premenopausal women has now almost reached that of the Caucasian population (Dunn 1977). The studies of special religious groups (Lyon et al. 1980, Phillips et al. 1980) also suggest the influence of cultural factors on the etiology of breast cancer. Moolgavkar et al. (1980) have shown how changes in incidence in different populations can be related to changes in successive birth cohorts.

The third line of evidence comes from population correlation studies associating breast cancer incidence and mortality with total dietary fat and other nutrient intake. Such correlations have been noted not only in populations of different countries (Drasar and Irving 1973, Armstrong and Doll 1975, Carroll 1975, Knox 1977) but also in populations within a country , as in Japan (Hirayama 1977) or the United States (Enig et al. 1978), though the latter report failed to find the correlation with animal fat that had been found in the international studies. Hirayama (1977) commented that increase in dietary fat intake appears to be the most striking of all the nutritional changes that have been noted in Japan in recent years. Gaskill et al. (1979) have evaluated age-adjusted breast cancer mortality and per capita demand for various foods by state within the United States. They found a positive correlation between breast cancer mortality and milk, table fats, beef, calories, protein, and fat and a negative correlation with egg consumption. Only the associations of milk and egg consumption with mortality from breast cancer remained significant, however, when age of first marriage (as an indicator of age at first birth) was controlled. These two associations also persisted after other demographic and dietary variables, including intake of fat, were controlled. This study thus suggested a special role for dairy products in the etiology of breast cancer. Hems (1978) found that age-standardized breast cancer mortality rates for women of 41 countries during 1970–71 were positively correlated with intake of total fat, animal protein, and animal calories, independently of other components of diet for 1964–66. Differences in childbearing appeared to contribute little to the variation of breast cancer mortality rates between countries. Hems (1980) subsequently evaluated changes of breast cancer mortality for women in England and Wales between 1911 and 1975 in relation to changes in the consumption of fat, sugar, and animal protein one to two decades earlier. The association was strongest for fat and sugar intake one decade earlier. The mortality changes were not related to changes in childbearing. He noted that the social class gradient in breast cancer mortality almost disappeared during the 1950s, rates declining for the upper classes but increasing for the lower. These changes could have resulted from the changes that occurred in the diet of the different classes in the early 1940s.

Schrauzer (1976) and Schrauzer et al. (1977) postulated an inverse relationship between mortality from breast and colon cancer and the consumption of cereals and seafoods. There appeared to be a direct correlation between these cancers and a high intake of fat, sugar, and meat (Schrauzer 1975). Schrauzer suggested that food consumption patterns reflected the selenium content of the diets consumed and postulated a negative correlation between selenium intake of population groups and their mortality from cancer.

The fourth indirect line of evidence comes from data that support the effect of certain risk factors for breast cancer, which are themselves probably nutritionally mediated. The most important of these are weight, height (and the related indices of body mass dependent on height and weight), and age of menarche.

Differentials in weight between breast cancer patients and controls were found in Taiwan (Lin et al. 1971) and in Sao Paulo, Brazil (Mirra et al. 1971). An association of breast cancer with both weight and height acting independently was found by de Waard and Baanders—Van Halewijn (1974) in a cohort study of postmenopausal women in the Netherlands. In a later study, de Waard et al. (1977) computed age-specific curves for different height and weight groups. There was a divergence of the curves in postmenopausal women and the heavier and taller women showed higher incidence levels. However, there appeared to be little independent effect for weight if there was an adjustment for its correlation with height; deWaard (1975) suggested that lean body mass may be the important variable. However, if height is critical (and it is critical to the calculation of lean body mass) and nutritional factors are relevant, they must begin to operate in adolescence or earlier, rather than in adult life (MacMahon 1975).

In a study of anthropometric variables in women with breast cancer, hospital controls without cancer, and women from the normal population, attending a mass miniature radiography unit, Brinkley et al. (1971) found a number of variables including biiliac dimension, weight, sitting height, and biacromial-biiliac ratio as statistically significant in discriminating the cases from the controls. They suggested that women with breast cancer tend to be more masculine in body type.

In a case-control study of 400 cases of breast cancer and 400 neighborhood controls, Choi et al. (1978) found hardly any effect of height but, in postmenopausal women, an effect of weight, as recalled 12 months before diagnosis of breast cancer and at the time of the menopause. The largest difference was in a small group of patients and controls age 70 or older. There were no differences between premenopausal patients and controls. Later Burch et al. (1981) attempted to replicate these findings in women with breast cancer age 65 or older and in controls drawn from the population but only found a small (and nonsignificant) weight differential and no greater effect in women age 70 or more.

Nevertheless, support for the hypothesis of deWaard has come from a study of 1,868 breast cancer patients and 3,391 controls (Paffenbarger et al. 1980). In premenopausal women, lowered risk of breast cancer with higher Quetelet's index was found. In contrast, in postmenopausal women a markedly higher risk of breast cancer associated with increased Quetelet's index was found. Although weight gain between age 20 and the time of interview showed little or no influence on breast cancer risk in the premenopausal women, it was strongly related to risk in postmenopausal women.

Further, in the long-term prospective study conducted by the American Cancer Society (Lew and Garfinkel 1979), a significant trend of increasing mortality from breast cancer with increasing weight index was found. For those with a weight index of 140% or more, there was a mortality ratio of 1.53 in relation to those 90–109% of average weight, in contrast to a mortality ratio of 0.82 for those with a weight index of less than 80% (the severely underweight).

Completely negative findings have also been reported for height and weight. Thus, in a case-control study of 179 newly diagnosed patients with breast cancer and age-matched controls from a population register, Adami et al. (1977) found no difference in the distributions of height and weight or for two different indices for overweight. Further, in a large case-control study using patients with other types of cancer as controls for patients with breast cancer, Wynder et al. (1978) failed to find an effect of weight. Soini (1977), in a case-control study of 122 patients with breast cancer and 534 controls who were 41–60 years of age and were from a breast cancer screening program, found no effect of height, weight, degree of overweight (Quetelet's index), or the product of weight and height. Further, in a population study in which height, weight, the product of height and weight, and body mass (weight per height^2) of females in selected municipalities were used to estimate the correlation of breast cancer incidence with the size of women, Hakama et al. (1979) failed to find any association with these variables. Nevertheless, seeking an effect of nutrition using indirect indicators at the population level is an insensitive approach, and, therefore, this study cannot be regarded as refuting the hypothesis.

As noted earlier, age at menarche is a risk factor for breast cancer, though the effect is relatively weak (MacMahon et al. 1973, Miller 1978). Women with an early age at menarche, especially prior to the age of 12, have the highest risk. There is evidence that body weight and food intake are related to early estrus of rats (Frisch et al. 1975), which supports the hypothesis that a critical body composition of fatness is essential for estrus in the rat, as it appears to be for menarche in the human female (Frisch and McArthur 1974). Hence, if the effect of diet and nutrition on breast cancer is mediated through a hormonal mechanism (Cole and Cramer 1977), this could account for the effect of age at menarche (Miller and Bulbrook 1980).

Petrakis et al. (1981) have investigated nipple aspirates of breast fluid from non-pregnant, healthy women. Cholesterol levels were found to be elevated above plasma levels and to increase with advancing age. Cholesterol epoxide, a carcinogen in animals, was detected in 7 of 17 women, most of whom had high levels of breast fluid cholesterol. Petrakis et al. (1981) hypothesized that high dietary fat may increase the level of cholesterol in breast fluid and produce local derivation of carcinogenic substances, such as cholesterol epoxide.

One of the difficulties of many of the studies performed to date is a failure of the investigators to consider the effect of multiple variables and their interrelationships. Gray et al. (1979), however, attempted in a population-type correlation analysis to evaluate the effect of total fat and animal protein consumption on breast cancer incidence and mortality internationally while controlling for height, weight, and age at menarche. Although this was a study at the "macro" population level, they found that a significant effect of the dietary variables persisted after controlling for the other factors. This suggests that, although some of the effects of diet on breast cancer may be mediated through effects on anthropometric and other risk factors, such as age at menarche, there are more direct effects as well.

The most conclusive evidence should come from dietary studies at the individual level, either of the case-control or cohort type. Difficulties with dietary methodology have tended to inhibit investigations of this type. So far no cohort studies and only four case-control studies have been reported.

One case-control study involved 77 breast cancer patients and corresponding controls (Phillips 1975). The cases were identified from two Adventist-operated hospitals. For each of these cases, two controls, when possible, were selected from hospitalized patients with hernia or osteoarthritis, and one control for each case was selected from the general Seventh-Day Adventist population. Five foods were associated with breast cancer: Fried foods, fried potatoes, hard fat (used for frying), dairy products except milk, and white bread. The relative risks ranged from 1.6 to 2.6, the risk for fried potatoes being the highest and highly significant.

The second case-control study covered four areas of Canada and involved 400 newly diagnosed breast cancer patients and 400 neighborhood controls (Miller et al. 1978). Three different approaches to assessment of diet were used: 24-hour recall, a 4-day diary, and a detailed, quantitative diet history. However, most of the results were derived from the diet history, which covered a 2-month period 6 months prior to the time of interview and thus prior to the point of diagnosis of the cases. The mean nutrient intake, as estimated by the dietary history for six nutrients (total calories, total fat, saturated fat, oleic acid, linoleic acid, and cholesterol), was greater for the cases than the controls. In a risk-ratio analysis, the incidence of breast cancer was most strongly associated in the premenopausal group with total fat intake and was also associated with saturated fat and cholesterol intake. In the postmenopausal group, the only consistent association made was with total fat intake. The risk ratios were low (1.6 for total fat in premenopausal women and 1.5 in postmenopausal women), and there was no apparent dose-response relationship. Using a weighted average for pre- and postmenopausal women, Miller (1978) computed an attributable risk of 27% for total fat intake.

However, in a reanalysis of these data, combining 24-hour recall and the diet history, Howe (1982) has found increasing risk with increasing consumption of saturated fat, significant at the $P = 0.02$ level. This analysis followed the suggestion of Marshall and Graham (1981) that increased precision would follow from calculating the means derived from two or more different relatively imprecise methods.

Lubin et al. (1981) reported the results of a case-control study in Northern Alberta involving 577 women, ages 30 to 80, with breast cancer and 826 disease-free women interviewed subsequently. The questionnaire included information on the frequency with which eight food items were usually consumed and on milk and butter intake. The major sources of animal fat and animal protein were represented. Significant increasing trends of risk with more frequent consumption of beef, pork, and sweet desserts were found. Elevated risks were also noted for the use of butter at the table and for frying with butter and margarine, as opposed to vegetable oils. Risk also increased significantly with increasing indices of consumption of animal fat and animal protein, but not with cholesterol intake.

Graham et al. (1982) have recently reported the analysis of food frequency questionnaires administered to 2,024 breast cancer patients and 1,463 hospital control patients without cancer at Roswell Park Memorial Institute from 1958 to 1965. No association of breast cancer with estimated consumption of animal fat or other dietary factors was reported. However, they used a relatively brief questionnaire not specifically designed to assess the effect of fat intake.

In an indirect attempt to assess the diet of women with breast cancer, Nomura et al. (1978), in the Japan-Hawaii cancer study, compared the diets of 86 Japanese men whose wives had developed breast cancer with those of 6774 men in Hawaii. These investigators assumed a similarity between the diet of husbands and wives. They found that the husbands of the breast cancer patients consumed more beef or meat, butter, margarine and cheese, and corn and frankfurters, and less Japanese foods than the control spouses.

Currently there are two case-control studies supported by the U.S. breast cancer task force in Israel and Hawaii and another case-control study in Recife, Brazil, (Kalache A., personal communication 1982) that are also investigating the association of diet and breast cancer. Further data from case-control studies will, therefore, be forthcoming.

One possible mechanism for the effect of high-fat diets in increasing the risk of breast cancer could be through serum cholesterol or plasma lipid levels or both. However, prospective studies of women who have had cholesterol levels determined have failed to find evidence of an association (Hiatt et al. 1982).

CONCLUSION

Miller and Bulbrook (1980) have pointed out that a population that achieved a 5-year reduction in age at first delivery might achieve a 30% reduction in incidence of breast cancer. They have also suggested that women should be informed that if they plan to have children, and other considerations do not interfere, they should have their first child by the age of 25. However, it seems unlikely at present that major inroads into the problem of breast cancer could be achieved by primary prevention concentrated on these aspects.

However, the two aspects that I have reviewed in this paper, the use of exogenous estrogens and diet, deserve far greater attention, especially the latter. There now seems little doubt that increased risk of breast cancer is a cogent reason for avoiding high dose and prolonged use of estrogens at the time of the menopause. Further, use of oral contraceptives should be avoided in premenopausal women age 45 or older and due caution exercised in contraceptive use in women with biopsy-proven benign breast disease, especially, I would suggest, in those with atypical hyperplasia.

As far as diet and nutrition are concerned, a number of different sources of information now support the association of high fat in the diet with risk of breast cancer. Although further work is desirable to clarify the association, the consistency of the evidence derived from the epidemiologic and experimental studies supports the possibility that the association is causal. Indeed, this evidence, together with similar evidence relating to colorectal and other cancers, has led a committee of the U.S. National Academy of Sciences (1982) to recommend a population reduction of dietary fat intake from the present level of 40% of available calories to 30% of calorie intake. This reduction seems achievable without a major disturbance in dietary habits, is unlikely to be hazardous, and, possibly after a period, will result in a reduction in the incidence of breast and other cancers affected by fat intake.

ACKNOWLEDGMENTS

This work was supported by the National Cancer Institute of Canada.

REFERENCES

Adami, H. O., A. Rimsten, B. Stenkvist, and J. Vegelius. 1977. Influence of height, weight, and obesity on risk of breast cancer in an unselected Swedish population. Br. J. Cancer 36:787–792.

Armstrong, B., and R. Doll. 1975. Environmental factors and cancer incidence and mortality in different countries, with special reference to dietary practices. Int. J. Cancer 15:617–631.

Bjarnson, O., N. Day, G. Snaedal, and H. Tulinius. 1974. The effect of year of birth on the breast cancer age incidence curve in Iceland. Int. J. Cancer 13:689–696.

Black, M. M., C. S. Kwon, H. P. Leis, and T. H. C. Barclay. 1980. Family history and oral contraceptives. Unique relationships in breast cancer patients. Cancer 46:2747–2751.

Boston Drug Collaborative Drug Surveillance Program. 1974. Surgically confirmed gall bladder disease, venous thromboembolism, and breast tumors in relation to postmenopausal estrogen therapy. N. Engl. J. Med. 290:15–19.

Brinkley, D., R. G. Carpenter, and J. L. Haybittle. 1971. An anthropometric study of women with cancer. Brit. J. Prev. Soc. Med. 25:65–75.

Brinton, L. A., R. N. Hoover, M. Szklo, and J. F. Fraumeni Jr. 1981. Menopausal estrogen use and risk of breast cancer. Cancer 47:2517–2522.

Buell, P. 1974. Changing incidence of breast cancer in Japanese-American women. JNCI 51:1479–1483.

Burch, J. D., G. R. Howe, and A. B. Miller. 1981. Breast cancer in relation to weight in women aged 65 years and over. Can. Med. Ass. J. 124:1326–1327.

Carroll, K. K. 1975. Experimental evidence of dietary factors and hormone-dependent cancers. Cancer Res. 35:3374–3383.

Carroll, K. K., and G. J. Hopkins. 1979. Dietary polyunsaturated fat versus saturated fat in relation to mammary carcinogenesis. Lipids 14:155–158.

Casagrande, J., V. Gerkins, B. E. Henderson, T. Mack, and M. C. Pike. 1976. Exogenous estrogens and breast cancer in women with natural menopause. JNCI 56:839–841.

Choi, N. W., G. R. Howe, A. B. Miller, V. Matthews, R. W. Morgan, L. Munan, J. D. Burch, J. Feather, M. Jain, and A. Kelly. 1978. An epidemiologic study of breast cancer. Am. J. Epidemiol. 107:510–521.

Cole, P., and D. Cramer. 1977. Diet and cancer of endocrine target organs. Cancer 40:434–437.

deWaard, F. 1975. Breast cancer incidence and nutritional status with particular reference to body weight and height. Cancer Res. 35:3351–3356.

deWaard, F., and E. A. Baanders van Halewijn. 1974. A prospective study in general practice on breast cancer risk in postmenopausal women. Int. J. Cancer. 14:153–160.

deWaard, F., J. P. Cornelis, K. Aoki, and M. Yoshida. 1977. Breast cancer incidence according to weight and height in two cities of the Netherlands and in Aichi prefecture, Japan. Cancer 40:1269–1275.

Drasar, B. S., and D. Irving. 1973. Environmental factors and cancer of the colon and breast. Br. J. Cancer 27:167–172.

Dunn, J. E. 1977. Breast cancer among American Japanese in the San Francisco Bay Area. Natl. Cancer Inst. Monogr. 47:157–160.

Enig, M. G., R. J. Munn, and M. Keeney. 1978. Dietary fat and cancer trends: A critique. Fed. Proc. 37:2215–2220.

Fasal, E., and R. S. Paffenbarger. 1975. Oral contraceptives as related to cancer and benign lesions of the breast. JNCI 55:767–773.

Frisch, R. E., D. M. Hegsted, and K. Yoshinaga. 1975. Body weight and food intake at early estrus of rats on a high fat diet. Proc. Natl. Acad. Sci. USA 72:4172–4176.

Frisch, R. E., and J. McArthur. 1974. Menstrual cycles: Fatness as a determinant of minimum weight for height necessary for their maintenance or onset. Science. 185:949–951.

Gaskill, S. P., W. L. McGuire, C. K. Osborne, and M. P. Stern. 1979. Breast cancer mortality and diet in the United States. Cancer Res. 39:3628–3637.

Graham, S., J. Marshall, C. Mettlin, T. Rzepka, T. Nemoto, and T. Byers. 1982. Diet in the epidemiology of breast cancer. Am. J. Epidemiol. 116:68–75.

Gray, G. E., M. C. Pike, and B. E. Henderson. 1979. Breast cancer incidence and mortality rates in different countries in relation to known risk factors and dietary practices. Br. J. Cancer 39:1–7.

Hakama, M., I. Soini, E. Kuosma, M. Lehtonen, and A. Aromaa. 1979. Breast Cancer incidence: Geographical correlations in Finland. Int. J. Epidemiol. 8:33–40.

Hems, G. 1978. The contributions of diet and childbearing to breast cancer rates. Br. J. Cancer 37:974–982.

Hems, G. 1980. Associations between breast cancer mortality rates, childbearing and diet in the United Kingdom. Br. J. Cancer 41:429–437.

Hiatt, R. A., G. D. Friedman, R. D. Bawol, and H. K. Ury. 1982. Breast cancer and serum cholesterol. JNCI 68:885–889.

Hirayama, T. 1977. Changing patterns of cancer in Japan with special reference to the decrease of stomach cancer mortality, *in* Origins of Human Cancer. Cold Spring Harbor Laboratory, Cold Spring Harbor, New York, pp. 55–75.

Hoover, R., A. Glass, W. D. Finkle, D. Azevedo, and K. Milne. 1981. Conjugated estrogens and breast cancer in women. JNCI 67:815–820.

Hoover, R., L. A. Gray, P. Cole, and B. MacMahon. 1976. Menopausal estrogens and breast cancer. N. Engl. J. Med. 295:401–405.

Jick, H., A. M. Walker, R. N. Watkins, D. C. D'Ewart, J. R. Hunter, A. Danford, S. Madsen, B. J. Dinan, and K. J. Rothman. 1980a. Oral contraceptives and breast cancer. Am. J. Epidemiol. 112:577–585.

Jick, H., A. M. Walker, R. N. Watkins, D. C. D'Ewart, J. R. Hunter, A. Danford, S. Madsen, B. J. Dinan, and K. J. Rothman. 1980b. Replacement estrogens and breast cancer. Am. J. Epidemiol. 112:586–594.

Kelsey, J. L., D. B. Fischer, T. R. Holford, V. A. LiVolsi, E. D. Moslow, I. S. Goldenberg, and C. White. 1981. Exogenous estrogens and other factors in the epidemiology of breast cancer. JNCI 67:327–333.

Knox, E. G. 1977. Foods and diseases. Brit. J. Soc. Prev. Med. 31:71–80.

Layde, P. M., L. A. Webster, P. A. Wingo, J. J. Schlesselman, and H. W. Ory. 1982. Long-term oral contraceptive use and the risk of breast cancer. (Abstract) Epidemic Intelligence Service Conference, 1982, Atlanta, Georgia.

Lees, A. W., P. E. Burns, and M. Grace. 1978. Oral contraceptives and breast disease in pre-menopausal Northern Albertan Women. Int. J. Cancer 22:700–707.

Lew, E. A., and L. Garfinkel. 1979. Variations in mortality by weight among 750,000 men and women. J. Chronic. Dis. 32:563–576.

Lin, T. M., K. P. Chen, and B. MacMahon. 1971. Epidemiologic characteristics of cancer of the breast in Taiwan. Cancer 27:1497–1504.

Lubin, J. H., P. E. Burns, W. J. Blot, R. G. Ziegler, A. W. Lees, and J. F. Fraumeni, Jr. 1981. Dietary factors and breast cancer risk. Int. J. Cancer. 28:685–689.

Lyon, J. L., J. W. Gardner, and D. W. West. 1980. Cancer risk and life-style: Cancer among Mormons from 1967–1975, *in* Cancer Incidence in Defined Populations, Banbury Report 4, J. Cairns, J. L. Lyon, and M. Skolnick, eds. Cold Spring Harbor Laboratory, Cold Spring Harbor, New York, pp. 3–27.

MacMahon, B. 1975. Formal discussion of breast cancer incidence and nutritional status with particular reference to body weight and height. Cancer Res. 35:3357–3358.

MacMahon, B., P. Cole, and J. Brown. 1973. Etiology of human breast cancer: A review. JNCI 50:21–42.

Marshall, J., and S. Graham. 1981. Use of two observations to reduce distortion in risk assessment. (Abstract) Am. J. Epidemiol. 114:443.

Meier, P., and R. L. Landau. 1980. Estrogen replacement therapy. JAMA 243:1658–1659.

Miller, A. B. 1978. An overview of hormone associated cancers. Cancer Res. 38:3985–3990.

Miller, A. B., and R. D. Bulbrook. 1980. Special report: The Epidemiology and Etiology of Breast Cancer. N. Engl. J. Med. 303:1246–1248.

Miller, A. B., A. Kelly, N. W. Choi, V. Matthews, R. W. Morgan, L. Munan, J. D. Burch, J. Feather, G. R. Howe, and M. Jain. 1978. A study of diet and breast cancer. Am. J. Epidemiol. 107:499–509.

Mirra, A. P., P. Cole, and B. MacMahon. 1971. Breast cancer in an area of high parity. Cancer Res. 31:77–83.

Moolgavkar, S. H., N. E. Day, and R. G. Stevens. 1980. Two-stage model for carcinogensis: Epidemiology of breast cancer in females. JNCI 65:559–569.

National Academy of Sciences. 1982. Diet, Nutrition, and Cancer. National Academy Press, Washington, D.C.

Nomura, A., B. E. Henderson, and J. Lee. 1978. Breast cancer and diet among the Japanese in Hawaii. Am. J. Clin. Nutr. 31:2020–2025.

Paffenbarger, R. S., J. B. Kampert, and H. G. Chang. 1980. Characteristics that predict breast cancer before and after the menopause. Am. J. Epidemiol. 112:258–268.

Petrakis, N. L., L. D. Gruenke, and J. C. Craig. 1981. Cholesterol and cholesterol epoxides in nipple aspirates of human breast fluid. Cancer Res. 41:2563–2565.

Pike, M. C., B. E. Henderson, J. T. Casagrande, I. Rosario, and G. E. Gray. 1981. Oral contraceptive use and early abortion as risk factors for breast cancer in young women. Br. J. Cancer 43:72–76.

Phillips, R. L. 1975. Role of life-style and dietary habits in risk of cancer among Seventh-Day Adventists. Cancer Res. 35:3513–3522.

Phillips, R. L., J. W. Kuzma, and T. M. Lotz. 1980. Cancer mortality among comparable members versus nonmembers of the Seventh-Day Adventist Church, *in* Cancer Incidence in Defined Populations, Banbury Report 4, J. Cairns, J. L. Lyon, and M. Skolnick, eds. Cold Spring Harbor Laboratory. Cold Spring Harbor, New York, pp. 93–102.

Ross, R. K., A. Paganini-Hill, V. R. Gerkins, T. M. Mack, R. Pfeffer, M. Arthur, and B. E. Henderson. 1980. A case-control study of menopausal estrogen therapy and breast cancer. JAMA 243:1635–1639.

Royal College of General Practitioners. 1981. Breast cancer and oral contraceptives: Findings in Royal College of General Practitioner's Study. Br. Med. J. 282:2089–2093.

Sartwell, P. E., F. G. Alethes, and J. A. Tonascia. 1977. Exogenous hormones, reproductive history and breast cancer. JNCI 59:1589–1592.

Schrauzer, G. N. 1975. Selenium and cancer. A review. Bioinorg. Chem. 5:275–281.

Schrauzer, G. N. 1976. Cancer mortality correlation studies. II. Regional associations of mortalities with the consumption of foods and other commodities. Med. Hypotheses. 2:39.

Schrauzer, G. N., D. A. White, and C. J. Schneider. 1977. Cancer mortality correlation studies. II. Statistical associations with dietary selenium intakes. Bioinorg. Chem. 7:23–34.

Soini, I. 1977. Risk factors of breast cancer in Finland. Int. J. Epidemiol. 6:365–373.

Trapido, E. J. 1981. A prospective cohort study of oral contraceptives and breast cancer. JNCI 67:1011–1015.

Vessey, M. P., K. McPherson, and R. Doll. 1981. Breast Cancer and oral contraceptives: Findings in the Oxford Family Planning Association contraceptive study. Br. Med. J. 282:2093–2094.

Vessey, M. P., K. McPherson, D. Yeates, and R. Doll. 1982. Oral contraceptive use and abortion before first term pregnancy in relation to breast cancer risk. Br. J. Cancer 45:327–331.

Wynder, E. L., F. A. MacGornach, and S. D. Stellman. 1978. The epidemiology of breast cancer in 875 United States caucasian women. Cancer. 41:2345–2354.

Current Controversies in Breast Cancer, edited
by F. C. Ames, G. R. Blumenschein, and E. D. Montague.
University of Texas Press, Austin © 1984.

Are Pre- and Postmenopausal Breast Cancer Separate Diseases?

David E. Anderson, Ph.D.

*Department of Genetics, The University of Texas
M. D. Anderson Hospital and Tumor Institute at Houston, Houston, Texas*

The age-specific incidence curve for breast cancer differs from the curves for other cancers in two important respects: 1) Rather than a steady increase over the entire age span it shows a steady increase only to about the time of menopause, then a decline for a few years, and finally a slow increase to old age; 2) western countries or those with a high incidence of breast cancer (e.g. United States, England) show steep increases in incidence after menopause in contrast to countries with inter-mediate incidence (e.g. Finland, Yugoslavia) that show little or no increase. Coun-tries with a low incidence of breast cancer (e.g. Japan, Taiwan) show decreases after menopause. One explanation for these pre- and postmenopausal differences within and among populations is that breast cancer is the consequence of two different etiologies (deWaard et al. 1964, 1969, Hakama 1969, Berndt and Landmann 1969). One etiological type is hypothesized as occurring primarily in the premenopausal period and is thought to be affected by estrogens of ovarian origin; the other type is thought to occur in the postmenopausal period and to be the consequence of es-trogens of adrenal origin (deWaard et al. 1964). DeWaard (1969) further hypothe-sized that the premenopausal type is prevalent in all populations, whether high- or low-incidence populations, while the postmenopausal type is more frequent in the affluent, high-incidence populations characterized by overnutrition.

This hypothesis of two etiologic types is still being debated (deWaard 1979, 1981, Manton and Stallard 1980a, b, Moolgavkar 1980). The role of estrogens is not in dispute nor are their ovarian or extraovarian origins, but the need to postulate a different role for ovarian and extraovarian estrogens in breast tissue is one area of debate; another is that the population differences in incidence of breast cancer at postmenopausal ages, which deWaard (1969) considered as evidence of environ-mental differences, are now attributed to cohort effects (Moolgavkar et al. 1979, 1980, Stevens et al. 1982).

The hypothesis has theoretical and practical importance because it could provide insight into possible etiologic mechanisms, which, in turn, would have bearing on the implementation of effective management and prevention practices. The purpose of the present report is to summarize recent evidence mainly from epidemiologic and genetic studies that relate to the two-disease hypothesis.

EPIDEMIOLOGIC FINDINGS

Risk Factors

A number of factors have been identified that increase a woman's risk of developing breast cancer, such as increasing age, prior breast cancer, prior benign disease, early age at menarche, late age at menopause, nulliparity, late age at first childbirth or pregnancy, increased weight and height, obesity, increased intake of dietary fat, a family history of breast cancer, and exposure to ionizing radiation (MacMahon et al. 1973, Levin and Thomas 1977, Petrakis et al. 1982).

If premenopausal breast cancer were to etiologically differ from postmenopausal breast cancer, then, conceivably, these risk factors could have different effects on the two types of breast cancer. Late age at menopause, for example, might be a risk factor only among patients developing their disease in the postmenopausal period and might have no effect among premenopausal patients. Several studies have investigated this type of possibility. No clear-cut results have as yet emerged. For example, an early age at menarche was identified as being a significant risk factor in premenopausal and not in postmenopausal patients by Stavraky and Emmons (1974) and Vakil and Morgan (1976); however, Choi et al. (1978) reported it to be more important in postmenopausal patients, and Adami et al. (1978), Wynder et al. (1978), and Paffenbarger et al. (1980) noted no important differences between premenopausal and postmenopausal patients. The results from studies investigating age at first pregnancy or at childbirth have been equally variable. Stavraky and Emmons (1974) and Vakil and Morgan (1976) reported that age at childbirth was a significant risk factor in postmenopausal women only, while Craig et al. (1974) and Wynder et al. (1978) found it to be a significant factor among premenopausal women, and Choi et al. (1978), Adami et al. (1978), Frankl (1980), and Paffenbarger et al. (1980) could detect no differences in risk between the premenopausal and postmenopausal women. The results for nulliparity as a risk factor have been similarly variable (Hems 1970, Vakil and Morgan 1976, Wynder et al. 1978, Frankl 1980, Paffenbarger et al. 1980), as they have for age at natural menopause (Hems 1970, Stavraky and Emmons 1974, Adami et al. 1978, Paffenbarger et al. 1980), lactation (Stavraky and Emmons 1974, Craig et al. 1974, Adami et al. 1978, Frankl 1980), and height and weight/height^2 index (deWaard et al. 1964, Stavraky and Emmons 1974, Vakil and Morgan 1976, Wynder et al. 1978, Choi et al. 1978). The results of studies investigating weight as a risk factor have been a bit more consistent; increased weight has been associated with increased risk primarily in postmenopausal patients according to Berndt and Landmann (1969), deWaard et al. (1964, 1969), Frankl (1980), and Paffenbarger et al. (1980), but no such effect was recorded by Vakil and Morgan (1976), Choi et al. (1978), or Wynder et al. (1978). The results of studies of parity as a risk factor were consistent only in that no pre-

and postmenopausal differences were detected by Stavraky and Emmons (1974), Adami et al. (1978), Choi et al. (1978), or Paffenbarger et al. (1980); nor were any detected for oral contraceptive use by Stavraky and Emmons (1974), Wynder et al. (1978), and Paffenbarger et al. (1980).

Some miscellaneous attributes have also been investigated. Hems (1970), for example, in a correlation study on international mortality rates, observed higher correlations between mean annual per capita intakes of total sugar and total fat and breast cancer mortality rates at late ages (65–69 years) than at early ages (40–44 years). In addition, a higher correlation was detected between the population frequencies of blood type A and breast cancer mortality rates at early than at late ages. Contrary findings were reported by Anderson (1971) and Anderson and Haas (1978), who observed a slightly higher frequency of type A only among breast cancer patients who were in the postmenopausal age groups. Blood type ss has also been implicated in breast cancer and notably among premenopausal patients, but this finding was not confirmed (Anderson, 1971, see Anderson 1976 for review). Blot et al. (1977) studied breast cancer mortality in 3,056 counties in the United States. An excess mortality in postmenopausal women was found in the northeastern states while the mortality among premenopausal women was more uniformly distributed over the country. Ovarian cancer mortality and fertility patterns were linked to breast cancer among premenopausal women, whereas German ethnicity, income, and colon cancer mortality were associated with breast cancer mortality in postmenopausal women.

The conclusions of each of the individual investigators, based on all of the risk factors that were evaluated, were as follows: Hems (1970), Craig et al. (1974), Vakil and Morgan (1976), and Choi et al. (1978) considered premenopausal breast cancer to differ from postmenopausal breast cancer. Stavraky and Emmons (1974), Adami et al. (1978), Wynder et al. (1978), Frankl (1980), and Paffenbarger et al. (1980), however, found no consistent differences between the premenopausal and postmenopausal forms of the disease.

The one clear fact to emerge from these various investigations is that the findings for any one risk factor or for all risk factors combined are highly variable. The results provide no convincing evidence of an association peculiar only to premenopausal breast cancer or to postmenopausal breast cancer. This absence of a differential effect could be construed as evidence against the hypothesis that premenopausal breast cancer differs from the postmenopausal form of the disease. However, other possibilities should also be considered. The majority of studies were based on relatively small sample sizes. The number of premenopausal patients, who were in the minority compared with postmenopausal patients in all studies, ranged from only 30 to 118 patients. Only two studies included 300 or more premenopausal patients (Wynder et al. 1978, Paffenbarger et al. 1980). Furthermore, the studies involved methodological differences. Some were case-control studies based on detailed interviews with patients and controls, others surveyed patients and controls using mailed questionnaires. Another correlated international breast cancer mortality with population parity rates, birth rates, etc. The sources of patients and sources and types of controls also differed, as did the criteria for classifying patients and controls into premenopausal and postmenopausal groups. Analytical differences were also involved. So, perhaps some of the variability in results could have stemmed from investigational differences. But, if so, this further suggests that if differences in risk factors do exist between premenopausal and postmenopausal breast cancer, they must be so small as to be virtually undetectable.

Family History

The epidemiologic studies also generated anamnestic data on family history of breast cancer. But unlike the results for the other risk factors, those relating to family history were relatively consistent. Of the eight studies providing such information, five reported higher frequencies of a positive family history of breast cancer in premenopausal than in postmenopausal patients (Berndt and Landmann 1969, Vakil and Morgan 1976, Wynder et al. 1978, Choi et al. 1978, Paffenbarger et al. 1980). In another study, a high frequency was also observed in premenopausal patients, but the study related to any type of breast disease, including breast cancer (Craig et al. 1974). Frankl (1980) detected no difference in the incidence of family history of breast cancer between pre- and postmenopausal patients. DeWaard et al. (1964) found the familial effect to be confined to postmenopausal patients. This finding was used as evidence to support the two-disease hypothesis, because the patients in the postmenopausal groups and with family histories of breast cancer were characterized by obesity, hypertension, and diabetes, thus suggesting adrenal involvement. Breast cancer patients without these characteristics and who were presumably premenopausal patients provided no evidence of a familial effect.

These findings of deWaard et al. (1964) have not been supported by genetic investigations, in which the familial occurrences of breast cancer were based on verified medical reports rather than on anamnestic data. The genetic studies have convincingly demonstrated that breast cancer patients with family histories of the disease are characterized by a significantly earlier average age at diagnosis than unselected breast cancer patients and that this age is generally prior to menopause. The patients with family histories of breast cancer also have a significantly higher frequency of bilaterality than unselected patients, and this excess frequency is much more pronounced in those with diagnoses prior to age 50 than after this age (Anderson 1971, 1977). These two characteristics have genetic significance since relatives of patients with premenopausal or bilateral disease have noticeably higher risks for the disease than relatives of patients with postmenopausal or unilateral disease. For example, the relatives of patients with premenopausal disease had a 3.1-fold higher risk than relatives of controls. Bilateral disease increased the risk to 5.4-fold, and both premenopausal and bilateral disease further increased the risk to 8.8-fold. In contrast, the risks for relatives of patients with postmenopausal or unilateral disease were only 1.2- to 1.5-fold higher than in control relatives (Anderson 1972).

The risks to relatives were also found to be influenced by the type of family history; i.e., the patient had a mother affected by breast cancer, or an affected sister, or an affected grandmother, aunt, etc. The risks were highest when the mother was affected, were lower when a sister was affected, and were lowest when a second-degree relative was affected. The disease was 5-fold more frequent in daughters of mothers with breast cancer than in controls of the same age (Anderson 1974). Subsequent studies showed lifetime probabilities of these daughters developing breast cancer to range from 27 to 32% (Anderson 1977). Disease in patients from these types of families generally developed in the premenopausal period and often bilaterally. When the patient's sister was affected, the risk to the remaining sisters was 2.7-fold higher than that of controls (Anderson 1974), which equated to lifetime probabilities of 11% to 14% (Anderson 1977). The disease in women from these types of families primarily developed postmenopausally and unilaterally. A later study showed that if the disease in both the patient and her affected mother or affected sister developed premenopausally and was associated with bilateral disease in the family, then the lifetime probability for the remaining sisters and daughters developing the disease increased to 50%, whereas when the disease occurred postmenopausally and unilaterally in both the patient and her affected relative, the lifetime risks for the remaining sisters and daughters reduced to lower levels. In fact, the lifetime risks for these women were little different from the expected 7% risk for the general population (Anderson 1982a,b). That a high risk is associated with premenopausal and/or bilateral disease has now been amply confirmed by others (Brinton et al. 1979, Bain et al. 1980, Black and Kwon 1980, Al-Jurf et al. 1981, see Anderson 1982b for review, as well as those summarized in the preceeding epidemiologic section). Adami et al. (1980, 1981) and Tulinius et al. (1982) have also described higher but nonsignificant risks for premenopausal patients.

MATHEMATICAL MODELS

Several mathematical models have been developed in an attempt to explain the clinical, epidemiologic, and genetic characteristics of breast cancer. Few, however, have addressed the issue of two diseases, in which one develops premenopausally and the other postmenopausally, as proposed by deWaard et al. (1964). Bross et al. (1968), for example, proposed a two-disease model to explain the growth and spread of breast cancer, but the two-disease concept related to tumor cells in Disease A having a doubling time less than 1.2 months and those in Disease B a longer interval.

DeLisi (1977) proposed a model that was based on clones of breast cells being distributed among three stages. Normal cells (stage I) were subject to transition into hyperplastic lesions (stage II) and, subsequently, to transformation into clinical malignancy (stage III), with the probability of these developments at each stage being small. This model was applied to cross-sectional incidence data from Norway, Sweden, Finland, Denmark, and Japan, and it provided close fits to observational data. In a general way, it also simulated the effects of menarche, menopause, and pregnancy on breast cancer risk. Rather than pointing to two diseases, however, the break in the incidence curves associated with menopause was considered to reflect a single disease in which growth of breast tissue was influenced by hormonal changes, presumably in ovarian hormones, at menopause. The effect of menopause was proposed to retard transformation of advanced hyperplasia into clinical malignancy (stage II to III), rather than to retard the transition of normal cells to hyperplastic ones (stage I to II).

A somewhat similar but more sophisticated model (in the sense that it incorporated more refined cell parameters) was proposed by Moolgavkar et al. (1980). Theirs was a two-stage model that allowed for the birth, growth, death, and differentiation of breast cells with time; this model also allowed for the transition of normal breast cells, with small probability, into initiated or intermediate cells and the subsequent transformation of some initiated cells into malignant cells. This model was similar in concept to, and in fact incorporated, the two-hit hypothesis of Knudson (1971) that had been proposed to explain heritable and nonheritable cancers.

Moolgavkar et al. (1980) applied their model to age-specific incidence data from six populations at high, medium, and low risk. After adjustment for temporal increases in the risk of breast cancer in all populations, the age-incidence curves were very similar in shape to one another and conformed closely to the shape of the curve generated by the model. The model simulated the differences in risk associated with age at menarche, age at first birth, and age at menopause. It also accommodated the effects of inherited susceptibility, irradiation of breast tissue, benign breast disease, and replacement estrogen therapy, the major aspects of the epidemiology of breast cancer. Like DeLisi (1977), Moolgavkar et al. (1980) saw no reason for postulating the existence of two distinct diseases. They considered breast cancer to be adequately explained by the concept of a single disease that originated from a single cell type under the influence of estrogens, and it mattered not whether the estrogens came from an ovarian or extraovarian source. The break in the age curve at menopause was attributed to involution of breast tissue caused by lessened estrogen stimulation. Their model accommodated the possibility that the incidence curve after menopause could increase or decrease depending on the availability of extraovarian estrogen to support the turnover of breast tissue.

This model has since been applied to lung cancer and has been discussed in relation to experimental carcinogenesis in animals and in relation to the genetics of carcinogenesis in humans by Moolgavkar and Knudson (1981). Day (1982) has used the model to determine whether the promoting effects of hormones on breast cancer are early- or late-stage effects.

Manton and Stallard (1980a) appear to be the only ones to have developed a model in which a premenopausal or a postmenopausal type of breast cancer was specifically assumed to underlie the age distribution of breast cancer mortality. Their model differed from the previous ones in that the parameters were not based on kinetic events of breast tissue but included representations of the time from tumor initiation to death, competing risk effects of other causes of death, and differential susceptibility to each of the two-disease components. Their two-disease model successfully predicted the 1969 age-specific probabilities of death from breast cancer for white women in the age range of 25 to 94 years. The parameter estimates further indicated that premenopausal disease involved seven stages, and postmenopausal disease four stages. The transition rate among the premenopausal stages was twice as rapid as for the postmenopausal stages. The estimates of variability in susceptibility indicated marked skewness for premenopausal disease. These findings suggested that the rapid, early increase in mortality in patients with premenopausal disease was concentrated in a group of highly susceptible individuals. The results were considered to be consistent with epidemiologic and genetic observations in indicating that individual susceptibility, whether influenced by oophorectomy, pregnancy, or family history, was most modifiable early in life.

Earlier, Knudson (1971) had advanced a two-hit model to explain the occurrence of heritable and nonheritable tumors. He hypothesized that all tumors were the consequence of two mutational events. The heritable and nonheritable tumors were identical except that the first mutational event in heritable tumors was genetically programmed; i.e., it was prezygotic, present in every cell including germ cells, and, thus, only a single, second mutational event was required for tumor development. In the nonheritable form, however, two infrequent mutational events were required for tumor development. Consequently, the heritable type would be early and multiple in occurrence in contrast to the nonheritable type, which would be late and single in occurrence.

Manton and Stallard (1980a) applied this proposal to their two-disease model; i.e., premenopausal disease was assumed to require one less event or stage than postmenopausal disease. This constraint led to results basically in keeping with those of their original model, except the prevalence estimate of familial or premenopausal disease increased markedly to 80%. Their original model had provided an estimate of 54%. Both values were noticeably higher than the 30% prevalence of familial breast cancer estimated under the concept of the two-hit model by Knudson et al. (1973), or the 20% prevalence reported by Hems (1970). In the Breast Cancer Detection Demonstration Project, 24% of 276,593 women reported a family history of breast cancer (Baker 1982). One possible explanation for Manton and Stallard's (1980a) higher estimates was that Knudson's (1971) two-hit model was based on heritable tumors being inherited in a dominant fashion; Manton and Stallard, however, considered their model to suggest a polygenic basis for premenopausal disease involving genetic-environmental interactions, while postmenopausal disease involved no genetic component. The lack of a genetic component in postmenopausal disease was contrary to the findings of deWaard et al. (1964), who observed a familial component only in postmenopausal breast cancer and none in premenopausal disease, a feature which they used to distinguish between the pre- and postmenopausal forms of the disease.

Manton and Stallard's (1980a) model has been criticized by Moolgavkar et al. (1980), who deemed it unlikely that ovarian estrogens were responsible for the development of breast cancer in seven stages and extraovarian estrogens responsible for its development in four stages. Furthermore, they saw no reason for ovarian and extraovarian estrogens having different effects on breast tissue, as was implied in the two-disease model of deWaard et al. (1964). Manton and Stallard (1980b) responded by emphasizing that their two-disease model fit the age-specific mortality data, while a single-disease model did not and that models with fewer than four stages failed to fit the data. Manton and Stallard (1980a) and Moolgavkar et al. (1980) criticized the model of DeLisi (1977) on the grounds that the effects of early pregnancy and genetic susceptibility were not realistically modeled, the model was applied to cross-sectional data that may have led to erroneous parameter estimates, and the parameters were difficult to interpret in biologic terms.

GENETIC STUDIES

The two-hit model of Knudson (1971) predicated that heritable tumors would be early and multiple in occurrence. This model has been applied to childhood cancers, namely, retinoblastoma, Wilms' tumor, neuroblastoma, and pheochromocytoma. Carriers of the genes for these diseases were, in fact, found to have an excess of multiple tumors and an early age at onset of disease when compared with patients with the nonheritable forms of the same tumors, as expected with the model. The model also appears to have applicability to adult cancer because they too occur in heritable and nonheritable forms, have early onset, and tend to be multiple or bilateral, as in breast cancer. Recent genetic observations provide added support for the two-hit model, but, at the same time, they provide support for the notion that breast cancer is a heterogeneous disease.

A 50% lifetime risk was reported in a previous section of this paper to apply to women from families with high frequencies of premenopausal and bilateral disease. A probability of this magnitude is highly suggestive of dominant inheritance for some cases of breast cancer. However, not one but at least three, and possibly four, different dominantly inherited clinical entities have now been described with these characteristics. The least frequent of these is the type first described by Li and Fraumeni (1969, 1975) and others. Lynch et al. (1978a) refer to the entity as SBLA syndrome because of the associated occurrence of sarcoma, breast cancer, brain tumor, leukemia, and adrenal neoplasms. Based on a review of published reports, breast cancer in this entity is diagnosed very early in life, at an average of about 35 years; it develops in over 50% of female gene carriers and is characterized by a bilaterality rate of 40–50%. The segregation ratio of the entity in sibships from an affected male or affected female parent has been estimated at 45.6 ± 11%, close to the 50% expected with dominant inheritance (Lynch et al. 1978a).

Another entity is Cowden's disease, which is clinically distinct from the SBLA syndrome. It is characterized by hamartomatous lesions of the skin and oral cavity occurring in association with tumors of the thyroid and breasts (see Brownstein et al. 1978, for references). Over 90% of female gene carriers develop breast tumors. These are first evident in patients at about 40 years of age, while the hamartomatous cutaneous lesions are generally detected in patients at about 30 years of age. Among the women with breast cancer, over 40% develop bilateral disease. The family histories in published reports strongly point to a dominantly inherited basis for this disorder.

The familial association of breast and ovarian cancer is another inherited entity (Lynch et al. 1978b, Fraumeni et al. 1975, King et al. 1980), which is also characterized by early onset and bilaterality (Anderson 1982a). The gene locus for this entity was recently reported by King et al. (1980) to be closely linked to the glutamate pyruvate transaminase (GPT) locus, which has been provisionally mapped to chromosome 10. In contrast, there was no evidence of linkage between the breast cancer susceptibility locus for the SBLA syndrome and the GPT locus or any genetic marker locus.

Still another entity and possibly the most frequent is one not involving any specific associated neoplasm; it is characterized by the familial aggregation of breast cancer. The breast cancers occurring in these types of families have later onset than in the other entities but still occur in the premenopausal period. The bilaterality rate is higher than expected, but not so high as that of the other entities. The breast cancer risks for relatives are of the same magnitude as in the entities involving associated neoplasms (Anderson, 1974).

In addition to these premenopausal, bilateral types, inherited forms of postmenopausal breast cancer or mixtures of pre- and postmenopausal disease have also been reported. One example is Muir's syndrome. This syndrome is characterized by sebaceous tumors developing in association with a variety of internal malignancies, of which cancer of the large bowel is most frequent (Anderson 1980). This disease is also dominantly inherited but differs from the other entities in that the breast cancer is much less frequent and occurs later, usually in the postmenopausal period. Pedigrees without features of Muir's syndrome, but showing postmenopausal breast cancer also have been described (Anderson 1976). A family basis for postmenopausal breast cancer occurring in association with obesity, hypertension, or diabetes was reported by deWaard et al. (1964), an association also observed by Anderson (1970).

COMMENT

The evidence bearing on the question of whether pre- and postmenopausal breast cancer represent one or two diseases is equivocal. Epidemiologic investigations have provided no clear-cut evidence supporting the two-disease hypothesis. Certainly no one risk factor or associated risk factors were consistently found to have different effects in women developing premenopausal versus postmenopausal breast cancer. At face value, the epidemiologic findings favor a one-disease concept.

Genetic studies, however, have provided some evidence of a difference between pre- and postmenopausal patients. Family histories of breast cancer were found more frequently in premenopausal than in postmenopausal patients. Furthermore, premenopausal patients had a higher frequency of bilateral disease, and their relatives had higher risks for developing breast cancer, particularly when the premenopausal patient had bilateral disease (Anderson 1972).

At least four distinct clinicogenetic entities, all inherited in a dominant fashion and characterized by premenopausal and bilateral disease, have now been identified (Anderson 1982a,b). The chromosomal location of one of these entities (breast and ovarian cancer) has been reported as being close to the GPT locus, which has been provisionally mapped to chromosome 10; another entity (SBLA syndrome) did not map to this locus or chromosome (King et al. 1980). In addition, some inherited postmenopausal types of breast cancer are also on record. The genetic evidence, therefore, points to a heterogeneous basis for familial breast cancer.

These hereditary forms are generally considered to constitute only a small fraction of all breast cancer occurrences. The exact fraction is unknown, but Knudson et al. (1973) arrived at an estimate of 30%, not too different from an estimate of 20% reported by Hems (1970) or the 24% noted in the Breast Cancer Detection Demonstration Project (Baker 1982). Manton and Stallard (1980a) provided an estimate of 54%. The fraction, therefore, may well be higher than has been previously assumed. Whatever the fraction may be, hereditary and nonhereditary or sporadic cancers are regarded as being pathologically identical (Moolgavkar and Knudson 1981). In fact, their only difference is that the first mutational event in heritable tumors is genetically programmed, and only a single second event is required for tumor development, whereas in the sporadic form two infrequent mutational events are required for tumor development (Knudson et al. 1973). As such, heritable tumors will be early and multiple in occurrence, while sporadic tumors will be later and single in occurrence, but pathogenetically they should be identical. If familial breast cancer is heterogeneous and if the heritable and sporadic tumors are pathogenetically similar, then it appears reasonable to assume that the sporadic type is also heterogeneous.

A heterogeneous basis for breast cancer has long been evidenced by the different clinical and pathologic types of breast cancer, i.e. lobular, papillary, Paget's, inflammatory, intraductal, mucoid, tubular, etc., and their different natural histories (Haagensen, 1971). The concept of a heterogeneous basis is now being extended to explain some of the variability in response to different therapeutic modalities (Canellos et al. 1982).

Thus, the long-standing evidence of different clinical and pathologic types and the genetic evidence pointing to variable risks and to different clinico-genetic types do not support the concept of a single disease as suggested by the multistage models of Moolgavkar et al. (1980) and DeLisi (1977) or the results from epidemiologic investigations. The available evidence is more in keeping with a heterogeneous disease, but more heterogeneous than implied in the two-disease proposals of deWaard et al. (1964) and Manton and Stallard (1980a).

One reason why breast cancer continues to be a controversial subject could be that the repeated attempts to explain the many vagaries of the disease are made on the basis of a single disease. For example, this approach might account for the lack of progress in understanding the role of hormones in breast cancer as suggested by Cole (1981). Subsequent studies, therefore, might lead to more progress if the concept of a single disease were replaced by the concept of a heterogeneous disease and if the disease were investigated according to its clinical, pathologic, and genetic subtypes or by whatever other classifications would serve to enhance the homogeneity of the patient material.

ACKNOWLEDGMENT

This investigation was supported in part by Grant Number GM19513, awarded by the National Cancer Institute, U.S. Department of Health and Human Services.

REFERENCES

Adami, H. O., J. Hansen, B. Jung, and A. Rimsten. 1981. Characteristics of familial breast cancer in Sweden: Absence of relation to age and unilateral versus bilateral disease. Cancer 48:1688–1695.

Adami, H. O., J. Hansen, B. Jung, and A. Rimsten. 1980. Familiality in breast cancer: A case-control study in a Swedish population. Br. J. Cancer 42:71–77.

Adami, H. O., A. Rimsten, B. Stenkvist, and J. Vegelius. 1978. Reproductive history and risk of breast cancer. Cancer 41:747–757.

Al-Jurf, A. S., L. F. Urdaneta, P. R. Jochimsen, and F. W. Stamler. 1981. Familial bilateral breast cancer. J. Surg. Oncol. 17:211–218.

Anderson, D. E. 1970. Genetic considerations in breast cancer, in Breast Cancer: Early and Late (The University of Texas M. D. Anderson Hospital and Tumor Institute at Houston, 13th Annual Clinical Conference, 1968). Year Book Medical Publishers, Chicago, pp. 27–35.

Anderson, D. E. 1971. Some characteristics of familial breast cancer. Cancer 28:1500–1504.

Anderson, D. E. 1972. A genetic study of human breast cancer. JNCI 48:1029–1034.

Anderson, D. E. 1974. Genetic study of breast cancer: Identification of a high-risk group. Cancer 34:1090–1097.

Anderson, D. E. 1976. Familial and genetic predisposition, in Risk Factors in Breast Cancer, B. A. Stoll, ed. William Heinemann Medical Books, Ltd., London, pp. 3–24.

Anderson, D. E. 1977. Breast cancer in families. Cancer 40:1855–1860.

Anderson, D. E. 1980. An inherited form of large bowel cancer: Muir's syndrome. Cancer 45:1103–1107.

Anderson, D. E. 1982a. Die familiare und genetische pradisposition bei erkrankungen der brust, in Die Erkrankungen der Weiblichen Brustdruse: Epidemiologie, Endokrinologie, Histopathologie, Diagnostik, Therapie, Nachsorge, Psychologie, H. Frischbier, ed. Georg Thieme Verlag, Stuttgart, pp. 1–6.

Anderson, D. E. 1982b. Familial predisposition, in Cancer Epidemiology and Prevention, D. Schottenfeld and J. F. Fraumeni, Jr., eds. W. B. Saunders, Philadelphia, pp. 483–493.

Anderson, D. E., and C. Haas. 1978. Genetic marker study in familial breast cancer, in Tumours of Early Life in Man and Animals, L. Severi, ed. (Proceedings of VIth Perugia Quadrennial International Conference on Cancer) Monteluce, Italy, pp. 537–549.

Bain, D., F. E. Speizer, B. Rosner, C. Belanger, and C. H. Hennekens. 1980. Family history of breast cancer as a risk indicator for the disease. Am. J. Epidemiol. 111:301–308.

Baker, L. H. 1982. Breast cancer detection demonstration project: Five-year summary report. CA 32:194–225.

Berndt, von H., and R. Landmann. 1969. Zwei epidemiologische typen des mammakarzinoms. Arch. Geschwulstforsch 33:157–168.

Black, M. M., and S. Kwon. 1980. Precancerous mastopathie: Structural and biological considerations. Pathol. Res. Pract. 166:491–514.

Blot, W. J., J. F. Fraumeni, Jr., and B. J. Stone. 1977. Geographic patterns of breast cancer in the United States. JNCI 59:1407–1411.

Brinton, L. A., R. R. Williams, R. N. Hoover, N. L. Stegens, M. Feinleib, J. F. Fraumeni, Jr. 1979. Breast cancer risk factors among screening program participants. JNCI 62:37–47.

Bross, E. D. J., E. Blumenson, N. H. Slack, and R. L. Priore. 1968. A two-disease model for breast cancer, in Prognostic Factors in Breast Cancer, A. P. M. Forrest and P. B. Kunkler, eds. The Williams and Wilkins Company, Baltimore, pp. 288–299.

Brownstein, M. H., M. Wolf, and J. B. Bikowski. 1978. Cowden's disease. Cancer 41:2393–2398.

Canellos, G. P., S. Hellman, and U. Veronesi. 1982. Occasional Notes: The management of early breast cancer. N. Engl. J. Med. 306:1430–1432.

Choi, N. W., G. R. Howe, A. B. Miller, V. Matthews, R. W. Morgan, L. Munan, J. D. Burch, J. Feather, M. Jain, and A. Kelly. 1978. An epidemiologic study of breast cancer. Am. J. Epidemiol. 107:510–521.

Cole, P. 1981. Estrogens and progesterone in human breast cancer, *in* Banbury Report 8: Hormones and Breast Cancer, M. C. Pike, P. K. Siiteri, C. W. Welsch, eds. Cold Spring Harbor Laboratory, Cold Spring Harbor, New York, pp. 109–113.

Craig, T. J., G. W. Comstock, and P. B. Geiser. 1974. Epidemiologic comparison of breast cancer patients with early and late onset of malignancy and general population controls. JNCI 53:1577–1581.

Day, N. E. 1982. Epidemiological evidence of promoting effects: The example of breast cancer. Carcinogenesis 7:183–199.

DeLisi, C. 1977. The age incidence of female breast cancer: Simple models and analysis of epidemiological patterns. Mathematical Biosciences 37:245–266.

deWaard, F. 1969. The epidemiology of breast cancer: Review and prospects. Int. J. Cancer 4:577–586.

deWaard, F. 1979. Premenopausal and postmenopausal breast cancer: One disease or two? JNCI 63:549–552.

deWaard, F. 1981. Body size and breast cancer risk, *in* Banbury Report 8: Hormones and Breast Cancer, M. C. Pike, P. K. Siiteri, and C. W. Welsch, eds. Cold Spring Harbor Laboratory, Cold Spring Harbor, New York, pp. 21–30.

deWaard, F., E. A. Baanders-van Halewijn, and J. Huizinga. 1964. The bimodal age distribution of patients with mammary carcinoma: Evidence for the existence of 2 types of human breast cancer. Cancer 17:141–151.

Frankl, G. 1980. Risk factors in breast cancer: Are they important, are they the same in pre- and post-menopausal breast cancer patients? Oncology 37:41–45.

Fraumeni, J. F. Jr., G. M. Grundy, E. T. Creagan, and R. B. Everson. 1975. Six families prone to ovarian cancer. Cancer 36:364–369.

Haagensen, C. D. 1971. Diseases of the Breast, 2nd ed. W. B. Saunders, Philadelphia, pp. 503–516.

Hakama, M. 1969. The peculiar age specific incidence curve for cancer of the breast: Clemmesen's hook. Acta Pathol. Microbiol. Immunol. Scan. 75:370–374.

Hems, G. 1970. Epidemiological characteristics of breast cancer in middle and late age. Br. J. Cancer 24:226–234.

King, M-C., R. C. P. Go, R. C. Elston, H. T. Lynch, and N. L. Petrakis, 1980. Allele increasing susceptibility to human breast cancer may be linked to the glutamate pyruvate transaminase locus. Science 208:406–408.

Knudson, A. G. Jr. 1971. Mutation and cancer: Statistical study of retinoblastoma. Proc. Natl. Acad. Sci. 68:820–823.

Knudson, A. G. Jr., L. C. Strong, and D. E. Anderson. 1973. Heredity and cancer in man. Progress in Medical Genetics, vol. IX. A. G. Steinberg and A. G. Bearn, eds. Grune & Stratton Inc., New York, pp. 113–158.

Levin, M. L., and D. B. Thomas. 1977. The epidemiology of breast cancer, *in* Breast Cancer. Alan R. Liss, Inc., New York, pp. 9–35.

Li, F. P., and J. F. Fraumeni, Jr. 1969. Soft-tissue sarcomas, breast cancer, and other neoplasms: A familial syndrome? Ann. Intern. Med 71:747–752.

Li, F. P., and J. F. Fraumeni, Jr. 1975. Familial breast cancer, soft-tissue sarcomas and other neoplasms. Ann. Intern. Med. 83:833–834.

Lynch, H. T., R. E. Harris, H. A. Guirgis, K. Maloney, L. L. Carmody, and J. F. Lynch. 1978a. Familial association of breast/ovarian carcinoma. Cancer 41:1543–1549.

Lynch, H. T., G. M. Mulcahy, R. E. Harris, H. A. Guirgis, and J. F. Lynch. 1978b. Genetic and pathologic findings in a kindred with hereditary sarcoma, breast cancer, brain tumors, leukemia, lung, laryngeal, and adrenal cortical carcinoma. Cancer 41:2055–2064.

MacMahon, F., P. Cole, and J. Brown. 1973. Etiology of human breast cancer: A review. JNCI 50:21–42.

Manton, K. G., and E. Stallard. 1980a. A two-disease model of female breast cancer: Mortality in 1969 among white females in the United States. JNCI 64:9–16.

Manton, K. G., and E. Stallard. 1980b. Multistage models for carcinogenesis. JNCI 65:215–216.

Moolgavkar, S. H. 1980. Multistage models for carcinogenesis. JNCI 65:215.

Moolgavkar, S. H., N. E. Day, and R. G. Stevens. 1980. Two-stage model for carcinogenesis: Epidemiology of breast cancer in females. JNCI 65:559–569.

Moolgavkar, S. H., and A. G. Knudson, Jr. 1981. Mutation and cancer: A model for human carcinogenesis. JNCI 66:1037–1052.

Moolgavkar, S. H., R. G. Stevens, and J. A. H. Lee. 1979. Effect of age on incidence of breast cancer in females. JNCI 62:493–501.

Paffenbarger, R. S. Jr., J. B. Kampert, and H. G. Chang. 1980. Characteristics that predict risk of breast cancer before and after menopause. Am. J. Epidemiol. 112:258–268.

Petrakis, N. L., V. L. Ernster, and M. C. King. 1982. Breast, *in* Cancer Epidemiology and Prevention, D. Schottenfeld and J. F. Fraumeni, Jr., eds. W. B. Saunders, Philadelphia, pp. 855–870.

Stavraky, K., and S. Emmons. 1974. Breast cancer in premenopausal and postmenopausal women. JNCI 53:647–654.

Stevens, R. G., S. H. Moolgavkar, and J. A. H. Lee. 1982. Temporal trends in breast cancer. Am. J. Epidemiol. 115:759–777.

Tulinius, H., N. E. Day, O. Bjarnason, G. Geirsson, G. Johannesson, M. A. Liceaga de Gonzalez, H. Sigvaldason, G. Bjarnadottir, and K. Grimsdottir. 1982. Familial breast cancer in Iceland. Int. J. Cancer 29:365–371.

Vakil, D. V., and R. W. Morgan. 1976. Pre- and postmenopausal breast cancer: Differences in risk factors, *in* Prevention and Detection of Cancer, Part 1, vol. 2, H. E. Nieburgs, ed. Marcel Dekker, Inc., New York, pp. 1539–1550.

Wynder, E. L., F. A. MacCornack, and S. D. Stellman. 1978. The epidemiology of breast cancer in 785 United States caucasian women. Cancer 41:2341–2354.

Current Controversies in Breast Cancer, edited
by F. C. Ames, G. R. Blumenschein, and E. D. Montague.
University of Texas Press, Austin © 1984.

Histologic Predictors of Breast Cancer: Epidemiologic and Statistical Aspects

William D. Dupont, Ph.D.,* and David L. Page, M.D.*†

*Departments of *Preventive Medicine and †Pathology, Vanderbilt University
Medical School, Nashville, Tennessee*

There is considerable evidence suggesting that benign breast disease is associated with an increased risk of breast cancer. Various authors have demonstrated that women who have undergone benign breast biopsy have a risk of developing breast cancer two to three times greater than that of women from the general population (Table 1). The lesions associated with these biopsies, however, show enormous morphologic and cytologic variability, suggesting that several distinct processes may be involved. In fact, the term fibrocystic disease that is usually applied to most benign breast lesions has little meaning other than "not cancer" (LiVolsi et al. 1978, Rogers and Page 1979, Love et al. 1982). For these reasons, it is of considerable interest to identify reproducible and prognostically meaningful categories of benign breast disease and to determine how breast cancer risk varies within these categories. In this paper, we will review the progress that has been made towards this goal and will discuss some of the histologic, epidemiologic, and statistical problems that make this a challenging and promising area of breast cancer research.

HISTOLOGIC CLASSIFICATION

Histologic abnormalities consist of cytologic changes within individual epithelial cells and variations of patterns formed by groups of these cells. Both of these changes vary in a spectrum from mild alterations through carcinoma. A major challenge in the development of any histologic classification scheme is to subdivide these continua into categories that are broad enough to be reliably diagnosed and yet fine enough to accurately reflect groupings with known malignant potential. In general, histologic patterns of cell groups are more easily identified and more readily reproduced than cytologic ones and have more practical relevance because they have been the standard of practice in surgical pathology of the breast. Nevertheless, cytologic atypia appears to have a parallel effect on breast cancer risk that is similar to its effect on cancer risk within the cervix. It is possible that cytologic atypia can be particularly helpful in classifying borderline lesions.

The epithelium of the female breast consists of lobular units that are connected to the nipple through a network of branching ducts. This structure is roughly analo-

Table 1. *Estimates of Breast Cancer Risk Associated with Benign Breast Biopsies*

Author, Date	Number of Patients	Length of Follow-up (Years)	Relative Risk
Hutchinson et al. (1980)	1356	13	2.2
Coombs et al. (1979)	647	12–20	3.0
Page et al. (1978)	925	18–25	1.4
Kodlin et al. (1977)	2931	7	2.7
Donnelly et al. (1975)	370	14	1.6
Davis et al. (1964)	284	13	1.7

gous to a grapevine: The base of the vine corresponds to the nipple and the grape bunches correspond to the lobular units. The individual grapes correspond to the acini, which are the milk-producing units of the breast. Each acinus secretes milk into a lumen, which drains ultimately into the duct system. The breast epithelium is under continual hormonal assault throughout the monthly menstrual cycle. It responds in a highly complex and individually variable fashion that makes it difficult to distinguish normal physiologic responses from abnormal ones. A strong argument can be made that many "lesions" currently diagnosed as "fibrocystic disease" are, in fact, within normal limits (Halter and Page 1980, Love et al. 1982).

Two often referenced systems for classifying breast lesions are those of Black and Chabon (1969) and Wellings et al. (1975). The system of Black and Chabon associates a two-character alpha-numeric code to each lesion. The first character is one of the letters A through D and indicates the location of the lesion within the breast. Location A refers to the primary ducts and the major interlobal subdivisions. Location B denotes the terminal interlobular ducts. Locations C and D form the lobules themselves. Location C refers to the intralobular ducts, while the D locations are the acini within the lobules. The second digit of the Black and Chabon system refers to the degree of proliferation within the lesion and may take the values 1 through 5: 1 indicating normal, 2 indicating hyperplasia, 3 and 4 indicating atypia, and 5 indicating in situ carcinoma. Their definition of proliferation depends on both morphologic and cytologic patterns but is perhaps based more on cytology.

The system of Wellings and Jensen (Wellings et al. 1975 and Jensen et al. 1976) supports the hypothesis that most lesions traditionally grouped within broad diagnostic categories of mammary dysplasia or fibrocystic disease arise either in the lobules or in the extralobular terminal ducts. [These categories include apocrine cysts, sclerosing adenosis, fibroadenomas, various forms of abnormal lobules, ductal carcinoma in situ (DCIS), and lobular carcinoma in situ (LCIS)]. Wellings et al. refer to a lobule and its associated terminal duct as a terminal ductal-lobular unit (TDLU) (Fig. 1). Their classification scheme includes two different types of atypical lobules (AL), denoted type A (ALA) and type B (ALB). ALA lesions advance toward DCIS as they increase in cell number and atypia. ALB lesions, on the other hand, progress towards LCIS. The ALA lesions are subdivided into five grades labeled, I, II, III, IV, V. These grades are based on both histologic and cytologic patterns and are clearly defined by Wellings and Jensen with the aid of many illustrations. They rep-

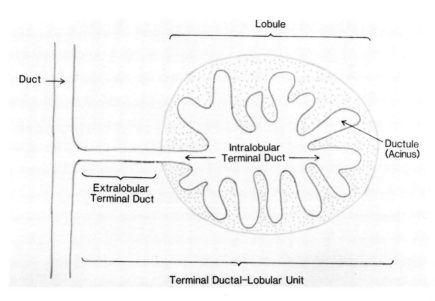

FIG. 1. Schematic diagram of the functional components of the breast epithelium.

resent increasing degrees of hyperplasia and atypia, with ALA-V denoting DCIS. The ALA-I category has also been described by Bonser et al. (1961) as columnar metaplasia. This category is unrecognized by the system of Black and Chabon (1969). Wellings and Jensen also more tentatively proposed a similar grading scheme from I through V for the ALB lesions.

We have been greatly influenced in our own classification scheme by the work of Wellings and Jensen and the concept of the TDLU. In order to facilitate interstudy comparisons, we record their diagnoses ALA-I through ALA-V. The ALA lesions have traditionally been referred to as ductal because the unfolded TDLU resembles a duct in the more extreme forms of this lesion. In view of their origin within the TDLU, however, we prefer to call them lesions of no specific type (NST), as they are neither "lobular" (ALB) nor apocrine.

We have found that the reproducibility of the classification of NST lesions can be enhanced by assessing each lesion according to both quantitative and qualitative factors. We recognize three quantitative subdivisions that describe these lesions' degrees of proliferation. These subdivisions are denoted mild, moderate, and florid. Any biopsy demonstrating an increase of two or more epithelial cells above the basement membrane will be recorded in one of these categories if the pattern of cellular relationships and cytologic criteria are other than those designated as lobular or apocrine (see below). Mild changes refer to increases in cell number that do not cross and do not tend to fill the involved spaces (analogous to ALA-II). When spaces seem to be both distended and filled with cells (small, irregular, cleared spaces separating some of the cells), the florid category is recorded. Moderate hyperplasia stands midway between the others and is characterized by cell groupings

Table 2. *Frequency of Lesions of NST* in a Consecutive Series of 3565 Benign Breast Biopsies*

Degree of Atypia	Proliferative Changes (%)				Total
	None	*Mild*	*Moderate*	*Florid*	
None	1896	909	408	136	3349
	(53.2)	(25.5)	(11.4)	(3.8)	(93.9)
Mild	15	19	63	39	136
	(0.42)	(0.53)	(1.77)	(1.09)	(3.81)
Advanced	6	2	14	58	80
	(0.17)	(0.06)	(0.39)	(1.63)	(2.24)
TOTAL	1917	930	485	233	3565
	(53.8)	(26.1)	(13.6)	(6.5)	(100.)

*No specific type.

that protrude into, and occasionally cross, the involved spaces. The NST lesions are also classified according to qualitative features associated with their degree of atypia. The most extreme form of atypia is that characterized by DCIS. This lesion is defined by the absence of a second cell population, smooth rounded spaces, and round, hyperchromatic, monotonous, evenly placed nuclei. Atypical NST lesions possess qualitative changes in which cellular patterns and cytologic features present some, but not all, of the characteristics of DCIS. Two subdivisions are recognized. Mild atypia includes less severe changes: A pattern often mimicking the type of epithelial hyperplasia frequently seen in gynecomastia. Advanced atypia of NST is a category of severely atypical epithelial hyperplasia of nonlobular type in which some but not all of the features of carcinoma in situ are present. The advantage of classifying NST lesions by both degree of proliferation and degree of atypia is that each degree of proliferation can be associated with each degree of atypia. The relative frequencies with which these different combinations occur are given in Table 2.

Our criteria for diagnosing LCIS are essentially identical to those of Foote and Stewart (1945). The LCIS is characterized by acini that are expanded and distorted by hyperplastic cells. These cells fill and distend the involved spaces. The cells themselves lack any organizational pattern and have specific cytologic features. We also recognize a less severe form of atypia with similar histology that coincides with ALB-III and/or ALB-IV of Wellings et al. (1975) and Jensen et al. (1976). We have not, however, been able to identify criteria for ALB-I or ALB-II that will permit reliable and reproducible classification.

We recognize a form of hyperplasia of apocrine type (Rogers and Page 1979). This characteristic and common alteration of mammary epithelium is usually seen in cystic spaces. When there is a single layer of these cells lining a space, simple apocrine change is recorded. The cells have a large amount of granular eosinophilic cytoplasm and tend to be columnar. There is frequently a rounded protrusion of cytoplasm from the luminal cytoplasmic border (apocrine snout). When these same cells form orderly tufts of cell groups protruding into the luminal space, the diagnosis of papillary apocrine change is recorded. This change is quantitated into three categories. In the mild category, there is no nuclear enlargement and no evidence of complexity of intercellular relationships (no arches or connections between the cells of each individual tuft). In the moderate category, touching of cells between tufts is seen with more complex protrusions of cell groups. In the severe catagory, delicate and prolonged archiform cell groupings are seen approaching the pattern of cribriform or micropapillary carcinoma in situ.

Diagnostic reliability and reproducibility is mandatory in any study of histologic risk factors. For the diagnostic category that produced the least agreement in our current study, two independent reviewers of slides concurred 93% of the time. Resolution of differences was done by discussion during a later simultaneous review using a dual viewing microscope and by reference to our atlas of microphotographs.

EPIDEMIOLOGY

Three basic methodologies have been applied to the epidemiologic evaluation of the cancer risk associated with benign breast lesions. These are the concurrent study, the retrospective case-control study, and the retrospective cohort study. The concurrent study attempts to implicate lesions as being premalignant by assessing the frequency with which they are found in association with invasive cancer. This association is usually contrasted with the prevalence of these lesions in noncancerous breasts obtained at autopsy. One of the most thorough studies of this type was that of Wellings et al. (1975), which we discussed in the previous section. These studies suggest that atypical proliferative breast lesions may be predictors of breast cancer. This evidence is strengthened by the morphologic similarities between these lesions and invasive cancer. Unfortunately, however, the concurrent nature of these studies precludes the conclusive proof that these lesions are true predictors of breast cancer. This is because the concurrent study cannot rule out the possibility that these lesions developed simultaneously with, or even after, the development of invasive cancer. For this reason, more rigorous methodologies must be used to address this problem.

The second approach is the retrospective case-control study. An example of this approach is the paper by Black et al. (1972), which found that women with hyperplasia had five times the risk of developing cancer than women lacking these changes. These studies evaluated previous benign biopsies in a group of breast cancer patients and in a suitable control group. By looking at the past biopsies of study patients, we can avoid the temporal problems associated with the concurrent study (Lilienfeld and Lilienfeld 1980). The Achilles' heel of these studies is the selection of the control group. Ideally, the case and control groups should be chosen to be representative of women with and without breast cancer. A certain amount of selection bias is permissible as long as it affects case and control selection equally. This, however, is particularly difficult to guarantee in studies of benign breast disease. There is considerable evidence that the rate of preclinical breast cancer growth is quite variable and that the interval between the onset of carcinoma and the development of unequivocal symptoms may be lengthy in some breast cancer patients (Fox 1979). This may lead to a case selection bias in favor of patients who present for biopsy because of relatives who developed cancer, or some other factor that leads them to be concerned about their breasts (Dupont et al. 1980). This in turn may lead to an overestimate of the cancer risks associated with benign lesions.

The third and most demanding approach to the assessment of breast cancer risk is the retrospective cohort study. In these studies, a consecutive sequence of patients who presented with benign breast lesions is identified for follow-up. This cohort of patients is then traced in order to determine their cancer outcome. Locating patients who have not been seen for several decades can be a very difficult and time-consuming process. However, when a high follow-up rate is obtained, this approach can provide as reliable risk estimates as those obtained in an observational study.

One factor that greatly enhances the reliability of retrospective cohort studies of benign breast disease is that histologic slides and paraffin-fixed tissues are routinely saved for later analysis. The consistent reanalysis of study biopsies without knowledge of subsequent cancer outcome is a critical requirement of these studies. It is the ability to perform such analyses that gives these studies the same credibility associated with true prospective studies. Indeed, they are often described as prospective studies in the literature.

The results of the cohort studies that have been published to date are quite variable (Table 3). Kodlin et al. (1977) studied 2,931 cases of benign breast lesions with an average follow-up of seven years. They reevaluated these lesions using the Black-Chabon grading system and found that relative risks varied from 2.3 for lesions of grade one or two to 6.0 for lesions of grade four. They also found that fibroadenomas had a relative risk of 7.0, while adenosis, fibrosing adenosis, or intraductal papilloma had a relative risk of 5.0. However, these latter diagnoses were not made by the investigators themselves but were taken from the original pathologists' reports. In our own first study (Page et al. 1978), we evaluated 925 women with a follow-up period of from 18–25 years. We found much lower overall risks than did Kodlin et al. (1977). Nevertheless, women with NST hyperplasia or papillary apocrine change had a relative risk of 1.8, while women with atypical lobular hyperplasia had a relative risk of 4.2. On the other hand, the risks associated with diagnoses obtained from the pathology reports in the study of Kodlin et al. (1977) were not confirmed by our first study.

Hutchinson et al. (1980) studied 1,356 women with an average follow-up of 13 years. All of the lesions were reanalyzed using a predefined classification scheme. Their discussion of their classification scheme, however, was brief, making it difficult to compare their results for proliferative lesions with those of the authors mentioned previously. They found that epithelial hyperplasia or papillomatosis was associated with a relative risk of 2.8. This risk was not appreciably affected by the presence or absence of atypia. However, the presence of calcification with epithelial hyperplasia or papillomatosis gave a relative risk of 5.3. They also found that fibroadenoma combined with fibrocystic disease was associated with a relative risk of 3.8. Preliminary results from our own study of proliferative disease are consistent

Table 3. *Recent Prospective Studies of Histologically Defined Benign Breast Disease*

Histologic Diagnosis	Number of Patients	Relative Risk
Hutchinson et al. (1980)		
Entire group	1356	2.2
Epithelial hyperplasia or papillomatosis	466	2.8
with atypia	33	2.9
without atypia	433	2.8
with calcification*	102	5.3
without calcification*	190	2.8
Fibroadenoma with fibrocystic disease	122	3.8
Page et al. (1978)		
Entire group	925	1.4
Atypical lobular hyperplasia	33	4.2
NST[†] hyperplasia	249	1.8
Papillary apocrine change	246	1.8
No hyperplasia	447	1.2
Fibroadenoma	189	1.3
Kodlin et al. (1977)		
Entire group	2931	2.7
Black-Chabon atypia score 4	49	6.0
Black-Chabon atypia score 3	262	2.4
Black-Chabon atypia score 1−2	2092	2.3
Fibroadenoma	849	7.0
Adenosis or fibrosing adenosis	177	5.0
Intraductal papilloma	80	5.0

*Women with main lesion type other than epithelial hyperplasia or papillomatosis excluded.
[†]No specific type.

with this result. They also found that nonproliferative fibrocystic disease was not associated with increased cancer risk, a result that agrees with the findings of Page et al. (1978).

Some additional results from the preceding three studies are summarized in Table 3. Comprehensive review papers on the epidemiology of benign breast disease and breast cancer have been written by Ernster (1981) and Kelsey (1979).

STATISTICS

The analysis of cohort study data is complicated by two factors. First, the cancer risk associated with a specific lesion depends not only on the proportion of women who develop cancer, but also on the time interval between the first benign biopsy and the cancer diagnosis. Second, the great majority of women will not develop breast cancer during the follow-up period. Our information on these women is censored since we do not know the future cancer outcome for these women. Traditional methods for analyzing these studies have been based on standard mortality ratios (see, for example, Breslow 1975). This technique has the advantage of conceptual and computational simplicity. It requires, however, the use of a standard reference population and the assumption that age-specific morbidity rates in the study group and reference population are proportional. The wide variability in relative risks associated with benign breast biopsies is undoubtedly due to the variation between the different study groups and their respective reference populations.

In the past decade, there has been an explosive growth in the development of survival analysis techniques, initiated by the landmark paper of Cox (1972). This methodology permits the modeling of follow-up time and outcome data in terms of multiple histologic and epidemiologic risk factors. A major advantage of this approach is that it permits the assessment of individual risk factors without reference to a standard population. Suppose that the i-th member of a cohort is cancer free at time t but is susceptible to developing cancer in the next small time interval Δt with probability $\lambda_i(t)\Delta t$. Then $\lambda_i(t)$ defines the hazard function for the i-th patient. This function can be thought of as the instantaneous force of morbidity acting on the i-th patient at time t. The Cox proportional hazards regression model assumes that $\lambda_i(t) = \lambda_o(t)\exp[z_{i1}\beta_1 + z_{i2}\beta_2 + , \ldots , + z_{ik}\beta_k]$, where $\lambda_o(t)$ is some unspecified baseline hazard; $z_{i1}, z_{i2}, \ldots, z_{ik}$ are the values of known risk factors associated with the i-th patient; and $\beta_1, \ldots, \beta_k$ are unknown parameters that determine the effect of their associated risk factors on the patient's cancer risk. An explanation of how this model is used to assess cancer risk is given in the Appendix.

The proportional hazards method is seminonparametric, since the baseline hazard function $\lambda_o(t)$ is unspecified by the model. However, the method does make the proportional hazards assumption that the relative risk between any two subgroups remains constant over time. The failure of this assumption can have a dramatic impact on the significance levels of the analyses. For example, Stablein et al. (1981) studied the survival data from a cancer chemotherapy trial in which the proportional hazards assumption failed. They found that the difference between treatment survival rates was not significant under the simple proportional hazards model ($P = .25$) but was unequivocably significant under a plausible model involving quadratic, time-dependent covariates ($P = .0096$).

The proportional hazards assumption is particularly vulnerable in studies in which age at initial biopsy is highly variable, because it is often more reasonable to assume that the difference in cancer hazard due to age remains constant over time. A number of options are available for dealing with this problem. The simplest approach is to define time t to be the patient's age instead of the time since the initial biopsy. This is the approach used by Hutchinson et al. (1980). While this approach neatly circumvents the proportional hazards problem with respect to age, it has the disadvantage of not allowing the patient's cancer risk to vary in response to the time that has elapsed since her initial biopsy. For example, under this model, two women both 60 years of age with identical risk factors are assumed to be at equal risk of developing breast cancer even though one patient had her benign biopsy at age 30 while the other's biopsy was at age 59.

Alternate approaches are to stratify the data by age or by other variables that violate the proportional hazards assumption, or to introduce time-dependent covariates. These approaches are described by Kalbfleisch and Prentice (1980). They all require verification of the adequacy of the underlying model assumptions. The first step in doing this is to examine the life table curves for the different subgroups using the unrestricted Kaplan-Meier method and the restricted survival curves generated by the model under consideration. If the restricted and unrestricted curves vary substantially, there is reason to suspect that the model assumptions are invalid. These assumptions may be checked graphically by plotting the log [-log()] of the baseline estimated survivorship curves for the proposed strata. Alternately, the Cox-Snell generalized ordered residuals can be plotted against the corresponding expected order statistics (Kay 1977, Cox and Snell 1968). The goodness-of-fit test, recently developed by Schoenfeld (1981), provides another promising method for evaluating the adequacy of the model.

CONCLUSIONS

In this paper, we have briefly outlined the anatomic, epidemiologic, and statistical problems that are involved in assessing the malignant potential of histologic predictors of breast cancer. This approach holds the promise of allowing us to identify women at high risk of developing breast cancer on the basis of histologic and epidemiologic risk factors. The studies that have been performed to date, however, have been somewhat disappointing in the lack of consistency of their conclusions. In order to rectify this, it will be necessary to describe the criteria for histologic diagnosis in sufficient detail to allow meaningful interstudy comparisons. Similarly, the recent developments in survival analysis hold great promise for the accurate risk assessment of various constellations of risk factors. However, in order to evaluate the appropriateness of the models selected for these techniques, it will be necessary to publish our analyses in greater detail than is customary for simpler statistical problems. It is our hope that through the interdisciplinary efforts of pathologists, epidemiologists, and statisticians, we will be able to make a valuable contribution to the clinical management of breast disease.

ACKNOWLEDGMENTS

This investigation was supported by Grant Number R01 CA31698-01A1 and contract number N01-CB-74098 awarded by the National Cancer Institute, U.S. Department of Health and Human Services.

APPENDIX

Suppose that we wished to examine the effect of fibroadenomas and family history of breast cancer on cancer risk. Let:

$$z_{i1} = \begin{cases} 1 & \text{if the i-th patient has fibroadenoma} \\ 0 & \text{otherwise} \end{cases}$$

Let z_{i2} be a similarly defined indicator function for family history, and let z_{i3} be the interaction indicator function for family history and fibroadenomas that equals 1 if and only if the patient has both risk factors. Then the simplest hazard regression model for these risk factors would be $\lambda_i(t) = \lambda_0(t)\exp[z_{i1}\beta_1 + z_{i2}\beta_2 + z_{i3}\beta_3]$. The method regresses z_{i1}, z_{i2} and z_{i3} against follow-up time and cancer outcome to obtain maximum likelihood estimates $\hat{\beta}_1$, $\hat{\beta}_2$ and $\hat{\beta}_3$ of β_1, β_2 and β_3, respectively. These parameter estimates are, in turn, used to provide relative-risk estimates by taking the ratio of the corresponding hazard function estimates. For example, patients with both risk factors have hazard $\lambda_0(t)\exp[\beta_1 + \beta_2 + \beta_3]$, while patients with neither have hazard $\lambda_0(t)$. Thus, the relative risk of patients having both family history and fibroadenoma compared to patients having neither of these risk factors is estimated by $\exp[\hat{\beta}_1 + \hat{\beta}_2 + \hat{\beta}_3]$. Note that it is necessary to include the interaction parameter β_3, since otherwise the model would imply that fibroadenoma and family history have a multiplicative effect on cancer risk.

REFERENCES

Black, M. M., and A. B. Chabon. 1969. In situ carcinoma of the breast. Pathology Annual 4:185–210.

Black, M. M., T. H. C. Barclay, S. J. Cutler, B. F. Hankey, and A. J. Asire. 1972. Association of atypical characteristics of benign breast lesions with subsequent risk of breast cancer. Cancer 29:338–343.

Bonser, G. M., J. A. Dossett, and J. W. Jull. 1961. Human and Experimental Breast Cancer. Pitman Medical Publishing Co., London.

Breslow, N. E. 1975. Analysis of survival data under the proportional hazards model. International Statistical Review 43:45–58.

Coombs, L. J., A. M. Lilienfeld, I. D. J. Bross, and W. S. Burnett. 1979. A prospective study of the relationship between benign breast diseases and breast carcinoma. Prev. Med. 8:40–52.

Cox, D. R. 1972. Regression models and life tables (with discussion). J. R. Stat. Soc. B 34:187–220.

Cox, D. R., and E. J. Snell. 1968. A general definition of residuals (with discussion). J. R. Stat. Soc. B. 30:248–275.

Davis, H. H., M. Simons, and J. B. Davis. 1964. Cystic disease of the breast: Relationship to carcinoma. Cancer 17:957–978.

Donnelly, P. K., K. W. Baker, J. A. Carney, and W. M. O'Fallon. 1975. Benign breast lesions and subsequent breast carcinoma in Rochester, Minnesota. Mayo. Clin. Proc. 50:650–656.

Dupont, W. D., L. W. Rogers, R. Vander Zwagg, and D. L. Page. 1980. The epidemiologic study of anatomic markers for increased risk of mammary cancer. Pathol. Res. Prac. 166:471–480.

Ernster, V. L. 1981. The epidemiology of benign breast disease. Epidemiologic Reviews 3:184–202.

Foote, F. W., and F. W. Stewart. 1945. Comparative studies of cancerous versus noncancerous breasts. Ann. Surg. 121:6–53, 197–222.

Fox, M. S. 1979. On the diagnosis and treatment of breast cancer. JAMA 241:489–494.

Halter, S. A., and D. L. Page. 1980. Premalignant breast disease, in Scientific Foundations of Oncology, Supplement, T. Symington, and R. L. Carter, eds. William Heinemann Medical Books Ltd., London, pp. 90–106.

Hutchinson, W. B., D. B. Thomas, W. B. Hamlin, G. J. Roth, A. V. Peterson, and B. Williams. 1980. Risk of breast cancer in women with benign breast disease. JNCI 65:13–20.

Jensen, H. M., J. R. Rice, and S. R. Wellings. 1976. Preneoplastic lesions in the human breast. Science 191:295–297.

Kalbfleisch, J. D., and R. L. Prentice. 1980. The Statistical Analysis of Failure Time Data. John Wiley and Sons, New York, pp. 89–98.

Kay, R. 1977. Proportional hazard regression models and the analysis of censored survival data. Applied Statistics 26:227–237.

Kelsey, J. L. 1979. A review of the epidemiology of human breast cancer. Epidemiologic Reviews 1:74–109.

Kodlin, D., E. E. Winger, N. L. Morgenstern, and U. Chen. 1977. Chronic mastopathy and breast cancer: A follow-up study. Cancer 39:2603–2607.

Lilienfeld, A. M., and D. E. Lilienfeld. 1980. Foundations of Epidemiology, 2nd edition. Oxford University Press, New York, pp. 191–225.

LiVolsi, V. A., B. V. Stadel, J. L. Kelsey, T. R. Holford, and C. White. 1978. Fibrocystic breast disease in oral-contraceptive users. A histopathological evaluation of epithelial atypia. N. Engl. J. Med. 299:381–385.

Love, S. M., R. S. Gelman, and W. Silen. 1982. Fibrocystic "disease" of the breast: A non-disease. N. Engl. J. Med 307:1010–1014.

Page, D. L., R. Vander Zwaag, L. W. Rogers, L. T. Williams, W. E. Walker, and W. H. Hartmann. 1978. Relation between component parts of fibrocystic disease complex and breast cancer. JNCI 61:1055–1063.

Rogers, L. W., and D. L. Page. 1979. Epithelial proliferative disease of the breast: A marker of increased cancer risk in certain age groups. Breast, Disease of the Breast 5:2–7.

Schoenfeld, D. 1981. The asymptotic properties of nonparametric tests for comparing survival distributions. Biometrika 68:316–319.

Stablein, D. M., W. H. Carter, Jr., and J. W. Novak. 1981. Analysis of survival data with non-proportional hazard functions. Controlled Clinical Trials 2:149–159.

Wellings, S. R., H. M. Jensen, and R. G. Marcum. 1975. An atlas of subgross pathology of the human breast with special reference to possible precancerous lesions. JNCI 55:231–273.

Current Controversies in Breast Cancer, edited
by F. C. Ames, G. R. Blumenschein, and E. D. Montague.
University of Texas Press, Austin © 1984.

Breast Cancer Screening Techniques

Herman I. Libshitz, M.D.

*Department of Diagnostic Radiology, The University of Texas M. D. Anderson Hospital and
Tumor Institute at Houston, Houston, Texas*

"In the usual course of breast cancer detection in clinical practice, it is very infrequent for the physician to be the first one to discover the lump. The woman most often presents herself in a symptomatic state." These words written by R. C. Hickey (Hickey 1957) of our institution, The University of Texas M. D. Anderson Hospital and Tumor Institute at Houston, are as true today, over a quarter century later, as when they were written. Over the years, many authors have pointed out the importance of detecting small lesions to improve survival rates in patients with breast cancer.

Berlin (1979) stated this most succinctly, "We must acknowledge that a palpable cancer is not an 'early' cancer." He also said that to find breast cancer before metastases have occurred requires screening of asymptomatic women. These sentiments have also been voiced by others including Duncan and Kerr (1976) who said: "It is therefore important to continue to develop and evaluate population screening programs and techniques that are safe, consistent, and precise enough to detect small cancers in the breast."

What then is screening? The U.S. Commission on Chronic Illness in 1957 defined screening as "the presumptive identification of unrecognized diseases or defects by the application of tests, examinations, or other procedures that can be applied rapidly. Screening tests sort out apparently well persons who probably have a disease from those who probably do not." Screening is performed in the belief that the detection of disease in an early or asymptomatic state will lead to appropriate treatment that, in turn, will lead to less mortality from the disease. Screening tests must, therefore, be painless, relatively inexpensive, acceptable to large populations, applicable to large populations, and reasonably safe. Similarly, screening tests can tolerate a moderately high false-positive rate, because additional diagnostic procedures will be performed, but can only tolerate a relatively low false-negative rate. It must also be appreciated that these tests are of no value if the detection threshold is not significantly lower than in the nonscreened population.

This last idea makes the question, "What size cancer is found?," the most important one in the evaluation of breast cancer screening techniques. If a possible screening method is not appropriately tested its use in place of a more sensitive test may significantly delay diagnosis and lead to an otherwise avoidable loss of life. The widespread use of a noninvasive "safe" test that does not lower the stage of lesions detected, does nothing but add unproductive expense to the cost of medical care.

What then are the breast cancer screening methods other than mammography that have been tried or proposed? These include: Thermography, ultrasonography, diaphonography, computed tomography, and physical examination. It is worth our spending a few minutes to consider thermography. In the early 1970s thermography of the breast appeared to be a technique that would be clinically useful. Thermography was particularly attractive because there is no ionizing radiation associated with it, and thus the possible risks of mammography, discussed by Dr. Moskowitz (1982, see pages 67 to 76, this volume), would be avoided. The true-positive rates for the detection of carcinoma of the breast by thermography were in the 75% to 85% range, and the false-positive rates were in the 15% to 40% range (Dodd 1977). It was hoped that an abnormal thermogram would be an adequate prescreener so that only those patients with abnormal thermograms would require mammography. It was recognized that an abnormal or asymmetrical thermogram was a nonspecific finding that could be caused by virtually any breast abnormality and would also be present in a significant number of women without breast abnormalities. Therefore, mammograms would be needed in all women with abnormal thermograms. Unfortunately, further experience with thermography reduced these hopes to disappointment.

It was realized that virtually all of the older reports concerning the efficacy of thermography dealt with symptomatic women and *not* a screening population. A report by Moskowitz et al. (1976) stated, "Thermography may well have a very limited role as a screening or prescreening modality for the detection of minimal or stage I breast cancers." Indeed, the likelihood of finding such small cancers was little better than chance. At about the same time, Johansson (1976) deemed thermography too insensitive and nonspecific to be used as a diagnostic method or a screening method for breast cancer. This was based on a high frequency of both false-negative and false-positive examinations.

Thermography was also included in the Breast Cancer Detection Demonstration Projects (BCDDP) in the mid 1970's. The results were also disappointing. Abnormal thermograms were present in only 42% of the breast cancers found at first screening (Beahrs et al. 1979). Even more disconcerting, thermography was *not* abnormal for two-thirds of the cases of breast cancer detected by mammography but not detected by physical examination. Based on these results at the BCDDP, the role of thermography as a possible alternative for mammography during screening was highly questionable, and its use was not required after the second year of screening.

Just as results in a symptomatic population do not necessarily indicate how well or poorly a particular method will do in the screening circumstance, accuracy rates do not always give the true measure of screening technique. Accepting the fact that approximately 5 in every 1000 women over age 40 will have breast cancer, let us assume that a screening examination, any screening examination, is performed. Let us then assume that all of these examinations are interpreted as being normal. The accuracy rate in this series would be 99.5% because, indeed, 995 of the thousand women would not have breast cancer. There are few examinations or techniques in medicine that offer an accuracy rate this high, but all of the cancers would be missed. To evaluate a screening technique, sensitivity, or the ratio of true-abnormal examinations to the total number of patients with abnormality, must be clearly stated in the results. Similarly, specificity, or the ratio of true-normal examinations to the total number of patients with abnormality, must be clearly stated in the results. Similarly, specificity, or the ratio of the true-normal examinations to the total number of patients with no abnormality, must be stated. If both of these values are not indicated in a report, one cannot measure the efficacy of the technique. If, for example, all of the 1000 examinations in the hypothetical series cited above were interpreted as abnormal, all five cancers would have been identified for a sensitivity rate of 100%. However, the specificity rate would be 0% as all the normals would be misinterpreted as abnormal.

Ultrasonography of the breast also does not entail the use of ionizing radiation. It is worth noting the following statement by Cole-Beuglet et al. (1981) regarding its use as a screening tool. "Insufficient data are available on tumors that are less than 2 cm in diameter to determine whether ultrasound mammography should be used as an initial imaging modality for breast examination." It is those cancers under 2 cm that are sought at screening, for these are the cancers most likely not to be palpable and most likely to be cured. Ultrasound, because of the physical limitations of the technique, presents difficulties in evaluating a fatty breast, the breast type more often present in older women in whom cancer is more often found. Ultrasound also cannot regularly identify the small microcalcifications that often are the only means of detecting very early cancer at mammography. These comments do not imply that there is no role for ultrasound of the breast in diagnostic problems, such as distinguishing a small or obscured cystic mass in the breast from a solid one that might represent a cancer. As yet, however, ultrasound examinations of the breast have not been shown to identify the small and more likely to be cured cancers in the screening circumstance.

Let us now consider briefly the other possible screening modalities. Diaphonography is a method of breast transillumination. It has yet to be proven effective in finding either very small cancers anywhere in the breast or cancers even of moderate to large size deep in the breast. There also have not been any trials of this modality in a broad-based, large population.

It is unlikely that computed tomography (CT) of the breast will find a place as a screening tool. The cost of CT units is quite high compared to that of conventional radiographic mammographic units. Fewer patients could be examined than with a conventional mammographic instrument. The radiation dose is also higher than that received with the use of conventional mammography, and it has been shown that cancers are better identified by CT when intravenous contrast is used, adding an additional risk to the procedure.

It is far too early to even comment as to whether or not nuclear magnetic resonance (NMR) will have any role to play in screening for breast cancer. NMR is a very new modality, and its role as a diagnostic tool has yet to be fully elucidated.

This then leaves the question of the role of physical examination in screening for breast cancer. Of the breast cancers found during the first 2 years at the BCDDP, 45% were found by mammography only (Beahrs et al. 1979). Another 47% were detected by both mammography and physical examination, and 4% were found by physical examination only. The difference in effectiveness in finding breast cancers is even more striking if one compares the cancers found at the first screening with those found at the second screening when most of the cancers prevalent in the population would have been eliminated. In the first screening, 43.9% of all cancers were found by mammography alone. In the second screening, 49.1% of all cancers were found by mammography alone. Thus, if one were to use only physical examination in screening, over 40% of all detectable cancers would be missed on the prevalent screen, and nearly 50% of all cancers would be missed in the subsequent incident screens. Any method that inherently misses such a high percentage of detectable cancers is not a satisfactory method to be used alone.

The combination of mammography and physical examination is today the most effective method of screening for breast cancer.

REFERENCES

Beahrs, O. H., S. Shapiro, and C. Smart. 1979. Report of the working group to review the NCI/ACS breast cancer detection demonstration projects. JNCI 62:641–709.

Berlin, N. I. 1979. Screening for breast cancer today. Prev. Med. 8:573–579.

Cole-Beuglet, C., B. B. Goldberg, A. B. Kurtz, C. S. Rubin, A. S. Patchefsky, and G. S. Shaber. 1981. Ultrasound mammography: A comparison with radiographic mammography. Radiology 139:693–698.

Dodd, G. D. 1977. Present status of thermography, ultrasound mammography in breast cancer detection. Cancer 39:2796–2805.

Duncan, W., and G. R. Kerr. 1976. The curability of breast cancer. Br. Med. J. 2:781–783.

Hickey, R. C. 1957. Cancer of the breast, 1661 patients. II. Considerations in the failure to cure after radical mastectomy. AJR 77:421–430.

Johansson, N. T. 1976. Thermography of the breast. Acta. Chir. Scand. (suppl) 460:3–91.

Moskowitz, M., J. Milbrath, P. Gartside, A. Zermeno, and D. Mandel. 1976. Lack of efficacy of thermography as a screening tool for minimal and stage I breast cancer. N. Engl. J. Med 295:249–252.

Current Controversies in Breast Cancer, edited
by F. C. Ames, G. R. Blumenschein, and E. D. Montague.
University of Texas Press, Austin © 1984.

Benefit-Versus-Risk Ratio of Mammographic Screening Techniques

Myron Moskowitz, M.D.

Department of Radiology, University of Cincinnati Medical Center, Cincinnati, Ohio

Before one can assess the benefit versus the risk of any procedure, one has to define the terms. When this is done, the level of scientific evidence that one will accept or that is necessary to buttress either side of the argument must be decided.

It is obvious that not all parameters on either side of the benefit-versus-risk equation are sufficiently objective to allow quantification. However, even for those that can be quantified and measured, the level of evidence acceptable may be in debate. If one demands for one side of the equation a level of scientific proof that will accept evidence only from a controlled prospective clinical trial, then it must follow that similar proof must be demanded of the other side of the equation.

For the purposes of this presentation, the benefit of mammography has been measured only in terms of potential deaths averted by early detection; and the risk marker is the potential oncogenic effect of ionizing radiation.

RISKS OF MAMMOGRAPHIC SCREENING

What are the risks associated with low-level ionizing radiation used for mammography? Ionizing radiation is a carcinogen. It has been amply demonstrated that for intermediate to high levels of radiation, from hundreds of rads up to the cell-killing threshold of therapeutic irradiation for malignancy, there is a linear response (insofar as breast cancer is concerned) with no reasonable plateau. However, whether the risk curve at very low levels is linear, less than linear, or supralinear, or quadratic is simply not known from the available data. Many models have been proposed.

A recent reanalysis of the Nova Scotia fluoroscopy series, reported by Dr. Anthony Miller (1982), strongly suggests that at low levels of radiation the shape of the curve is not linear but quadratic, suggesting a threshold response. Furthermore, the reanalysis of this patient population failed to demonstrate any excess risk at any dose level for women receiving their initial irradiation at age 40 or older.

The Japanese data (Beir Report 1972, Fabrikant 1981, and McGregor et al. 1977), which probably contain the only series of patients large enough to be statistically significant, indicated rather clearly a dichotomy in risk for those Japanese women who were over age 40 at the time of initial radiation as compared to females who were aged 10 to 19 at the time of initial radiation. The risk of the women who were younger at initial irradiation was at least twice that of the women who were older. Similarly, in the work reported from Sweden by Baral (1977), the same age dichotomy was observed. In Rochester women who received x-ray therapy for post-partum mastitis, the average age of the patients was about 27 (Shore et al. 1977). In this patient population, an excess risk similar to that of females aged 10 to 19 was demonstrated. This population did contain a number of women aged 37 to 39. However, it must be remembered that this was a postpartum population of patients whose breasts were highly metabolically active and under an intense hormonal proliferative stimulus. Considering that proliferating tissue is more sensitive to radiation than resting tissue, it is not surprising that pregnancy confers a similar status to the breast as menarche does.

Though it is not known how the radiation risk curve operates at low diagnostic levels, it can be assumed that the appropriate risk model is a straight-line, no-threshold approach. This may be overly conservative, but it has been used in subsequent calculations.

BENEFITS OF MAMMOGRAPHIC SCREENING

Thus far this presentation has primarily concerned the estimate of risk associated with ionizing radiation. As shown, the estimate of risks at low levels of ionizing radiation is questionable. Quality evidence emanating from a controlled trial concerning risk is lacking. On the other hand, there are hard data emanating from a controlled clinical trial of screening for breast cancer that strongly indicate a distinct benefit associated with screening for breast cancer, as measured in terms of mortality reduction.

The above mentioned study, the Health Insurance Plan of New York (HIP) controlled trial of screening, was carried out in the 1960s. Mammography and physical examination were the basic screening tools. Although this program has been discussed in abundant detail elsewhere, certain salient points are necessary to review here.

During the appropriate time intervals, 299 cancers were detected in the screened group, and 285 cancers occurred in the control group. Thus, screening did not significantly increase the number of cancers in any meaningful way. It only resulted in some degree of downstaging.

Early results demonstrated a 35% reduction in breast cancer mortality for women screened. However, closer analysis revealed that this benefit was limited to women over age 50 at the time of entry into the program. Long-term follow-up has demonstrated a truly important observation. (One must keep in mind that screening was only offered for 4 years.) At 10 and 14 years after screening, follow-up studies, investigating all breast cancer deaths that developed in the cohort since screening, showed a persistent mortality difference of about 20% in the study group when compared to the control group.

It must be emphasized that this was a mortality analysis of a controlled trial and, therefore, free of the problems of length bias and lead-time bias that would be present in a survival analysis of this group. One would have expected the mortality benefit to be vitiated by new cases that might appear shortly after cessation of screening. This has occurred, obviously to some extent, but for the benefit to last as long as it has is truly remarkable.

Further, this mortality reduction has been shown in follow-up studies to be equal in women less than age 50 at entry as well as in women over age 50 at entry. The differences when broken down by age are not statistically significant; however, a) the trend lines are identical, and b) mortality reduction has appeared in younger women at the time one would expect as a result of screening.

The observation, therefore, emerging from HIP is that a population of women over age 40 who were offered screening by physical examination and mammography have had a significant reduction in mortality compared to a control group.

This mortality reduction occurred *despite* the following: 1) one-third of the women offered screening were *never* screened; 2) only 44% of all cancers occurring in the women offered screening were detected; 3) while early survival (or case fatality rate) was better for patients in the study than for those in the control group, the long-term survival curves continue to show closure; 4) more recent population-based trials of screening in Sweden, Holland, and Canada (Tabar, personal communication, Andersson 1980, Andersson et al. 1979, and Rombach, 1980) as well as the study of self-selected women in the ACS-NCI Breast Cancer Detection Demonstration Projects (BCDDP) (Baker, 1982) suggest that during the initial year of screening HIP detected only about one-half to one-third the number of prevalent cancers that probably were present; 5) an inconsequential number of minimal cancers were recognized in HIP, and an equal number apeared in both study and control groups.

This information suggests that the mortality-reducing effect of screening in HIP was very likely related, at least in part, to something other than those cancers identified and treated. It is possible that either in situ lesions or precursor lesions removed at biopsy and unrecognized may have accounted for the benefit demonstrated in that study. Until a blinded pathology review of the benign biopsies in study and control groups is performed, this will have to remain a hypothesis. The empiric observation that mortality reduction occurred following screening intervention will simply have to be accepted, though the reason for this reduction remains unclear.

While only a few small cancers were found in the HIP study, it has been clearly shown by the BCDDP that at least 30% of cancers detected in younger women can be detected while less than 1 cm in size. The BCDDP at the University of Cincinnati Medical Center has found that for women age 35 to 45 approximately 60% of the cancers were detected while either less than 5mm in size or wholly intraductal or in situ lobular (Moskowitz 1981, 1983). Further, while only 60% of the cancers that could have been found by screening were detected in HIP, in The University of Cincinnati Medical Center BCDDP about 90% of the cancers were detected by screening. In the BCDDP as a whole, only 20% to 25% of the cancers occurred between screens. Thus it would seem that one of the major deficiencies of breast cancer screening as performed by HIP has been corrected in the past 20 years.

While it appears, therefore, that smaller cancers can be detected in younger women today, the question remains whether screening automatically confers a mortality benefit on the population so evaluated?

BEHAVIOR OF SMALL BREAST CANCERS

Before answering this question, one must determine whether it is possible to predict the behavior of these small lesions that are diagnosed by pathologists. One might equally ask whether it is possible to predict the biologic behavior of any lesion that is diagnosed by a pathologist. Do all breast cancers inexorably proceed to metastasis and eventually cause the patient's death, and if so, do they all do so at an equal rate? While all large cancers were once small, do all small cancers become large?

There are those, such as Maurice Fox (1979), who claim that, in point of fact, many so-called cancers determined as such by pathologists are biologically inert and are never a cause of death in patients. On the other hand, there are the biologic predeterminists, such as Baum (1977), who claim that all breast cancer is inevitably disseminated from its inception, and the outcome is foreordained. Surely the truth must lie somewhere between these extremes.

It is obvious to any clinician who has dealt with this disease that the natural history is a variegated one. Some tumors are very rapidly growing, explosive lesions; others are relatively slow-growing and indolent; the vast majority lie somewhere between these extremes of biologic aggressiveness. It has been said that approximately 50% of patients with breast cancer can be expected to die of it (U.S. Department of Health, Education, and Welfare 1972). According to the work of Bloom and Fields (1971), histologic grading and stage are reasonable predictors of both long- and short-term survival rates.

For example, their work suggests that, at least in part, survival is proportional to tumor size at the time of diagnosis. That is to say, patients with low-grade or slow-growing tumors smaller than 1.25 cm in maximum diameter have a three to four times better chance of surviving 5 years than do patients with a tumor of the same growth rate but with a size of 5 cm. Furthermore, regardless of grade, patients with stage I tumors have a better prognostic outlook at 5, 10, 15, and 20 years. In patients with stage I cancer, survival at 5, 10, and 15 years is essentially the same regardless of histologic grade. Prognosis for patients with stage II or higher tumors is progressively worse at 5, 10, and 15 years with increasing histologic grade. Thus, it seems important to detect breast cancer at a smaller size no matter what its growth rate, but for the patients harboring more undifferentiated, rapidly growing tumors the imperative is even greater to find the lesions when they are stage I or smaller.

The following questions concerning the biological activity of smaller lesions less than 5mm in size or those that are wholly intraductal or in situ lobular have also been investigated: Do they have the same spectrum of biologic activity as large lesions? How many of these lesions are obligate neoplasia, i.e., if left alone will go on to present as clinically detectable lesions? How many of these lesions are, in fact, not true lesions, but nonobligate preneoplastic lesions?

It is very difficult, but not impossible, to reasonably answer these questions. If one is dealing with a lesion that is potentially curable by local resection, then biopsy might be curative. Therefore, by following a group of patients who have been diagnosed and, perhaps, treated by biopsy, one can never determine the fate of that lesion. The risk of such patients for developing second tumors can only be quantified. Such risk has been determined by numerous investigators (for example: Black 1976, Buzanowski-Konakry 1975, Egger and Müller 1977), and they have, indeed, documented that these patients have a high risk of developing a second tumor.

However, the 10- to 25-year long-term actuarial survival for patients treated for minimal breast cancer by mastectomy has been reported to be 90% to 95%. The next question to be answered is whether there is any way to determine what would have happened to such lesions if not discovered and treated while in situ.

One way to evaluate the natural history of these lesions is to examine a population of women during active screening to determine the rate of breast cancers and the fraction of those cancers that are minimal, and then to observe that same population over a period of time without any screening intervention. If the minimal breast cancers are unreal, or would never have presented in the patient's lifetime, their lead time can be taken to be infinity. This being the case, the subsequent incidence of cancer occurring in the unscreened population would be reduced by the number of excess cases found during screening.

The BCDDP at The University of Cincinnati Medical Center has followed 6,000 women, ages 35 to 49, during 3 years of active screening and found 24 cancers, 58% of which were minimal. When screening was suddenly curtailed in this group, observation over the next 3 years revealed the expected short-term drop in annual incidence, followed by a rise, so that at the end of 3 years of observation the total number of cancers was exactly that observed during the screening interval. The only difference was that instead of 14 minimal cancers, there were only 5; instead of 20% stage II cancers, there were 58%, or 14 incurable lesions found. These data strongly suggest that the early natural history of the disease is as previously envisioned.

Another way to evaluate the potential clinical significance of these tiny lesions is to determine if the overall detection rate in the approximately 280,000 women in the overall BCDDP is in excess of what one would expect.

Seidman previously predicted from the demographic data collected on all of the participants in the BCDDP that the incidence rate of breast cancer in the self-selected screened women would probably be about 25% more than the national incidence. This would result from women enlisting themselves in the screening program based on known factors of risk such as family history, obesity, previous biopsy, etc. The data are now available on which one can test this model.

Because the prevalence year of any screening process will tend to be biased heavily towards symptomatic women (i.e., women with a lump), it is best to eliminate the prevalence year from consideration of the determination of the annual incidence rates. Rather it is better to go to a stable period and continue observation over a reasonable period of time so that fluctuations in incidence will have evened out. Therefore the annual breast cancer incidence has been examined in the approximately 280,000 screened women enrolled in the BCDDP beginning 2.5 years after entry, by age at entry. Data from this project represent all cases detected at screening as well as all cases not detected by screening within 12 months of a previously negative screen. The excess number of cancers in the BCDDP in annual incidence ranges from 13% to a high of 29%, yielding an average of 23% excess. Thus, the model of Seidman (1977) accurately predicts the annual incidence rate that would be expected in this BCDDP population based on known demographic and risk features alone.

It would seem very unlikely, therefore, that there is any significant excess in number of total cancers detected as a result of the screening process.

Even in The University of Cincinnati Medical Center BCDDP in which the rate of small tumors was 150% greater than the BCDDP as a whole ($P<.0000001$), the average annual incidence of breast cancer, including interval cancers, was 2.63 per thousand. The average annual incidence in the overall BCDDP was 2.45 per thousand. Thus, it would appear that an excess number of breast cancers, vis-à-vis the overall BCDDP and, by inference, vis-à-vis the national expected average, did not occur in the BCDDP at The University of Cincinnati Medical Center.

It has been previously demonstrated that the rate of detection of intraductal carcinomas at The University of Cincinnati Medical Center is anywhere from two to three times that rate found in certain other screening centers that did not pursue an aggressive approach (Moskowitz 1979). The total number of cancers, however, detected in these centers was virtually identical. Therefore, the data that are currently available indicate quite clearly that the early biology of breast cancer is as it has been classically hypothesized. Tiny cancers do grow to be big ones, and they appear to do so within a reasonably short time interval. In situ lobular carcinoma seems to be a less aggressive lesion than intraductal carcinoma, but since the in situ lobular carcinomas constitute a small fraction of the total cancers found, they do not create a problem in screening or in evaluation of the significance of minimal breast cancer.

A question of primary concern is whether an improvement in mortality will occur as a result of this early detection? Both the breast cancer mortality experience in The University of Cincinnati Medical Center BCDDP and the survival experience have been investigated. The survival experience included the evaluation of all cancers found during the prevalence year, all cancers that occurred between screens, all cancers detected as a result of screening, as well as all cancers that have been found in this patient population since screening has stopped or since the patient dropped out of the program. In some cases, this represented cancers appearing as late as 5 years after the last screen.

Of interest was the survival of women over as well as under age 50 at the time of entry into the screening program. Early HIP data demonstrated no benefit for screening in women under age 50 at the time of entry. Shapiro (1977) interpreted this to mean that there was a difference in the biology of tumors in younger women that precluded demonstration of a benefit. Our screening demonstrated equal improvement in 7-year survival for both younger and older women.

This raises the question of whether mortality reduction can be demonstrated in younger women. As indicated earlier, there are data now from a controlled trial that strongly suggest mortality reduction in this group. If self-selected women from The University of Cincinnati Medical Center BCDDP are compared with self-selected women from the HIP study, then added evidence for mortality benefit can be ascertained. While this approach is less than ideal, it does, to some extent, control the major bias of self selection. This comparison was made between women, ages 40 to 49, in the University of Cincinnati Medical Center BCDDP and self-selected women in HIP in the same age group at entry. The general mortality from causes other than breast cancer for these two populations was very similar, almost identical.

Breast cancer mortality in these two groups was also compared. When those patients who entered the program with a history of prior treatment for breast cancer were eliminated, there was a statistically and clinically significant difference in breast cancer mortality outcome between these two patient populations. In HIP, 13 deaths occurred in 46,615 person years of observation. At 5 years of follow-up, no deaths due to breast cancer were observed in the University of Cincinnati Medical Center BCDDP population of younger women. Based on HIP, seven deaths would have been expected to occur. The difference is statistically significant.

BENEFIT-VERSUS-RISK MODELS

Several benefit-versus-risk models for breast cancer are worthy of comment here. The model by Chiachierrini (1977) of the Bureau of Radiologic Health is of interest because it demonstrates the relationship between changing imaging doses and various assumed levels of benefit. His model assumes a modified absolute radiation risk and 100% participation of the women. For women age 40 to 44 if there is a magnitude of benefit of screening on the order of 30% (the same benefit demonstrated in HIP for women over the age of 49), then for 100,000 women screened annually for 5 years and receiving .5 rad, about 25 deaths would be averted; receiving .3 rad, about 30 deaths; and receiving .1 rad, about 40 deaths. If the mortality reduction were as small as 10%, 10 deaths would be averted if each patient received .1 rad. On the other hand, if screening were begun at age 45 to 49, for a 30% reduction in mortality, 50 net deaths would be averted if amount of absorption was .5 rad; .3 rad, approximately 60 deaths; and if .1 rad, approximately 70 deaths would be averted. (It should be parenthetically noted that today we can screen with mammography at an annual dose of .1 rad to .2 rad.)

Eddy (1980) has developed a rather extensive risk-versus-benefit model. His model assumes annual mammography and physical examination for life at an average dose of 1 rad per year. He also assumes that the magnitude of the benefits demonstrated in HIP for women over age 50 can be extended to younger women. With these basic assumptions and other detailed mathematical calculations and corrections, for annual screening of a population of women aged 35 at entry, he makes the following estimations:

If there were no assumed risk, the increase in life expectancy as a result of such screening would be 96.9 days. If the worst case risk assumption is made, the average increase in life expectancy would be 88.4 days. If the worst risk estimate were doubled, the net increase in life expectancy to this population would be 77.1 days.

In contrast, he estimates that for women over age 50 at entry, if there were no assumed risk, screening could be expected to add approximately 60.5 days; with the assumed worst risk, 60.2 days would be added; and if the worst risk were doubled, 59.8 days would be added.

The model that was developed by Fox and Moskowitz (1978) was based on the data generated from the Cincinnati and Milwaukee BCDDP. The model was to estimate the benefit versus the risk attributable only to the mammographic contribution to the screening process. This model accounted for self-selection bias, the presence of asymptomatic women, and interval cancer rates of 25%. An absolute 10-year survival rate of 80% was assumed for patients with minimal breast cancer, and national 10-year survival data for all other stages was used.

Furthermore, the benefits assessed in this model were limited to those cases detected by mammography alone. Not included were benefits to those patients with breast cancer detected by physical examination either alone or in conjunction with mammography. The influences of either of these modalities on the other could not be ruled out or evaluated.

Therefore, the results predicated in this model seem to be reasonably conservative. One of the key estimates necessary to establish this model was the prediction of the prevalence of the disease in the screened population and, from this, the mean detection lead time. These lead times were then compared with those gained from a randomly selected population-based screen in Falun, Sweden (Tabar and Dean 1982). The Fox and Moskowitz model for women under age 50 predicted a mean detection lead time of 2.1 ± .05 years; in the Swedish study, 2.52 years seemed to be gained for the same aged population. For women aged 55 to 64, the Fox and Moskowitz model predicted a mean detection lead time of 3.2 ± .06 years; in the 55 to 69-year age group in the Swedish study, 3.27 years appeared to be gained. The Fox and Moskowitz model projected a mean detection lead time of 4.7 ± 1.3 years for women age 65 to 74; in the 60- to 69-year age group in the Swedish screen, there appeared to be a mean detection lead time of 4.52 years. Therefore, for this major parameter of the Fox and Moskowitz model, the ability to predict lead time seemed to be correct.

But do the minimal breast cancers detected by screening behave as similar sized and staged cancers detected in the course of usual case finding? As previously indicated, no evidence exists to support the opinion that the cancers found by screening are indolent or not "real" cancers. To date, these cancers do not appear to be more aggressive, in terms of the tendency to metastasize or cause death, than similar sized and staged lesions detected outside of screening. At this writing, with 100%

follow-up of patients in the University of Cincinnati Medical Center BCDDP with minimal breast cancer, none have died.

This model estimates that for women who begin radiation at age 35 or older and receive an absorbed dose of 1 rad per year and five annual screens the added benefit of mammography benefit versus risk at a patient age of 35 to 44 can be estimated as 5.5 ± 2.9. For women aged 45 to 54, it is 11.2 ± 4.0. For those 55 to 64 years of age, the benefit-versus-risk ratio is 40 ± 14.7. If the absorbed dose is on the order of .2 rad, as is currently the dose received by patients at the University of Cincinnati Medical Center, each of these benefit-versus-risk ratios increases by approximately fivefold. If, as seems extremely likely from the recent data reported by Miller (1982), there is no risk to patients receiving radiation in the 35-or-older age group at this dose level, then the point is, indeed, moot. Again, these estimates apply only to the added independent benefit of mammography, i.e. those cases detected by mammography alone. If mammography in some way contributed to the detection of those cases found by both physical examination and mammography, the benefit versus risk indicated above would increase almost by an order of magnitude.

SUMMARY

For those who would demand a controlled clinical trial and absolute proof that screening for breast cancer favorably alters the outcome, one must admit that this has only been demonstrated in HIP. For those who are willing to accept some lesser quality of proof and who must deal with this problem on a day-to-day basis, the evidence suggests that a significant mortality reduction can be achieved even for women under age 50 if the disease is interdicted at a truly early phase. It must be concluded further that this early phase can be found today. Whether we have the desire, or the financial resources, or the necessary drive to pursue this goal is another question.

ACKNOWLEDGMENTS

This investigation was supported in part by Grant Number NCI CN 55310 awarded by the National Cancer Institute, U.S. Department of Health and Human Services, and Grant Number DPBC-11 awarded by the American Cancer Society.

REFERENCES

Andersson, I. 1980. Mammographic Screening for Breast Carcinoma: A Cross-Sectional Randomized Study of 45–69 Year-Old Women. Litos Retrtryck, Malmo, Sweden.

Andersson, I., L. Andrén, J. Hilldel, L. Linell, U. Ljungqvist, and H. Pettersson. 1979. Breast cancer screening and mammography: A population-based randomized trial with mammography as the only screening mode. Radiology 132:273–276.

Baker, L. 1982. Breast cancer detection demonstration project: Five-year summary report. CA 32:226–230.

Baral, E., L. E. Larsson, and B. Mattson. 1977. Breast cancer following irradiation of the breast. Cancer 40:2910.

Baum, M. 1977. The curability of breast cancer, *in* Breast Cancer Management, Early and Late, B. A. Stoll, ed. Wm. Heinimann Medical Books, Ltd., Great Britain, p. 3.

BEIR Report, Advisory Committee on the Biological Effects of Ionizing Radiation. 1972. The effects on populations of exposure to low levels of ionizing radiation. National Academy of Sciences, National Research Council, Washington, D.C.

Black, M. M. 1976. Structural, antigenic, and biological characteristics of precancerous mastopathy. Cancer Res. 36:2596–2604.

Bloom, H. J. J., and J. R. Fields. 1971. Impact of tumor grade and host resistance in survival of women with breast cancer. Cancer 28:1580.

Buzanowski-Konakry, K., E. G. Harrison, Jr., and W. S. Payne. 1975. Lobular carcinoma arising in fibroadenoma of the breast. Cancer 35:450–456.

Chiacchierini, R. P., and F. E. Luden. 1977. The issues: Benefit-risk in mammography, *in* Proceedings of the Eighth Annual Conference on Radiation Control. U.S. Department of Health, Education, and Welfare, (FDA) 77-8021, Washington, D.C., pp. 209–229.

Eddy, D. M., 1980. Screening for Cancer: Theory, Analysis, and Design. Prentice-Hall, Englewood Cliffs, New Jersey.

Egger, H., and S. Müller. 1977. Das Fibroadenom der Mamma. Dtsch. Med. Wochenschr. 102:1495–1500.

Fabrikant, J. I. 1981. The BEIR III report: Origin of the controversy. AJR 136:209–214.

Fox, M. S. 1979. On the diagnosis and treatment of breast cancer. JAMA 241:489–494.

Fox, S. H., M. Moskowitz, E. L. Saergen, G. Kereiakes, S. Milbrath, and M. W. Goodman. 1978. Benefit/risk analysis of aggressive mammographic screening. Radiology 128:350–365.

McGregor, D. H., C. E. Land, K. Choi, S. Tokuoka, P. I. Lui, T. Wakabayashi, and G. W. Beebe. 1977. Breast cancer incidence among atomic bomb survivors: Hiroshima and Nagasaki, 1950–1969. JNCI 59:799–811.

Miller, A. B., and R. D. Bulbrook. 1982. Screening, detection, and diagnosis of minimal breast cancer. Report of the Fourth Meeting of the U.I.C.C. Multidisciplinary Project on Breast Cancer, March, 1982. Lancet 1:1109–1111.

Moskowitz, M. 1981. Mammographic screening: Significance of minimal breast cancers. AJR 136:735–738.

Moskowitz, M. 1983. Minimal breast cancer redux. Radiol. Clin. North Am. (in press).

Moskowitz, M. 1979. Screening is not diagnosis. Radiology 133:265–268.

Rombach, J. J. 1980. Breast Cancer Screening: Results and Implications for Diagnostic Decision Making. Stafleu's Scientific Pub. Co., Alphen Aan Den Rijm, Brussels.

Seidman, H. 1977. Screening for breast cancer in younger women: Life expectancy gains and losses. An analysis according to risk indicator groups. CA 27:66–87.

Shapiro, S. 1977. Evidence on screening for breast cancer from a randomized trial. Cancer 39:2772–2782.

Shore, R. E., L. H. Hempelmann, E. Kowaluk, P. S. Mansur, B. S. Pasternak, R. E. Albert, and G. E. Houghie. 1977. Breast neoplasms in women treated with x-rays for acute postpartem mastitis. JNCI 59:813–822.

Tabar, L., and P. B. Dean. 1982. Mammographic parenchymal patterns: Risk indicator for breast cancer? JAMA 247:185–189.

U.S. Department of Health, Education, and Welfare. 1972. End Results in Cancer, (NIH) 73-272, Washington, D.C.

MINIMAL BREAST CANCER

Current Controversies in Breast Cancer, edited
by F. C. Ames, G. R. Blumenschein, and E. D. Montague.
University of Texas Press, Austin © 1984.

Minimal Breast Cancer: Definition and Prognosis

H. Stephen Gallager, M.D.

*Department of Pathology, The University of Texas M. D. Anderson Hospital and
Tumor Institute at Houston, Houston, Texas*

The concept of minimal breast cancer was an outgrowth of the development of mammography, and the histories of the two are intimately intertwined. Sporadic reports of radiographic imaging of the breast began to appear as far back as the first decade of the 20th century. In the following 40 years, the pioneering work of Warren (1930), Leborgne (1953), and Gershon-Cohen and Strickler (1938) clearly demonstrated the potential of the technique. It was the work of Egan (1960), however, that finally demonstrated that the method was capable of high diagnostic accuracy and, furthermore, that it could detect carcinoma in the absence of a palpable mass. There followed a multi-institutional study (Clark et al. 1965) that demonstrated that Egan's results could be duplicated by other radiologists with a minimum of training. This firmly established mammography as a diagnostic modality in breast disease.

By this time, the mammographic signs of carcinoma were well known, but the pathologic processes responsible for the changes were only vaguely understood. The presence of calcification, for example, was known to be associated with a high incidence of carcinoma, but the pathologic mechanism that produced calcification was unknown. Local skin thickening, often seen over invasive carcinomas, was assumed to be the result of edema, but this remained unproved. Increased prominence of ductal markings was another frequent sign of carcinoma for which no pathologic correlation existed.

In an effort to find explanations of these and related phenomena, a correlated mammographic-histopathologic study of the breast was undertaken in 1962. The stated objective of this study was to establish correlations between mammographic and histopathologic findings in breast cancer and thereby to contribute to improvement in the sensitivity and specificity of mammography. Surgical specimens from patients who had mastectomies following preoperative mammograms were subjected to subserial whole-organ sectioning. In each case, histologic diagnosis was established by trephine needle biopsy only. In this way, the tumor and the surrounding mammary tissue were maintained in a relatively intact state. To prepare each specimen, the axillary contents were first removed and scouted for lymph nodes in the usual manner. The breast itself was divided into three large blocks, each 5–7 cm thick. The plane of sectioning was chosen by reference to the preoperative mammograms. Giant sections 12 to 15 μm thick were cut at 1-mm intervals across the entire specimen. Each breast yielded a set of 80 to 200 whole-mount sections. These, when viewed in order, gave a three-dimensional overview of the breast and its contents that could be directly compared with the mammogram. During a period of 12 years, 209 specimens were studied in this way. All but a few contained invasive carcinomas, mostly 2–4 cm in diameter.

Ultimately, the objectives of this study were achieved and the results have been published (Gallager and Martin 1969 a, b, 1970). As work progressed, however, it was realized that by study of changes in ducts and lobules adjacent to invasive masses a clearer understanding of early breast cancer was emerging. It was noted, for example, that epithelial hyperplasia, epithelial atypia, and noninvasive carcinoma were almost universally present in breasts containing invasive masses. These epithelial alterations were not sharply distinct but, rather, formed a continuous spectrum of alteration. Multiplicity of invasive masses was commonplace, occurring in 37% of specimens. In over 90% of cases, invasion could be related to foci of intraductal carcinoma. Invasive masses almost always occurred in relation to ducts containing intraductal carcinoma.

Based on the data acquired from the study, an understanding of the natural history of breast cancer gradually evolved. Epithelial hyperplasia was regarded as a preneoplastic lesion in the sense that it invariably precedes carcinoma, although it may have other outcomes. The frequent coexistence of the lesions of fibrocystic disease and carcinoma in the same breast was explained on the basis of common origin of both lesions from epithelial hyperplasias of various kinds. Carcinoma, it was postulated, originates in the epithelium of mammary ducts and lobules. Intraepithelial extension probably precedes invasion. The concomitance of noninvasive and invasive carcinoma in the same breast was regarded as evidence of the relatively long duration of the preinvasive stage of mammary carcinoma, which may be a matter of months to several years. Only after invasion has occurred do dissemination and metastasis take place.

In its earliest phases, the behavior of breast carcinoma follows a predictable sequence. Once invasive growth has become established, however, behavior becomes more random. There may be secondary mass formation, intramammary lymphatic spread, extension to local structures, metastasis to regional lymph nodes, or systemic dissemination. The relationships among these various phenomena become complex and difficult to predict.

An obvious corollary to this model of natural history is that there exists a stage in the development of breast carcinoma in which invasion is either nonexistent or of near-microscopic dimension, and that in this stage simple methods of treatment might be expected to provide control or even cure. It was to characterize this stage that the concept of minimal breast cancer was proposed (Gallager and Martin 1971). The term was defined histopathologically as including noninvasive carcinoma, either ductal or lobular, and invasive carcinoma having a volume no greater than that of a sphere 0.5 cm in diameter (0.065 cm^3). This upper limit of volume was established by estimating the probability of axillary nodal metastasis in a series of mammographically measurable invasive carcinomas, then extrapolating to a volume at which the probability of positive axillary nodes was less than 10%. The term "minimal breast cancer" was carefully chosen to distinguish this pathologically defined group of lesions from "early" breast cancer and "occult" breast cancer. Early breast cancer, a vague term at best, is usually intended to mean carcinoma without axillary or other metastases, and an occult breast carcinoma is one that is asymptomatic, nonpalpable, and detectable only by mammography. Most, but not all, minimal breast cancers are both early and occult. A few metastasize to axillary nodes, and a few are palpable because of superficial location or produce symptoms such as nipple discharge.

It was considered appropriate to include noninvasive and microinvasive carcinomas together under a single term because they represent phases in a progression toward invasive carcinoma and because the actual point of initial invasion is difficult to establish. It is well known that there is a small incidence of axillary metastasis among noninvasive carcinomas. While this may be an artifact of inadequate sampling, two specimens from patients with involved axillary nodes have been studied by subserial whole-organ sectioning, and in neither was there any malignant lesion other than noninvasive intraductal carcinoma. Ozzello (1971) has shown by electron microscopy that ducts have naturally occurring gaps in their basal laminae through which malignant cells may protrude or escape into adjacent tissue. It must be concluded, therefore, that extremely early invasion is difficult or impossible to recognize by light microscopy alone and that carcinomas believed to be noninvasive by routine study may actually be invasive at an ultrastructural level.

At the time the concept of minimal breast cancer was first proposed, it was predicted that 5-year survivals within the group would exceed 90%, that the rate of axillary node metastasis would be less than 10%, and that the rate of bilaterality, especially subsequent bilaterality, would be high. These estimates were, of course, based on entirely hypothetical considerations. No group of cases fitting the definition had at that time been studied. Since then, four reports have appeared describing retrospective analyses of patients with minimal breast cancer (Wanebo et al. 1974, Frazier et al. 1977, Peters et al. 1977, Nevin et al. 1980). Together, the four reports analyze 484 patients. The series are similar in that patients were accrued between 1960 and 1976, 60% of patients were recruited after 1970, and median age at diagnosis was 52 years. Most of the lesions were either discovered by patients or discovered accidently during surgery for nonmalignant disease. Mammographic screening apparently played little part in the selection of this population. There was no consistency in treatment. Most patients had mastectomies of some sort but some were treated by local excision with or without radiation therapy.

The disease-free survival rate for all evaluable patients (average follow-up of 5.3 years) was 96.8%. There was no difference in survival rate among the three types of lesions included within the definition. Involved axillary nodes were found in 5.5% of the 415 patients who had these nodes surgically removed. The rate of nodal involvement for microinvasive carcinoma, 13.3%, was considerably higher than for intraductal carcinoma (1.7%) or lobular carcinoma in situ (2.8%). Interestingly, survival did not differ between positive-node and negative-node groups. This may be because many of the reported metastases were micrometastases less than 2 mm in diameter, which are known to have little effect upon prognosis.

Bilateral breast carcinoma, either simultaneous or subsequent, occurred in 21% of the 429 patients for whom data are available. The rate was greater among patients with lobular carcinoma in situ (42.4%). It was not, however, negligible in those with intraductal carcinoma (13.4%) or microinvasive carcinoma (9.9%). Bilaterality was found most frequently in series in which contralateral blind biopsy was done routinely at the time of mastectomy. Among patients whose contralateral biopsies were negative, subsequent contralateral carcinomas were extremely rare.

It has been suggested that minimal breast cancer represents an indolent form of carcinoma that never becomes life threatening. There is abundant evidence that this is not true. In a long-term follow-up study of patients with lobular carcinoma in situ treated by biopsy only (Rosen et al. 1978), the incidence of subsequent invasive carcinoma was nine times the expected number, and breast cancer deaths were 11 times the number anticipated. In two similar studies of intraductal carcinoma, 28% of patients subsequently developed invasive carcinoma (Betsill et al. 1978, Page et al. 1982). Moskowitz (1981) has reviewed the experience in a mammographic screening center, in which a particularly aggressive approach was applied. The threshold for recommendation of biopsy was intentionally set at a low level. About 40% of the carcinomas detected at this center were minimal carcinomas. Moskowitz points out that if minimal carcinomas were indolent lesions, the rate of cancer detection after the initial or prevalence year should have been greater than that expected. This was not the case, nor was the detection rate different from that found in screening centers employing higher thresholds, where the proportion of minimal breast cancer was lower. These data strongly imply that detection and treatment of minimal breast cancer is capable of reducing the incidence of more advanced disease and that minimal breast cancer is, as originally conceived, a stage in progression to invasive carcinoma and not a special kind of cancer.

Despite advances in mammography and mammographic screening programs, detection of minimal breast cancer remains largely a matter of chance. Most are found as a result of biopsy of some vaguely palpable abnormality that may or may not be related to the malignant process. Mammography clearly is capable of detecting some cases through indirect signs, particularly the presence of characteristic calcification. The sensitivity of mammography in detecting minimal breast cancer remains unknown, but some suggestive evidence is available from the recent 5-year summary report of the American Cancer Society and National Cancer Institute Breast Cancer Detection Demonstration Project (Baker 1982). In that study, 3557 carcinomas were detected by the screening centers. Of these, 1112 were minimal carcinomas. During the same period there were 744 carcinomas apparently missed by screening. If one makes the most unfavorable assumption that all of the interval carcinomas were minimal at the time of screening and escaped the screen, the sensitivity of mammography in the detection of minimal carcinoma is 60%.

There is presently insufficient information to indicate what form of treatment may be most appropriate for minimal breast cancer. Radical, modified radical, and extended simple mastectomies all produce high rates of disease-free survival. Whether partial mastectomy alone, radiation alone, or a combination of the two would be equally effective cannot be determined from available data. Any type of mastectomy may ultimately prove to be overtreatment for minimal breast cancer, but it is premature to suggest routine application of a less multilating procedure. As methods of detection improve, it is to be expected that there will be further accumulation of experience with this lesion and that some rational answer to the treatment question can be supplied.

REFERENCES

Baker, L. H. 1982. Breast cancer detection demonstration project: Five-year summary report. CA 32:194–225.

Betsill, W. L., P. P. Rosen, P. H. Leiberman, and G. F. Robbins. 1978. Intraductal carcinoma: Long-term follow-up after treatment by biopsy alone. JAMA 239:1863–1867.

Clark, R. L., M. M. Copeland, R. L. Egan, H. S. Gallager, H. Geller, J. P. Lindsay, L. C. Robbins, and E. C. White. 1965. Reproducibility of the technique of mammography (Egan) for cancer of the breast. Am. J. Surg. 109:127–133.

Egan, R. L. 1960. Experience with mammography in a tumor institution. Radiology 75:894–900.

Frazier, T. G., E. M. Copeland, H. S. Gallager, D. D. Paulus, and E. C. White. 1977. Prognosis and treatment in minimal breast cancer. Am. J. Surg. 133:697–701.

Gallager, H. S., and J. E. Martin. 1969a. The study of mammary carcinoma by correlated mammography and subserial whole organ sectioning: Early observations. Cancer 23:855–873.

Gallager, H. S., and J. E. Martin. 1969b. Early phases in the development of breast cancer. Cancer 24:1170–1178.

Gallager, H. S., and J. E. Martin. 1970. The pathology of early breast cancer, *in* Breast Cancer Early and Late, Year Book Medical Publishers, Chicago, pp. 37–50.

Gallager, H. S., and J. E. Martin. 1971. An orientation to the concept of minimal breast cancer. Cancer 28:1519–1526.

Gershon-Cohen, J., and A. Strickler. 1938. Roentgenologic examination of the normal breast: Its evaluation in demonstrating early neoplastic changes. AJR 40:189–201.

Leborgne, R. 1953. The Breast in Roentgen Diagnosis. Impresora Uruguay, Montevideo.

Moskowitz, M. 1981. Mammographic screening: Significance of minimal breast cancer. AJR 136:735–738.

Nevin, J. E., G. Pinzon, T. J. Moran, and J. T. Baggerly. 1980. Minimal breast cancer. Am. J. Surg. 139:357–359.

Ozzello, L. 1971. Ultrastructure of the human mammary gland, *in* Pathology Annual, S. C., Sommers, ed. Appleton-Century-Crofts, New York, pp. 1–59.

Page, D. L., W. D. DuPont, L. W. Rogers, and M. Landenberger. 1982. Intraductal carcinoma of the breast: Follow-up after biopsy alone. Cancer 49:751–758.

Peters, T. G., W. L. Donegan, and E. A. Burg. 1977. Minimal breast cancer: A clinical appraisal. Ann. Surg. 186:704–710.

Rosen, P. P., P. H. Leiberman, D. W. Braun, Jr., C. Kosloff, and F. Adair. 1978. Lobular carcinoma in situ of breast: Detailed analysis of 99 patients with average follow-up of 24 years. Am. J. Surg. Pathol. 2:225–251.

Wanebo, H. J., A. G. Huvos, and J. A. Urban. 1974. Treatment of minimal breast cancer. Cancer 33:349–357.

Warren, S. L. 1930. A roentgenologic study of the breast. AJR 24:113–124.

Current Controversies in Breast Cancer, edited
by F. C. Ames, G. R. Blumenschein, and E. D. Montague.
University of Texas Press, Austin © 1984.

Detection of Minimal Breast Cancer

David D. Paulus, M.D., F.A.C.R.

*Department of Diagnostic Radiology, The University of Texas M. D. Anderson Hospital
and Tumor Institute at Houston, Houston, Texas*

The most consistently accurate means available for detecting small nonpalpable breast cancers is mammography.* High survival rates reflect the importance of detecting breast cancer in early stages of development. Approximately 85% of patients survive 5 years when their breast cancers are diagnosed in early stages. Patients with minimal breast cancer, as defined by Martin and Gallager, have a 5-year survival rate of 96.6% (H. S. Gallager, personal communication). Frazier et al. (1977) projected by actuarial analysis a 20-year survival rate of 93.2% for a group of 176 patients with minimal breast cancer.

POTENTIAL OF MAMMOGRAPHY IN DETECTION OF MINIMAL BREAST CANCER

A summary of the 5-year results of the NCI/ACS breast cancer screening program by 29 regional centers or Breast Cancer Detection Demonstration Projects (BCDDP) clearly demonstrates the capability of mammography, when properly applied, to detect breast cancer in early or minimal stages of development. During this period, 280,222 women were screened one or more times by physical examination and mammography. There were a total of 3,557 cancers detected, including 533 cancers of unknown size. Thirty-eight percent of the cancers of known size (3,024) were under 1 cm in diameter, of which 68% were noninvasive and 32% were in women under the age of 50.

Mammography alone detected 43.6% of all cancers of known size (3,024), 58.4% of cancers under 1 cm in diameter, and 60.4% of noninfiltrating cancers. These groups of patients will have the best prognoses and the highest survival rates. Physical examination alone, when mammograms were negative, detected 8.7% of all cancers of known size, 6.6% of cancers under 1 cm in diameter, and 5.6% of noninfiltrating cancers.

Mammography and physical examination were both positive in 48.5% of all cancers of known size and in 35% of cancers under 1 cm in diameter (infiltrating and

---

* "Mammography" as used in this text includes xeromammography and film mammography using current low-dose and film or screen techniques.

noninfiltrating cancers). Overall, mammography had a true-positive detection rate of 92% for all cancers of known size and 93.4% for all cancers under 1 cm in diameter.

Although mammography has generally been regarded as less accurate among premenopausal women because of their greater breast density, mammography alone detected 36.9% of all cancers in the 40- to 49-year age group of women who had mammograms; physical examination alone detected 9.6% of all cancers, and both mammography and physical examination were positive in 52% and unknown in 1.5% of all cancers. Mammography had a true-positive cancer detection rate of 88.9% in this age group.

Seventy percent of the invasive cancers under 1 cm in diameter and 73% of in situ cancers with microcalcifications were detected by mammography alone in the BCDDP. In essence, a large number of cancers, particularly small, minimal, and easily curable ones, would have been missed had mammography not been used. The increase in detection of breast cancer by mammography alone from 20% in the early literature to over 40% at present documents an improvement in both mammogram quality and in the interpretive abilities of radiologists.

RADIOGRAPHIC CHANGES IN BREAST CANCER DETECTION

Minimal or noninvasive cancers are, with few exceptions, small and usually cause minimal or vague radiographic changes. In many patients, only an indeterminate or suspicious diagnosis can be made. The radiographic changes of a typical breast cancer include mass, surrounding fibrotic response with distorted tissue, nipple and skin retraction, skin thickening, and sometimes enlarged axillary nodes exceeding 1.5 to 2 cm in diameter. These changes are easily diagnosed clinically and radiographically. Unfortunately, they often indicate advanced cancer that has spread beyond the breast.

Conversely, the radiographic changes of minimal or noninvasive breast cancer include increased vascularity, increased breast density, locally dense stroma, local stromal distortion, enlarged or prominent ducts, and punctate or clustered calcifications. Although none of these changes are specific, any may occur in minimal breast cancer. Detection of one or more of these changes should increase the clinician's suspicion that a minimal breast cancer is present.

IMPORTANCE OF CALCIFICATIONS IN
BREAST CANCER DETECTION

Numerous linear, irregular, or punctate calcifications, particularly when localized or clustered, are excellent radiographic markers of breast disease. Benign calcifications are more common than malignant calcifications, in part because benign breast disease is more common than malignant disease. The presence of localized or clustered punctate calcifications should always be viewed as indicators of possible early or minimal breast cancer. In 1977, Mohr reported that 32% of 290 biopsy specimens from carcinomas of the breast contained calcifications. Hoeffken and Lanyi (1977), in the histologic examination of 212 patients with clustered microcalcifications, found that 27% (58/212) had cancer, and of these 70.7% (41/58) had noninvasive carcinoma.

In 1,481 consecutive breast specimens, Koehl et al. (1970) determined the incidence of calcifications of 450 malignant lesions; 62% (277) of the specimens had clusters of calcifications. This included 32 lobular carcinomas in situ, of which 25 (78%) were shown to have clustered calcifications on histologic examination. In the same series, various other benign pathologies also had significant percentages of histologically demonstrated calcifications.

In 1974, Wolfe analyzed 462 breast carcinomas in which 50.9% (244) were associated with calcifications visible on mammograms. Of 139 clinically occult carcinomas, 74% were associated with calcifications visible on mammograms, half of them without an associated mass.

In 1980, Egan et al. reported their study of 721 breasts containing mammographically detected calcifications without accompanying masses. The women had been followed from 4 to 16 years. Of 337 patients with clustered calcifications, 205 eventually had biopsies, and 78 (23%) of these proved to have malignant tumors. Of the 78 malignancies, 58% were noninvasive. The remaining 386 patients had both scattered and clustered calcifications. Of these, 265 patients eventually underwent biopsy, and 14% (37) of these were proved to have malignant tumors while 54% (20/37) had noninvasive tumors.

The location of calcifications in carcinoma was reviewed by Koehl et al. in 1970. Calcifications in duct cell carcinoma were located in the central necrotic debris of the intraductal portions of carcinomas, in small acini of infiltrating carcinomas, in the dense hyalinizing stroma of tumor, and in adjacent noncancerous lobules of ducts, that is, not within carcinoma. The last location is of considerable importance because it indicates that local areas of severe benign disease or proliferative change, i.e., "fertile gardens" for growth, can be identified radiographically and may have an increased incidence of malignant disease. The calcifications seen in lobular carcinoma in situ were usually in normal lobules adjacent to the carcinoma.

Mammography is the only diagnostic modality at present that can consistently detect microcalcifications not associated with a tissue mass in breast cancer. Preoperative needle localization based on the preliminary mammographic appearances is helpful to the surgeon in the precise and efficient excision of these suspicious areas. Following preoperative needle placement in the breast, confirmatory mammogram images are taken, properly labeled, and immediately sent with the patient to surgery. Following surgical excision of the area, specimen radiography confirms that the entire abnormal or suspicious area has indeed been removed.

CASE ILLUSTRATION

In 1969, a 44-year-old woman had a right radical mastectomy for breast cancer 8 years prior to her admission to the hospital for evaluation of a questionable lump in

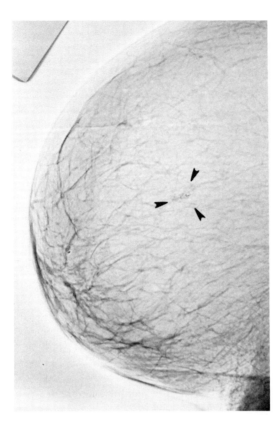

FIG. 1. Initial positive-mode xeromammogram (mediolateral projection) reveals a cluster of punctate, irregular calcifications in the lateral aspect of the left breast (between arrowheads), radiographically considered indeterminate with suspicion of possible early malignancy. No mass or increased glandular density is evident.

the left breast. She had also been treated and followed for chronic lymphocytic leukemia. Physical examination revealed no dominant mass, but a questionable nodule was present under the left nipple. The right breast was unremarkable.

Xeromammograms of the left breast revealed a 1-cm cluster of tiny calcifications in the upper outer quadrant 11 cm from the nipple (away from the area of clinical concern) and 2 cm under the skin surface (Figs. 1 and 2). No mass or other abnormal change was associated with the calcifications, which were considered indeterminate and suspicious for possible intraductal (noninvasive) carcinoma. There was a suggestion of benign subareolar nodularity without evidence of malignancy.

Because the area of the breast that contained the suspicious calcifications was negative for tumor on physical examination, preoperative needle localization was performed in the mammographic suite immediately prior to excisional biopsy (Fig. 3). A biopsy specimen radiograph was taken before and after sectioning of the specimen to ensure removal of the calcifications and to localize them for the pathologist (Figs. 4 and 5).

Histological examination revealed intraductal carcinoma of the breast (noninvasive comedo carcinoma). Well-differentiated lymphocytic lymphoma was found in the breast parenchyma (in random sections of a large generous specimen and not

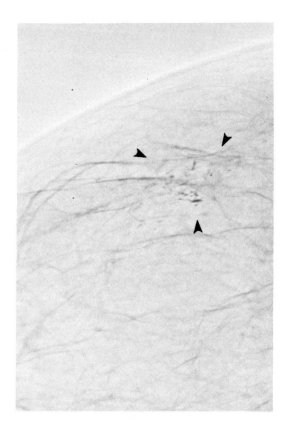

FIG. 2. Positive-mode xeromammogram (coned craniocaudad projection) shows the cluster of punctate calcifications (between arrowheads) to lie superficially in the lateral aspect of the left breast.

related to the intraductal carcinoma). An extended simple mastectomy of the left breast 2 weeks later revealed focal residual intraductal carcinoma. Fourteen axillary lymph nodes were negative for metastatic carcinoma, but well-differentiated lymphocytic lymphoma was present in several lymph nodes. Well-differentiated lymphoma is the tissue manifestation of chronic lymphocytic leukemia.

VALUE OF MAMMOGRAPHY WITH PALPABLE MASSES AND PRIOR TO BREAST SURGERY

Mammography is performed prior to breast surgery for confirmation of the clinical suspicion or diagnosis, to detect an unsuspected cancer, and as a survey of the opposite breast. Routine mammography is performed on patients who have clinically indeterminate breast masses that are to undergo biopsy. The mammogram may indicate either greater or less suspicion than the clinical examination. In both cases, however, the information obtained is valuable to the surgeon in scheduling the proper surgical procedure and in discussing the various treatment alternatives with the patient. Mammography is helpful in the evaluation of nonpalpable axillary lymph nodes. It may be even more important in the evaluation and detection of un-

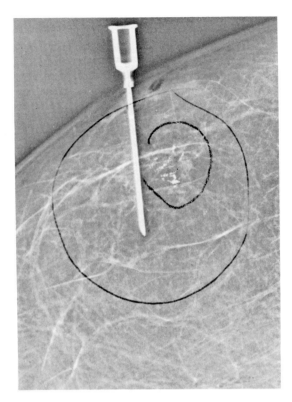

FIG. 3. Negative-mode xeromammogram (craniocaudad projection) for preoperative needle localization immediately prior to surgery. Needle localization images are always made with negative-mode xeroradiography to avoid the toner deletion zone that occurs around the needle in the positive mode, which might obscure the cluster of calcifications. All images are carefully labeled with a wax crayon to indicate direction, i.e., medial, lateral, superior, and inferior, and are sent with the patient directly to surgery.

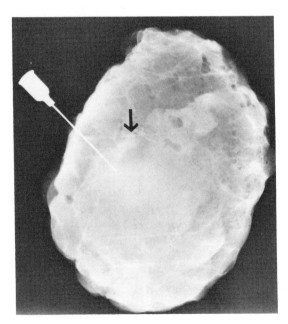

FIG. 4. Initial specimen radiograph of excised breast tissue taken immediately after resection (with localization needle in place) confirms removal of the cluster of calcifications (arrow). Failure to visualize the radiographically suspicious area in the specimen would necessitate further tissue resection and repeat specimen radiography.

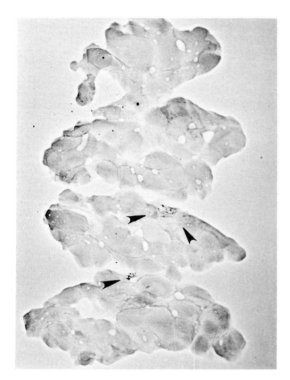

FIG. 5. Radiographs made after slicing the initial specimen into smaller pieces allow more precise localization of the excised tissue containing the calcifications (arrows) for the pathologist and ensure that the most suspicious areas of the specimen will be examined histologically. Pathologic diagnosis was intraductal (noninvasive) carcinoma of the breast.

suspected lesions in a breast with a known lesion or in the contralateral, presumably negative, breast.

Even with clinically obvious carcinoma, preoperative mammography can determine the tumor size, location, and the extent of involved breast, as well as evaluate and detect abnormalities in the contralateral breast. The contralateral breast, if clinically and radiographically negative, should be examined to establish a baseline for future follow-up examinations.

The detection and treatment of early or minimal breast cancer requires the concerted and cooperative efforts of the surgeon, the diagnostic radiologist, the radiotherapist, and the pathologist to preserve its high survival rate. The radiologist, through the use of mammography, plays a vital role in the detection and localization of these minimal cancers.

REFERENCES

Baker, L. H. 1982. Breast cancer detection demonstration project: Five-year summary report. Ca 32:194–225.

Dodd, G. D. 1981. Radiation detection and diagnosis of breast cancer. Cancer 47:1766–1769.

Egan, R. L., M. B. McSweeney, and C. W. Sewell. 1980. Intramammary calcifications without an associated mass in benign and malignant diseases. Radiology 137:1–7.

Frazier, T. G., E. M. Copeland, H. S. Gallager, D. D. Paulus, and E. C. White. 1977. The prognosis and treatment of minimal breast cancer. Am. J. Surg. 133:697–701.

Gallager, H. S., and J. E. Martin. 1971. An orientation to the concept of minimal breast cancer, 1971. Cancer 28:1505.

Hoeffken, W. and M. Lanyi. 1977. Mammography. W. B. Saunders Company, Philadelphia, pp. 257–275.

Koehl, R. H., R. E. Snyder, R. P. Hutter, and F. W. Foote. 1970. The incidence and significance of calcifications within operative breast specimens. Am. J. Clin. Pathol. 53:3–14.

Mohr, H. J. 1977. Moglichkeiten und widrigheiten in der fruhdiagnostik des mammakarginomas. Arch. Geschwulslforch 47:583.

Wolfe, J. N. 1974. Analysis of 462 breast carcinomas. AJR 121:846.

Current Controversies in Breast Cancer, edited
by F. C. Ames, G. R. Blumenschein, and E. D. Montague.
University of Texas Press, Austin © 1984.

Radiation Therapy for Minimal Breast Cancer

Eleanor D. Montague, M.D.

*Department of Radiotherapy, The University of Texas M. D. Anderson Hospital and
Tumor Institute at Houston, Houston, Texas*

The definition of minimal breast cancer proposed by Gallagher and Martin (1969) includes either ductal or lobular noninvasive carcinoma or invasive carcinoma having a volume no greater than that of a sphere 0.5 cm in diameter. It is estimated, through correlation of mammographically measurable primary tumors and incidence of axillary node metastasis, that the probability of axillary metastasis is less than 10% in these three histopathologic entities.

This article describes the results of treatment at The University of Texas M. D. Anderson Hospital and Tumor Institute at Houston of a small number of patients who had minimal breast cancer. These patients were treated by mastectomy alone or by tumor excision followed by irradiation. Patients who had small-volume invasive and noninvasive cancer are analyzed together.

MATERIALS

From 1955 through 1979, 138 patients who had minimal breast cancer were treated at UT M. D. Anderson Hospital: 12 were treated with biopsy excision (2 had local recurrences), 4 were treated with mastectomy and had positive lymph nodes (2 received postoperative irradiation), and 122 were treated with mastectomy alone and had histologically negative lymph nodes. Twenty patients who also had cancer in the other breast were also treated with mastectomy alone. Forty other patients were treated during this same time with tumor excision and irradiation. Table 1 shows the distribution of pathology in these patients, noting that noninvasive intraductal carcinoma was frequently described in the surgical specimen along with invasive cancer. Of these 40 patients, four had conservation surgery and bilateral irradiation for simultaneous bilateral breast cancer. All patients had clinically palpable breast masses in the early years; more recently, occult tumors have been detected roentgenographically. Tables 2 and 3 show the surgical procedures employed; patients were treated with classical radical mastectomy in the first decade of this review.

Patients with invasive breast cancer have always had axillary dissection when radical mastectomy has been performed. In recent years, less radical surgery has been performed for noninvasive disease, with the extended simple mastectomy

Table 1. *Primary Pathologic Diagnosis and Treatment of Patients with Minimal Breast Cancer (1955–1979)*

Pathology	Mastectomy	Excision and XRT
Invasive*	44 (11[†])	9 (2)
Noninvasive intraductal	68 (9)	30 (2)
Lobular in situ	10	1

*50% of patients with invasive carcinoma had accompanied diagnosis of intraductal noninvasive carcinoma.
[†]Number of patients with bilateral breast cancer.

Table 2. *Type of Mastectomy (1955–1979)*

Mastectomy	No. Patients
Classical radical	51
Modified radical	25
Simple mastectomy and dissection of the lateral axilla	39
Simple mastectomy alone*	7

*⁵⁄₇ patients had lobular carcinoma in situ.

Table 3. *Conservation Surgical Procedure and Irradiation (1955–1979)*

Surgical Procedure	No. Patients
Excision	32
Segmental mastectomy alone	4
Segmental mastectomy and dissection of the lateral axilla	4

being performed more frequently. Most surgeons will perform a simple mastectomy for lobular in situ carcinoma.

RADIATION WITH CONSERVATION SURGERY

Axillary dissection was not performed in patients treated with irradiation until after 1974; thus, the status of the axilla was determined clinically.

Invasive Breast Cancer

Supervoltage irradiation with ^{60}Co following excision biopsy began to be used in 1955 at UT M. D. Anderson Hospital, and gradually evolved into the present technique. Any patient who had invasive cancer without axillary dissection received ^{60}Co irradiation to the breast and adjacent chest wall, axilla, supraclavicular, and internal mammary areas. The entire breast was irradiated through medial and lateral tangential portals, generally without bolus. During the last 7 years, using open and wedged-filtered fields, 5,000 rad in 5 weeks has been given, plus an additional 1,000-rad tumor dose, usually with electrons, to the site of the excised tumor in the breast. The 5,000-rad tumor dose to the axilla and supraclavicular areas was delivered through the anterior supraclavicular-axillary field and the posterior axillary field opposing the low and central axilla. The internal mammary nodes were irradiated through a direct field for a 4,500-rad dose in 5 weeks (Fletcher 1980). The technique used after 1974 was to remove the primary lesion with segmental mastectomy and perform a dissection of the lateral axilla. Histologic confirmation of the axillary status permits a better definition of areas to be irradiated; if the axilla is negative and if the invasive cancer is located in the outer half of the breast, only the breast need be irradiated; if in the central or inner portions of the breast, then the breast and internal mammary chain are irradiated. The rare patient with positive axillary lymph nodes would have the entire breast, supraclavicular, and internal mammary chain areas irradiated.

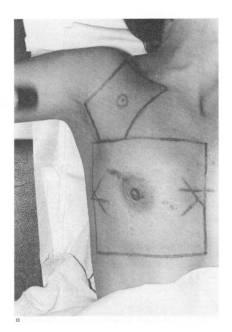 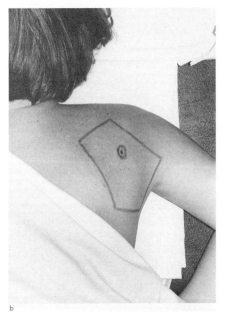

FIG. 1A and B. The patient had noninvasive intraductal carcinoma removed from the upper outer quadrant of the right breast. The surgeon advised an extended simple mastectomy, which the patient refused. Treatment portals provide the equivalent of the surgery and include the breast and low and central axilla for a 5,000-rad tumor dose in 5 weeks (25 fractions) with ^{60}Co. (Reproduced from Fletcher et al. 1980, with permission of Lea and Febiger.)

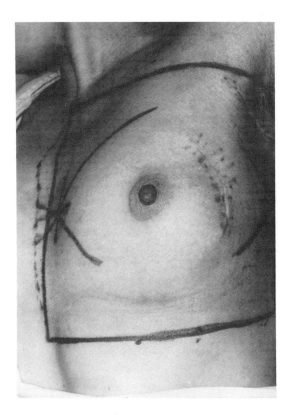

FIG. 2. The patient had a noninvasive intraductal carcinoma removed from the upper outer quadrant of the left breast. The surgeon advised a simple mastectomy. Treatment portals with ^{60}Co provide the equivalent of the surgery; a 5,000-rad tumor dose in 5 weeks (25 fractions) was delivered.

Noninvasive Cancer

Prior to 1970, eight patients with noninvasive cancer were treated with radiotherapy not only to the breast but also to the axillary, supraclavicular, and internal mammary chain lymph nodes. From 1970 to 1979, four patients were treated with radiotherapy to the breast and axilla (Figures 1a and 1b) (because the referring surgeon would have performed an extended simple mastectomy dissecting the lateral axilla), and 18 patients (including the one with lobular in situ carcinoma) received radiation only to the breast (Figure 2). Figure 3 shows the infraclavicular electron beam portal used to treat breast tissue above the margin of the tangential fields if the tumor bed is marginally within the tangents or if there are multiple sites of disease in the upper half of the breast.

RESULTS

Table 4 shows that two patients have experienced recurrences: One patient had a recurrence in the breast, and another patient treated by mastectomy only had a supraclavicular recurrence, which was controlled by irradiation. The latter patient had

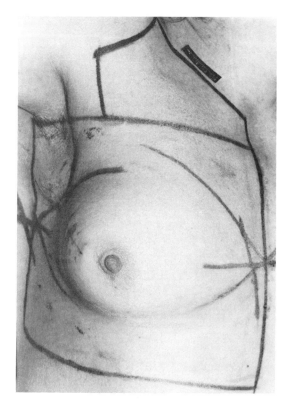

FIG. 3. The patient had a 2.0-cm upper outer quadrant mass with microcalcifications on xeromammography. A lateral axillary dissection in continuity with excision of the primary tumor removed 10 histologically negative lymph nodes; noninvasive intraductal carcinoma was found. Cobalt-60 tangential fields delivered a 5,000-rad tumor dose to the breast using 1:1 open and wedged fields. A 7-MeV electron beam was used to deliver a 4,500-rad tumor dose to the breast tissue above the tangential portals and below the clavicle. No boost was delivered to the excision site, since the disease was noninvasive and widely excised. The patient is free of disease in January, 1981. (Reproduced from Montague et al. 1982, with permission of Masson Publishers.)

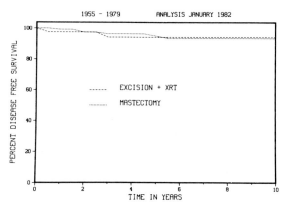

FIG. 4. Ten-year disease-free survival of patients treated with mastectomy or conservation surgery and irradiation.

a medially located invasive primary tumor, for which no elective irradiation had been given.

There is no difference between the 10-year disease-free survival rates for patients treated with mastectomy or conservation surgery and irradiation (Figure 4).

The cosmetic results of conservation surgery and irradiation improved as the surgical and radiotherapeutic techniques became more refined and as the irradiated volume was lessened. When only the breast is treated, there are no junction lines, and little or no fibrosis is noted in the breast after a 5,000-rad tumor dose (Figure 5). Since the lymph nodes are rarely positive in minimal breast cancer, it is the unusual patient who requires irradiation to the larger volume of the breast and the supraclavicular and internal mammary chain nodes; the dissected axilla is not irradiated unless extranodal disease is identified.

DISCUSSION

Considerable experience has been accumulated concerning the control of breast cancer with postoperative irradiation after radical or modified radical mastectomy and in patients with advanced local-regional disease treated with simple or simple extended mastectomy and irradiation; a dose of 4,500–5,000 rad controls 90% of potential subclinical disease (Fletcher 1974, Fletcher 1980). Although mastectomy

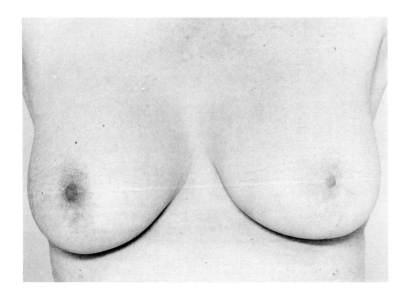

FIG. 5. The patient had a 1.0-cm upper outer quadrant noninvasive carcinoma of the left breast excised; ^{60}Co irradiation was given through medial and lateral tangential fields for a 5,000-rad tumor dose in 5 weeks (25 fractions). She remains well with good cosmetic result 7 years later.

Table 4. *Local Recurrence in Patients with Minimal Breast Cancer Treated with Conservation Surgery and Irradiation (XRT) or Mastectomy Alone (1955–1979)**

Site	Excision and XRT (40 patients)	Mastectomy Alone (122 patients)
Breast	1[†]	–
Axilla	–	–
Supraclavicular	–	1[‡]
Parasternal	–	–

*Adapted from Montague et al., 1982.
[†]No evidence of disease 5 years after radical mastectomy.
[‡]No evidence of disease 4 years after irradiation.

for minimal breast cancer is very successful, there is now evidence that conservation surgery and irradiation are equally successful. Additional evidence has been provided by the clinical trial reported by Veronesi (1981), in which 80% of the patients had tumors less than 2 cm in diameter, and in which patients treated with quadrantectomy and irradiation did as well as patients treated with radical or modified radical mastectomy.

The current National Surgical Adjuvant Breast/Bowel Project (NSABP) clinical trial in stage I and stage II breast cancer is attempting to define the least radical, effective treatment for breast cancer: All patients have axillary dissection, and the primary treatment is randomized to segmental mastectomy alone, segmental mastectomy and irradiation of the breast, or total mastectomy (Fisher et al. 1980). The outcome of the trial should help define the minimal effective treatment for patients with minimal breast cancer as well.

ACKNOWLEDGMENTS

This investigation was supported in part by Grant Number CA06294 awarded by the National Cancer Institute, Department of Health and Human Services.

REFERENCES

Fisher, B., C. Redmond, and E. R. Fisher. 1980. The contribution of recent NSABP clinical trials of primary breast cancer therapy to an understanding of tumor biology: An overview of findings. Cancer 46:1009–1025.

Fletcher, G. H. 1974. Radiation therapy and subclinical disease, *in* Neoplasia of Head and Neck. Year Book Medical Publishers, Inc., Chicago, pp. 19–38.

Fletcher, G. H. 1980. Textbook of Radiotherapy, 3rd edition. Lea and Fibger, Philadelphia, pp. 527–579.

Gallager, H. S., and J. E. Martin. 1969. The study of mammary carcinoma by mammography and whole organ sectioning. Cancer 23:855.

Montague, E. D., W. J. Spanos, Jr., F. Ames, M. Romsdahl, G. H. Fletcher, S. R. Schell, and
M. J. Oswald. 1983. Conservative treatment of noninvasive or small-volume invasive breast
cancer, *in* Breast Carcinoma: Current Diagnosis and Treatment, S. Feig, ed. Masson Publishers,
New York, pp. 429–432.

Veronesi, U., R. Saccozzi, M. Del Vecchio, A. Banfi, C. Clemente, M. De Lena, G. Gallus, M.
Greco, A. Luini, E. Marubini, F. Rilke, B. Salvadori, A. Zecchini, and R. Zucali. 1981. Comparing radical mastectomy with quadrantectomy, axillary dissection, and radiotherapy in patients with small cancers of the breast. N. Engl. J. Med. 305:6–11.

RADIATION/SURGERY FOR OPERABLE BREAST CANCER

Current Controversies in Breast Cancer, edited
by F. C. Ames, G. R. Blumenschein, and E. D. Montague.
University of Texas Press, Austin © 1984.

The Place of Radical Surgery for Stages I and II Breast Cancer

Frederick C. Ames, M. D.

Department of General Surgery, The University of Texas M. D. Anderson Hospital and Tumor Institute at Houston, Houston, Texas

For many years, radical mastectomy and modified radical mastectomy have been the two most used operations for the primary surgical treatment of breast cancer. In recent years, however, there has developed a growing shift toward the use of lesser surgical procedures that involve little or no axillary dissection or that leave the breast intact. The use of these less extensive procedures as alternatives to radical surgery for treatment of breast cancer has been given wide media coverage and is common knowledge among the lay public. Unfortunately, little attention has been given to the criteria for patient selection necessary to make the use of such lesser surgical procedures safe and effective. As a result, there often is confusion among both the public as well as the medical community about the proper place of these alternatives to radical surgery in the treatment of patients who have stage I and stage II breast cancer. The issue is far more complex than just considering what the alternatives to radical surgery might be. It is equally important to realize that all patients with breast cancer, even within a given clinical stage, are not necessarily alike. Breast cancers range from early lesions that are often curable by almost any form of treatment to multifocal or advanced lesions that demand the most aggressive combination of therapies for any chance of patient survival. Even among patients with clinical stage I or stage II disease, the tumors may range in size up to 5 cm in diameter, and the lymph nodes found with metastases may easily number four or more. Thus, even within the group with the clinical stage II disease are found patients who present a difficult challenge for the therapist in terms of both survival and local control. Under these circumstances, with relatively larger tumors and multiple positive lymph nodes, the use of lesser surgical procedures as primary therapy with preservation of the breast is, at present, speculative and may even be dangerous. In addition, it is debatable whether even somewhat smaller tumors in awkward locations or in small breasts are suitable for breast preservation. Therefore, even if one accepts that a lesser operation on either the breast or the axilla is an appropriate alternative for some stage I and stage II breast cancers, such may not be the case for all patients in these clinical groups. Conversely, modified radical mastectomy is an appropriate surgical treatment for virtually any stage I or stage II breast cancer patient (Baker et al. 1979, Robinson 1976). This discussion will out-line the criteria used in selecting the optimal primary therapy for patients with stage I or stage II breast cancer at The University of Texas M. D. Anderson Hospital and Tumor Institute at Houston, with emphasis on factors that favor the use of modified radical mastectomy.

SEGMENTAL MASTECTOMY

Factors in Favor

The sole advantage of conservation surgery for breast cancer patients is that the breast remains intact. Although the initial hospitalization may be somewhat shorter by up to 7 days in our hospital, this initial saving of time and expense is offset by the cost and inconvenience of the mandatory 5 weeks of radiation therapy required after conservation surgery.

Factors Not in Favor

There are several factors militating against the use of segmental mastectomy (Table 1). In terms of medical risk to the patient from the surgical procedure, seg-mental mastectomy with axillary staging is no more safe than modified radical mas-tectomy in experienced hands. Both procedures, in fact, are quite safe, although segmental mastectomy mandates the use of radiation therapy, which may itself of-fer some medical risks to certain patients. Omitting the axillary staging procedure certainly shortens the surgical procedure, the hospitalization, and the long-term complications of slight arm edema, but it also ignores the possibility of axillary nodal metastasis and the potential need for considering adjunctive chemotherapy.

While the survival statistics offered for segmental mastectomy and radiation therapy are quite good and appear to be equal to those of standard therapy in the form of modified radical mastectomy (Fisher et al. 1977, Harris et al. 1978, Mon-tague et al. 1983, Veronesi et al. 1981), we admit that our experience with the seg-mental procedure involves several hundred patients with a follow-up period of only 5 to 10 years, in contrast to many more patients treated over a much longer period with modified radical mastectomy. Another unfavorable factor in the use of segmen-tal mastectomy with radiation is that the surgical margins are less certain, especially if a biopsy has been done with significant breast disturbance or without prebiopsy mammography. As a result, the pathologic stage may be unreliable in regard to both the tumor stage or the axillary nodal stage. As the size of the tumor increases rela-tive to the size of the breast, and as the tumor is found closer to the nipple, it be-comes more difficult to obtain an adequate surgical margin without compromising the cosmetic result. Thus, if the cosmetic result is not satisfactory, the sole reason for not performing modified radical mastectomy is lost; conversely, if a proper sur-gical margin is not achieved, the safety of the procedure is threatened. Similarly, as less axillary tissue is dissected, the cosmetic appearance of the breast is improved,

Table 1. *Segmental Mastectomy and Radiation for Stages I and II Breast Cancer: Factors Not in Favor*

Survival based on limited experience
Risk of surgery no less than mastectomy
Surgical margin less certain
    (May not be known with prior biopsy)
Pathological stage may be unreliable
        T-stage with outside excision[*]
        N-stage with incomplete dissection[*]
Cosmesis may alter surgical margin
        With increasing tumor size[*]
        With tumor near nipple[*]
        With less axillary dissection[*]
XRT[†] Mandatory—adds time and a question of increasing risk
Complications in follow-up
        Long-term control less certain[*]
Safe effects of XRT[†] less certain

---

[*]Especially with stage II disease.
[†]XRT = irradiation.

but at the expense of less reliable axillary staging information (Fisher et al. 1981). The use of segmental mastectomy mandates the use of radiation therapy which may have long-term effects not completely understood at present. Physicians may face special problems in follow-up of patients having received conservation surgery and irradiation because the diseased breasts of these patients are often of a different consistency and firmness, especially in the area of the surgical scar and radiation field overlap.

MODIFIED RADICAL MASTECTOMY

Factors in favor

In contrast to the limited information we have on the advantages and disadvantages of segmental mastectomy, we have a great deal of experience with modified radical mastectomy (Table 2) and know what we can expect in terms of optimal survival and medical risk when it is used (Baker et al. 1979, Eilber et al. 1982, Robinson 1976). Since no adjunctive treatment is mandated by its use, we also know that it is safe and expeditious treatment for older or medically impaired patients (Hunt et al. 1980). Modified radical mastectomy effects maximal tumor reduction, and there is less worry about tumor size, location, surgical margin, or multiplicity of tumors. The problem of a surprise pathologic upstaging, usually due to discovery of axillary nodal metastases involving multiple lymph nodes, can easily be managed by prompt chemotherapy with no compromise of local control. Radiation therapy is easily used as desired, either shortly after surgery or after adjunctive chemotherapy, and is quite well tolerated (Tapley et al. 1982). Currently, there is little disability from the procedure, even when radiation therapy is used, and follow-up examination of the chest wall and axilla is straight forward. The 10- and 20-year

Table 2. *Modified Radical Mastectomy for Stage I and II
Breast Cancer: Factors in Favor*

Known optimal survival
Low medical risk
Expeditious–radiation therapy not mandatory
Maximal tumor reduction
    Surgical margin no problem
    Complete tumor and axillary staging
        Size and location of tumor little problem*
        Multiple foci no problem*
        Surprise upstaging no problem*
        Prompt chemotherapy easy*
Compatible with radiation therapy as desired
Regional follow-up easy
Little disability
Long-term effects well known
Reconstruction straight forward

---

*Especially with stage II disease.

aftereffects of modified radical mastectomy are well known. In addition, breast reconstruction, especially utilizing myocutaneous flaps, is becoming more refined and is more widely available to patients, partly offsetting the disadvantage of the loss of the breast.

Factors Not in Favor

The factors not in favor of modified radical mastectomy as the surgical treatment for stage I and stage II breast cancer are few. Aside from the obvious disadvantage of the loss of the breast, there may be a slightly greater incidence of mild arm edema than with segmental mastectomy and axillary staging. Because of the more full axillary dissection with modified radical mastectomy, hospitalization is 3 to 7 days longer than required for segmental mastectomy; however, the cost of longer hospitalization is more than offset by the cost and inconvenience of the necessary radiation therapy used when segmental mastectomy is done.

SELECTION OF TREATMENT

Stage I Breast Cancer

Candidates for Modified Radical Mastectomy

Patients with tumors smaller than 2 cm in diameter and with clinically negative axillae are all candidates for treatment by modified radical mastectomy. Patients who are older, at higher medical risk, or who want quick one-stage treatment without any assumption of uncertainties or potentially added risk are especially suitable for treatment by modified radical mastectomy. In addition, patients who have

Table 3. *Surgical Treatment of Stage I Breast Cancer*
(T Less Than 2 cm, N_0)*

Modified radical suitable for all
Segmental mastectomy and radiation therapy:
    Possible alternative for solitary lesion away from nipple
    Accurate clinical assessment essential

*T = tumor; N = nodes.

already received mastectomy of the other breast or who stand a great chance of contralateral disease because of tumor biology or family history are generally considered most suitable for treatment by modified radical mastectomy. When a significant breast disturbance has been created by biopsy prior to referral and exact tumor size is uncertain, especially when no mammogram was obtained prior to biopsy, the patients are placed in stage II category or are left unstaged and are not considered as stage I patients.

Candidates for Segmental Mastectomy plus Radiation

Patients with solitary lesions not near the nipple may be considered candidates for segmental mastectomy with axillary sampling and radiation therapy (Table 3). In this category patients who have minimal breast and tumor disturbance from outside biopsy may be included, as long as we are quite comfortable with their staging based on the available information and physical examination. At present, a reexcision of the biopsy scar in the form of a segmental mastectomy is indicated and is carried out together with the lateral axillary dissection for staging purposes. A recent review of a 2-year experience in our hospital with this technique has shown that approximately half of such patients have been found to have residual cancer in the reexcision specimen and that even in T1 lesions 19% had axillary metastases. It was also found that by taking all the nodes in the lateral axillary compartment (lateral to the pectoralis minor muscle), 75% of the specimens revealed 10 to 20 lymph nodes, which provided not only accurate pathological staging of the axilla but very acceptable cosmetic and functional results as well.

Stage II Breast Cancer

Candidates for Modified Radical Mastectomy

For these patients with tumors over 2 cm in diameter or who have clinically positive axillary lymph nodes, modified radical mastectomy is the standard form of therapy (Table 4). Patients who either prefer or would benefit from quick single-stage therapy with the assumption of the least amount of risk and uncertainty are especially suitable for treatment by modified radical mastectomy. In addition, when the primary tumor approaches 4 to 5 cm in size and the palpated axillary disease

Table 4. *Surgical Treatment Stage II Breast Cancer*

Modified radical suitable for all
Segmental mastectomy and radiation therapy possible alternative for:
    Solitary lesion away from nipple
    Generally tumor < 3–4 cm
    Limited axillary disease clinically determined
        Single + node < 2–3 cm
           (with 4 + nodes found at surgery use chemotherapy before
           radiation therapy; increasing concern about margin)
        Accurate clinical assessment essential

suggests more than limited involvement (1 to 3 positive nodes) and when the overall disease stage actually approaches stage III, it becomes more difficult to achieve both a good cosmetic result and an adequate surgical margin. Of potentially greater worry is the need for prompt chemotherapy in these patients with relatively more advanced disease. Following segmental mastectomy in such patients, the use of immediate adjunctive chemotherapy increases the fear of inadequate local control because of delayed radiation therapy. In such cases, modified radical mastectomy gives a far superior surgical margin with maximum tumor reduction. Patients with marked disturbance of the breast are generally excluded from this group unless there is clear evidence that the tumor size places the patient in this category. The area of breast disturbance must be able to be excised with the standard modified radical mastectomy incision.

Candidates for Segmental Mastectomy and Radiation

For patients with relatively earlier stage II lesions measuring less than 3 or 4 cm in greatest diameter and who have very modest clinical axillary involvement, segmental mastectomy with lateral axillary sampling and radiation therapy may be an appropriate alternative to modified radical mastectomy (Montague et al. 1983). When such therapy is used, however, occasional surprise pathologic upstaging following surgery will be encountered, which may pose added risks unless very careful case selection has been practiced to insure adequate surgical margins if adjunctive chemotherapy is thought advisable prior to radiation therapy. Overall, when accurate clinical assessment of the tumor, the breast, and the axilla are not possible or do not indicate the presence of stage I or low stage II disease, modified radical mastectomy is favored as the surgical treatment of choice; in such a setting, segmental mastectomy with radiation therapy is not considered an equally safe and appropriate alternative.

SUMMARY

Lesser surgical procedures that preserve the breast and employ radiation therapy may be suitable alternatives for the treatment of selected patients who have stage I and stage II breast cancer. Patient acceptance seems quite favorable, but the number of factors that actually favor such treatment are few and relate largely to the cosmetic appearance of the preserved breast rather than to any effects on survival or even function. Radiation therapy is mandatory, and the potential risks assumed with this form of treatment are several and may be magnified by a larger tumor, an inappropriate location, inadequate surgical margin, or surprise pathologic upstaging after surgery. Overall, modified radical mastectomy gives quick, effective, one-step surgical treatment for almost any stage I or stage II breast cancer, as well as maximum tumor reduction and complete pathologic staging, and does not mandate the use of any other adjunctive treatment. Only patients who have easily assessed, relatively smaller, solitary, appropriately located stage I or early stage II tumors should be offered breast preservation with radiation therapy.

REFERENCES

Baker, R. R., A. Montague, and J. Childs. 1979. A comparison of modified radical mastectomy to radical mastectomy in the treatment of operable breast cancer. Ann. Surg. 189:553.

Eilber, F. R., C. A. Milne, E. C. White, and C. M. McBride. 1982. Early carcinoma of the breast: Evaluation of regional therapy and features influencing prognosis. South Med. J. 75:9–13.

Fisher, B., E. Montague, C. Redmond, and other NSABP investigators. 1977. Comparison of radical mastectomy with alternative treatments for primary breast cancer: A first report of results from a prospective randomized clinical trial. Cancer 39:2827–2839.

Fisher, B., N. Wolmark, M. Bauer, C. Redmond, and M. Gebhardt. 1981. The accuracy of clinical nodal staging and of limited axillary dissection as a determinant of histologic nodal status in carcinoma of the breast. Surg. Gynecol. Obstet. 152:765–772.

Harris, J. R., M. B. Levene, and S. Hellman. 1978. Results of treating stages I and II carcinoma of the breast with primary radiation therapy. Cancer Treat. Rep. 62:985–991.

Hunt, K. E., D. E. Fry, and K. I. Bland. 1980. Breast carcinoma in the elderly patient: An assessment of operative risk, morbidity, and mortality. Am. J. Surg. 339–342.

Montague, E. D., W. J. Spauss, Jr., F. Ames, M. Romsdahl, S. Schell, G. H. Fletcher, and M. J. Oswald. 1983. Conservation surgery and irradiation for the treatment of clinically favorable breast cancer, *in* Breast Cancer: Current Diagnosis and Treatment, R. McClelland and S. A. Feig eds., Mason Co., New York (in press).

Robinson, G. N. 1976. The primary surgical treatment of carcinoma of the breast: A trend toward modified radical mastectomy. Mayo Clin. Proc. 51:433.

Tapley, N. D., W. J. Spauss, Jr., G. H. Fletcher, E. D. Montague, S. Schell, and M. J. Oswald. 1982. Results in patients with breast cancer treated by radical mastectomy and postoperative radiation with no adjuvant chemotherapy. Cancer 49:1316–1319.

Veronesi, U., R. Saccozzi, M. Del Vecchio, A. Banfi, C. Clemente, M. DeLena, G. Gallus, M. Greco, A. Lvini, E. Marubini, G. Muscolino, F. Rilke, B. Salvadori, A. Zecchini, and R. Zucali. 1981. Comparing radical mastectomy with quadrantectomy, axillary dissection, and radiotherapy in patients with small cancers of the breast. N. Engl. J. Med. 305:6–11.

Current Controversies in Breast Cancer, edited
by F. C. Ames, G. R. Blumenschein, and E. D. Montague.
University of Texas Press, Austin © 1984.

The Treatment Philosophy, Technique, and Results of Primary Radiation for Early Breast Cancer at the Joint Center for Radiation Therapy

Jay R. Harris, M.D., and Samuel Hellman, M.D.

*The Joint Center for Radiation Therapy, Department of Radiation Therapy,
Harvard Medical School, Boston, Massachusetts*

Primary radiation therapy for early breast cancer refers to the use of conservative surgery combined with radiation therapy as an alternative to mastectomy. For this technique to be a useful alternative, three objectives must be achieved:

1. a high level of local tumor control
2. good cosmetic and function results
3. effective integration with adjuvant systemic therapy.

Local tumor control is the primary objective of local treatment. Long-term follow-up of effective local treatment has shown that a significant proportion of patients with early breast cancer remain free of recurrence and can be considered cured. As a philosophy of treatment, we view primary radiation therapy as a radical approach, one designed to provide a high level of local tumor control. In contrast, a conservative approach would accept a higher rate of local recurrence based on the view that maximizing local tumor control is not critical for survival. At present, the evidence favoring the radical-versus-conservative approach is inconclusive. As a result, it appears prudent to accept the radical approach, since incorrectly accepting the radical approach will not result in increased mortality from breast cancer. In contrast, if the conservative view is incorrectly accepted, an increased mortality from breast cancer would be seen.

The results of mastectomy in treating early breast cancer are well known and indicate that initial recurrence in approximately 10% to 15% of patients develops locally (Fisher et al. 1970, Valagussa et al. 1978). The chief objection to mastectomy is the psychological effect of amputating the female breast, an organ that has great importance for sexual identity in our culture. The goal of primary radiation therapy is, therefore, to provide not only equally high levels of local tumor control but also good cosmetic and functional results.

Although we stress that local tumor control is the primary objective of local treatment, it is clear that local treatment is itself limited. Many patients with apparently localized breast cancer manifest metastases in the years following local treatment. This suggests that occult distant disease is present in many patients who have early breast cancer. Attempts at enlarging the scope of local treatment, such as using postoperative irradiation or performing more aggressive surgical procedures, have done little to improve the cure rate. It is now generally acknowledged that therapeutic improvements in the cure rate will be achieved primarily through the use of effective adjuvant systemic therapy. The results of combination chemotherapy with such drugs as cyclophosphamide, methotrexate, 5-fluorouracil (5-FU), Adriamycin, vincristine, and prednisone for reducing the recurrence rate have been encouraging, but further follow-up will be required to assess fully its effect on the cure rate. At present, however, adjuvant systemic therapy using these agents has become standard therapy in this country for "young" women considered to be at "high risk." There is not yet general agreement on the definition of "young" or "high risk," but all premenopausal and many otherwise healthy postmenopausal women with histologically positive axillary nodes are candidates for adjuvant systemic therapy.

There are two considerations pertinent to the integration of primary radiation therapy and adjuvant systemic therapy. One is the identification of patients to receive adjuvant therapy, and the other is the sequencing of these two modalities. As noted above, involvement of axillary lymph nodes is one of the conventional determinants of high risk. Because of this, axillary node evaluation has become important when using primary radiation therapy. The results of axillary node evaluation also affect the radiation therapy technique. This will be discussed in detail below. The optimal sequencing of radiation therapy and chemotherapy has not been determined. This article will also discuss this aspect of primary radiation therapy.

The Joint Center for Radiation Therapy was founded in July 1968, and we have treated breast cancer patients with primary radiation therapy since that year. Our technique of treatment has evolved through reviews of our treatment results and the introduction of axillary dissection. In the early years of our institution, we used a conventional three-field technique similar to that employed for postoperative irradiation. Two opposed tangential fields were used in irradiating the breast, lower axilla, and internal mammary lymph nodes. A separate anterior field was used for the upper axilla and supraclavicular region. Patients were treated using a 4-MV linear accelerator after excisional biopsy or, in some cases, incisional biopsy. The doses used varied considerably during these early years. The breast and draining lymph node areas received between 4,400 rad in 5 weeks and 6,000 rad in 6 weeks, given either four or five times a week. In some patients, a supplementary "boost" of approximately 2,000 rad was given to the primary tumor area using ^{192}Ir interstitial implantation. In general, implantation was performed in patients whose tumors extended close to the margins of resection.

The external-beam technique required elevating the head and shoulders of the patient to make the sternum parallel to the treatment couch. The couch turntable angle was kept at 0° and the tangential fields were opposed at 180°. The inferior edge of the anterior field was matched to the superior edge of the tangential fields on the patient's skin.

In 1976, we found that patients treated by excisional biopsy had better local tumor control than similar patients treated by incisional biopsy (Levene et al. 1977). Since then, we have recommended that an excisional biopsy be performed in all patients as part of primary radiation therapy. Excisional biopsy refers to a resection of the primary tumor mass but does not necessarily indicate that microscopic margins are negative. Many of the patients, in fact, had tumor that, on microscopic analysis, was found to extend to the resection margin. We have not found mammography useful in verifying the adequacy of excision except in those cases in which the primary tumor demonstrates microcalcifications. We have found post-biopsy mammograms useful in a number of instances for detecting residual microcalcifications. For these patients, we recommend reexcision prior to irradiation.

In 1978, we performed a detailed cosmetic evaluation on our patients treated by primary radiation therapy (Harris et al. 1979). On the basis of this review, three principal treatment factors were identified that influenced the cosmetic outcome: 1) the extent of the biopsy procedure; 2) the time/dose factors of the radiation therapy; and 3) the radiation therapy technique. It was our belief that the cosmetic result was often unsatisfactory following a wide resection of the primary tumor. Since the likelihood of local tumor control was high in patients treated merely by excisional biopsy, we concluded that a wide resection was, in general, not advisable. It was also found that increasing doses of external beam radiation to the entire breast were associated with greater degrees of fibrosis and retraction of the treated breast. Patients who received 6,000 rad in 6 weeks by external-beam irradiation all had significant retraction and fibrosis, while patients who received 4,500–5,000 rad in 5 weeks did not usually show significant changes. In addition, ^{192}Ir implantation following external beam irradiation did not appear to diminish the cosmetic result. Following this review, we have treated patients with 4,600 rad to the entire breast in 23 fractions over 4.5 weeks. (A tumor-minimum-dose is specified as 1.5 cm from the deep intersection of the tangential fields.)

A number of technical features were also found to be important to achieving good cosmetic results. Skin changes secondary to treatment were infrequent in these patients, and this was related to the use of supervoltage radiation and the absence of bolus. Some of our early patients were treated without tissue compensators for the tangential fields, and these patients had more retraction and fibrosis than patients treated with tissue compensators. Using a 4-MV linear accelerator, large dose inhomogeneities are seen if tissue compensators are not used for the tangential fields. Finally, we observed that a number of these patients had developed a localized area of fibrosis or skin change at the matchline between the anterior field and the tangential fields. This match-line effect was seen in patients who had otherwise excellent cosmetic results. An analysis of the problem revealed that even when adjacent fields are perfectly aligned on skin, areas of dose overlap can be created at depth because of beam divergence. To correct this problem, a modified three-field technique for breast treatment was designed (Svensson et al. 1980). This technique creates a vertical match plane at the match line. By the use of appropriate shielding blocks on all fields and setting the proper turntable and collimator angles, the tangential fields can be precisely matched to the anterior field. The original modification involved the use of a "hanging block" at the superior edge of the tangential fields. A recent, more convenient modification (Figure 1) has been developed using mounted shielding blocks (Siddon et al. 1983). The use of the modified three-field treatment technique has resulted in diminished match-line effects in our patients and an improvement in the cosmetic result.

In 1978, we first examined our treatment results to assess the importance of delivering a boost radiation dose to the primary tumor region (Harris et al. 1978). This boost dose was typically given by interstitial implantation at our institution. As noted above, patients undergoing interstitial implantation typically had close margins of resection and were, therefore, thought to be at a higher risk of local recurrence than patients not undergoing interstitial implantation. Despite this, we found that none of the 32 patients undergoing implantation had local recurrences compared to seven of the 103 patients not undergoing implantation. Subsequent analyses have supported this observation that local tumor control is improved by the use of boost radiation to the primary tumor region. In our most recent review of 255 patients treated between July 1968 and December 1978 (Harris and Hellman 1983), recurrence in the breast was classified either as: 1) true recurrence, occurring directly within the primary tumor region; 2) marginal miss, occurring within the primary tumor region but at the edge of a boost volume; or 3) elsewhere in the breast, occurring at a site distinctly separate from the primary tumor region. We examined the relationship between radiation dose delivered to the primary tumor region by the combination of whole-breast irradiation and a local boost, and the likelihood of a true recurrence in patients undergoing excisional biopsy. Eight of the 90 patients (9%) who received less than 6,000 rad to the primary tumor region developed true recurrences, compared to none of the 154 patients who received 6,000 rad or greater. These results indicate that for patients treated by excisional biopsy and 4,600 to 5,000 rad in 23 treatments over 5 weeks to the entire breast, a boost dose to the primary tumor area improves local tumor control.

We recognize that the importance of a boost dose may depend on the extent of the surgery for the primary tumor. As noted above, patients described here typically had resections of only a small rim of adjacent breast tissue. In some institutions, patients undergo a larger surgical procedure, such as resection of an entire segment or quadrant of the breast. Our results do not necessarily apply to patients treated by these more extensive procedures. The importance of a boost dose in these patients has not been determined. It should be noted, however, that even in the quadrantectomy experience reported from Milan, the primary tumor region received an additional orthovoltage boost of 1,000 rad (Veronesi et al. 1981).

The optimal technique for delivering a radiation boost to the primary tumor area is a matter of controversy. This boost can be delivered either by interstitial implantation, external-beam photons, or electron beam. Our approach has been to deliver an additional 2,000–2,200 rad to the primary tumor area using interstitial [192]Ir. Whenever feasible, a two-plane implant is used, and the involved quadrant is implanted. The technique used is similar to that described at Creteil (Pierquin et al. 1980). In selected circumstances, we prefer to use electron-beam irradiation. For example, in

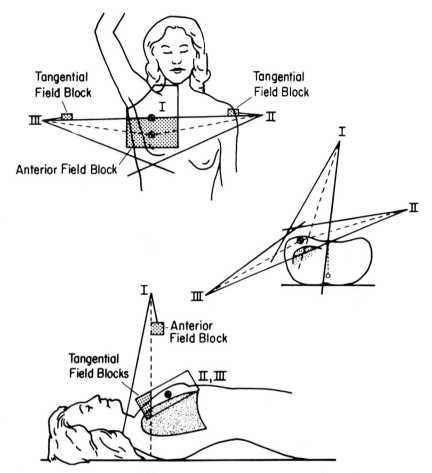

FIG. 1. Joint Center for Radiation Therapy treatment technique for primary radiation therapy (reproduced from Siddon et al. 1983, with permission of Pergamon Press).

a patient with a small primary tumor located in the upper inner quadrant of the breast, an implant can be difficult to perform because of inadequate breast tissue, and an electron-beam boost is preferred. In general, we have favored the use of interstitial implantation as a boost because of its improved skin sparing and the potential biologic advantages of continuous low-dose and low-rate irradiation.

In 1981, in collaboration with the Department of Pathology at the Beth Israel Hospital, we investigated the relationship of microscopic findings within the excisional biopsy specimen to the likelihood of a relapse in the treated breast (Connolly et al. 1983). The findings from this study help to clarify the need for a radiation boost in patients treated by excisional biopsy. We identified three pathologic features associated with an increased risk of breast relapse: 1) moderate or marked intraductal involvement within the primary tumor; 2) the presence of intraductal carcinoma in the breast tissue adjacent to the primary tumor; and 3) high proliferative activity within the tumor, as demonstrated by either poor nuclear grade or frequent mitoses. Our analysis revealed that the increased risk of relapse was confined to the small subset of patients whose tumors demonstrated all three features. Patients in this high-risk category had a 5-year breast relapse rate of 39%, compared to 4% for patients whose tumors demonstrated none, one, or two of these features. The dose of radiation delivered to the primary tumor region influenced the likelihood of breast relapse. For the high-risk patients who received 6,000 rad or greater to the primary tumor area, breast relapse was 16%, compared to 52% for patients who received less than 6,000 rad. Furthermore, the two breast relapses that occurred in patients who received 6,000 rad or greater were marginal misses and not true recurrences. These preliminary results required further follow-up and confirmation by other investigators, but suggest the following conclusions:

1. A small subset of patients who are at high risk of local recurrence if a boost to the primary tumor region is not given can be identified by the pathologic features of the excisional biopsy specimen.

2. Since two of the high-risk patients who received greater than 6,000 rad developed marginal misses, a generous volume boost should be considered for these high-risk patients.

It is also possible that further pathologic studies may identify patients who do not require radiation boosts to the primary tumor region. Since we have only 27 low-risk patients who did not receive boosts, we believe it is premature to abandon the routine use of boosts in low-risk patients.

Beginning in the late 1970s, axillary dissection was introduced as a part of primary radiation therapy for patients with early breast cancer. The purpose of the axillary dissection is to identify patients at high risk for distant relapse who should be considered for adjuvant systemic therapy. The extent of the axillary dissection to be performed has been a matter of controversy. The more limited the dissection, the greater the likelihood of a false-negative result. Conversely, the more extensive the dissection, the greater the likelihood of breast and arm edema. In reviewing the results of axillary dissection at our institution, we concluded that a lateral axillary dissection was preferred (Rose et al. 1983). A lateral dissection removes all of the nodes from level I and those nodes from level II located lateral to the axillary vein. The dissection is performed through a separate incision horizontally placed in the axilla, and an average of 10–15 nodes are recovered. For the most part, axillary node involvement by breast cancer is sequential. Level III involvement is rarely seen in the absence of involvement in levels I or II. As a result, the false-negative rate is low using this procedure. In addition, complications secondary to a lateral dissection are uncommon.

The results of axillary dissection also provide useful information for treatment planning by primary radiation therapy. For patients who have lateral primary tumors and negative dissections, it is reasonable to treat only the breast itself, since involvement of the internal mammary nodes (IMNs) or the upper axillary nodes is uncommon. For patients who have medial or central primary tumors and negative dissections, treatment of the IMNs is of debatable value and has never been shown to improve survival in this subgroup. Since 10% to 15% of these patients will have involvement of the IMNs, we believe it is reasonable to treat this area if no increased risk of complications is obtained. In practice, patients at our institution are treated if the IMNs can be included without a significant increase in lung and heart irradiation. The location of the IMNs is determined using lymphoscintigraphy (Rose et al. 1979). Two tangential fields are used to treat the lower IMNs and breast, and an anterior field is used to treat the upper IMNs, axillary apex, and supraclavicular node area. The boundaries of this anterior field are drawn to avoid irradiation of the dissected portion of the axilla. The lateral border of the anterior field is placed at the coracoid process or at the clip placed by the surgeon at the most medial extent of the axillary dissection. For patients who have positive axillary nodes, irradiation of the dissected portion of the axilla is also avoided unless extensive involvement is noted or the dissection is believed to be inadequate.

The optimal integration of adjuvant systemic therapy and radiation therapy is an unresolved issue at our institution. Initially, patients received systemic therapy at the completion of radiation therapy. This approach has been criticized because of the delay in initiating systemic therapy and the possible difficulties prior irradiation may cause in delivering full-dose chemotherapy. For this reason, we now administer systemic therapy promptly. Questions about the number of cycles to be given prior to starting radiation therapy and whether to use chemotherapy and radiation therapy concomitantly have not been settled.

Our most recently reviewed results in treating patients with stages I and II breast cancer are shown in Figures 2 and 3. We treated 255 patients who had invasive breast cancer between July 1968 and June 1978. Eleven of these patients were also treated for an opposite breast cancer, so that a total of 266 patients were available for analysis of local tumor control. Figure 2 shows the actuarial curve for local tu-

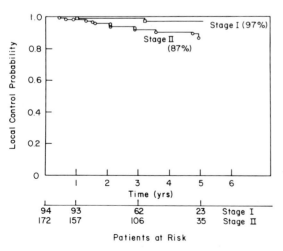

FIG. 2. Actuarial local tumor control by stage (Joint Center for Radiation Therapy series).

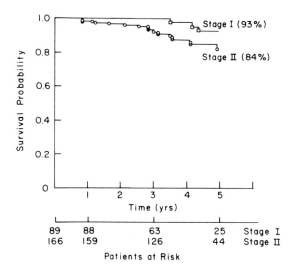

FIG. 3. Actuarial survival by stage (Joint Center for Radiation Therapy series).

mor control by stage. The 5-year rate of local tumor control was 97% for patients with stage I and 87% for those with stage II disease. Figure 3 shows the actuarial curve for survival by stage. The 5-year survival rate was 93% for patients with stage I and 84% for those with stage II disease.

The available treatment results using primary radiation therapy for patients with early breast cancer are encouraging. Retrospective studies such as ours, as well as two recent prospective randomized clinical trials, have provided support for the view that primary radiation therapy is equivalent to mastectomy. Because of the long natural history of the disease, further follow-up will be required to confirm this view. Based on the available results, however, we believe it is unlikely that properly delivered primary radiation therapy will result in a significant survival disadvantage compared to mastectomy. As a result, we offer primary radiation therapy to women with early breast cancer as an alternative to modified radical mastectomy.

REFERENCES

Connolly, J., S. Schnitt, J. R. Harris, S. Hellman, and R. Cohen. 1983. Pathological correlates to local tumor control following primary radiation therapy in patients with early breast cancer, *in* Alternatives to Mastectomy, J. R. Harris, S. Hellman, and W. Silen, eds. J. B. Lippincott Co., Philadelphia (in press).

Fisher, B., N. H. Slack, P. J. Cavanaugh, B. Gardner, R. G. Ravdin, and other cooperating investigators. 1970. Postoperative radiotherapy in the treatment of breast cancer: Results of the NSABP clinical trial. Ann. Surg. 172:711–730.

Harris, J. R., and S. Hellman. 1983. Primary radiation therapy for early breast cancer: The experience at the Joint Center for Radiation Therapy, *in* Alternatives to Mastectomy, J. R. Harris, S. Hellman, and W. Silen, eds. J. B. Lippincott Co., Philadelphia (in press).

Harris, J. R., M. B. Levene, and S. Hellman. 1978. Role of radiation therapy in the primary treatment of carcinoma of the breast. Semin. Oncol. 5:403–416.

Harris, J. R., M. B. Levene, G. Svensson, and S. Hellman. 1979. Analysis of cosmetic results following primary radiation therapy for stages I and II carcinoma of the breast. Int. J. Radiat. Oncol. Biol. Phys. 5:257–261.

Levene, M. B., J. R. Harris, and S. Hellman. 1977. Treatment of carcinoma of the breast by radiation therapy. Cancer 39:2840–2845.

Pierquin, B., C. Maylin, R. Owen, Y. Otmezguine, M. Raynal, W. Mueller, and S. Hannoun. 1980. Radical radiation therapy of breast cancer. Int. J. Radiat. Oncol. Biol. Phys. 6:17–30.

Rose, C. M., W. D. Kaplan, A. Marck, W. D. Bloomer, and S. Hellman. 1979. Parasternal lymphoscintigraphy: Implications for treatment of internal mammary nodes in breast cancer. Int. J. Radiat. Oncol. Biol. Phys. 5:1849–1853.

Rose, C. M., L .E. Botnick, R. Goodman, J. R. Harris, P. Findlay, M. Richter, W. Silen, and S. Hellman. 1983. The role of limited axillary dissection in the treatment of breast cancer by primary irradiation, *in* Alternatives to Mastectomy, J. R. Harris, S. Hellman, and W. Silen, eds. J. B. Lippincott Co., Philadelphia (in press).

Siddon, R. L., B. A. Buck, J. R. Harris, and G. K. Svensson. 1983. Three-field technique using tangential field cover blocks. Int. J. Radiat. Oncol. Biol. Phys. (in press).

Svensson, G. K., B. E. Bjarngard, R. D. Larsen, and M. B. Levene. 1980. A modified three-field technique for breast treatment. Int. J. Radiat. Oncol. Biol. Phys. 6:689–694.

Valagussa, P., G. Bonadonna, and U. Veronesi. 1978. Patterns of relapse and survival following radical mastectomy. Cancer 41:1178.

Veronesi, U., R. Saccozzi, M. Del Vecchio, A. Banfi, C. Clemente, M. De Lena, G. Gallus, M. Greco, A. Luini, E. Marubini, G. Muscolino, F. Rilke, B. Salvadori, A. Zecchini, and R. Zucali. 1981. Comparing radical mastectomy with quadrantectomy, axillary dissection, and radiotherapy in patients with small cancers of the breast. N. Engl. J. Med. 305:6–11.

Current Controversies in Breast Cancer, edited
by F. C. Ames, G. R. Blumenschein, and E. D. Montague.
University of Texas Press, Austin © 1984.

Breast Carcinoma: Experience of the Curie Institute

R. Calle, M.D.,* J. P. Pilleron, M.D.,† J. R. Vilcoq, M.D.,*
P. Schlienger, M.D.,* and J. C. Durand, M.D.†

*Departments of *Radiotherapy and †Surgery, Curie Institute, Paris, France*

At the Curie Institute, patients with operable breast cancer, for many years, had been treated by breast conservation methods using either irradiation alone or as adjunctive therapy to minimal surgical procedures.

In 1936, Baclesse et al. (1939) proved by histologic examinations that tumor control could be achieved by adequate irradiation. Baclesse et al. (1960) treated 100 cases by lumpectomy and irradiation and more than 400 cases by exclusive irradiation (Baclesse 1965). Unfortunately, with the 200 kv that was used at the time, cosmetic results were poor and, in some cases, severe complications occurred. With the advent of megavoltage, cosmetic results were greatly improved, radiation sequelae became minimal, and salvage mastectomy was much easier to perform.

Since 1960, at the Curie Institute, conservation treatment with megavoltage, either with or without lumpectomy (Calle et al. 1978, Calle and Pilleron 1979), has been used for patients with invasive breast carcinoma. These conservation methods have been used in hopes that long-term survival comparable to that obtained by mastectomy would be achieved and that, at the same time, breast preservation with good cosmetic results would be possible.

Depending on the size of the primary tumor and clinical findings in the axillae, patients were referred for either of the two treatment alternatives. Generally, lumpectomy followed by irradiation was performed for patients with early breast carcinoma while radiation alone was used for more locally advanced cancers.

From 1960 to 1976, 1,280 operable breast cancers have been managed by conservative treatment. Patients were considered to have operable disease if they had primary tumors equal to or less than 7 cm, not fixed to the chest wall, without "peau d'orange," skin infiltration, or ulceration, and with clinically negative axillary nodes or with clinically positive mobile nodes. Patients who were older than 70 or had bilateral tumors or other primary tumors, excluding those of the skin, were not included in this study.

In all patients, histologic confirmation of an invasive carcinoma was obtained by lumpectomy or drill biopsy.

Actuarial results were drawn using Kaplan-Meier estimates (Kaplan & Meier

Table 1. *Distribution of Patients Receiving Conservation Treatments by Tumor Stage and Nodal Disease*

	N_0/N_1a	N_1b	Total
T_1	172		172 (13%)
T_2	507	162	669 (52%)
T_3 ($\leq$ 7 cm)	218	221	439 (34%)
Total	897 (70%)	383 (30%)	1280

1958), and comparison between curves was assessed using the Log Rank Test (Peto et al. 1977).

The tumors were staged according to the TNM Classification of the International Union Against Cancer (TNM Classification des Tumeurs Malignes 1979) (Table 1). Radiation sequelae have been classified as follows: Minimal—tolerable or transient; moderate—undeniable but acceptable; and severe—with definite handicap. Cosmetic results have been graded as follows: Excellent to good—no or minimal fibrosis or skin telangiectasia; good to fair—fibrosis or telangiectasia or both involving less than one-half of the breast with no significant distortion of the breast; and poor—fibrosis or telangiectasia or both involving more than one-half of the circumference of the breast with or without distortion of the breast.

IRRADIATION AFTER LUMPECTOMY

Tumors less than or equal to 3 cm and not associated with clinically pathologic nodes were treated by lumpectomy and adjunctive irradiation. In these patients, a lumpectomy incision was made directly over the tumor. An oblong piece of tissue, including the tumor and 2 cm of normal tissue, was excised. Hemostasis was complete. If the tumor was detected only by microcalcifications, then the surgical specimen was x-rayed.

Since 1974, with the advent of adjuvant chemotherapy, we have modified our protocol. We now perform lumpectomy and axillary dissection. If the nodes are found to be negative, only the breast is irradiated; if the nodes are positive, then the breast, as well as the homolateral lymphatics, is irradiated. Systemic adjuvant chemotherapy is given to patients with more than one positive axillary node.

Postoperative radiotherapy with ^{60}Co is started 7 to 10 days after lumpectomy. A tumor dose of 5,000 rad is administered over 5 weeks to the entire gland and to the regional lymph nodes if found to be negative. A booster dose of 1,000 rad is then delivered in 1 week by reduced fields to the tumor bed and to the lower axillary nodes (Calle et al. 1973, Vilcoq et al., in press).

Of the 268 patients who underwent this treatment and had a minimum follow-up of 5 years, 240 (90%) were alive and free of disease (NED). Of these 240, 226 (94%) had breast preservation (Table 2).

One hundred forty-three patients had a minimum follow-up of 10 years, and 111

Table 2. *Lumpectomy + Irradition: 5-and 10-Year Results*

	No. of Cases	Alive NED*	Alive NED with Breasts Preserved
5 years	268	240 (90%)	226 (94%)
10 years	143	111 (78%)	99 (89%)

*NED = no evidence of disease.

Table 3. *Relapse after Lumpectomy + Irradiation in 268 Patients: 5-Year Results*

	No. of Cases	Alive NED* at 5 years
Local mammary recurrence	16[†] (6%)	11[‡] (69%)
Local axillary recurrence	4 (1.5%)	3[§] (75%)
False local recurrence	2	2
Supraclavicular node recurrence	2	
Distant disease	16 (6%)	
Second primary	1	
Intercurrent illness	1	
Lost to follow-up	2	
	44	16

*NED = no evidence of disease.
[†]One patient refused secondary surgery.
[‡]Breast preserved in one patient by limited secondary surgery: Lumpectomy and axillary dissection.
[§]Breast preserved in one patient by limited secondary surgery: Axillary dissection alone.

(78%) were alive and free of disease. Of these 111, 99 (89%) kept their breasts. Twenty patients (7.5%) had mammary or axillary recurrence (Table 3). Nineteen of the 20 patients had secondary surgery: Seventeen had radical or modified radical mastectomy, one had lumpectomy with axillary dissection, and one had axillary dissection alone. One patient refused surgery. Of the 19 patients treated by salvage surgery, 14 (74%) are alive and free of disease with a minimum follow-up after surgery of 5 years. Two other patients had mastectomy for false recurrences and remained in good condition.

Over 95% of those whose breasts were preserved had acceptable cosmetic results at 5 years (Table 4); only two of the 240 patients who were alive at 5 years developed severe radiation sequelae (Table 5).

EXCLUSIVE IRRADIATION WITHOUT PRIOR LIMITED SURGERY

This method is applied to patients with tumors between 3 and 7 cm with or without clinically involved axillae (N_0, N_1a, N_1b) or with tumors equal to or less than 3

Table 4. *Cosmetic Results at 5 Years Among 567 Patients Who Received Conservation Treatment Alive NED* with Breast Preserved*

	Lumpectomy + Irradiation (226 cases)	Exclusive Irradiation (341 cases)
Excellent to good	68%	42%
Good to fair	28%	46%
Poor	4%	12%

*NED = no evidence of disease.

Table 5. *Moderate and Severe Radiation Sequelae in 950 Patients Who Received Conservation Treatment and are Alive NED* at 5 Years*

	Lumpectomy + Irradiation (240 cases)	Exclusive Irradiation (710 cases)
Moderate	41	121
Severe	2	18
	43	139

*NED = No evidence of disease.

cm but with clinically involved axillae (N_1b). Following drill biopsy for pathologic examination, a dose of 5,500 to 6,000 rad in 5.5 to 6 weeks is given to the entire breast and lower axillae and 5,000 rad to the remaining homolateral lymphatics. At the completion of these doses, clinical and mammographic evaluation is performed to determine the regression of the tumor. The patients are then divided in two groups:

The first group includes patients in whom tumors have not significantly regressed. Mastectomy with axillary dissection is performed 2 or 3 months after evaluation. In some exceptional cases, mastectomy is performed 4 to 6 months afterwards. This group is, in essence, similar to patients who receive preoperative irradiation in moderate doses followed by mastectomy.

The second group includes patients in whom the tumor has significantly regressed. Irradiation is continued through reduced portals using either ^{60}Co or electron-beam therapy to the primary tumor and lower axillary nodes. A total dose of about 8,000 rad is given to the primary tumor and 6,000 to 7,000 rad to the lower axillary lymph nodes. Salvage surgery is only performed for local-regional recurrence. The technique of irradiation is as previously described (Calle et al. 1973, Vilcoq et al., in press).

A total of 1,012 patients were treated by this method with a minimum follow-up of 5 years. Survival in patients receiving irradiation without prior surgery is plotted according to the TNM classification in Figure 1. Survival of patients whose breasts

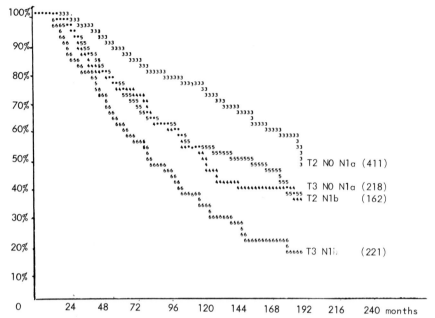

FIG. 1. Survival, according to the TNM (tumor, nodes, metastasis) Classification, in patients who received irradiation only without prior surgery.

were conserved after exclusive irradiation is shown in Figure 2. Breast conservation was significantly better for patients with T_2 and N_0 classification.

Of 1,012 patients, 456 (45%) had mastectomy for persistent disease after irradiation, 5,000–6,000 rad, and 556 (55%) had irradiation alone (Table 6).

Of the 456 patients who had persistent disease, the 5-year absolute disease-free survival rate was 75% (344 of 456). The majority of failures were due to distant disease.

Of the 556 patients who had irradiation alone, 65% (366 of 556) survived 5 years. One hundred twenty-nine patients (23%) had mammary or axillary recurrences or both. Of the 129 patients with local-regional recurrence, 111 (86%) had salvage surgery, which was generally modified or radical mastectomy. Of the 111 who underwent salvage surgery, 57 (51%) were alive and disease free at 5 years.

Eighty percent of patients had acceptable cosmetic results at 5 years (Table 4); of the 710 patients alive at 5 years, 18 had severe sequelae (Table 5).

OVERALL RESULTS

The disease-free survival and percentage of breast preservation in the entire series of 1,280 patients receiving conservation treatment is shown in Table 7. Seventy-four percent of all patients considered to be surgically operable were alive and free of disease at 5 years, and two-thirds had preserved breasts.

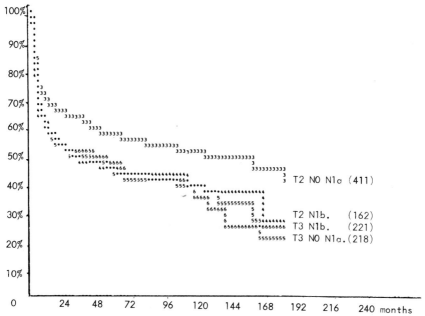

FIG. 2. Survival, according to the TNM (tumor, nodes, metastasis) Classification, in patients whose breasts were conserved after exclusive irradiation.

Table 6. *Five-Year Results for Patients Initially Receiving Exclusive Irradiation*

Treatment	Absolute Survival	
	N.E.D.*	Alive N.E.D. with breasts preserved
Irradiation and surgery for persistent disease[†]	456	344 (75%)	18 (0.05%)
Radical irradiation alone[‡]	556	366 (65%)	323 (88%)
	1,012	710 (70%)	341 (48%)

*NED = no evidence of disease.
[†]Generally modified or radical mastectomy except for some cases with limited surgery.
[‡]Surgery only performed in case of local-regional recurrence.

Table 7. *Five- and 10-Year Disease-Free Survival in 1,280 Patients Receiving Conservation Treatment*

	No. of Patients	Alive NED*	Alive NED with Breast Preservation
5 years	1,280	950/1,280 (74%)	567/950 (60%)
10 years	606	328/606 (54%)	213/328 (65%)

*NED = No evidence of disease.

COMMENTS

The present retrospective analysis clearly demonstrates that lumpectomy with or without axillary dissection followed by moderate doses of irradiation is justified. This method appears to be the treatment of choice for small, operable, invasive breast carcinoma (with classifications of T_1, T_2, N_0, N_1a). The 5- and 10-year results are equivalent to those obtained by standard surgical procedures, yet the percentage of patients with breast preservation is high, around 90% at 10 years.

Cosmetic results are very good, and occurrence of incapacitating sequelae is the exception. With an adequate technique of irradiation, the rate of local recurrence is 7.5% at 5 years, and half of the recurrences appear in local sites other than the primary (Vilcoq et al. 1981); these local-regional recurrences can be salvaged successfully by secondary surgery. Our results have been confirmed by other authors (Harris and Hellmann 1981, Montague et al. 1979, Veronesi et al. 1981, Pierquin et al. 1980, Amalric et al. 1982).

Lumpectomy with or without axillary dissection followed by irradiation has had a definite place in the treatment of early invasive breast carcinoma.

Exclusive irradiation has also been used as treatment for patients with lesions considered to be locally advanced. In these series, at 5 years, 45% of patients, because of lack of tumor regression underwent surgery and received only what we considered to be a preoperative dose of irradiation. This was done purposely in order to avoid long-term poor cosmesis in patients who appear to have relatively radioresistant tumors. The remaining 55% of patients completed their planned course of radical irradition; 23% suffered local-regional recurrence and required salvage surgery. The difference in 5-year survival rates between this group of patients and those receiving preoperative radiation doses, 65% versus 75%, respectively, is not statistically significant. According to the TNM (TNM Classification des Tumeurs Malignes 1979) classification, the percentage of breast preservation is significantly high for lesions classified as T_2, N_0. It is perhaps possible to obtain a high percentage of breast conservation by giving radiation doses of more than 8,000 rad or using interstitial implant, but we prefer to avoid excessive irradiation to obtain acceptable cosmetic results.

Breast conservation treatment requires a close cooperation of the radiotherapist, the surgeon, and the patient. It should be practiced only by experienced radiotherapists and by surgeons who are familiar with secondary surgery in heavily irradiated breasts.

ACKNOWLEDGMENTS

The authors are grateful to Bernard Asselain and Charles Picco for statistical assistance and to Chantal Gautier for her secretarial assistance.

REFERENCES

Amalric, R., F. Santamaria, and F. Robert, I. Seigle, C. Altschuler, J. M. Kurty, J. M. Spitalier, H. Brandone, Y. Ayme, J. F. Pollet, R. Burmeister, and R. Abed. 1982. Radiation therapy with or without primary limited surgery for operable breast cancer. A 20-year experience at the Marseille Cancer Institute. Cancer 49:30–34.

Baclesse, F. 1965. Five-years results in 431 breast cancers treated solely by roentgen rays. Ann. Surg. 161:103–104.

Baclesse, F., A. Ennuyer, and J. Cheguillaume. 1960. Est-on autroisé à pratiquer une tumorectomie simple suivie de radiothérapie en cas de tumeur mammaire? J. Radiol. 41:137–139.

Baclesse, F., G. Gricouroff, and A. Tailhefer. 1939. Essai de reontgenthérapie du cancer du sein suivie d'opération large. Résultats histologiques. Bull. Cancer 28:729–743.

Calle, R., G. H. Fletcher, and B. Pierquin. 1973. Les bases de la radiothérapie curative des épithéliomas mammaires. J. Radiol. 54:929–938.

Calle, R., and J. P. Pilleron. 1979. Radiation therapy, with or without lumpectomy for operable breast cancer: Ten years results. Breast. Diseases of the Breast 5:2–6.

Calle, R., J. P. Pilleron, P. Schlienger, and J. R. Vilcoq. 1978. Conservative management of operable breast cancer. Ten years experience at the Foundation Curie. Cancer 42:2045–2053.

Harris, J. R., and S. Hellmann. 1981. Primary radiation therapy for breast cancer. Annu. Rev. Med. 32:387–404.

Kaplan, E. L., and P. Meier. 1958. Nonparametric estimation from incomplete observations. J. Am. Statis. Ass. 53:457–481.

Montague, E. D., A. E. Guitteriez, and J. L. Barker. 1979. Conservation surgery and radiation for the treatment of favorable breast cancer. Cancer 43:1058–1061.

Peto, R., M. C. Pike, P. Armitage, N. E. Breslow, D. R. Cox, S. V. Howard, N. Nantel, K. McPherson, J. Peto, and P. G. Smith. 1977. Design and analysis of randomized clinical trials requiring prolonged observation of each patient. Br. J. of Cancer 35:1–39.

Pierquin, B., R. Owern, and C. Maylin. 1980. Radical radiation therapy for breast cancer. Int. J. Radiat. Oncol. Biol. Phys. 6:17–24.

TNM Classification des Tumeurs Malignes. 1979. Union Internationale Contre le Cancer, Geneve, 1972, pp. 47–53.

Veronesi, U., R. Saccozi, M. Del Vecchio, A. Banfi, C. Clemente, M. De Lena, G. Gallus, M. Greco, A. Luini, E. Marubini, G. Muscolino, F. Rilke, B. Salvadori, A. Zecchini, and R. Zucoli. 1981. Comparing radical mastectomy with quadrantectomy, axillary dissection and radiotherapy in patients with small cancers of the breast. N. Engl. J. Med. 2:6–11.

Vilcoq, J. R., R. Calle, and P. Schlienger. 1983. Irradiation techniques for the conservative treatment of localized breast cancer, *in* Conservative Management of Breast Cancer: New Surgical and Radiotherapeutic Techniques, J. Harris, S. Hellman, and W. Silen, eds. J. B. Lippincott Co., Philadelphia, pp. 213–224.

Vilcoq, J. R., R. Calle, P. Stacey, and N. A. Ghossein. 1981. The outcome of treatment by tumorectomy and radiotherapy of patients with operable breast cancer. Int. J. Radiat. Oncol. Biol. Phys. 7:1327–1332.

Current Controversies in Breast Cancer, edited
by F. C. Ames, G. R. Blumenschein, and E. D. Montague.
University of Texas Press, Austin © 1984.

Conservation Surgery and Irradiation in Stages I and II Breast Cancer: The M. D. Anderson Experience

Sylvia R. Schell, M.D.

Department of Radiotherapy, The University of Texas M. D. Anderson Hospital and Tumor Institute at Houston, Houston, Texas

During recent years, gradual but important changes have occurred in the treatment of patients with breast cancer. There has been a trend toward more conservative surgical procedures followed by radiation therapy in breast cancer patients with clinically favorable breast cancer. There is ample data to support the position that the combined approach of conservation surgery and postoperative irradiation is as effective as the radical mastectomy (Harris et al. 1981, Montague et al. 1979, Vilcoq et al. 1981). This paper will review the results of treatment in patients with stages I and II breast cancer treated with conservation surgery and postoperative irradiation compared to patients treated with radical mastectomy.

METHODS

Between 1955 through 1979, 535 patients were treated with radical mastectomy alone, and 225 patients were treated with conservation surgery and radiotherapy. The patient distribution is shown in Tables 1 and 2. Patients with positive lymph nodes treated with radical mastectomy were candidates to receive postoperative irradiation (peripheral lymphatic irradiation with or without chest wall irradiation) but, for a variety of reasons, did not.

Patients suitable for breast conservation and radiotherapy were carefully selected according to the criteria outlined in Table 3; some patients were considered unsuitable if suboptimal cosmetic results were a strong possibility, i.e., in patients with very small breasts or with retroareolar tumors, in which segmental resection would have resulted in severe breast deformity, or in patients with very pendulous breasts in whom the irradiated volume would be excessive, thereby increasing the incidence of late complications. Because there was a higher failure rate for those patients having excision of a primary tumor prior to referral (8.1%) to The University of Texas M. D. Anderson Hospital and Tumor Institute at Houston compared to those undergoing excision at this hospital (2.8%), a reexcision of the primary site has been performed whenever possible (Montague et al. 1983a). This difference in control

Table 1. *Patients with Clinically Favorable Stages I and II Breast Cancer Treated with Radical Mastectomy: 1955–1979*

	T_1	T_2
Total no. patients*	222	313
N_0 histologic	203	241
N_1 histologic	19	72

*Stage I: 203 patients; Stage II: 335 patients.

Table 2. *Patients with Clinically Favorable Stages I and II Breast Cancer Treated with Conservation Surgery and Radiotherapy: 1955–1979*

	T_1	T_2
Total no. patients*	103	122
N_0 clinical	70	45
N_0 histologic	33	19
N_1 clinical		24
N_1 histologic		34

*Stage I: 103 patients; Stage II: 122 patients.

Table 3. *Criteria for Patient Selection for Conservation Surgery and Irradiation**

Primary tumor:
    Single focus ≤4 cm, or multiple foci grouped within a
                    radius ≤4 cm
    No grave signs
Axilla:
    Negative
    or
    Small mobile low nodes

*Adapted from: Montague et al. 1983.

has probably been related to the fact that in most instances the referring surgeons were preparing the patient for a radical mastectomy, so that tumors were not completely excised.

TREATMENT TECHNIQUE

The areas to be irradiated were determined by the location of the primary tumor and histologic status of the axilla (Table 4). The breast was treated with tangential open and wedge fields with ^{60}Co, for a total tumor dose of 5,000 rad in 5 weeks (25 fractions) followed by a boost of 1,000 rad (5 fractions) to the area of the primary,

Table 4. *Areas to be Irradiated Following Excision and Axillary Dissection**

Histologic Status of Nodes	Radiotherapy Fields	
	Outer Quadrant Primary	Central or Inner
T₁ (−)	breast	breast, internal mammary chain
(+)	breast, supraclavicular and subclavicular axillary apex, internal mammary chain	breast, supraclavicular and subclavicular apex, internal mammary chain
T₂ (−)	breast	breast, supraclavicular nodes and subclavicular apex, internal mammary chain
(+)	breast, supraclavicular and subclavicular axillary apex, internal mammary chain	breast, supraclavicular and subclavicular axillary apex, internal mammary chain

* Indications for whole axilla irradiation: Patients without an axillary dissection or with inadequate axillary dissection (<10 nodes), fixed nodes, ⩾3.0 cm or extranodal disease.

usually given with the electron beam (6–13MeV). A boost of 1,500–2,000 rad with an iridium implant was given in patients with positive or unknown margins or in patients who required boosts to large volumes.

In patients without axillary dissection, a 5,000-rad tumor dose in 5 weeks (25 fractions) was given to the axilla through an anterior supraclavicular field, including the subclavicular axillary apex, and a posterior axillary field, including the low and central axilla. Patients undergoing a lateral dissection of the axilla were not required to receive posterior axillary field irradiation, unless the nodes were ⩾3cm or showed evidence of extranodal disease. The internal mammary chain was irradiated through a direct appositional field for a total tumor dose of 4,500 rad in 5 weeks (25 fractions). Patients with positive nodes with central or inner quadrant tumors received a boost of 500-rad tumor dose to the first three intercostal spaces. The supraclavicular field received 5,000 rad in 5 weeks (25 fractions). A combination of photons and electrons was used for treatment to the internal mammary and supraclavicular nodes in order to minimize the dose to underlying vital structures (Fletcher et al. 1980).

RESULTS

Prior to 1974, only clinical staging of the axilla was available to determine extent of disease. After 1974, dissection of the axilla was performed to provide histologic data regarding nodal status. Initially, patients underwent a complete axillary dissection; however, this procedure had a high incidence of complications manifested by arm edema and retrograde breast edema; therefore, the dissection has been limited to the lateral axilla (lateral to the pectoralis minor muscle), resulting in fewer complications.

In this study, there was no difference in the local-regional control in patients treated with excision and irradiation compared to those treated with radical mastec-

Table 5. *Breast Cancer Stage I ($T_1 > .5$-2 cm N_0) Local-Regional Recurrences**
in Patients Treated with Conservation Surgery and Irradiation or Radical Mastectomy:
1955–1979[†]

| | Excision & Irradiation | | Radical-Mastectomy |
	N_0 Clinical	N_0 Histologic	N_0 Histologic
No. of patients	70	33	203
Breast or chest wall	5	2	5
Axilla	1	–	1
Supraclavicular	–	–	3
Parasternal	–	–	1
% of patients with recurrence	7.1% (5/70)	6% (2/33)	4.4% (9/203)
	6.8% (7/103)		

*A patient may have more than one recurrence.
[†]Adapted from Montague et al. 1983.

Table 6. *Breast Cancer Stage II (T_2N_0 or $T_1T_2N_1$) Local-Regional Recurrences* in Patients*
Treated with Conservation and Irradiation or Radical Mastectomy: 1955–1979[†]

| | Excision & Irradiation | | Radical-Mastectomy |
	Clinical	Histologic	Histologic
No. of patients	69	53	332
Breast or chest wall	3	2	16
Axilla		1	5
Supraclavicular			9
Parasternal			3
% of patients with recurrence	4.4% (3/69)	5.6% (3/53)	8.4% (28/332)
	4.9% (6/122)		

*A patient may have more than one recurrence.
[†]Adapted from Montague et al. 1983.

tomy alone (Tables 5 and 6), but a difference did exist in the pattern of failure: Patients receiving radiotherapy had no recurrences in the supraclavicular and parasternal (internal mammary chain) areas (Montague et al. 1983b).

Figures 1–3 show the disease-free 10-year survival rates. There was no statistically significant survival benefit to patients treated with radical surgery as compared to those treated with conservation surgery and irradiation.

Because of concern relative to radiocarcinogenesis, an analysis was performed of patients with stages I and II bilateral breast cancer treated from 1948–1976 to determine if irradiation used in treatment of the first breast predisposed the other breast to the development of cancer. As can be seen in Table 7, patients who were treated with combined surgery and radiation therapy for the first breast have had no greater incidence of second breast cancer than patients treated with surgery alone (Schell et al. 1982).

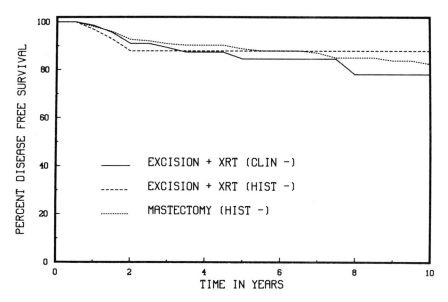

FIG. 1. Disease-free survival by treatment for histologically (HIST) and clinically (CLIN) negative stage I breast cancer (1955–1979). (XRT = radiation therapy)

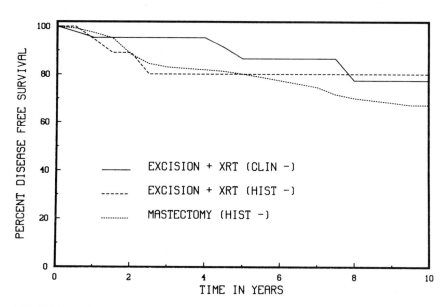

FIG. 2. Disease-free survival by treatment for histologically (HIST) and clinically (CLIN) negative stage II breast cancer (1955–1979). (XRT = radiation therapy)

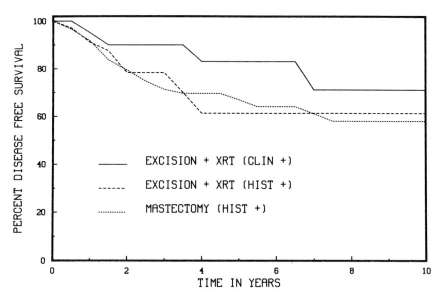

FIG. 3. Disease-free survival by treatment for histologically (HIST) and clinically (CLIN) positive stage II breast cancer (1955–1979). (XRT = radiation therapy)

Table 7. *Stages I & II ($T_1N_0T_2N_1$) Bilateral Breast Cancer: Consecutive Presentation: 1948–1976**

Treatment for First Breast Primary		Number of Patients Developing Second Breast Primary (%)		
Surgery only		30/409	(7.3%)	
Peripheral lymphatic irradiation		27/553	(4.9%)	
Peripheral lymphatic + electron beam chest wall		7/321	(2.2%)	
Irradiation of chest	Simple mastectomy	5/228	(2.2%)	57/1673 (3.4%)
wall with	Wedge excision	0/98	----	
tangential	Preoperative and			
portals	radical			
	mastectomy	18/473	(3.8%)	

*Adapted from Schell et al. 1982.

DISCUSSION

Breast cancer patients treated with conservation surgery and radiation for clinically favorable breast cancer require careful selection and assessment by a team of physicians, consisting of a surgeon and a radiotherapist in consultation with a radiologist and a pathologist. Both the surgeon and radiotherapist must provide careful follow-up examinations (both clinical and roentgenographic) and must continually refine both surgical and radiotherapy techniques in order to achieve optimal results.

REFERENCES

Harris, J. R., L. Bormick, W. D. Bloomen, J. T. Chaffey, and S. Hellman. 1981. Primary radiation therapy for early breast cancer: The experience at the Joint Center for Radiation Therapy. Int. J. Radiat. Oncol. Biol. Phys. 7:1549–1552.

Fletcher, G. H., E. D. Montague, N. duV. Tapley, and J. L. Barker. 1980. Radiotherapy in the management of nondisseminated breast cancer, *in* Textbook of Radiotherapy, 3rd edition, G. H. Fletcher, ed. Lea & Febiger, Philadelphia, pp. 527–579.

Montague, E. D., A. E. Gutierrez, J. L. Barker, N. duV. Tapley, and G. H. Fletcher. 1979. Conservation surgery and irradiation for the treatment of favorable breast cancer. Cancer 43: 1058–1061.

Montague, E. D., D. D. Paulus, and S. R. Schell. 1983a. Selection and follow-up of patients for conservation surgery and irradiation, *in* Frontiers in Radiation Therapy and Oncology, vol. 17, J. M. Varth, ed. Karger, Switzerland, pp. 124–130.

Montague, E. D., S. R. Schell, M. M. Romsdahl, and F. C. Ames. 1983b. Conservation surgery and irradiation in clinically favorable breast cancer: The M. D. Anderson Experience, *in* Conservative Management of Breast Cancer: New Surgical and Radiotherapeutic Techniques, J. Harris, S. Hellman, and W. Silen, eds. J. B. Lippincott Co., Philadelphia, pp. 53–59.

Schell, S. R., E. D. Montague, W. J. Spanos, Jr., N. duV. Tapley, G. H. Fletcher, and M. J. Oswald. 1982. Bilateral breast cancer in patients with initial stage I and II disease. Cancer 50: 1191–1194.

Vilcoq, J. R., R. Calle, P. Stacey, and N. A. Ghossein. 1981. The outcome of treatment by tumorectory and radiotherapy of patients with operable breast cancer. Int. J. Radiat. Oncol. Biol. Phys. 7:1327–1332.

ADJUNCTIVE THERAPY

Current Controversies in Breast Cancer, edited
by F. C. Ames, G. R. Blumenschein, and E. D. Montague.
University of Texas Press, Austin © 1984.

The Enigma Of Breast Cancer

Gilbert H. Fletcher, M.D.

*Department of Radiotherapy, The University of Texas M. D. Anderson Hospital and
Tumor Institute at Houston, Houston, Texas*

In 1969, Sir John Bruce, Professor of Surgery at the University of Edinburgh, published an article entitled "The Enigma of Breast Cancer" (Bruce 1969). It was based on the fact that radical mastectomy alone, extended radical mastectomy, simple mastectomy, or tumorectomy with radiotherapy produced identical 5-year survival rates. He concluded that variations on the local-regional methods of treatment did not affect the occurrence of distant metastasis.

At the middle of this century, after investigating breast cancer mortality since 1900, some epidemiologists reached the conclusion that survival rates of patients with breast cancer were not affected by any treatment at all (McKinnon 1951, Park and Lees 1951); in their study, the 5-year survival rate was used as an index. Other authors have constructed mathematical models of the behavior of breast cancer and have concluded that the same proportion of patients at any time during follow-up experience failure, so that eventually all patients will die from breast cancer (Cutler and Axtell 1963). Other studies have indicated that less than 15% of breast cancer patients with positive axillary lymph nodes will be free of disseminated disease (Bross and Blumenson 1971, Lipsett 1981).

This essay will analyze the incidence of failures and survival rates in patients treated at the The University of Texas M. D. Anderson Hospital and Tumor Institute at Houston since 1963 without adjuvant chemotherapy. A review of the present status of systemic treatment will also be made.

ADJUVANT RADIOTHERAPY CLINICAL TRIALS

Since 1948, at UT M. D. Anderson Hospital patients with histologically positive axillary nodes or lesions located in the center or inner quadrants of the breast have received postoperative irradiation to the peripheral lymphatics, that is, the apex of the axilla and the supraclavicular and internal mammary chain nodes (Fletcher 1980). Until 1963, elective irradiation of the chest wall was not performed. In 1963, when the electron beam became available, chest wall irradiation was performed electively in patients with a high incidence of involved nodes in the axilla or with grave signs of the primary tumor, consisting of a primary lesion more than 5 cm in diameter or pathological evidence of skin, perineural, or lymphatic invasion

(Haagensen 1971). Initially, to be eligible for chest wall irradiation, patients had to have at least 50% of the nodes involved, but later eligibility was lowered to 20% (Tapley 1976).

In the National Surgical Adjuvant Breast Project (NSABP) trial of placebo versus triethylenethiophosphoramide (Thio-TEPA), the incidence of failures up to 10 years, according to the histological status of the axillae in the patients receiving placebo, has been widely accepted as baseline data (Fisher et al. 1975b). The conclusion was drawn that since 86% of the patients with four or more positive nodes suffered recurrence, this extent of axillary involvement always indicates dissemination of the disease. The data are used for comparison with the UT M. D. Anderson Hospital data (Tapley et al. 1982) (Table 1). The incidence of failures at 10 years is much less in the UT M. D. Anderson Hospital series for patients with positive nodes and, within that group, also less for patients with one to three positive nodes and four or more positive nodes. There are no data after 10 years in the NSABP publication, but in the UT M. D. Anderson Hospital series there were eight failures after 10 years and seven before 15 years. Figure 1 shows the cumulative failure rate.

Table 2 shows the 10-year disease-free survival rates for UT M. D. Anderson Hospital and the NSABP patients. Although there is a higher incidence of patients with positive axillary nodes in the UT M. D. Anderson Hospital series, the overall survival rate is 54% in this group versus 46% in the NSABP group. In the UT M. D. Anderson Hospital series, 44% of the patients with positive axillary nodes and 33% of those with four or more positive axillary nodes were alive, disease free, at 10 years versus 24.9% and 13.4%, respectively, in the NSABP series. In a series of patients with positive axillary nodes, 90% of whom had received irradiation to the peripheral lymphatics, a 50% disease-free rate at 10 years has been obtained

Table 1. *Comparison of Treatment Failure Rates Between MDAH* Pts. with Radical Mastectomy and Postoperative Irradiation and NSABP† Pts. with Radical Mastectomy Alone‡*

	Treatment Failures (TF)					
	At 10 Years				After 10 Years§	
	MDAH		NSABP‖		MDAH	NSABP
Node status	%	No. Pts.	%	No. Pts.	No. TF	
Negative	22.1	131	24.1	170	0	no data
Positive	57.7#	392	76.1#	163	8	no data
1-3	48.0¶	173	64.5¶	76	6	no data
≥4	65.3	219	82.2**	87	2	no data

*UT M. D. Anderson Hospital.
†National Surgical Adjuvant Breast Project.
‡No adjuvant chemotherapy in both groups.
‖Trial between 1958–1962.
§523 patients with 10 years minimum follow-up time.
 189 patients with 15 years minimum follow-up time.
#$P < .005$.
¶$P < .02$.
**$P < .005$.

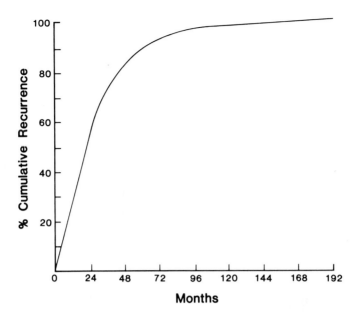

FIG. 1. The cumulative rate of failure for patients treated with radical mastectomy and postoperative radiotherapy from 1963 through 1977 (analysis 1981). Cumulative failure rate increases rapidly during first 5 years of follow-up.

Table 2. *10-Year Disease-Free Survival Rates by Axillary Node Status in MDAH* Pts.*
Treated with Radical Mastectomy and Postoperative Irradiation and NSABP[†] Pts.
Treated with Radical Mastectomy Alone[‡]

| | Disease-Free Survival Rate | | | |
| | MDAH | | NSABP | |
Node Status	No. of Pts.	% (10 years)	No. of Pts.	% (10 years)
Negative	260	79	205	64.9
Positive	660[§] (71.1%)[‖]	44[#]	185 (49.2%)[‖]	24.9
1-3	324	56	88	37.5
≥ 4	336	33	97	13.4
Overall group	920	54%	390	45.9%

*UT M. D. Anderson Hospital.
[†]National Surgical Adjuvant Breast Project.
[‡]No adjuvant chemotherapy.
[§]Average number of nodes per pt. with positive nodes is 6.6.
[‖]% of pts. with positive nodes.
[#]68% is the expected survival rate in general mortality tables for the group given their age, race, and sex.

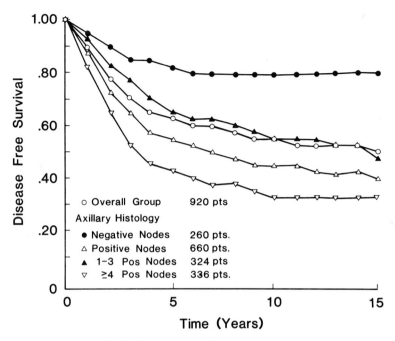

FIG. 2. Disease-free survival of patients treated with radical mastectomy and postoperative radiation (survival curves according to Berkson-Gage method). The percentage of patients with positive axillary nodes is 71.1%, and the mean number of positive nodes in patients with positive nodes is 6.6. (Reproduced from Tapley et al. 1982, with permission of J. B. Lippincott Co.)

(Cody et al. 1982). Figure 2 shows that after 10 years there is a flattening of the survival curves, indicating that patients alive free of disease at 10 years have a very low risk of dying later from the disease. That flattening of the survival curve had already been observed by Haagensen (1971).

Table 3 classifies the incidence of local-regional failures by various treatment modalities. There is only a 9% incidence of local-regional failures in the patients receiving irradiation to the peripheral lymphatics and chest wall, although 87% of the patients had positive axillary nodes. The average number of positive axillary nodes in these patients with positive nodes was 9.6. In similar series of patients with heavy involvement of the axillary nodes, the incidence of local-regional failure is between 30–40% (Haagensen 1971, Spratt 1967).

Since the publication of the Manchester Clinical Trial investigating radical mastectomy with or without peripheral lymphatic irradiation, it has been considered that, since the survival rates were not improved by postoperative irradiation of the peripheral lymphatics, recurrences can be as well treated when they appear (Paterson and Russell 1959b). This has not been substantiated in various studies of the results of irradiation for gross recurrences (Bedwinek et al. 1981, Chu et al. 1976, Madoc-Jones et al. 1976).

Table 3. *Local-Regional Recurrences in Pts. Treated with Radical or Modified Radical Mastectomy Alone or with Postoperative Irradiation (XRT) (1955–1976)*

	Radical Mastectomy Alone (441 Pts.)	XRT to Peripheral Lymphatics (535 Pts.)	XRT to Peripheral Lympathics and Chest Wall (449 Pts.)
Percent of pts. with histologically positive nodes	14%	59%*	87%*
Percent of pts. with local-regional recurrences	7.5% (33/441)	12% (62/535)	9% (44/449)

*Average number of positive nodes for pts. with positive nodes: Peripheral lymphatic—3.7; peripheral lymphatic and chest wall—9.6.

ADJUVANT CHEMOTHERAPY CLINICAL TRIALS

In almost all the prospective randomized clinical trials of adjuvant chemotherapy, only one subset of the total patient population is affected. In the Thio-TEPA-versus-placebo study, only premenopausal women with four or more positive axillary nodes statistically benefited from Thio-TEPA (Fisher et al. 1975b). Although the statistical significance appears to be great, simple calculation shows that a very small number of patients of the 414 who were randomized to receive the drug have been statistically cured (Table 4). In the clinical trial of melphalan (L-PAM) versus placebo, the patients who benefited were premenopausal patients with one to three positive nodes; 8 patients were cured out of a total of 179 who received the drug (Fisher et al. 1975a, Fisher et al. 1979). In the cyclophosphamide, methotrexate, and 5-fluorouracil (CMF)-versus-placebo clinical trial, only the patients who received Level I dose (85% of the planned dose), 17% of the total number of patients who were randomized to receive the drug, benefited; 11 of these patients were cured (Bonadonna 1981). Table 5 summarizes the data for the three trials. When related to the total number of patients, the results are clinically insignificant.

In a clinical trial of cyclophosphamide given in the week immediately after mastectomy, there were better survival rates in all patients, pre- and postmenopausal, but the same amount of cyclophosphamide given 3 weeks after mastectomy was without effect (Nissen-Meyer et al. 1978). This introduces the interesting speculation that when a tumor has reached a certain volume, the drugs may not penetrate, as experimentally shown in spheroids (West et al. 1980). Furthermore, it has been shown that hypoxic cells, which exist in a significant volume of aggregates of cancer cells, are less sensitive to some of the chemotherapeutic agents (Rose et al. 1980). In the 1950s, studies showed tumor cells in the circulating blood of cancer patients, with an increase of tumor cells circulating during surgical procedures (Cruz et al. 1956). Therefore, chemotherapy should theoretically be given imme-

Table 4.* *Number of Pts. Cured by Thio-TEPA in 414 Pts. Who Received the Drug*

At 5 Years	
Premenopausal with $\geq$ 4 positive nodes	
56.6%[†] of 23 pts. survived	13
Only 24.3%[†] of 23 pts. would have survived without Thio-TEPA	5
Number of pts. surviving at 5 years because of Thio-TEPA	8

At 10 Years	
Premenopausal with $\geq$ 4 positive nodes	
34.8%[†] of 23 pts. survived	8
Only 13.5%[†] of 23 pts. would have survived without Thio-TEPA	3
Number of pts. surviving at 10 years because of Thio-TEPA	5

*Reproduced from Fletcher 1976, with permission of Pergamon Press, Inc.
[†]Percentages are calculated from life table plots of probability of survival.

Table 5. *Breast Cancer: Disease-Free Survival Data*

	Total Pts. Randomized to Receive Drugs	Results
Thio-TEPA vs. placebo	414	premenopausal pts. with $\geq$ 4 positive nodes—5 more pts. in Thio-TEPA group (23 pts.) alive at 10 years.
L-PAM vs. placebo	179	premenopausal pts. with 1-3 positive nodes—8 more pts. in L-PAM group (32 pts.) disease free at 4 years.
CMF vs. placebo	449	11 more pts. in Level I* CMF group (78 pts.) alive at 5 years.

*Receiving 85% of planned dose.

diately after the mastectomy, before the cells that make a distant implant have multiplied to produce a spheroid.

It has been repeatedly stated that, on theoretical grounds, polychemotherapy should be superior to single-agent chemotherapy, but the benefit of multidrug therapy has not been shown in all trials (Cohen et al. 1981). It is often stated that radiation therapy interferes with the dosage tolerated for chemotherapy, but that is not a universal experience as reported in the CMF study in Milan (DeLena et al. 1981).

OTHER CLINICAL TRIALS

Since the middle 1950s, there have been clinical trials of elective ovarian irradiation. In the Manchester trial, the results at 5 years are very close to statistical significance (P = .06) (Paterson et al. 1959a). A trial of ovarian elective irradiation and prednisone has shown benefit in premenopausal women (Meakin et al. 1977). On occasion, the permanent cure of a patient with disseminated breast cancer has been observed with hormonal therapy only (Kennedy et al. 1976).

SIGNIFICANCE OF AXILLARY INVOLVEMENT

The presence of histologically positive nodes in the axillary specimen is considered to darken the prognosis significantly and to be an indication for adjuvant chemotherapy. In patients with clinically negative axillary nodes in the NSABP clinical trial of radical mastectomy alone versus simple mastectomy and radiation versus simple mastectomy alone, the incidence of patients having had no treatment to the axilla, who later developed an axillary failure, is approximately one-third of the expected one, according to the incidence of histologically positive axillary nodes in the patients who were randomized to receive radical mastectomy (Fisher 1977). It shows that not all patients with histologically positive axillary nodes will develop clinical manifestation of the disease in the axilla. Studies of the prognostic significance of axillary involvement have shown that in patients with aggregates of diseased nodes, no more than 1.3 mm in diameter in one study or 2 mm in another study, the failure and survival rates are not affected (Fisher et al. 1978, Huvos 1971).

DISCUSSION

The study of breast cancer has led to various theories and assumptions concerning factors affecting survival. The data presented in this essay do not agree with some of them. It is not correct that almost all patients with positive axillary nodes die from distant metastasis, since approximately 50% have been shown to be alive free of disease at 10 years; it is also not correct that all patients with four or more positive nodes will die from disseminated disease because approximately one-third have been shown to be alive free of disease at 10 years. Although a 10-year disease-free survival is not to be equated absolutely with cure, it is close to it. Small aggregates (up to 2 mm in diameter) of cancer in the axillary nodes seem not to influence prognosis.

The assumption, based on no data, that gross recurrences can be as well treated when they appear is not correct, because in a significant number of patients the recurrent disease cannot be controlled by irradiation at the time of recurrence. This stands to reason because a gross recurrence has more malignant clonogens, some of them hypoxic, whereas when irradiation is given electively, one is dealing with subclinical disease.

ACKNOWLEDGMENTS

This investigation was supported by Grant Numbers CA6294 and CA16672, awarded by the National Cancer Institute, U.S. Department of Health and Human Services.

REFERENCES

Bedwinek, J. M., B. Finberg, J. Lee, and M. Ocwieza. 1981. Analysis of failures following local treatment of isolated local-regional recurrence of breast cancer. Int. J. Radiat. Oncol. Biol. Phys. 7:581–585.

Berkson, J., and R. P. Gage. 1950. Calculation of survival rates for cancer. Mayo Clin. Proc. 25:270–286.

Bonadonna, G., and P. Valagussa. 1981. Dose-response effect of adjuvant chemotherapy in breast cancer. N. Engl. J. Med. 304:10–15.

Bross, I. D. J., and L. E. Blumenson. 1971. Predictive design of experiments using deep mathematical models. Cancer 28:1637–1646.

Bruce, J. 1969. The enigma of breast cancer. Cancer 24:1314–1318.

Chu, F. C. H., F. Lin, J. H. Kim, S. H. Huh, and C. J. Garmatis. 1976. Locally recurrent carcinoma of the breast. Cancer 37:2677–2681.

Cody, H. S., S. S. Bretsky, and J. A. Urban. 1982. The continuing importance of adequate surgery for operable breast cancer: Significant salvage of node-positive patients without adjuvant chemotherapy. CA 32(4):242–256.

Cohen, E., E. F. Scanlon, J. A. Caprini, M. P. Cunningham, M. A. Oviedo, B. Robinson, and J. L. Knox. 1981. Follow-up adjuvant chemotherapy and chemoimmunotherapy for stage II and III carcinoma of the breast. Cancer 1754–1761.

Cruz, E. P., G. O. McDonald, and W. H. Cole. 1956. Prophylactic treatment of cancer: The use of chemotherapeutic agents to prevent tumor metastasis. Surgery 40:291.

Cutler, S. J., and S. J. Axtell. 1963. Partitioning of a patient population with respect to different mortality risks. Am. Statis. Assoc. J. 701–712.

De Lena, M., M. Varini, R. Zucali, D. Rovine, G. Viganolti, P. Valagussa, V. Veronesi, and G. Bonadonna. 1981. Multimodal treatment for locally advanced breast cancer: Results of chemotherapy-radiotherapy versus chemotherapy-surgery. Cancer Clin. Trials 4:229–236.

Fisher, B., B. Carbone, S. G. Economou, R. Frelick, A. Glass, H. Lerner, C. Redmond, M. Zelen, P. Band, D. L. Katrych, W. Wolmark, and E. R. Fisher. 1975a. 1-Phenylalanine mustard (L-PAM) in the management of primary breast cancer. A report of early findings. N. Engl. J. Med. 292:117–122.

Fisher, B., N. Slack, D. Katrych, and N. Wolmark. 1975b. Ten-year follow-up results of patients with carcinoma of the breast in a cooperative clinical trial evaluating surgical adjuvant chemotherapy. Surg. Gynecol. Obstet. 140:528–534.

Fisher, B., E. Montague, C. Redmond, and other NSABP investigators. 1977. Comparison of radical mastectomy with alternative treatments for primary breast cancer. A first report of results from a prospective randomized clinical trial. Cancer 39:2827.

Fisher, B., B. Sherman, H. Rockette, C. Redmond, R. Margolese, and E. R. Fisher. 1979. 1-Phenylalanine mustard (L-PAM) in the management of premenopausal patients with primary breast cancer: Lack of association of disease-free survival with depression of ovarian function. Cancer 44:847–857.

Fisher, E. R., S. Swamidoss, C. H. Lee, H. Rockette, C. Redmond, and E. R. Fisher. 1978. Detection and significance of occult axillary node metastases in patients with invasive breast cancer. Cancer 42:2025.

Fletcher, G. H. 1976. Reflections on breast cancer. Int. J. Radiat. Oncol. Biol. Phys. 1:769–779.

Fletcher, G. H. 1980. Textbook of Radiotherapy, 3rd ed., Lea & Febiger, Philadelphia, pp. 527–583.

Haagensen, C. D. 1971. Disease of The Breast, 2nd ed., W. B. Saunders Co., Philadelphia.

Huvos, A. G., R. V. P. Hutter, and J. Berg. 1971. Significance of axillary macrometastases and micrometastases in mammary cancer. Ann Surg 173:44–46.

Jackson, S. M. 1966. Carcinoma of the breast: The significance of supraclavicular lymph node metastases. Clin. Radiol. 17:107–114.

Kennedy, B. J., A. Tellenjen, S. Kennedy, and N. Havenrick. 1976. Psychological response of patients cured for advanced cancer. Cancer 38:2184–2191.

Lipsett, M. B. 1981. Postoperative radiation for women with cancer of the breast and positive axillary lymph nodes. Should it continue? N. Engl. J. Med. 304:112–114.

Madoc-Jones, H., A. J. Nelson, III, and E. D. Montague. 1976. Evaluation of the effectiveness of radiotherapy in the management of early nodal recurrences from adenocarcinoma of the breast. Breast 2:31.

McKinnon, N. E. 1951. Breast cancer: The fallacy of comparison of dissimilar groups in appraising treatment. Can. J. Public Health 42:88–94.

Meakin, J. W., W. E. C. Allt, L. A. Beale, T. C. Brown, R. S. Bush, R. M. Clark, P. S. Fitzpatrick, N. V. Hawkins, R. D. Lenkin, T. L. Pringle, and W. D. Rider. 1977. Ovarian irradiation and prednisone following surgery for carcinoma of the breast, *in* Adjuvant Therapy of Cancer, S. E. Salmon and S. E. Jones, eds. Elsevier/North Holland, Amsterdam, Holland, pp. 95–99.

Nissen-Meyer, R., K. Kjellgren, K. Malmio, B. Mansson, and T. Norin. 1978. Surgical adjuvant chemotherapy. Results with one short course with cyclophosphamide after mastectomy for breast cancer. Cancer 41:2088–2098.

Park, W. W., and J. C. Lees. 1951. The absolute curability of cancer of the breast. Surg. Gynecol. Obstet. 93:129–152.

Paterson, R., and M. H. Russell. 1959a. Clinical trials in malignant disease: Part II—Breast cancer: Value of irradiation of ovaries. J. Fac. Radiol. (Lond.) 10:130–133.

Paterson, R., and M. H. Russell. 1959b. Clinical trials in malignant disease: Part III—Breast Cancer: Evaluation of postoperative radiotherapy. J. Fac. Radiol. (Lond.) 10:175–180.

Rose, C. M., J. L. Millar, J. H. Peacock, T. A. Phelps, and T. C. Stephens. 1980. Differential enhancement of melphalan cytotoxicity in tumor and normal tissues by misonidazole. Cancer Management 5:520–527.

Spratt, J. S. 1967. Locally recurrent cancer after radical mastectomy. Cancer 20:1051.

Tapley, N. duV., ed. 1976. Clinical Applications of the Electron Beam. John Wiley & Sons, New York, pp. 199–231.

Tapley, N. duV., W. J. Spanos, Jr., G. H. Fletcher, E. D. Montague, S. Schell, and M. J. Oswald. 1982. Results in patients with breast cancer treated by radical mastectomy and postoperative irradiation with no adjuvant chemotherapy. Cancer 49:1316–1319.

West, G. W., R. Weichselbaum, and J. B. Little. 1980. Limited penetration of methotrexate into human osteosarcoma spheroids as a proposed model for solid tumor resistance to adjuvant chemotherapy. Cancer Res. 40:3665–3668.

Current Controversies in Breast Cancer, edited
by F. C. Ames, G. R. Blumenschein, and E. D. Montague.
University of Texas Press, Austin © 1984.

Prognostic Factors in Stage I Breast Cancer

Cornelis J. H. Van de Velde, M.D., Ph.D.,* Geoffrey G. Giacco,
M.S.,† and H. Stephen Gallager, M.D.‡

*Department of Surgery, University Hospital Leyden, The Netherlands, and Departments
of †Patient Studies and ‡Pathology, The University of Texas M. D. Anderson Hospital and
Tumor Institute at Houston, Houston, Texas*

Over the past ten years, there has been a distinct increase in the number of breast cancer patients whose lesions are discovered at an early stage. It has been estimated that at least half of the patients currently presenting for initial treatment have stage I disease (Hutter, 1980). The recent report from the American Cancer Society and National Cancer Institute Breast Detection Demonstration Project (Baker 1982) implies that there may be a further increase in such patients as a result of screening efforts. The national five-year survival rate for patients with stage I breast cancer is 73%, but excess mortality within this group extends at least to 20 years. It seems reasonable to assume that recurrence in this situation, and particularly late recurrence, is the result of activation of micrometastatic deposits of tumor, usually in systemic locations. There is mounting evidence that adjuvant chemotherapy can inhibit this activation (Bonadonna and Valagussa 1981) and that the observed improvement in survival is real and not simply a prolongation of time to recurrence.

For these reasons, it is increasingly desirable to develop criteria that allow the selection of those patients most in need of adjuvant chemotherapy. The existence of reliable standards would also protect from possible complications those patients for whom treatment would be of little value.

In an attempt to determine what factors are important, we have carried out a retrospective study of a relatively large number of carefully stratified patients with stage I breast cancer whose mastectomies were performed 10 or more years ago. The influences of a wide variety of factors, both clinical and pathologic, have been examined. This paper is a preliminary report of the analysis of these data.

MATERIAL AND METHODS

A list of 537 consecutive patients with breast cancer clinically staged as $T_1N_0M_0$ and initially treated between 1960 and 1969 was obtained from the records of the University of Texas M. D. Anderson Hospital and Tumor Institute at Houston. Excluded from this group were patients who had preoperative radiation therapy or who were treated by radiation therapy only, those whose surgical procedure included no axillary dissection, those with only noninvasive or microinvasive carcinoma, those who had had prior contralateral breast carcinomas, and those few for whom data were incomplete. The remaining group, on which this study is based, consisted of 207 patients with pathologic stage $T_1N_0M_0$ carcinomas. All of the patients had invasive carcinomas 1 cm or more in diameter. Treatment was uniform, following the protocol then standard at UT M. D. Anderson Hospital. Follow-up was complete for 10 years or more for all patients.

Data extracted from the clinical records included age, sex, race, parity, menstrual status, and family history of breast carcinoma. The Quetelet index of obesity was calculated from the patient's recorded height and weight. Laterality and location of the tumor within the breast were noted from both clinical and mammographic information. Sizes of invasive masses, determined by clinical and pathologic examinations, were obtained from the records; in addition, measurements in three dimensions were taken from preoperative mammograms. All histologic material was reviewed. The characteristics recorded included the nature of the tumor border, the histologic type of tumor, the histologic and nuclear grades, and the presence of necrosis, vascular involvement, lymphocytic infiltration, and multicentricity.

Each recorded factor was individually analyzed for its influence on the recurrence rate. In addition, combinations of factors were similarly analyzed. Appropriate tests of statistical significance were applied.

RESULTS

No statistically significant relationships were found between any of the clinically determined factors and the recurrence rate. There were some differences between individual decade age groups, but these showed no consistency and probably represented artifact due to the small sizes of groups at the extremes. Age, race, menstrual status, parity, family history, and history of previous benign disease all were insignificant.

Interestingly, there was no difference in prognosis between patients with breast carcinomas in outer quadrants and those with central or medial lesions. All of the patients in the latter group, however, received postoperative radiation therapy to the internal mammary and supraclavicular regions. Without concurrent controls, however, it cannot be stated with assurance that the application of radiation therapy accounted for the lack of difference.

Tumor size, as mentioned above, was measured in three ways. The measurements of greatest diameter, determined clinically, mammographically, and pathologically, correlated well with one another. The medians for clinical and mammographic measurement were 132% and 116%, respectively, of the mean pathologic measurement. No single measurement showed any relationship to prognosis. Determination of mass volume, however, proved to be prognostically significant. The recurrence rate among patients with masses having volumes less than 10 cm^3 was 18.1%; that among patients with larger masses was 35.9% ($P = 0.045$).

As in most such series, invasive ductal carcinoma made up approximately 70% of all histologic tumor types. An additional 13.5% of tumors consisted of invasive lobular carcinomas and carcinomas of mixed cellularity in which there was an invasive lobular component. Unexpectedly, patients in this group showed a recurrence rate almost double that of other histologic types. Specifically, the recurrence rate for lobular and mixed carcinomas was 48.4% as compared to 27.6% for the other types ($P = 0.034$). This difference seemed to be independent of other variables. As anticipated, mucinous, medullary, and comedo carcinomas were associated with favorable prognoses, but the numbers of cases in these categories were too small for differences to be meaningful.

Tumor grade in this study was determined both by the histologic method of Bloom and Richardson (1957) and by the nuclear grading of Black and Speer (1957). There was general agreement between the two systems. Invasive lobular carcinomas were considered routinely to be of intermediate grade. Mixed lobular and ductal carcinomas were considered to be grade 2 unless the ductal component of the tumor was of higher grade. The presence of a favorable tumor grade conferred a distinct advantage in freedom from recurrence. The recurrence rate was 17.6% for patients with grade 1 tumors and 34.9% for those with tumors of higher grade ($P=0.014$). The number of high-grade tumors was not sufficient to establish a distinction between recurrence rates of grade 2 and 3 tumors.

Multiplicity of invasion in a single breast was found in 10.1% of the patients. The phenomenon was distinctly more frequent among patients with high-grade carcinomas. As in other studies (Egan 1982), multicentricity was found to be an unfavorable prognostic indicator. The recurrence rate in these patients was 39.8% as compared to 29.0% for patients with single invasive tumor sites ($P = 0.04$). When both high tumor grade and multicentricity were present, the difference was accentuated (47.4% versus 21.8%, respectively, $P = 0.013$).

Neoplastic involvement of intramammary lymphatic vessels proved to be of no significant prognostic value. The majority of patients with this finding had tumors of high or intermediate grades, but even among patients with both phenomena there was no influence on recurrence. It is perhaps noteworthy that 79% of initial recurrences in this group developed either in the lung or in bone.

Other factors studied showed no association with survival.

DISCUSSION

This study has demonstrated that it is possible to identify subsets of patients with negative axillary nodes within which the likelihood of recurrence is relatively high. The elimination of variables other than those related to the tumor itself permits fairly clear-cut conclusions concerning prognosis, although factors found to be of no significance in this study might assume greater meaning if a larger series were studied. Since the incidence of recurrence in patients without involved lymph nodes is relatively low, extension of the study to a larger population would be desirable.

Relationships between prognosis and tumor volume, tumor grade, and multicentricity have been recorded by others. The apparent unfavorable influence of invasive lobular carcinoma, however, is contrary to what has been found in comparable studies (Rosen et al. 1981) and requires further investigation.

REFERENCES

Baker, L. H. 1982. Breast cancer detection demonstration project: Five-year summary report. CA 32:194–225.

Black, M. M., and F. D. Speer. 1957. Nuclear structure in cancer tissue. Surg. Gynecol. Obstet. 105:97–102.

Bloom, H. J. G., and W. W. Richardson. 1957. Histologic grading and prognosis in breast cancer. Br. J. Cancer 11:359–377.

Bonadonna, G., and P. Valagussa. 1981. Dose-response effect of adjuvant chemotherapy in breast cancer. N. Engl. J. Med. 304:10–15.

Egan, R. L. 1982. Multicentric breast carcinomas. Clinical-radiologic-pathologic whole organ studies and 10-year survival. Cancer 49:1123–1130.

Hutter, R. V. P. 1980. The influence of pathologic factors on breast cancer management. Cancer 46:961–976.

Rosen, P. P., P. E. Saigo, D. W. Braun, Jr., E. Weathers, and A. De Palo. 1981. Predictors of recurrence in stage I ($T_1N_0M_0$) breast cancer. Ann. Surg. 193:15–25.

Current Controversies in Breast Cancer, edited
by F. C. Ames, G. R. Blumenschein, and E. D. Montague.
University of Texas Press, Austin © 1984.

Adjunctive Therapy in Breast Cancer: The Stockholm Experience

Arne Wallgren, M.D., Ulla Glas, M.D., Lars-Erik Strender, M.D.,
Leif Karnström, B.A., Bo Nilsson, B.Sc., and participating
investigators from the Stockholm Breast Cancer Group

*Stockholm-Gotland Oncologic Center, Radiumhemmet,
Karolinska Hospital, Stockholm, Sweden.*

In Stockholm there has been a long tradition of a joint preoperative evaluation of breast tumor patients by surgeons and radiotherapists. The cytologist later became an important member of the team. More than 90% of clinically detected breast cancers are diagnosed by means of fine needle aspiration cytologic biopsy. In 1976, the team approach to breast cancer evaluation and treatment was formalized when the so-called oncologic center for the Health Service Region of Stockholm and Gotland was established. An oncologic center is not a center in the physical sense but a pooling of all resources for cancer care within the health service region. A central office runs the regional cancer registry and also serves as the administrative office for clinical trials.

In 1971, a clinical trial on preoperative and postoperative radiotherapy was initiated at the Radiumhemmet, the oncologic department of the Karolinska Hospital, in cooperation with five surgical departments in Stockholm. The entry of patients was closed in November 1976 when a management program for breast cancer was established within the oncologic center. This program also included clinical trials on adjuvant cytotoxic and endocrine treatment. These have been performed as multicenter studies in which the oncologic and surgical departments of the region cooperate.

PREOPERATIVE AND POSTOPERATIVE RADIOTHERAPY

The design and early results of this trial have been reported previously (Wallgren et al. 1978, Wallgren et al. 1980, Strender et al. 1981). Premenopausal women and those postmenopausal women less than 71 years of age with operable breast cancer were accepted if their cancers were clearly diagnosed preoperatively by means of fine-needle aspiration biopsy. A total of 960 patients were included in the study, 316 of whom were randomly chosen to receive preoperative radiotherapy, 323 chosen to receive postoperative radiotherapy, and 321 patients to receive surgery alone. The surgical treatment in all three groups consisted of modified radical mastectomy. The radiotherapy was given in only one institution. The aim was to deliver a dose of 4,500 rad in 5 weeks to the internal mammary, the supraclavicular, and the axillary lymph node regions as well as to the breast and the entire width of the chest wall. An analysis of the actual doses given revealed that the dose in the ipsilateral internal mammary lymph nodes was considerably lower in patients treated postoperatively than in those treated preoperatively due to differences in treatment techniques. The difference was especially pronounced during the latter half of the study period (Strender et al. 1981).

Result

The result of the trial on preoperative and postoperative radiotherapy when the patients had been followed-up for 57–124 months are summarized in Tables 1–4.

Preoperative and postoperative radiotherapy decreased the recurrence rate to the same extent (Table 1). This was mainly due to a reduction of local and regional recurrences (Table 2) in both pre- and postmenopausal women. There was no indication that radiotherapy increased the frequency of distant metastasis (Table 2).

In previous reports with shorter follow-up, preoperative radiotherapy was found to increase the survival significantly (Wallgren et al. 1978, Wallgren et al. 1980, Strender et al. 1981). Though the ratio of death rates indicated an advantage for the preoperatively irradiated patients compared to those treated only surgically in this study, the difference was not statistically significant (Table 3). In patients with inner

Table 1. *Ratio of Recurrence Rates for Irradiated Patients to that of Surgical Controls*

Treatment Group	No. of Patients	No. of Failures	Ratio of Recurrence Rates
Preoperative radiotherapy	316	104	0.67 (0.53–0.86*)
Postoperative radiotherapy	323	96	0.63 (0.49–0.80)
Surgery only	321	135	1.00

*Within parentheses are shown the 95% confidence limits.

Table 2. *Number of Patients with Recurrent Disease According to Site of Recurrence*

Treatment Group	Local and Regional	Distant	All Failures
Preoperative radiotherapy	25	100	104
Postoperative radiotherapy	23	94	96
Surgery only	83	110	135

Table 3. *Ratio of Mortality Rates of Irradiated Patients to that of the Surgical Controls.*

Treatment Group	No. of Patients	No. of Deaths	Ratio of Mortality Rates
Preoperative radiotherapy	316	90	0.85 (0.64−1.13*)
Postoperative radiotherapy	323	89	0.85 (0.64−1.13)
Surgery only	321	102	1.00

*Within parentheses are shown the 95% confidence limits.

Table 4. *Ratio of Mortality Rates of Patients with Inner Quadrant Tumors Treated with Radiotherapy to That of Surgical Controls.*

Treatment Group	No. of Patients	No. of Deaths	Ratio of Mortality Rates
Preoperative radiotherapy	74	17	0.70 (0.37−1.32*)
Postoperative radiotherapy	58	14	0.76 (0.39−1.47)
Surgery only	70	22	1.00

*Within parentheses are shown the 95% confidence limits.

quadrant tumors, who might benefit most from treatment of involved internal mammary lymph nodes, the decrease of the death rate for those receiving radiotherapy was even more pronounced than for those with central or outer quadrant tumors, but not statistically significant (Table 4).

Conclusions

The conclusions are that preoperative and postoperative radiotherapy to the same extent reduced the frequency of local and regional recurrences and, thus, increased the recurrence-free survival of breast cancer patients. The improved survival for patients with inner quadrant tumors that was observed when the internal mammary lymph nodes were "adequately" irradiated could support the hypothesis that local control of the disease might improve the survival for subsets of patients. Similar findings have been reported from the Oslo trial (Høst and Brennhovd 1977) and from the Guy's Hospital trial on breast cancer conserving treatment (Hayward 1981). In other large trials, however, no indication of an improved survival was found after irradiation of the internal mammary lymph nodes (Cancer Research Campaign 1980, Fisher et al. 1981). The question of whether adequate irradiation of the internal mammary lymph nodes will improve survival in patients with inner quadrant tumors is still considered controversial (Canellos et al. 1982), and a definite answer can only be reached from an adequately planned clinical trial.

ADJUNCTIVE CYTOTOXIC AND ENDOCRINE TREATMENT IN OPERABLE BREAST CANCER

In 1976 trials were initiated to study the merits of systemic treatment, cytotoxic chemotherapy, and tamoxifen in breast cancer.

Cytotoxic Therapy

Cytotoxic therapy was studied in patients with a high likelihood of relapse, i.e. those with nodal involvement or with tumors exceeding 3 cm in diameter. Their controls were treated with postoperative radiotherapy since this gave the best recurrence-free survival in the above-mentioned trial.

The chemotherapy consisted of methotrexate, 40 mg/m^2 intravenously (I.V.) administered on days 1 and 8 and 5-fluorouracil, 600 mg/m^2 I.V. administered on days 1 and 8 of each course. Initially, chlorambucil, 10–15 mg, was given orally on days 1–8 but was replaced by cyclophosphamide, 100 mg/m^2 given orally on days 1–14. Twelve courses were given in 1–1.5 years. Because of side effects, approximately 70% of postmenopausal and 90% of premenopausal patients completed their 12 courses.

The trial is still open. At the present time 178 premenopausal and 288 postmenopausal patients are included in the study. The end point of this study is death.

After a mean follow-up of 31 months, there has been no significant difference in recurrence-free survival between the groups receiving radiotherapy and chemotherapy. In the group receiving radiotherapy, 62 of 225 patients have experienced recurrent disease. In the group receiving chemotherapy, the corresponding figures are 71 of 241 patients. Chemotherapy did not control local and regional disease to the same extent as radiotherapy, but, at least in the premenopausal women cytotoxic chemotherapy significantly decreased the rate of distant metastasis.

Adjuvant Tamoxifen

All postmenopausal patients with operable disease irrespective of nodal status were also randomized to receive tamoxifen, 40 mg daily, for 2 years. Thus, the postmenopausal patients with a high risk of relapse were included in a 2 × 2 factorial study on both cytotoxic chemotherapy versus radiotherapy and on the use of tamoxifen. At the present time, 522 postmenopausal patients with a low risk of recurrence, i.e. without lymph node involvement and with tumors 3 cm or less, and 306 women with a high risk of relapse are included in the study. The early results of this trial show that tamoxifen reduces the risk of recurrence irrespective of other treatment (Wallgren et al. 1981). This improvement was thus seen in patients who were also treated with adjunctive cytotoxic chemotherapy or with radiotherapy. The improvement was established during the 2 years of treatment. Thereafter, no further reduction of recurrence was seen. Because of the low frequency of side effects, longer treatment with tamoxifen might be attempted to determine if this would further decrease the rate of recurrence.

CONCLUSIONS

The three studies of adjunctive treatment in breast cancer show that radiotherapy, cytotoxic chemotherapy, and tamoxifen treatment increase the recurrence-free survival in women with operable breast cancer. The side effects and the costs of these treatment modalities are very different. Even if the patient is not cured, an increased time interval until recurrence is of great importance to her if the side effects are acceptable. The survival benefits of the adjunctive treatments are likely to be less pronounced than their effects on duration of recurrence-free survival. Definite therapeutic recommendations can only be made when the magnitude of the possible survival benefits is known.

ACKNOWLEDGMENTS

These investigations were supported by grants from King Gustaf V Jubilee Fund.

REFERENCES

Cancer Research Campaign (King's/Cambridge) Trial for early breast cancer. 1980. Lancet 2:55–60.

Canellos, G. P., S. Hellman, and U. Veronesi. 1982. The management of early breast cancer. N. Engl. J. Med. 306:1430–1432.

Fisher, B., N. Wolmark, C. Redmond, M. Deutsch, E. R. Fisher, and participating NSABP investigators. 1981. Findings from NSABP protocol No B-04: Comparison of radical mastectomy with alternative treatments. II. The clinical and biological significance of medial-central breast cancers. Cancer 48:1863–1872.

Hayward, J. L. 1981. The surgeon's role in primary breast cancer. Breast Cancer Research and Treatment 1:27–32.

Høst, H., and L. O Brennhovd. 1977. The effect of postoperative radiotherapy in breast cancer. Int. J. Radiat. Oncol. Biol. Phys. 2:1061–1067.

Strender, L. E., A. Wallgren, J. Arndt, O. Arner, J. Bergström, B. Blomstedt, P. O. Granberg, B. Nilsson, L. Räf, and C. Silfverswärd. 1981. Adjuvant radiotherapy in operable breast cancer: Correlation between dose in internal mammary nodes and prognosis. Int. J. Radiat. Oncol. Biol. Phys. 7:1319–1325.

Wallgren, A., O. Arner, J. Bergström, B. Blomstedt, P. O. Granberg, L. Karnström, L. Räf, and C. Silfverswärd. 1978. Preoperative radiotherapy in operable breast cancer. Results in the Stockholm breast cancer trial. Cancer 42:1120–1125.

Wallgren, A., O. Arner, J. Bergström, B. Blomstedt, P. O. Granberg, L. Karnström, L. Räf, and C. Silfverswärd. 1980. The value of preoperative radiotherapy in operable mammary carcinoma. Int. J. Radiat. Oncol. Biol. Phys. 6:287–290.

Wallgren, A., W. Baral, U. Glas, M. Kaigas, L. Karnström, B. Nordenskjöld, N. O. Theve, N. Wilking, and C. Silfverswärd. 1981. Adjuvant breast cancer treatment with tamoxifen and combination chemotherapy in postmenopausal women, *in* Adjuvant Therapy of Cancer III, S. E. Salmon and S. E. Jones, eds. Grune & Stratton, New York, pp. 345–350.

Current Controversies in Breast Cancer, edited
by F. C. Ames, G. R. Blumenschein, and E. D. Montague.
University of Texas Press, Austin © 1984.

Adjunctive Hormonal Therapy for Stage II Breast Cancer

Bernard Fisher, M.D. *

Department of Surgery, University of Pittsburgh, Pittsburgh, Pennsylvania, and National Surgical Adjuvant Breast and Bowel Project, Pittsburgh, Pennsylvania*

The National Surgical Adjuvant Breast and Bowel Project (NSABP) has been conducting clinical trials in sequential fashion to evaluate various regimens of adjuvant chemotherapy in women who have primary breast cancer and positive axillary lymph nodes. In 1972, an initial trial was begun to determine the worth of 1-phenylalanine mustard (P). When patient accrual was completed in that trial, a second trial was initiated. It compared P with the combination of P and 5-fluorouracil (F). Findings revealed that PF decreased the incidence of treatment failure and prolonged survival in more subgroups of patients than did P. A third study that compared PF with the combination of PF and methotrexate demonstrated no advantage from the addition of methotrexate. When sufficient evidence accumulated indicating that tamoxifen (T) exerts an antitumor effect in patients with metastatic breast cancer, its evaluation in primary disease became justified (Cole et al. 1971, Ward 1973, Lerner et al. 1976). Consequently, a new NSABP trial was begun to determine whether the addition of T to PF would enhance the disease-free survival (DFS) and overall survival (S) achieved with PF. The findings from this prospective randomized clinical trial involving 1891 women have been reported (Fisher et al. 1981, Fisher et al. 1983). It was observed that the benefit from the addition of T to PF was related to the age of patients and to the estrogen receptor (ER) levels of their tumors. This presentation provides a brief overview of the more pertinent observations from patients having an average follow-up time of 40 months.

METHODS

The details of patient selection, experimental design, drug administration, and tumor receptor analysis have all been previously documented (Fisher et al. 1981, Fisher et al. 1975). This trial was conducted in women undergoing treatment at 68 institutions in the United States and Canada that are members of the NSABP.

*See Appendix I for a list of NSABP institutions and principal investigators participating in Protocol B-09.

Women with one or more axillary lymph nodes histologically verified as positive and who had radical mastectomies (conventional or modified) were eligible for study if they fulfilled specific criteria identical to those used in prior NSABP trials of adjuvant therapy. They were separated into groups according to age ($\leq$ 49 years and $\geq$ 50 years) and number of positive lymph nodes (one to three nodes and $\geq$ four nodes). There were 1891 patients randomized to receive either PF or PFT between January 1, 1977, and May 16, 1980. The two treatment groups were found to be similar in age, location and size of tumor, duration of symptoms, and degree of nodal involvement. Tumor specimens were assayed for both ER and PR content with the sucrose-density gradient, dextran-coated charcoal titration with Scatchard analysis, or dextran-coated charcoal with a single saturating dose. In this report, both receptor levels are reported as fmoles/mg of cytosol protein.

The dose of P in both treatment groups was 4 mg/m^2 of body-surface area given daily by mouth for the first 5 days of each cycle; F (300 mg/m^2 was given intravenously on each of the same 5 days. Each cycle was repeated every 6 weeks 17 times for approximately 2 years. The dose of T in the PFT treatment group was 10 mg by mouth twice a day for the entire 2 years of therapy. Treatment was begun no sooner than 2 weeks and no later than 4 weeks after surgery. Doses were modified according to the presence and degree of hematologic and gastrointestinal toxicity.

Table 1. *Disease-Free Survival and Survival at 3 Years in Patients with ER or PR Levels < 10 fmoles**

Group	No. Patients PF	No. Patients PFT	% DFS PF	% DFS PFT	P† Value	% S PF	% S PFT	P† Value
ER								
All patients	299	315	54 (176)‡	60 (192)	0.38	74 (159)	70 (185)	0.56
$\leq$ 49 years	153	170	57 (92)	57 (105)	0.66	80 (77)	68 (98)	0.03
$\geq$ 50 years	146	145	50 (84)	63 (87)	0.09	68 (82)	72 (87)	0.34
PR								
All patients	260	282	56 (147)	55 (161)	0.34	79 (125)	70 (155)	0.003
$\leq$ 49 years	107	120	60 (66)	44 (75)	0.02	87 (49)	64 (69)	<0.001
$\geq$ 50 years	153	162	53 (81)	64 (86)	0.33	73 (76)	75 (86)	0.74

* Abbreviations are as follows: ER = estrogen receptor; and PR = progesterone receptor; DFS = disease-free survival; S = Survival; P = 1-phenylalanine mustard; F = 5-fluorouracil; T = tamoxifen; P = probability.
† Summary two-sided chi-square test, adjusted for number of positive lymph nodes.
‡ ( ) = No. of patients followed to 3 years.

The actuarial life-table method was used to summarize the distribution of treatment failure and patient survival. Statistical significance of the differences between the life-table distributions was assessed by a summary chi-square or log-rank test. Levels of significance shown relate to a two-sided test.

RESULTS

Findings Related to Tumor ER or PR

No overall benefit in DFS or S has resulted from the addition of T to PF when the tumor ER or PR level was $<$ 10 fmoles (Table 1). Neither patients $\leq$ 49 nor those $\geq$ 50 years old demonstrated an advantage from the three drugs, although in those $\geq$ 50 years there was some improvement (P = 0.09) in DFS. Of particular note is the observation that PFT-treated patients $\leq$ 49 years old with tumor ER levels $<$ 10 fmoles have a significantly decreased survival (P = 0.03). When their tumor PR levels were $<$ 10 fmoles, both DFS and S were significantly decreased (P = 0.02 and $<$ 0.001, respectively). Findings in patients with one to three or $\geq$ four positive lymph nodes were similar to those noted for all patients in the age group being considered.

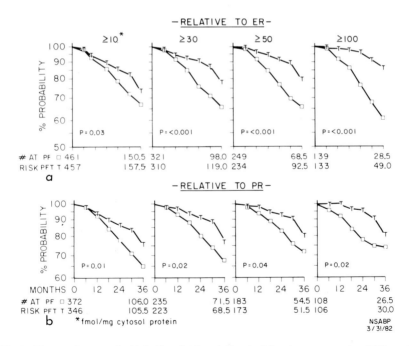

FIG. 1. Disease-free survival of all patients relative to (a) estrogen-receptor (ER) and (b) progesterone-receptor (PR) levels (P = 1-phenylalanine mustard; F = 5-fluorouracil; T = tamoxifen).

Table 2. *Disease-Free Survival and Survival at 3 Years in Patients ≥ 50 Years of Age With ER or PR Levels ≥ 10 fmoles**

Receptor Level fmol	No. Patients		% DFS		P†
	PF	PFT	PF	PFT	Value
ER					
≥ 10	299	300	66 (168)‡	78 (153)	0.002
≥ 30	229	228	63 (132)	81 (116)	<0.001
≥ 50	191	184	63 (107)	82 (94)	<0.001
≥ 100	119	116	58 (60)	91 (49)	<0.001
PR					
≥ 10	212	195	64 (115)	79 (96)	<0.001
≥ 30	125	131	66 (67)	84 (52)	<0.001
≥ 50	102	102	69 (50)	87 (36)	0.001
≥ 100	57	63	71 (25)	86 (20)	0.003

*Abbreviations are as follows: ER = estrogen receptor; PR = progesterone receptor; DFS = disease-free survival; S = Survival; P = 1-phenylalanine mustard; F = 5-fluorouracil; T = tamoxifen; P = probability.
†Summary two-sided chi-square test, adjusted for no. of positive nodes.
‡( ) = No. of patients followed to 3 years.

The DFS of all patients having tumor ER or PR levels ≥ 10 fmoles was significantly better in PFT-treated patients (Figure 1). Moreover, as levels of tumor ER increased, so did the benefit. Findings in that regard with PR were less pronounced.

The beneficial results from PFT observed in patients who had receptor-positive tumors (≥ 10 fmoles) was due to findings in those ≥ 50 years of age. In those patients, either overall (Table 2) or in both nodal subgroups, PFT prolonged the DFS and the advantage was greater the higher the tumor ER level.

Patients ≤ 49 years old with tumor ER or PR ≥ 10 fmoles demonstrated no benefit from PFT, and there was no evidence that higher tumor receptor levels in those patients would affect these results. The difference between the findings in the two age groups is exemplified by the complete lack of an advantage from PFT in those ≤ 49 years old with ≥ four positive nodes (Figure 2) and the remarkable benefit in those ≥ 50 years old with ≥ four positive nodes (Figure 3).

At present, no survival advantage has been demonstrated for any group or subgroup of patients who have received PFT.

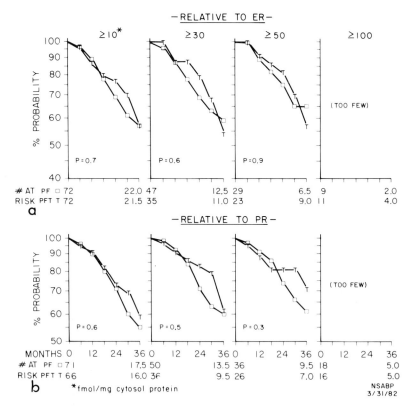

FIG. 2. Disease-free survival of patients ≤ 49 years old with ≥ four positive lymph nodes relative to (a) estrogen-receptor (ER) and (b) progesterone-receptor (PR) levels (P = 1-phenylalanine mustard; F = 5-fluorouracil; T = tamoxifen).

Findings Related to ER and PR

Findings have indicated the advantage of knowing both ER and PR values. In patients ≤ 49 years old, the disadvantage in DFS and S following PFT therapy observed when both ER and PR are in the range of 0–9 fmoles is not present if the PR is ≥ 10 fmoles, even though the ER is 0–9 fmoles (Table 3). Also, when there is a low PR (0–9) in the presence of an ER ≥ 10 fmoles, the negative effect of PFT is evident; however, when both receptors are ≥ 10 fmoles, the disadvantage from PFT is not present.

Evaluations of patients ≥ 50 years old with respect to ER *and* PR indicates an advantage from PFT in DFS when both ER and PR are ≥ 10 fmoles. Of greater importance is the observation that findings from patients 50–59 years old differ from those in patients 60–70 years old. The findings of those in the younger decade are intermediate between those seen in patients ≤ 49 years old and in those 60–70 years old. Survival results are poorer on PFT when PR levels are low, particularly if

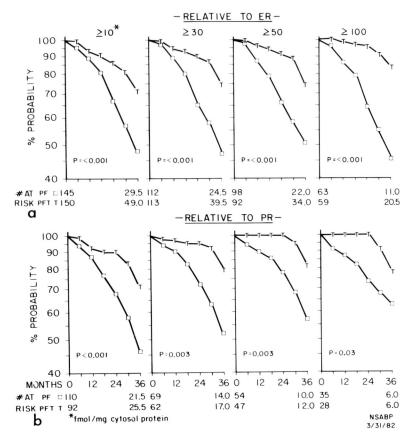

FIG. 3. Disease-free survival of patients ≥ 50 years old with ≥ four positive lymph nodes relative to (a) estrogen-receptor (ER) and (b) progesterone-receptor (PR) levels (P = 1-phenylalanine mustard; F = 5-fluorouracil; T = tamoxifen).

ER levels are low, whereas among patients 60–70 years old there is an advantage from PFT regardless of the receptor levels (Table 4).

COMMENTS AND CONCLUSION

The overall results after 3 years show that the addition of T to PF significantly enhances the DFS of patients who have breast cancer and positive nodes. The benefit is limited to women ≥ 50 years old and is associated with the ER and PR content of tumors. Of particular interest was the observation that patients ≤ 49 years of age had lower DFS and S on PFT when their tumor ER or PR levels were 0–9 fmoles. It is important to emphasize that the results from this seemingly deleterious response, while poorer than findings from PF-treated patients, were no worse than those observed in untreated controls. A variety of explanations for this observation have

Table 3. *Relation of Tumor ER and PR Levels to Disease-Free Survival and Survival at 3 Years in Patients ≤ 49 Years Old**

ER and PR (fmol)		No. Patients		% DFS		P† Value	% S		P† Value
		PF	PFT	PF	PFT		PF	PFT	
0-9	0-9	70	86	50 (40)‡	47 (53)	0.42	86 (27)	62 (49)	0.003
0-9	≥ 10	51	52	61 (33)	65 (28)	0.98	78 (29)	73 (25)	0.95
≥ 10	0-9	34	34	76 (24)	37 (22)	0.03	93 (20)	70 (20)	0.01
≥ 10	≥ 10	106	95	66 (60)	72 (49)	0.27	86 (52)	90 (46)	0.49

* Abbreviations are as follows: ER = estrogen receptor; PR = progesterone receptor; DFS = disease-free survival; S = survival; P = 1-phenylalanine mustard; F = 5-fluorouracil; T = tamoxifen; *P* = probability.
† Summary two-sided chi-square test adjusted for no. of positive lymph nodes.
‡ ( ) = No. of patients followed to 3 years.

Table 4. *Relation of Tumor ER and PR Levels to Disease-Free Survival at 3 Years in Patients 50−59 and 60−70 Years of Age**

ER and PR (fmol)		50−59 Years					60−70 Years				
		No. Patients		% DFS		P† Value	No. Patients		% DFS		P† Value
		PF	PFT	PF	PFT		PF	PFT	PF	PFT	
0-9	0-9	45	49	60 (24)‡	48 (31)	0.46	38	32	24 (23)	60 (12)	0.02
0-9	≥ 10	25	25	59 (12)	83 (13)	0.15	12	6	Too few		−
≥ 10	0-9	42	42	62 (19)	66 (24)	0.94	27	37	71 (14)	85 (17)	0.54
≥ 10	≥ 10	95	97	64 (54)	73 (43)	0.02	79	66	67 (42)	91 (26)	0.04

* Abbreviations are as follows: ER = estrogen receptor; PR = progesterone receptor; DFS = disease-free survival; P = 1-phenylalanine mustard; F = 5-fluorouracil; T = tamoxifen; *P* = probability.
† Summary two-sided chi-square test adjusted for no. of positive lymph nodes.
‡ ( ) = No. of patients followed to 3 years.

been considered, and findings from ancillary studies have failed to support any that have been suggested. The most likely reason that younger patients with receptor-poor tumors have inferior results following PFT therapy is that the usual advantage from chemotherapy observed in that age group has been nullified by altered drug metabolism and no benefit accrues from the use of T. In the older age group with tumors having high receptor content, a similar inhibition of PF action may occur, but T is able to exert a beneficial effect because receptor levels are higher than in younger patients. Whether similar findings would occur if T were administered alone or in conjunction with other adjuvant chemotherapy regimens is unknown.

These data support the importance of knowing both the ER and PR content of tumors. They indicate that the effects of T are more closely related to the PR than ER levels of tumors. The results of multivariate analyses carried out in this study and reported elsewhere in detail support this conclusion (Fisher et al. 1983).

The information also suggests that there may be justification for a more prolonged administration of T; the increased rate of failure in the second half of the third year suggests this. Current NSABP studies are examining the effects of using T for more than 2 years.

ACKNOWLEDGMENTS

This investigation was supported by Grant Number U10-CA-12027 and Contract Number CA-U10-34211, awarded by the National Cancer Institute, U.S. Department of Health and Human Services, and by Grant Number RC-13, awarded by the American Cancer Society.

REFERENCES

Cole, M. P., C. T. A. Jones, and I. D. H. Todd. 1971. A new anti-oestrogenic agent in the late breast cancer: An early clinical appraisal of ICI46474. Br. J. Cancer 25:270–275.

Fisher, B., P. Carbone, S. G. Economou, R. Frelick, A. Glass, H. Lerner, C. Redmond, M. Zelen, P. Band, D. L. Katrych, N. Wolmark, E. R. Fisher, and other cooperative investigators. 1975. 1-phenylalanine mustard (L-PAM) in the management of primary breast cancer: A report of early findings. N. Engl. J. Med. 292:117–122.

Fisher, B., C. Redmond, A. Brown, D. L. Wickerham, N. Wolmark, J. Allegra, G. Escher, M. Lippman, E. Savlov, J. Wittliff, and E. R. Fisher, with the contributions of D. Plotkin, D. Bowman, J. Wolter, R. Bornstein, R. Desser, R. Frelick, and other NSABP investigators. 1983. The influence of tumor estrogen and progesterone receptor levels on the response to tamoxifen and chemotherapy in primary breast cancer. J. Clin. Oncol. (in press).

Fisher, B., C. Redmond, A. Brown, N. Wolmark, J. Wittliff, E. R. Fisher, D. Plotkin, D. Bowman, S. Sachs, J. Wolter, R. Frelick, R. Desser, N. LiCalzi, P. Geggie, T. Campbell, E. G. Elias, D. Prager, P. Koontz, H. Volk, N. Dimitrov, B. Gardner, H. Lerner, H. Shibata, and other NSABP investigators. 1981. Treatment of primary breast cancer with chemotherapy and tamoxifen. N. Engl. J. Med. 305:1–6.

Lerner, H. J., P. R. Band, L. Israel, and B. S. Leung. 1976. Phase II study of tamoxifen: Report of 74 patients with stage IV breast cancer. Cancer Treat. Rep. 60:1431–1435.

Ward, H. W. C. 1973. Anti-oestrogen therapy for breast cancer: A trial of tamoxifen at two dose levels. Br. Med. J. 1:13–14.

APPENDIX I

Participants in Protocol No. B-09

Institution	*Principal Investigator*
Albany Regional Cancer Center, Albany NY	Thomas J. Cunningham
Albert Einstein College of Medicine, Bronx, NY	Herbert Volk
Albert Einstein Medical Center, Philadelphia, PA	Stanley N. Levick/
	Ajit M. Desai
Allentown Hospital, Allentown, PA	David Prager
Berkshire Medical Center, Pittsfield, MA	Jesse Spector/
	Harvey Zimbler
Billings Interhospital Oncology Project,	David B. Myers
Billings, MT	
Boston University, Boston, MA	Peter J. Deckers/
	Merrill I. Feldman
Camden-Clark Hospital, Parkersburg, WV	Nikunj Shah
Chicago Medical School, Chicago, IL	Ediz Ezdinli
Cross Cancer Institute, Edmonton, Alberta	Sandy Paterson
Dekalb General Hospital, Decatur, GA	S. Angier Wills
Denver General Hospital, Denver, CO	George E. Moore
Downstate Medical Center (SUNY), Brooklyn, NY	Bernard Gardner
Ellis Fischel State Cancer Hospital, Columbia, MO	William G. Kraybill
Geisinger Medical Center, Danvill, PA	Philip Breen/
	James Evans
Group Health Medical Center, Seattle, WA	Roberts Bourdeau
Gulf Coast Community Hospital, Panama City, FL	William Gregory Bruce
Gulf Coast Oncology, Pensacola, FL	Allan Patton
Hahnemann Medical College, Philadelphia, PA	Isidore Brodsky
Harbor/UCLA Medical Center, Torrance, CA	David State/
	M. Michael Shabot
Hennepin County Medical Center,	Claude R. Hitchcock
Minneapolis, MN	
Highland Hospital, Rochester, NY	Sidney Sobel
Jefferson Hospital, Philadelphia, PA	Arthur Weiss
Jefferson Medical College, Philadelphia, PA	Harvey Brodovosky
Kaiser Permanente, Harbor City, CA	Eugene Pollack
Kaiser Permanente, Portland, CA	Andrew Glass
Kaiser Permanente, San Diego, CA	Thomas Campbell
Lahey Clinic, Boston, MA	Richard Oberfield
Letterman Army Medical Center, San	David Gandara
Francisco, CA	
L'Hotel-Dieu De Quebec	Louis Dionne
Louisiana State University, New Orleans, LA	Isidore Cohn/
	Robert Beazley
Louisiana State University, Shreveport, LA	Leonard Goldman/
	Don M. Morris
Lynn Hospital, Lynn, MA	Lester Tobin
Maimonides Medical Center, Brooklyn, NY	Anthony Critselis
Manitoba Cancer Foundation, Winnipeg, Manitoba	David Bowman
Marin General Hospital, San Rafael, CA	Peter D. Eisenberg
Martin Luther Hospital, Anaheim, CA	Jack Brook
Medical College of Virginia, Richmond, VA	Walter Lawrence
Medical College of Wisconsin, Milwaukee, WI	William Donegan
Memorial Cancer Research Foundation, Culver	David Plotkin
City, CA	

Michael Reese Hospital, Chicago, IL
Michigan State University, East Lansing, MI

Montefiore Hospital & Medical Center, Bronx, NY
Montreal General Hospital, Montreal, Quebec
Mount Sinai Medical Center, Cleveland, OH

Newark Beth Israel Hospital, Newark, NJ
Ottawa Civic Hospital, Ottawa, Canada

Pennsylvania Hospital, Philadelphia, PA
Royal Victoria Hospital, Montreal, Quebec
Rush Presbyterian–St. Luke's Medical Center,
    Chicago, IL
South Nassau Communities Hospital,
    Oceanside, NY
St. Luc Hospital, Montreal, Quebec

St. Luke's Hospital, Kansas City, MO
St. Michael's Hospital, Toronto, Canada
St. Vincent's Hospital, New York, NY
Texas Tech Medical School, Amarillo, TX
Tom Baker Cancer Center, Calgary, Alberta
Tufts University–New England Medical Center,
    Boston, MA
Tulane University, New Orleans, LA
Naval Regional Medical Center, Oakland, CA
University Hospital of Florida, Jacksonville, FL
University of California, San Diego, CA
University of Chicago, Chicago, IL
University of Florida, Jacksonville, FL
University of Hawaii, Honolulu, HI
University of Illinois, Chicago, IL
University of Iowa, Iowa City, IA
University of Louisville, Louisville, KY
University of Maryland, Baltimore, MD
University of North Carolina at Chapel Hill, NC
University of Pennsylvania, Philadelphia, PA
University of Pittsburgh, Pittsburgh, PA
University of Texas Health Center at San
    Antonio, TX
University of Vermont, Burlington, VT
Valley Hospital, Ridgewood, NJ
Washington Regional Medical Center,
    Fayetteville, AR
Washington University, St. Louis, MO
West Suburban Hospital, Oak Park, IL
White Memorial Medical Center, Los Angeles, CA
Wilmington Medical Center, Wilmington, DE

Wuestoff Memorial Hospital, Rockledge, FL

Richard Desser
Nikolay Dimitrov/
Leif Suhrland
Richard G. Rosen
John MacFarlane
Richard Bornstein/
Jeffrey L. Ponsky
Frederick B. Cohen
James Devitt/
Rebecca McDermot
Harvey Lerner
Henry Shibata
Steven Economou/
Janet Wolter
Nicholas LiCalzi

Roger Poisson/
Sandra Legault-Poisson
Paul Koontz
Leo Mahoney
Thomas Nealon
Edwin Savlov
L. Martin Jerry
Leo Stolbach/
David R. Parkinson
Carl Sutherland
Michael A. Crucitt
Luis F. Urdaneta
Yosef Pilch
Donald L. Sweet
Neil Abramson
Noboru Oishi
Tapas K. Das Gupta
Peter Jochimsen
Joseph C. Allegra
E. George Elias
Robert L. Capizzi
John Glick
Bernard Fisher
A. B. Cruz/
J. Bradley Aust
Roger Foster
Hugh Auchincloss
Arthur Hoge/
James H. Bledsoe
Marc Wallack
Everett Nicholas
Matthew Tan
Robert Frelick/
Timothy Wozniak
Edward W. Knight

Current Controversies in Breast Cancer, edited
by F. C. Ames, G. R. Blumenschein, and E. D. Montague.
University of Texas Press, Austin © 1984.

Adjuvant Therapy for Stage II or III Breast Cancer: UT M. D. Anderson Hospital Experience

Aman U. Buzdar, M.D.,* Terry L. Smith, B. S.,† George R. Blumenschein, M.D.,*·Gabriel N. Hortobagyi, M.D.,* Hwee-Yong Yap, M.D.,* Evan M. Hersh, M.D.,‡ and Edmund A. Gehan, Ph.D.†

*Departments of * Internal Medicine, † Biomathematics, and ‡ Clinical Immunology and Biologic Therapy, The University of Texas M. D. Anderson Hospital and Tumor Institute at Houston, Houston, Texas*

Since 1974, a combination of fluorouracil, doxorubicin and cyclophosphamide (FAC) has been evaluated in patients with operable breast cancer following regional therapy at The University of Texas M. D. Anderson Hospital and Tumor Institute at Houston. The FAC regimen was selected for the adjuvant studies because, in our experience, this combination results in higher objective response rates in advanced breast cancer. In this article, we present the results of two FAC studies.

PATIENTS AND METHODS

Between 1974 and 1977, 222 patients were treated on the first FAC protocol (75-23 study). In this study, most patients had routine postoperative irradiation, and all patients received nonspecific immunotherapy with bacillus Calmette-Guerin (BCG). The chemotherapy was administered at 4-week intervals. Between 1977 and 1980, 238 patients were treated on the second FAC protocol (77-30 study). All patients in the second study were randomized to FAC alone or FAC+BCG, and intervals between the courses were reduced to 3 weeks. In the latter part of the study (May 1978), patients were also randomized to receive or not receive irradiation. Patients were eligible for these studies if breast cancer was technically resectable and if they had no definite evidence of disseminated disease on staging. The study population consisted of patients with UICC stage II, III, or IV disease (patients with T_4 or N_3 lesions). Chemotherapy doses were identical in the two studies. Total dose of doxorubicin was limited to 300 mg/m^2, after which patients were switched to the maintenance phase of therapy (Table 1). At the end of 2 years all treatment was discontinued. The results of the initial trial were compared to results of therapy in a group of historical control patients seen at our institution between 1971 and 1973. The details of the control group have been previously reported (Buzdar, et al. 1981).

Table 1. *Chemotherapy Regimen**

FAC Regimen
5-Fluorouracil: 400 mg/m² I.V., days 1 & 8
Doxorubicin: 40 mg/m² I.V., day 1, for a total of 300 mg/m²
Cyclophosphamide: 400 mg/m² I.V., day 1
Maintenance Therapy
5-Fluorouracil: 500 mg/m² P.O., days 1 & 8
Methotrexate: 30 mg/m², I.M., days 1 & 8
Cyclophosphamide: 500 mg/m², P.O., day 2

*Abbreviations are as follows: FAC = 5-fluorouracil, doxorubicin, and cyclophosphamide; I.V. = intravenously; P.O. = by mouth; I.M. = intramuscularly.

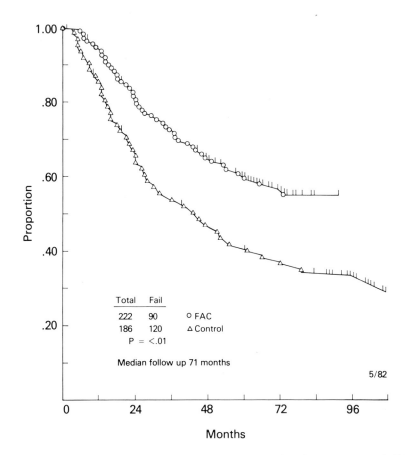

Total	Fail	
222	90	○ FAC
186	120	△ Control
P = <.01		

Median follow up 71 months

5/82

FIG. 1. Disease-free survival from surgery of all patients treated on the 75-23 protocol. (FAC = 5-fluorouracil, doxorubicin, cyclophosphamide)

RESULTS

At the time of this analysis, the median follow-up time was 71 months for the 75-23 study and 39 months for the 77-30 study. The disease-free survival rate of all patients in the 75-23 study was compared to that of the control group (Figure 1). An estimated 60% of the patients in the FAC group and 35% in the control group were free of disease after 6 years. The difference in disease-free survival rates between the two groups was statistically significant ($P < .01$). Figure 2 shows the disease-free survival rate of patients with stage II disease. The estimated disease-free survival rate of patients with stage II disease after 6 years was 67% and 38% for the FAC and control groups, respectively, and these differences were highly significant ($P < .01$). In Table 2 the estimated disease-free survival rate at 6 years is shown for patients with stage II disease according to number of involved nodes and age. The disease-free survival rates of FAC patients with 1–3 and 4–10 positive nodes were

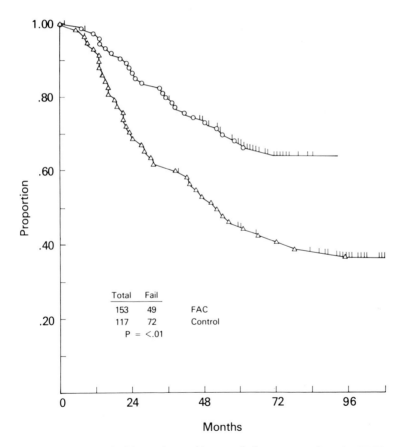

FIG. 2. Disease-free survival for patients with stage II disease treated on the 75-23 protocol. (FAC = 5-fluorouracil, doxorubicin, and cyclophosphamide)

Table 2. *Disease-Free Survival of Pts. with Stage II Disease*

| | Estimated % Disease-Free at 6 yrs. | | |
	FAC*	Control	P†
No. of Positive Nodes			
1−3	70	42	.01
4−10	69	41	<.01
> 10	46	29	.16
Age			
50 yrs.	68	31	<.01
≥50 yrs.	62	45	<.01

*FAC = Fluorouracil, doxorubicin, and cyclophosphamide.
†P = probability.

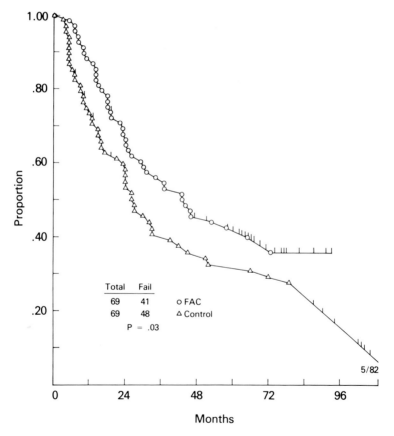

FIG. 3. Disease-free survival of patients with stage III disease (patients with T_4 or N_3 classifications were included) treated on the 75-23 protocol. (FAC = 5-fluorouracil, doxorubicin, and cyclophosphamide)

similar, but patients with ≥ 10 positive nodes had a disease-free survival rate similar to that of patients with stage III disease. The disease-free survival rates of FAC patients with 1–3 positive nodes and 4–10 positive nodes were significantly superior to those of the control group, but for patients with > 10 positive nodes disease-free survival was not significantly different at the $P = .05$ level ($P = .16$). Figure 3 shows the disease-free survival rate of patients with stage III disease (including T_4 or N_3). There was modest improvement in the disease-free survival rate of FAC-treated patients compared to that of the control group ($P = .03$).

Figure 4 shows overall survival rate of all patients. An estimated 68% of the patients treated with FAC are alive after 6 years, compared to 51% in the control group ($P < .01$).

Patients randomized to receive FAC and FAC+BCG in the 77-30 study are compared in Table 3. The distribution of patients was similar between the two groups

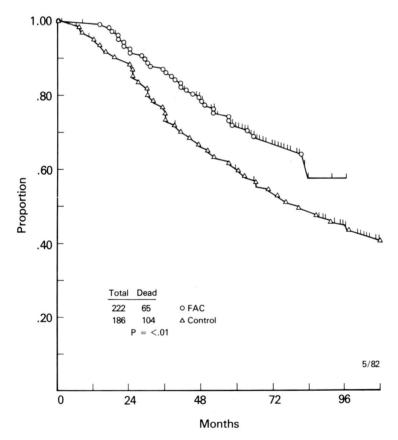

FIG. 4. Survival from surgery of all patients treated on the 75-23 protocol. (FAC = 5-fluorouracil, doxorubicin, cyclophosphamide)

Table 3. *Comparison of Pts. Treated with FAC Alone or FAC+BCG**

Characteristics	No BCG No. Pts. (%)	BCG No. Pts. (%)	P
Total	127	111	
Age			
<50 years	56 (44)	55 (50)	
≥50 years	71 (56)	56 (50)	.48
Menopause status			
Premenopausal	56 (44)	55 (50)	
Perimenopausal and postmenopausal	71 (56)	56 (50)	.48
Stage of disease			
II	77 (61)	66 (60)	
III	33 (26)	27 (24)	.82
IV	17 (13)	18 (16)	
Size of lesion (cm)			
<3	28 (22)	26 (23)	
3–5	69 (54)	57 (51)	.90
>5	30 (24)	28 (25)	
No. involved nodes			
≤3	42 (33)	33 (29)	
4–10	48 (38)	45 (40)	.84
>10	36 (29)	34 (31)	

*Abbreviations are as follows: FAC = 5-flourouracil, doxorubicin, and cyclophosphamide; BCG = bacillus Calmette Guerin; P = probability.

Table 4. *Disease-Free Survival of FAC and FAC+BCG Groups**

Characteristics	No. Pts.	No. Recurrences	Estimated % Disease-Free at 3 yrs.	P (2-tailed test)
FAC	127	33	75	
FAC + BCG	111	33	70	.44
<50 yrs. old				
FAC	56	17	69	
FAC + BCG	55	12	77	.60
>50 yrs. old				
FAC	71	11	79	
FAC + BCG	56	21	60	.10

*Abbreviations are as follows: FAC = 5-fluorouracil, doxorubicin, and cyclophosphamide; BCG = bacillus Calmette Guerin; P = probability.

according to age, menopausal status, stage of disease, size of the primary tumor, and number of involved nodes. There were no significant differences in the overall disease-free survival of FAC versus FAC+BCG groups (Table 4). Disease-free survival of FAC and FAC+BCG groups was also compared according to age. Disease-free survival of patients <50 years old was similar for the two subgroups, but patients ⩾ 50 years old receiving FAC+BCG had a disease-free survival rate inferior to that of the FAC group; these differences were not significant at the $P = .05$ level.

Seventy-five patients in the 77-30 study did not receive postoperative irradiation. Pretreatment characteristics of patients treated with postoperative irradiation were compared to patients who did not receive irradiation (Table 5). Distributions of characteristics were similar within the two groups. The disease-free survival rate at 3 years is shown in Table 6. The overall disease-free survival rates of patients treated with or without postoperative irradiation were similar. There were no differ-

Table 5. *Comparison of Pts. Treated With or Without Postoperative Irradiation*

Characteristics	No Irradiation No. Pts.(%)	Irradiation No. Pts.(%)	P*
Total	75	163	
Age			
<50 years	38 (51)	73 (45)	.48
⩾50 years	37 (49)	90 (55)	
Menopause status			
Premenopausal	39 (52)	72 (44)	.32
Perimenopausal and postmenopausal	36 (48)	91 (56)	
Stage of disease			
II	49 (65)	94 (58)	
III	15 (20)	45 (28)	.43
IV	11 (15)	24 (14)	
Size of lesion (cm)			
<3	17 (23)	37 (23)	
3–5	43 (57)	83 (51)	.53
>5	15 (20)	43 (26)	
No. of involved nodes			
⩽3	24 (32)	51 (31)	
4–10	33 (44)	60 (37)	.44
>10	18 (24)	52 (32)	

* P = probability.

Table 6. *Disease-Free Survival According to Irradiation Status*

	Estimated % 3 yrs. Disease-Free		
	No Irradiation	Irradiation	P*
All patients	68	73	.79
Stage			
II	76	80	68
III (includes T_4 or N_3	62	65	.9

* P = probability.

Table 7. *Site of First Recurrence by Irradiation Status*

	No Irradiation	Irradiation
Site	No. Pts.(%)	No. Pts.(%)
Local-regional	7 (9)	3 (2)
Systemic	16 (21)	39 (23)
Opposite breast	0	2 (1)
Total	23 (30)	43 (26)

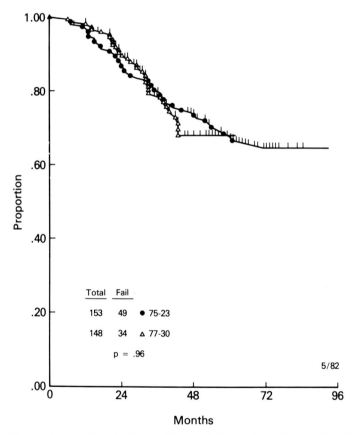

FIG. 5. Disease-free survival of patients with stage II disease treated with FAC on the 75-23 and 77-30 protocols.

ferences in disease-free survival rates between the two groups according to stage of disease. The sites of initial relapse in patients treated with or without postoperative irradiation are shown in Table 7. Local-regional recurrence rates were 2% versus 9% for patients treated with or without irradiation, respectively. The incidence of systemic relapses was similar between the two groups.

The disease-free survival rates of patients with stage II and stage III disease in the two studies were compared. The disease-free survival rates of patients with stage II disease treated in the 75-23 study versus those treated in the 77-30 study were similar (Figure 5). The disease-free survival rate of patients with stage III (includes T_4 or N_3 patients) disease treated in the 77-30 study was somewhat greater than that of the 75-23 study patients (Figure 6). The disease-free survival rate of all FAC patients according to stage of disease is illustrated in Figure 7. Patients with stage II

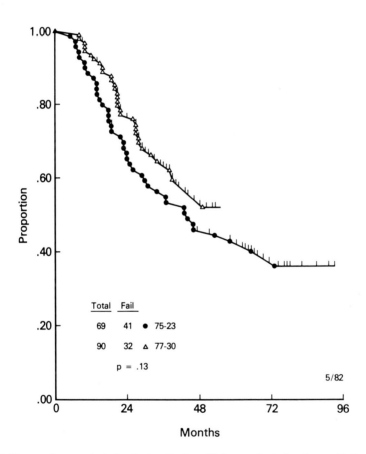

FIG. 6. Disease-free survival of patients with stage III disease (including those with T_4 or N_3 classifications) treated with FAC on the 75-23 and 77-30 protocols.

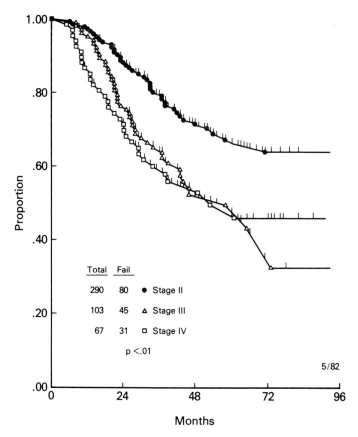

FIG. 7. Disease-free survival of FAC-treated patients according to stage of disease.

Table 8. *Toxicities of Adjuvant FAC* Studies*

Characteristics	75-23 Study No. Pts.(%)	77-30 Study No. Pts.(%)	P†
Fever during neutropenia	7 (3)	13 (5)	.3
Hematuria	1 (<1)	3 (1)	.6
Doxorubicin skin infiltration	5 (2)	5 (2)	.9
Congestive heart failure	4 (2)	4 (1.6)	.9

* FAC = 5-fluorouracil, doxorubicin, and cyclophosphamide.
† P = probability.

Table 9. *Cardiotoxicity**

Patient No.	Age	Interval Between Last Doxorubicin Dose & Symptoms (Months)	Risk Factors	Symptoms	Status	Last Follow-up From Symptoms
1	56	12	XRT (R), CoPD	SOB, no increased cardiac size, no CHF, ejec. 5	alive, asymptomatic	72+ months
2	55	1	XRT (R)	increased cardiac size, SOB, ejec. 74	alive, asymptomatic	26+ months
3	47	6	XRT (L), hypertension	increased cardiac size, no CHF	dead, metastasis	20 months
4	68	1	XRT (L), increased cardiac size, diabetic	CHF	dead CHF	5 months
5	49	7	XRT (R), Pvc EKG	SOB, CHF	dead CHF	21 months
6	44	27	acute MI 27 months after doxorubicin	CHF	dead CHF	13 months
7	51	7	XRT (R)	Pvc on EKG, no CHF	alive, asymptomatic	29+ months
8	56	5	QT interval prolonged	Pvc	alive, asymptomatic	40+ months

* Abbreviations are defined as follows: XRT = irradiation; R = right sided; CoPD = chronic obstructive lung disease; SOB = shortness of breath; CHF = congestive heart failure; Ejec. = ejection fraction; L = left sided; Pvc = premature ventricular contraction; MI = myocardial infarction; QT = cardiac output.

disease had a significantly superior disease-free survival rate than that of patients with stage III or stage IV disease. The disease-free survival rates of patients with stage III or stage IV disease were similar.

TOXICITY

The toxicity of the FAC treatment is summarized in Table 8. The myelosuppressive toxicity was acceptable, with 17% of patients experiencing granulocytopenia $< 1,000/mm^3$. Median lowest absolute granulocyte count was between 1,000 and $3,000/mm^3$ in 73% of patients; 10% had lowest absolute granulocyte counts $> 3,000/mm^3$. The median lowest platelet count of $< 100,000/mm^3$ was seen in 5% of patients. Infectious complications were observed in 3% to 5% of patients in the two studies, and the toxicity of the two treatment protocols was similar.

Two percent of the patients had congestive heart failure, and information on these eight patients is shown in Table 9. Three patients died of congestive heart failure, and one patient who had myocardial dysfunction subsequently died of metastatic disease. Four patients improved with symptomatic care and were alive at 26 to 72 months following the last dose of doxorubicin. The incidence of congestive heart failure was approximately 3% in the control population; none of those patients had had doxorubicin therapy.

The occurrence of second malignant neoplasms among control and FAC-treated patients is shown in Table 10. The incidence of second malignancy was similar between the two patient populations. The time distribution of the second malignancies is illustrated in Figure 8. At present, there is no evidence of increased risk of second neoplasms among FAC-treated patients.

Table 10. *Type of Second Malignant Neoplasm*

Type*	FAC†	Control
Leukemia	2	3
Melanoma	1	1
Renal	1	–
Head & neck	–	2
Gynecological	–	3
Gastrointestinal	1	1
Lung	–	1

*Second primary breast cancers were not considered in the analysis. There were four patients (.9%) in the FAC group and three patients (2%) in the control group who developed primary breast cancer in the contralateral breast.
†FAC = 5-fluorouracil, doxorubicin, and cyclophosphamide.

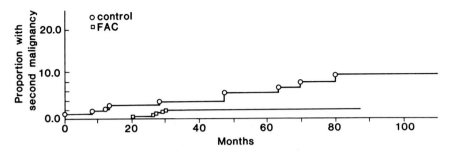

FIG. 8. Time distribution of second malignancies between the FAC and control groups. (FAC = 5-fluorouracil, doxorubicin, and cyclophosphamide)

DISCUSSION

The data from these studies show that FAC chemotherapy can significantly prolong the disease-free survival and overall survival of high-risk breast cancer patients. There was significant improvement in the disease-free survival of patients with stage II disease with ≤ 10 positive nodes. In patients with stage III disease and in patients with stage II disease with > 10 positive nodes, there was modest improvement in the disease-free survival rate. In our first study, all patients received nonspecific immunotherapy with BCG, and most had routine postoperative irradiation. It was not possible to evaluate the effects of these two treatment modalities on disease-free survival rates in this study, but the second study was designed to do so. Results showed that the addition of BCG did not offer any therapeutic benefit. Among patients ≥ 50 years age, those receiving FAC+BCG had somewhat inferior disease-free survival rates, although differences were not statistically significant. Routine postoperative irradiation had no demonstrable influence on disease-free survival. In contrast to some earlier reports, the efficacy of FAC chemotherapy was not reduced by routine postoperative irradiation (Nissen-Meyer et al. 1978, Cooper et al. 1979).

Altering the treatment schedules to 3-week intervals in the second study did not improve the therapeutic efficacy of the regimen in patients who had favorable prognoses; however, there was some suggestion that chemotherapy given at more frequent intervals could improve disease-free survival in patients with stage III disease. Additional follow-up is needed to determine the true impact of altering of the treatment schedule in this group of patients. The toxicity of the treatment has been acceptable, and there has been no increased risk of other malignancies. The risk of doxorubicin-induced cardiotoxicity at this dose level has been extremely low and delayed onset of congestive heart failure has not been observed during long-term follow-up.

ACKNOWLEDGMENTS

This study was supported in part by Grant Number 1-CB-33888 awarded by the National Cancer Institute, U.S. Department of Health and Human Services.

The authors would like to thank Vickie E. Richard for assisting in preparation of this manuscript.

REFERENCES

Buzdar, A. U., T. L. Smith, G. R. Blumenschein, G. Hortobagyi, E. Hersh, and E. Gehan. 1981. Adjuvant chemotherapy with fluorouracil, doxorubicin, and cyclophosphamide (FAC) for stage II or III breast cancer: 5-year results, *in* Adjuvant Therapy of Cancer III, S. E. Salmon and S. E. Jones eds. Grune & Stratton, New York, pp. 427–434.

Cooper, G., J. F. Holland, and O. Glidewell. 1979. Adjuvant chemotherapy of breast cancer. Cancer 44:793–798.

Nissen-Meyer, R., K. Kjellgren, K. Malmio, B. Mansson, and T. Norin. 1978. Surgical adjuvant chemotherapy results with one short course with cyclophosphamide after mastectomy for breast cancer. Cancer 41:2088–2098.

IMAGING AND TUMOR MARKERS

Current Controversies in Breast Cancer, edited
by F. C. Ames, G. R. Blumenschein, and E. D. Montague.
University of Texas Press, Austin © 1984.

Imaging For Staging and Follow-Up of Breast Cancer

Richard H. Gold, M.D.

*Skeletal Radiology Section, Center for the Health Sciences, University of California
at Los Angeles, Los Angeles, California*

What imaging procedures should be part of the pretreatment evaluation of a patient with breast cancer? There is general agreement that chest roentgenograms, including posteroanterior and lateral views, are essential. Controversy exists, however, regarding the usefulness of other imaging tests such as radionuclide bone and liver scans and, to a lesser extent, even mammography. The efficacy of these procedures for both staging and follow-up will be discussed. The various imaging procedures for the detection of liver metastases in the follow-up of breast cancer patients will also be evaluated and compared.

MAMMOGRAPHY

Bilateral mammography plays an important role in the preoperative evaluation of the woman with suspected breast cancer. Indeed, in its *Manual for Staging of Cancer* (1978), the American Joint Committee on Cancer has listed mammography as a optional staging procedure. Mammography is useful not only to investigate the clinically obvious lesion that is soon to receive definitive pathologic evaluation, but also to evaluate both breasts and, in particular, the contralateral one for signs of clinically occult cancer. Should ominous mammographic findings be detected in an area other than the one scheduled for biopsy, the mammographer can perform a needle localization of the suspicious area. The clinically occult lesion, together with the clinically obvious one, can then undergo biopsy without the risk and expense of repeated surgery and additional anesthesia.

For patients who are to be treated by mastectomy, the detection of additional lesions in the involved breast may be of only limited value. But when primary radiation therapy or limited resection and radiation therapy are the treatments of choice, the detection of multicentric lesions in the involved breast may result either in alteration of the radiotherapeutic approach or in a change of the decision to perform radiation therapy to one favoring mastectomy.

A mammogram of the contralateral breast is not only useful in the detection of clinically occult cancer, it also serves as a baseline for future mammographic examinations. Subsequent comparison may permit detection of subtle features of early cancer that might otherwise go unrecognized.

Although mammography may lead to the detection of a nonpalpable carcinoma only a few millimeters in diameter within a fatty breast, radiographically dense, dysplastic tissue may obscure even a large carcinoma in mammograms. A "negative" mammogram, therefore, can never replace the biopsy of a suspicious lesion detected by physical examination.

What of the suspicious lesion detected by mammography that is not palpable? In that situation the radiologist, surgeon, and pathologist must cooperate in a team effort to confirm the diagnosis. Preoperative needle localization is followed by excision biopsy and subsequent radiography of the pathologic specimen. Specimen radiography not only confirms that the lesion has actually been excised, but also permits localization within the specimen of the most suspicious area, from whence the pathologist may obtain material for his permanent histologic sections.

Patients who have been treated by mastectomy should receive a yearly follow-up mammographic examination of the contralateral breast because it is at increased risk. Patients who have been treated by lesser surgical procedures or radiation therapy, or both, should also have yearly follow-up mammograms of the treated breast to search for new or recurrent tumor.

RADIONUCLIDE BONE SCANNING

A number of indications for bone scanning have been advocated for the patient with breast cancer (Waxman 1981). The increasing use of the two-stage surgical procedure, in which a biopsy specimen is obtained and permanent histologic sections are evaluated prior to definitive treatment, has made many of these indications more valid today than ever before. They include: (1) staging of the clinically asymptomatic patient with breast cancer; (2) examination of the patient with persistent pain that is thought to be skeletal in origin despite equivocal or negative radiographs; (3) determination of the extent of skeletal metastases when radiographs are abnormal; (4) evaluation of areas that are difficult to study by conventional radiographic techniques, such as the sternum and scapula; (5) differentiation of pathologic from traumatic fracture by disclosing additional sites of involvement not detected in radiographs; (6) planning of radiation treatment portals; (7) determination of response to hormonal, chemical, or radiation therapy; (8) periodic evaluation of the asymptomatic patient who is clinically free of disease.

The recent surge of interest in radionuclide bone imaging is attributable not only to its expanded role in the diagnosis of skeletal abnormalities, but also to significant technological improvements in both scanning agents and imaging equipment. Perhaps the most important contribution of bone scanning is its ability to detect metastatic disease far earlier than is possible with radiography. Up to 50% of a volume of adult cancellous bone must be destroyed before changes become visible in standard radiographs (Borak 1942). In 1968, Greenberg et al. reported that metastases to bone led to changes in ^{67}Ga and ^{85}Sr bone scans 1 to 4 months before their radiographic changes became apparent. A significant breakthrough in radionuclide bone scanning occurred in the early 1970s with the introduction of ^{99m}Tc agents. These agents result in low radiation doses since they do not emit beta rays and have a half-life of only 6 hours. When phosphonates are labeled with technetium, the isotope is taken up by chemisorption onto the phosphorus groups of calcium hydroxyapatite, the basic crystal of bone. Although the exact mechanism by which such isotopes are deposited remains unknown, increased blood flow to bone and areas of abnormal bone turnover are known to accelerate their accumulation. Among the various compounds that have been labeled with ^{99m}Tc, the disphosphonates are the ones most readily cleared from the blood pool. This results in low blood and extraskeletal activity and an improved image, permitting greater diagnostic accuracy.

The bone scan is the most sensitive noninvasive method for detecting metastasis to bone from nonosseous primary malignancies (O'Mara 1974) and, in general, has replaced the radiographic metastatic bone survey. The scan has the additional advantage of presenting the complete skeleton in a single image. Almost 80% of osseous metastases are found in the axial skeleton (Krishnamurthy et al. 1977).

False-Positive Scans

Bone scans, while extremely sensitive to localized abnormalities in the skeleton, are nonspecific as to the cause of the increased radionuclide uptake. In fact, at least one-third of solitary abnormalities detected in the bone scans of patients with primary malignant disease have been shown to result from benign processes or normal variations (Corcoran et al. 1976). Table 1 highlights these nonmalignant causes of increased radionuclide activity.

Recognition of the normal scan image and its variations is important if interpretive errors, which may be responsible for false-positive diagnoses, are to be avoided. In the normal skull the isotope is generally distributed over the entire cranium, and commonly accumulates in normal paranasal sinuses. Hyperostosis frontalis interna leads to a bilaterally symmetrical increase in isotope accumulation within the frontal bones, a finding that can be verified in anteroposterior and lateral skull radiographs. Localized accumulations may also be noted within the jaws in association with dentures, dental problems, or recent dental procedures.

In the neck, localized anterior accumulation of isotope occurs frequently and may represent calcification in the thyroid cartilage, activity in the thyroid gland itself, or degenerative changes in the cervical spine. An accentuated uptake is often present in the normal sternum, the sternoclavicular joints, and the sternomanubrial joint. Uptake in costochondral junctions may be prominent, and accentuated uptake may also occur in the acromioclavicular joints and in the tips of the scapulae. Normal sacroiliac joints typically manifest prominent but symmetrical uptake. Similarly, bilaterally symmetrical accumulations of isotope in the juxta-articular regions of the long bones is not unusual, and commonly accompanies acute osteoporosis.

Many benign disorders result in positive scans: Benign cartilage tumors, arthritides, Paget's disease, fibrous dysplasia, bone infarct, osteomyelitis, and soft tissue inflammation. Previous surgery or fracture may be associated with increased uptake of isotope for as long as 1 to 3 years after the incident. Bone scans performed up to

Table 1. *Nonmalignant Causes of Increased Activity in Radionuclide Bone Scans*

Normal Structures
  Base of the skull
  External occipital protuberance
  Paranasal sinuses
  Inferior tip of scapulae
  Spinous processes of vertebrae
  Sternum
  Sternoclavicular joints
  Sternomanubrial joint
  Costochondral junctions
  Calcified thyroid cartilage
  Thyroid
  Sacroiliac joints
Benign Soft Tissue Abnormalities
  Calcific tendinitis
  Cellulitis
  Injection site of scan agent
  Myositis ossificans
  Operative site
Benign Osseous Abnormalities
  Benign cartilage tumors
  Bone infarct
  Fibrous dysplasia
  Healing fractures
  Hyperostosis frontalis interna
  Hypertrophic pulmonary osteoarthropathy
  Inflammatory arthritis
  Metabolic bone disease
  Osteoarthritis
  Osteoid osteoma
  Osteomyelitis
  Paget's disease
  Spondylosis and degenerative disc disease
  Surgical or biopsy site

several months after mastectomy may reveal increased isotope accumulation in the region of the shoulder and upper chest on the ipsilateral side.

Many published reports on the value of bone scans in patients with breast cancer are difficult to evaluate because some scans were classified not as positive or negative, but rather as suspicious. The rate of such suspicious findings has varied from 1% (Lentle et al. 1975) to 14% (Hammond et al. 1978). In some series such suspicious findings were considered as negative (Campbell et al. 1976, Davies et al. 1977), while in others they were considered as positive (Hammond et al. 1978) and, in all likelihood, included a number of false-positives.

It is obvious that many of the false-positive scans resulted from review of the scan independently of the review of corresponding radiographs. If the scans and radiographs had been concomitantly reviewed and correlated, it is likely that the problem of false-positives could have been resolved to a significant extent.

To improve specificity, we have found it useful to correlate the foci of increased activity with selected radiographs of the same sites. At the UCLA Center for the Health Sciences the scan is immediately reviewed by a member of the Division of Nuclear Medicine. If there are no recent radiographs of the "hot spots," the patient is sent to the Division of Diagnostic Radiology, where appropriate radiographs of the foci of increased activity are performed. An anteroposterior radiograph of the pelvis is obtained for every patient to decrease false-negative scans caused by radio-nuclide activity in the superimposed urinary bladder that obscures pelvic lesions. Bladder activity can be diminished if the patient voids just prior to being scanned. The scan and radiographs are subsequently reviewed in a correlative conference attended by experts in nuclear medicine and skeletal radiology, and a single comprehensive diagnostic impression is recorded.

There are several advantages to this combined routine: It eliminates excessive, inappropriate, and inadequate radiographic examinations, thereby reducing both radiation dose and financial burden; the referring clinician receives a single definitive opinion rather than two sometimes vague reports that may conflict; and, by performing the two examinations in close proximity, the need for a return visit to obtain corroborative radiographs is obviated.

When a patient with breast cancer manifests a focus of increased radionuclide activity that cannot be explained by a radiographically evident benign abnormality, it must be assumed to be a metastatic lesion until proved otherwise. Three alternatives are available to determine the origin of the scan abnormality: (1) repeat the scan (and the radiograph if the scan is still "hot") in 4 to 6 weeks; minor trauma may result in a "hot spot," and the radiographic changes not be evident for weeks (e.g., stress fracture), or the scan may resolve without any radiographic change ever appearing; (2) follow the abnormal scan site with radiographs alone—radiographic changes of metastatic breast carcinoma may be delayed as long as 18 months from the time of the earliest scan abnormality (Galasko 1969); (3) perform a percutaneous needle biopsy, a relatively innocuous and productive procedure, especially useful when an immediate therapeutic decision must be made.

False-Negative Scans

Rarely, at sites of extremely aggressive metastases, the scan, instead of manifesting increased activity, shows deficits in isotope accumulation. Such "cold" or photopenic metastases are found most often in association with lung or breast carcinoma or soft tissue sarcoma. (Well-defined regions of decreased isotope accumulation in the absence of metastases may also occur in radiation therapy fields). Accumulation in the urinary bladder obscures abnormal isotope activity in portions of the ischial and pubic bones and the sacrum.

In diffuse metastatic disease, the isotope accumulation may occasionally be so uniform as to give a false-negative impression. One clue to the true state of affairs is the presence of a greater than normal intensity of isotope uptake in the skeleton, producing a so-called superscan. Another clue is the absence of activity in the kidneys, bladder, and soft tissues.

Value of Preoperative Bone Scan

The value of routine bone scanning in asymptomatic patients with known primary malignant disease is debatable. It might be argued, for example, that the use of bone scans as screening procedures for metastasis must be guided by the same principle that applies for any other screening procedure: There must be a reasonably high likelihood of finding a significant number of positive cases in asymptomatic patients. An equally effective opposing argument, however, might stress the usefulness of the scan as a baseline with which future scans could be compared to detect evolving metastases as near to their inception as possible.

Preoperatively, patients with stage III disease show a consistent and significant increased incidence of positive bone scans. In a study by McNeil et al. (1978), the yield of bone scanning was zero of 37 patients in stage I, 4% in stage II, and 16% in stage III. McNeil (1978) concluded that preoperative bone scans in patients with clinical stage III breast cancer revealed significant numbers of unsuspected metastases, but that the value of bone scans in patients with stage I or stage II disease lay primarily in providing a baseline evaluation. Baker (1977) reported that 10 of 41 patients (24%) with stage III disease had evidence of bone metastasis detected by preoperative bone scan, whereas only one of 64 patients with stage I or stage II breast cancer had a positive scan. Galasko (1977) reported that of 50 patients with advanced mammary carcinoma, metastases were demonstrated radiographically in 25 (50%). The same group of 50 patients was studied by bone scanning and 36 (72%) had positive scans. Numerous lesions that went undetected in the radiographs were detected in the scans. Thus, the need for preoperative bone scans in patients with clinical stage III disease has been well established.

Preoperative bone scanning of women with stage I or stage II breast cancer, however, has yielded a wide variation in results from different institutions. Hoffman and Marty (1972), Citrin et al. (1976), and Sklaroff and Sklaroff (1976) reported an incidence of positive bone scans in patients with stage I or stage II breast cancer of 40%, 14%, and 14%, respectively. Conversely, Baker (1977) indicated that of 64 patients with stage I or stage II breast cancer, bone scans were positive for metastasis in only one, an incidence of 1.5%. Gerber et al. (1977) performed bone scans on 122 women with biopsy-proved breast carcinoma. Only two of his 110 patients with stage I or stage II disease had preoperative scan abnormalities interpreted as bone metastases. But of 55 women with normal preoperative scans, 20 had changes suggestive of bone metastases on subsequent scans, most within 24 months of surgery. Five of the 23 women with potential surgical cures (negative lymph nodes at surgery) had bone metastases within 2 years of their operations.

The diversity of opinion regarding the usefulness of bone scans in stage I or stage II disease may reflect variations within these stages (Brady and Croll 1979). According to the TNM classification proposed by the American Joint Committee on Cancer (1978), patients with stage I disease have lesions classified as T_1, N_0, M_0. Patients with stage II disease have lesions classified as T_1, N_1, M_0 or T_2, N_1, M_0. Thus, stage I and stage II actually represent a diversity of tumor sizes and nodal involvement. The size of the tumors may vary from one too small to palpate and detected only by mammography to one as large as 5 cm. A patient with stage II disease may even have moveable homolateral axillary lymph nodes that are considered clinically to contain metastases. Consider, for example, a hypothetical patient who is clinically stage II and has a T_2 lesion 5 cm in diameter that manifests poorly differentiated histology and is located in the medial hemisphere of the breast. The patient also has moveable, firm, enlarged homolateral axillary lymph nodes. The yield of occult metastases in a group of such patients could be considerable.

What is the significance of a positive bone scan? Lee (1981) summarized 17 reports published between 1972 and 1978 that included all available follow-up information on patients who had breast cancer and positive bone scans. Overall, 73% of the patients with positive scans eventually developed some kind of metastasis. However, about 20% had nonosseous recurrence. Indeed, two series revealed that more patients developed nonosseous than osseous metastases. Overall, only half of the patients with positive bone scans harbored or later developed bone metastases.

Some physicians have advocated that patients with stage I or II disease should have baseline scans at the time of their initial treatment, with serial scans then being performed at 6-month or yearly intervals. Subsequent scans could then be compared to the baseline, permitting the detection of subtle increases in activity that could indicate early metastases. Other physicians have reasoned that a scan is necessary only to evaluate skeletal symptoms, and that if the scan is then reviewed along with radiographs of sites of abnormally increased activity, the sensitivity and specificity of the scan will be increased, obviating the need for a baseline scan.

In summary, a routine preoperative bone scan for stage I breast cancer patients produces negligible immediate benefits, but may serve a useful purpose as a baseline. Clinical stage II breast cancer is a "grey area" and may include patients with large primary tumors and axillary nodal involvement, implying a greater chance for the occurrence of skeletal metastases and, hence, a significant yield in bone scans. Patients with clinical stage III or IV disease have a greater chance of harboring metastases and should have an extensive diagnostic evaluation, including bone scans, prior to definitive treatment. Cogent arguments in favor or against the use of bone scans in the initial workup of stage I and some stage II patients were presented respectively by Waxman (1981) and Lee (1981), who summarized the pertinent data from the literature.

Value of Follow-up Bone Scan

The bone scan is valuable for monitoring the progression or regression of metastatic disease. In the early stage of healing, metastatic lesions may undergo a paradoxical increase in activity, but this will eventually diminish and may even return to normal. The bone scan is particularly useful in evaluating the response of blastic metastases that, on healing, may become even more sclerotic in radiographs, giving a false x-ray impression of progression.

The Bone Scan as a Predictor of Prognosis

Hammond et al. (1978) investigated 36 patients with breast cancer who were treated with postoperative adjuvant chemotherapy. Among the 20 patients whose second bone scans were unchanged compared to their initial studies, there was no clinical recurrence after a mean follow-up of 20 months. In contrast, among the 16 patients whose subsequent bone scans had changed, there were six with recurrences (mean follow-up of 43 months). These authors concluded that changes in serial bone scans could be used to identify a group of patients at high risk for early recurrence. Five of the patients with recurrent lesions, however, came from the 10 patients with stage III disease, and only one came from the 26 with stage I or stage II disease. This implies that clinical information regarding the stage of disease at the time of initial examination could foretell subsequent relapses better than routine or serial bone scans. Moreover, one of the six patients with recurrence actually had disappearance of a focal scan abnormality between the first and subsequent scans. Thus, an improvement in scan findings occurred while the disease actually progressed. The clinicopathologic characteristics of the primary tumor and the extent of involvement of the axillary nodes led to a more accurate prediction of prognosis than the bone scan.

IMAGING HEPATIC METASTASES

A wealth of imaging modalities is currently available to evaluate the liver for metastatic disease. The ^{99m}Tc sulfur colloid liver scan is relatively inexpensive, easily accessible, and, understandably, the most popular screening examination for patients with possible liver metastases. To be imaged, however, the metastases must be 2 cm or greater in size. Because the yield of true-positive pretreatment liver scans is even smaller than that of bone scans, it is generally recommended that they be reserved for patients with pertinent symptoms, abnormal liver chemistries, or hepatomegaly.

Unfortunately, false-positive interpretations are relatively common, and result from anatomic variations, defects caused by normal juxtahepatic structures, alterations in reticuloendothelial cell activity, and blood flow unrelated to mass lesions. In one series of 234 patients with breast cancer studied with routine preoperative liver scans, 11 (5%) abnormal scans were obtained (Wiener and Sachs 1970). But eight of the 11 abnormal scans were found to represent false-positive evaluations, so that ultimately only 1% of the scans yielded true evidence of metastatic disease. The significant number of false-positives implies that histologic confirmation may be essential before definitive primary therapy is abandoned.

Although one recent review reported no significant difference in the accuracy of liver scans as compared with computed tomography (CT) and ultrasound (Ashare 1980), most investigators believe that both ultrasonography and CT are more specific than the radionuclide scan, and that CT is the most sensitive, albeit the most costly, of the imaging modalities (Friedman and Esposito 1980, Yeh and Rabinowitz

1980). A promising, but still experimental, innovation in CT liver scanning has been the introduction of a new contrast agent, EOE 13, currently undergoing clinical trials. The agent consists of a 53% concentration of iodinated ester of poppyseed oil. Upon intravenous infusion in experimental animals, the material was taken up by the Kupffer cells of the liver and transferred to the hepatocytes within 24 hours. Tumor cells did not take up the material. The resultant CT scans showed striking enhancement of the liver parenchyma, permitting lower density intrahepatic tumor masses as small as 4mm to be visualized. A report of 10 patients scanned both with and without EOE 13 revealed that the agent improved the visualization of liver metastasis in eight of them (Vermess et al. 1980).

Ultrasonography is also useful in the evaluation of intrahepatic metastatic disease. Detection of lesions as small as 2 cm is possible. Inexpensive, innocuous, and relatively simple to perform, ultrasound is also an excellent modality to follow the progress of liver metastases during treatment. It can also be effectively used to localize larger lesions for biopsy or aspiration.

SUMMARY

The initial work-up of patients with breast cancer in the various clinical stages is summarized in Table 2. This work-up combines clinical practicality with cost-effectiveness, and highlights those parts related to imaging. Although a bone scan in stage I disease is unlikely to produce immediate benefit, it may prove invaluable as a baseline to enhance the detection of subtle changes that could represent metastases in a subsequent scan. Nevertheless, it is impossible to evaluate the usefulness of any baseline procedure without measuring it against its cost. Whereas the cost of a bone scan in some communities may run as high as 400 dollars, too high perhaps to justify its use as simply a baseline indicator, the cost in other communities is below 150 dollars, making it eminently cost-effective. Selected radiographs of sites of increased radionuclide activity and an anteroposterior radiograph of the pelvis should

Table 2. *Initial Work-Up of Patients With Breast Cancer*

Work-Up of Clinical Stage I Disease in Patients with No Symptoms of Metastasis
Chest radiographs (posteroanterior and lateral views)   Mammogram of both breasts   Complete blood count   Screening blood chemistry panel (such as SMA-12)   Bone scan (baseline), cost permitting   Liver scan (recommended only if symptoms, hepatomegaly, or abnormal liver function tests suggest the presence of metastases)
Work-Up of Clinical Stage II Disease
As above
Work-Up of Clinical Stage III or Stage IV Disease
As above, with the addition of liver scan

be correlated with the scan to permit a single comprehensive diagnostic impression. Although the ^{99m}Tc sulfur colloid scan remains popular, ultrasonography and computed tomography are advancing at a rapid pace and may soon replace the radionuclide scan in the detection of liver metastases. The technique for chest radiography should provide sufficient image latitude to detect small parenchymal densities. We have found a high kilovoltage technique (130 to 150 kVp) to be ideal for this purpose.

ACKNOWLEDGMENT

I gratefully thank Mrs. Darryl Bailey for her help in the preparation of the manuscript.

REFERENCES

American Joint Committee on Cancer Staging and End-Results Reporting. 1978. Manual for Staging of Cancer, 2nd ed., 1983. J. B. Lippincott Co., Philadelphia, pp. 127–133.

Ashare, A. B. 1980. Radiocolloid liver scintigraphy. A choice and an echo. Radiol. Clin. North Am. 18:315–319.

Baker, E. R. 1977. The indications for bone scans in the preoperative assessment of patients with operable breast cancer. Breast 3:43–45.

Borak, J. 1942. Relationship between the clinical and roentgenological findings in bone metastases. Surg. Gynecol. Obstet. 75:599–604.

Brady, L. W., and M. N. Croll. 1979. The role of bone scanning in the cancer patient. Skeletal Radiol. 3:217–222.

Campbell, D. J., A. J. Banks, and G. D. Oates. 1976. The value of preliminary bone scanning in staging and assessing the prognosis of breast cancer. Br. J. Surg. 63:811–816.

Citrin, D. L., C. M. Furnival, R. G. Bessent, W. R. Grieg, G. Bell, and L. H. Blumgart. 1976. Radioactive technetium phosphate bone scanning in preoperative assessment and follow-up of patients with primary cancer of the breast. Surg. Gynecol. Obstet. 143:360–364.

Corcoran, R. J., J. H. Thrall, R. W. Kyle, R. J. Kaminski, and M. C. Johnson. 1976. Solitary abnormalities in bone scans of patients with extraosseous malignancies. Radiology 121: 663–667.

Davies, C. J., P. A. Griffiths, B. J. Preston, A. H. Morris, C. W. Elston, and R. W. Blamey. 1977. Staging breast cancer: Role of bone scanning. Br. Med. J. 2:603–605.

Friedman, M. L., and F. S. Esposito. 1980. Comparison of CT scanning and radionuclide imaging in liver disease. CRC Critical Reviews in Diagnostic Imaging, CRC Press, Inc., Boca Raton, pp. 143–189.

Galasko, C. S. B. 1969. The detection of skeletal metastases from mammary cancer by gamma camera scintigraphy. Br. J. Surg. 56:757–764.

Galasko, C. S. B. 1977. The role of skeletal scintigraphy in detection of metastatic breast cancer. World J. Surg. 1:295–298.

Gerber, F. H., J. J. Goodreau, P. T. Kirchner, and W. J. Fouty. 1977. Efficacy of preoperative and postoperative bone scanning in the management of breast carcinoma. N. Engl. J. Med. 297:300–303.

Greenberg, E. J., D. A. Weber, R. Pochaczevsky, P. J. Kenny, W. P. L. Myers, and J. S. Laughlin. 1968. Detection of neoplastic bone lesions by quantitative scanning and radiography. J. Nucl. Med. 9:613–620.

Hammond, N., S. E. Jones, S. E. Salmon, D. Patton, and J. Woolfenden. 1978. Predictive value of bone scans in an adjuvant breast cancer program. Cancer 41:138–142.

Hoffman, H. C., and R. Marty. 1972. Bone scanning. Its value in the preoperative evaluation of patients with suspicious breast masses. Am. J. Surg. 124:194–199.

Krishnamurthy, G. T., M. Tubis, J. Hiss, and W. H. Blahd. 1977. Distribution pattern of metastatic bone disease. A need for total body skeletal image. JAMA 237:2504–2506.

Lee, Y.-T. N. 1981. Bone scans are of sufficient accuracy and sensitivity to be part of the routine work-up prior to definitive surgical treatment of cancer: Opposed, *in* Medical Oncology—Controversies in Cancer Treatment, M. B. Van Scoy-Mosher, ed. G. K. Hall, Boston, pp. 53–68.

Lentle, B. C., P. E. Burns, H. Dierich, and F. I. Jackson. 1975. Bone scintiscanning in the initial assessment of carcinoma of the breast. Surg. Gynecol. Obstet. 141:43–47.

McNeil, B. J. 1978. Rationale for the use of bone scans in selected metastatic and primary bone tumors. Semin. Nucl. Med. 8:336–345.

McNeil, B., P. D. Pace, E. B. Gray, S. J. Adelstein, and R. E. Wilson. 1978. Preoperative and follow-up bone scans in patients with primary carcinoma of the breast. Surg. Gynecol. Obstet. 147:745–748.

O'Mara, R. E. 1974. Bone scanning in osseous metastatic disease. JAMA 229:1915–1917.

Sklaroff, R. B., and D. M. Sklaroff. 1976. Bone metastases from breast cancer at the time of radical mastectomy as detected by bone scan: 8 year follow-up. Cancer 38:107–111.

Vermess, M., J. L. Doppman, P. Sugarbaker, R. I. Fisher, D. C. Chatterji, J. Luetzeler, G. Grimes, M. Girton, and R. H. Adamson. 1980. Clinical trials with a new intravenous liposoluble contrast material for computed tomography of the liver and spleen. Radiology 137:217–222.

Waxman, A. D. 1981. Bone scans are of sufficient accuracy and sensitivity to be part of the routine work-up prior to definitive surgical treatment of breast cancer: In favor, *in* Medical Oncology—Controversies in Cancer Treatment, M. B. Van Scoy-Mosher, ed. G. K. Hall, Boston, pp. 69–76.

Wiener, S. N., and S. H. Sachs. 1970. An assessment of positive liver scanning in patients with breast cancer. Arch. Surg. 113:126–127.

Yeh, H., and J. G. Rabinowitz. 1980. Ultrasonography and computed tomography of the liver. Radiol Clin. North Am. 18:321–338.

Current Controversies in Breast Cancer, edited
by F. C. Ames, G. R. Blumenschein, and E. D. Montague.
University of Texas Press, Austin © 1984.

Radiographic Evaluation of Bony Metastases of Breast Cancer

Herman I. Libshitz, M.D.,* and Gabriel N. Hortobagyi, M.D.†

From the Departments of *Diagnostic Radiology and †Internal Medicine, The University of Texas M. D. Anderson Hospital and Tumor Institute at Houston, Houston, Texas

Approximately 70% of patients with metastatic breast cancer develop osseous metastases during their clinical course. Of these, about 20% have only bony metastatic disease (Barry 1981). While criteria are available and generally accepted for evaluation of metastases in soft tissues, there has been considerable discussion about the criteria for evaluation of response of bony metastases (International Union Against Cancer 1977). Indeed, many, if not most, therapeutic reports clearly exclude patients with bony metastases alone and do not consider the clinical course of these metastases when other "measurable" metastases are present. In an attempt to develop a reproducible and uniform method of evaluating the response of bony metastases to chemotherapy and to guide subsequent therapeutic interventions, the study herein described was undertaken (Libshitz and Hortobagyi 1981).

MATERIALS AND METHODS

The population studied consisted of 50 consecutive patients with metastatic breast cancer with known bony metastases. None had received prior systemic chemotherapy or hormonal therapy. All were treated with combination chemotherapy programs consisting of 5-fluorouracil, Adriamycin, cyclophosphamide, and methotrexate (or other therapeutically equivalent programs) (Blumenschein et al. 1980, Hortobagyi et al. 1979a,b). Evaluation included a baseline radionuclide bone scan and radiographic skeletal survey and at least one bone scan and skeletal survey 3 months after initiation of chemotherapy.

The patient population averaged 51.2 years of age (range 29 to 69 years). Twenty-six patients were premenopausal, 21 were postmenopausal, and three were perimenopausal. The perimenopausal patients were included with the postmenopausal group for purposes of tabulation. There was an average of 11 studies of the skeleton (one baseline and 10 follow-up examinations). The average length of follow-up was 29.1 months (range three to 81 months).

To make the study as objective as possible, neither questionable metastases, questionable response, nor questionable worsening during therapy were recorded. Definite change had to be present. Only changes seen on bone radiographs were considered in evaluation of response. Scan findings and biochemical tests were not considered at the evaluation of radiographic findings. Findings of these examinations were later correlated with the radiographic findings.

All studies performed within a 7-day period were considered as having been performed at the same time, so that examinations made to evaluate a specific question would not be counted as separate studies. Fractures in a bone were not considered metastases unless a definite metastatic component could be identified in the bone or developed subsequently in the same area of bone. Similarly, fractures that subsequently involved bone were not considered evidence of progression of disease.

Metastases were classified as osteolytic, mixed, or blastic or as presenting first as fractures. To be considered either lytic or blastic, the lesions had to be purely so. Those neither purely lytic nor purely blastic were recorded as mixed.

RESULTS

Osseous metastases were identified in 44 of 50 patients (88%) at pretreatment evaluation. Lytic metastases were present in 26 of the 44 (59%); mixed metastases were present in 11 patients (25%); blastic metastases in four patients (7%); and fractures in three patients (7%). Bone metastases were identified in follow-up studies in the other six patients. In this group, two patients each had mixed and blastic metastases, and two patients had fractures.

All subsequent radiographs were evaluated as to whether there was healing, no response, or worsening of osseous metastases. Of the 44 patients in whom metastatic disease was identified in the initial study, 29 had definite evidence of a response to treatment. Twenty-five of the 29 had evidence of response on the first follow-up study. The average duration to response was 2.9 months. The longest duration was 5 months.

The metastases identified in follow-up studies were seen at an average of 8 months after initiation of therapy.

EVALUATION OF RESPONSE

Lytic Lesions

Evaluation of therapeutic response was easiest with lytic lesions. The first evidence of response was the development of a sclerotic rim around the lytic lesion (Figure 1). If healing continued, there was gradual centripetal filling-in of the lytic defect (Figure 2). Further healing, when it occurred, resulted in an almost uniformly blastic appearance. This filling-in occurred over several months to a year. Despite the filling-in, the trabecular pattern remained abnormal when compared to areas of normal bone. With progressive healing, the blastic appearance would gradually fade, and bone density and trabecular pattern would return to normal or nearly normal.

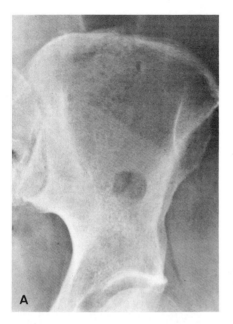 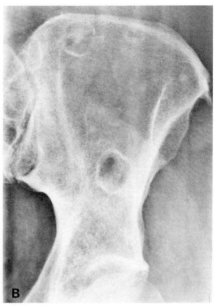

FIG. 1. Sclerotic Rim. **A.** Radiograph of the left ilium demonstrating a lytic metastatic lesion. **B.** Sclerotic rims are seen demarcating the lesion seen in Figure 1A as well as other metastases not identifiable on the original radiograph. (Reproduced from Libshitz 1981, with permission of Skeletal Radiology).

Similar sclerotic rims could also be identified about previously undetected lytic lesions. Changes of this sort should not be confused with worsening of disease.

Identification of worsening was easy when lytic areas increased in diameter or if new lytic lesions developed. Worsening was more difficult to determine when a response to therapy occurred. Increase in diameter of the lytic rim indicated worsening. Similarly, increase in the diameter or area of a filled-in lesion indicated worsening. Occasionally, focal destruction of the lytic rim could be identified, which also signaled worsening (Figure 3). The most difficult distinction was between fading of a filled-in blastic area and focal destruction of such a blastic region. Evidence of alteration in other areas often made this distinction easier.

Mixed Lesions

Mixed lesions can be thought of as lytic lesions in which some response—either development of a sclerotic rim or some filling-in (Figure 4)—has occurred spontaneously. Such lesions can be followed in the same way as lytic lesions in which response has occurred. Development of new mixed lesions after initiation of therapy are the cause of some difficulty in evaluation of response. Because these could represent therapeutic response in previously undetected lesions, primary attention

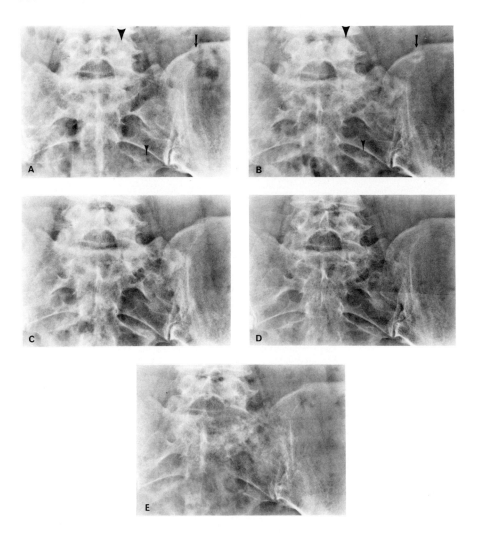

FIG. 2. Progression of healing. **A.** Radiograph of the sacrum, L-5, and medial left ilium. Lytic metastases are present in the pedicle of L-5 (large arrowhead), superior aspect of the left ilium (arrow), superior aspect of the left sacral wing (partially obscured by bowel gas), and the third sacral strut on the left (small arrowhead). **B.** Three months after initiation of chemotherapy, healing is identified. A sclerotic rim is seen in the pedicle of L-5 (large arrowhead) and the superior aspect of the left ilium (arrow). Sclerotic changes are also seen in the left sacral wing and in the third sacral strut on the left (small arrowhead). **C.** Six months after Figure 2B was taken and 9 months after initiation of therapy, further healing is present. The blastic response of filling-in is seen in the pedicle of L-5 and in the superior aspect of the left ilium. Further blastic repair is seen in the left sacral wing and in the third sacral strut on the left. **D.** Twenty-seven months after the initiation of chemotherapy, all of the previously identifiable areas of metastases now appear virtually normal. **E.** Two years after Figure 2D was taken and 4.5 years after initiation of chemotherapy, recurrent metastatic disease is present throughout the sacrum and the pedicle of L-5. (Reproduced from Libshitz 1981, with permission of Skeletal Radiology).

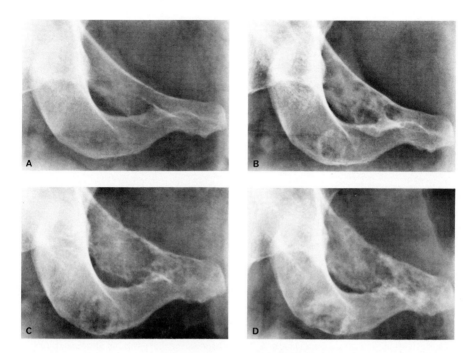

FIG. 3. Recrudescence of metastases. **A.** Radiograph of the right ischium and pubis showing lytic metastatic disease in both. **B.** A sclerotic rim is seen demarcating a lytic lesion in the ischium as well as lesions in the pubis 5 months after initiation of chemotherapy. **C.** Five months after Figure 3B was taken, destruction of the sclerotic rim in the ischium and obvious recrudescence in the pubis is seen. **D.** Two months after Figure 3C was taken, following a change in therapy, a sclerotic rim is again seen. This sclerotic rim is larger than the one seen in Figure 3B. (Reproduced from Libshitz 1981, with permission of Skeletal Radiology).

should be placed on the initial lesions in this circumstance. Because response so consistently occurs centripetally in these lesions, increase in the area of a given lesion signals worsening.

Blastic Lesions

Blastic lesions are the most difficult to evaluate. Not only are blastic lesions less frequent, but response occurs more slowly. The fading of originally blastic lesions is similar to that of lytic or mixed lesions that are healing and have become blastic. Focal lytic change in blastic areas must be distinguished from this fading as it signals worsening (Figure 5). Increase in the area of blastic change also indicates worsening.

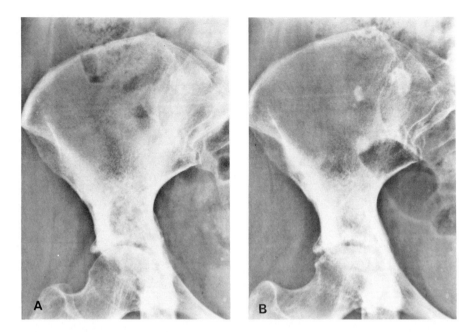

FIG. 4. Response in mixed metastases. **A.** Radiograph of the ilium and hip showing the initial presentation of mixed metastasis above the acetabulum. Possible lesion in the medial aspect of the ilium is partially obscured by bowel. **B.** Following chemotherapy, some filling-in of the supra-acetabular metastasis is noted. Additional blastic areas that also represent response to therapy are now obvious elsewhere in the ilium. (Reproduced from Libshitz 1981, with permission of Skeletal Radiology).

DISCUSSION

The natural variability of the radiographic appearance of bony metastases of breast cancer can make evaluation difficult. One cannot begin such an evaluation without knowing whether or not the patient has received therapy. If the patient has received therapy, one must also know what kind of therapy. Without prior studies for comparison, it would be impossible to distinguish the initial appearance of mixed or blastic lesions from lytic lesions that have responded to therapy. Similarly, prior radiotherapy to a given area can delay response and inhibit extent of response to chemotherapy or hormonal therapy. The radiologist must be aware of the current clinical status of the patient, the current therapy as well as prior therapy, and the locations of lesions identified on bone scans.

Despite these difficulties, the response of bony metastatic disease does follow a definite pattern. Once a baseline appearance is established and the therapeutic status of the patient known, most patients are evaluable. The changes in lytic, mixed, and blastic metastases can be thought of as a continuum, shown in Table I. Response of lytic disease goes through definite stages from a rim of sclerosis, to gradual filling-

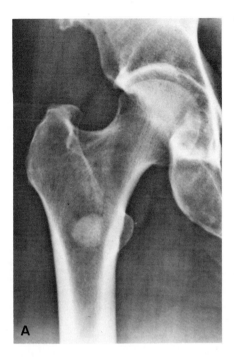 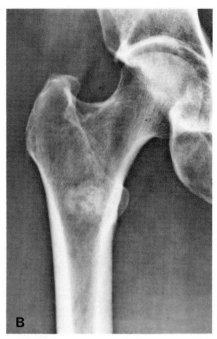

FIG. 5. Recrudescence in a blastic lesion. **A.** Well-defined blastic lesion in the right femur 9 months after initiation of chemotherapy that was not apparent on the initial examination. **B.** Increase in the area of the blastic lesion as well as focal areas of lucency 7 months after Figure 5A was taken. Either change would be indicative of recrudescence. (Reproduced from Libshitz 1981, with permission of Skeletal Radiology).

in, to a blastic appearance, to uniform fading of the blastic area. The response in mixed lesions can be thought of as starting at the sclerotic rim and then responding in the same manner. Blastic disease can be considered to begin at the uniformly blastic stage and then to uniformly fade with healing. This sequence of events is in keeping with prior reports of response following radiotherapy (Adair 1932, Bouchard 1945, Wulff 1939).

Worsening of disease also follows several basic patterns. In lytic disease, increase in size of lytic lesions or development of new lytic lesions signals worsening. Focal or generalized destruction of the sclerotic rim also indicates worsening. In addition, an increase in diameter of the sclerotic rim signals worsening. This can be thought of as a response of the metastatic disease that is unable to keep up with the destructive component. Worsening of filled-in or blastic lesions is manifested by focal areas of lytic destruction. An increasing area of blastic change also represents worsening. The latter observation can be thought of as a metastatic focus in which response does not quite keep up with metastatis but in which some response continues to occur.

Table 1. *Healing of Bony Metastases of Breast Cancer*

Lytic	Mixed	Blastic
Pure lytic	-------	-------
Rim of sclerosis	rim of sclerosis	-------
Filling in	filling in	-------
Uniformly blastic	uniformly blastic	uniformly blastic
Uniform fading	uniform fading	uniform fading

The preceding discussion indicates that defining the area or volume of the metastatic disease is important. The extent of disease is demarcated by the sclerotic rim or blastic area. This volume should *not* increase; repair should occur within this defined region. Also important to note is that evidence of healing can occur in regions not identified as diseased in pretreatment studies. This evidence should not be interpreted as a sign of progression of disease. It is felt, though it cannot be stated categorically, that evidence of response should be identified within six months of initiation of therapy; usually identification occurs within three to four months.

It is also important to note that changes can occur slowly (over many months) so that comparison with just the immediately preceding radiographs is not always adequate. Quite often multiple previous studies, including those of multiple bones, have to be reviewed to reach the correct conclusion. Flat bones are generally easier to evaluate than either long bones or vertebrae. One must also keep in mind that while multiple osseous metastases usually respond similarly, variance in the response of different metastases can occur. This is particularly true if radiotherapy has been given to a particular region.

That radionuclide bone scans and radiography are complimentary in identifying bony metastases is evidenced by the six patients in this study who did not have radiographic signs of bony disease on their initial evaluation, but in whom metastases were identified in bone scans. We believe that the initial evaluation of the breast cancer patient should include both a bone scan and a skeletal survey. Baseline studies with both imaging techniques should be available so that abnormalities on radiographs not due to metastases but that cause positive bone scans can be properly evaluated. Similarly, those lesions not evident on bone scans can be identified.

The findings in this group of patients receiving radiography and radionuclide bone scan have been correlated (Hortobagyi et al., unpublished observation). Approximately 30% of all lesions were detected by only one modality (radiography only, 11%; scan only, 19%). There were 149 anatomic areas involved by metastatic disease. Bone scans had a false-positive detection rate of 21% and a false-negative detection rate of 15%. The false-positive detection rate for radiography was 3%, and the false-negative rate 28%. These data indicate that bone scans are more sensitive but less specific than radiographs.

We believe that radiography is the method of choice in following therapeutic response once osseous metastases have been identified. There were 34 patients in this series who had evaluable nonosseous metastatic disease as well as osseous disease. Response in the nonosseous metastases correlated with evidence of improvement of bone lesions in 91% of the radiographs; this response correlated with evidence of improvement in only 57% of the bone scans. There was agreement between clinical and radiographic evidence of progression in 81% of the patients; in 72% of the patients bone scans and clinical findings correlated.

REFERENCES

Adair, F. E. 1932. The treatment of metastatic and inoperable mammary cancer: With a discussion of certain distinct types of metastasis. AJR 27:517–531.

Barry, W. F., S. A. Wells, C. E. Cox, and D. E. Haagensen, Jr. 1981. Clinical and radiographic correlations in breast cancer patients with osseous metastases. Skeletal. Radiol. 6:27–32.

Blumenschein, G. R., G. N. Hortobagyi, S. P. Richman, J. U. Gutterman, C. K. Tashima, A. U. Buzdar, M. A. Burgess, R. B. Livingston, and E. M. Hersh. 1980. Alternating noncross-resistant combination chemotherapy and active nonspecific immunotherapy with BCG or MER-BCG for advanced breast carcinoma. Cancer 45:742–749.

Bouchard, J. 1945. Skeletal metastases in cancer of the breast: Study of the character, incidence and response to roentgen therapy. AJR 54:156–171.

Hortobagyi, G. N., J. U. Gutterman, G. R. Blumenschein, C. K. Tashima, M. A. Burgess, L. Einhorn, A. U. Buzdar, S. P. Richman, and E. M. Hersh. 1979a. Combination chemoimmuno-therapy of metastatic breast cancer with 5-fluorouracil, Adriamycin, cyclophosphamide and BCG. Cancer 44:1955–1962.

Hortobagyi, G. N., G. R. Blumenschein, C. K. Tashima, A. U. Buzdar, M. A. Burgess, R. B. Livingston, M. Valdivieso, J. U. Gutterman, E. M. Hersh, and G. P. Bodey. 1979b. Ftorafur, Adriamycin, cyclophosphamide, and BCG in the treatment of metastatic breast cancer. Cancer 43:398–405.

International Union Against Cancer. 1977. Assessment of response to therapy in advanced breast cancer. Br. J. Cancer 35:292–298.

Libshitz, H. I., and G. N. Hortobagyi. 1981. Radiographic evaluation of therapeutic response in bony metastases of breast cancer. Skeletal. Radiol. 7:159–165.

Wulff, H. B. 1939. Radiological treatment of skeletal metastases in mammary cancer. Acta. Radiol. 20:40–68.

Current Controversies in Breast Cancer, edited
by F. C. Ames, G. R. Blumenschein, and E. D. Montague.
University of Texas Press, Austin © 1984.

Experience with Tumor Marker Profile Testing in Breast Cancer

Herbert A. Fritsche, Ph.D.,* Gabriel N. Hortobagyi, M.D.,† Bailey
A. Birdsong, M.D.,* Frank J. Liu, M.D.,* and George R.
Blumenschein, M.D.†

*Departments of * Laboratory Medicine and † Internal Medicine, The University of Texas
M. D. Anderson Hospital and Tumor Institute at Houston, Houston, Texas*

The clinical usefulness of carcinoembryonic antigen (CEA) as a tumor marker for breast cancer has been well established. In those breast cancer patients who demonstrate elevated levels of serum CEA, falling CEA values indicate response to therapy, while CEA values that continue to rise suggest recurrence or progression of the disease (Mughal et al. 1983, Falkson et al. 1982, Chatal et al. 1981, and Lamerz et al. 1980).

In an attempt to increase the number of patients who could benefit from serial monitoring, we have investigated the usefulness of calcitonin and the BB isoenzyme of creatine kinase (CK-BB) as tumor markers for breast cancer. These two markers were selected for study on the basis of preliminary reports on their potential usefulness (Bezwoda et al. 1981, Schwartz et al. 1979), the presence of calcitonin receptors on breast cancer cell lines in culture (Martin et al. 1980, Findlay et al. 1982), and our previous experience with these two markers for monitoring patients with oat cell cancer of the lung (Fritsche and Valdivieso 1982).

MATERIALS AND METHODS

In our study of these markers, CEA, calcitonin, and CK-BB were combined into a test profile that was used to monitor 50 patients with breast cancer during their therapy. The response of the markers was then correlated with the clinical course of the patients to determine their usefulness in detecting recurrence or progressive disease and for assessing the patient's response to therapy. The duration of follow-up of these patients ranged from 4 months to 27 months, and during this period approximately 300 determinations of the tumor-marker profile was made.

Calcitonin, CEA, and CK-BB were assayed with radioimmunoassay procedures using commercially available reagents. The CEA procedure was a modification of the Z-gel method (Roche Diagnostics, Nutley, N.J.) in that perchloric acid extraction was not used and a second antibody was substituted for the Z-gel (Fritsche et al. 1980). The CK-BB marker was determined with the "CK-BB Quant" assay (Mallinckrodt, Inc., St. Louis, Mo.), and calcitonin was determined with the "Calcitonin II" kit (Immuno Nuclear, Stillwater, Minn.). The upper limit of normal for each marker was determined in our laboratory with blood samples from healthy donors. The upper limit of normal for CEA was dependent upon the use of tobacco, 6.0 ng/ml for nonsmokers and 10.0 ng/ml for smokers. The age, sex, race, and smoking status did not appear to have any effect upon the normal range for CK-BB and calcitonin (CK-BB, 0–8.0 ng/ml; calcitonin, 30–120 pg/ml).

RESULTS

Table 1 shows the status of the breast cancer patients and the incidence of each tumor-marker abnormality when the 50 patients were entered into the study. Thirty-one of the 50 patients were demonstrating their first or second relapse with either local recurrence or metastasis. Seven of the 31 patients had a tumor-marker profile determined before therapy was initiated, while 24 of the 31 patients were entered into the marker study after therapy has been started. Nineteen of the 50 patients showed no clinical evidence of disease (NED) at the time of entry into the study.

Approximately 40%, or 12, of the patients with relapse had a marker abnormality, while only one of the 19 patients in the NED group showed an elevated tumor marker. In the group of patients with recurrence or distant metastasis, single elevations of markers occurred in 10 patients, and multiple marker abnormalities occurred only twice: Once with CEA and CK-BB and once with CEA and calcitonin. The marker abnormality in the one NED patient was due to CK-BB, and this case will be discussed in more detail later. During the follow-up of these 50 patients, 27 of them developed progression of their disease, five responded to therapy with either a partial or complete remission, and 18 patients remained disease free.

Table 1. *Status of 50 Patients and Initial Marker Values at Time of Patient Entry**

| | With Recurrence of Disease | | NED After First or Second Recurrence |
	TMP Before Therapy	TMP During Therapy	
No. of patients	7	24	19
Fraction with elevated markers	2/7	10/24	1/19
CEA elevated	1/7	8/24	0/19
CK-BB elevated	1/7		1/19
Calcitonin elevated	0/7		0/19
CEA and CK-BB		1/24	
CEA and calcitonin		1/24	

*Abbreviations are as follows: TMP = tumor marker profile; NED = no evidence of disease; CEA = carcinoembryonic antigen; CK-BB = BB isoenzyme of creatine kinase.

Normal Marker Variation and False Positives

The tumor-marker data obtained from the 18 NED patients who remained disease free were analyzed first for several reasons. First, these patients served as a "control" group and demonstrated the normal variation of the markers. This data was helpful for establishing the criteria for defining clinically significant changes in the marker values. Second, a study of disease-free patients, many of whom were on adjuvant chemotherapy, can help to define any effect of drugs on the circulating level of the markers and identify those benign conditions that may also influence the marker values. For the most part, the markers were generally quite stable during the follow-up of the NED patients. However, some of these patients showed sporadic elevations of the marker as shown in Figure 1. The marker profile of this NED patient is one example in which all three of the markers showed a sporadic elevation at about the same time, in March and April of 1981. The precision of the tumor-marker assays at values below the upper limit of normal had a coefficient of variation in the range of 7–10%, so this variation was not due to statistical variation. In

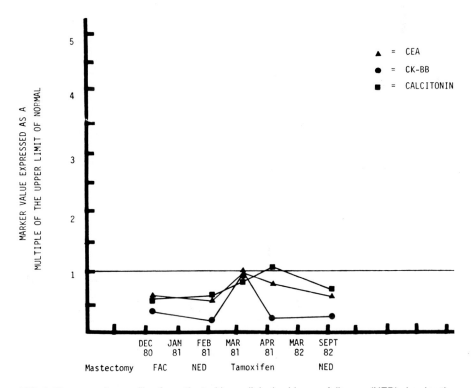

FIG. 1. Tumor-marker profile of a patient with no clinical evidence of disease (NED) showing the normal variation of the markers. (FAC = 5-fluorouracil, Adriamycin, and cyclophosphamide; CEA = carcinoembryonic antigen; CK-BB = BB isoenzyme of creatine kinase)

such cases, the sporadic elevation may slightly exceed the upper limit of normal. This type of transient elevation occurred more frequently with CK-BB than with calcitonin and even less frequently with CEA. The variation was defined as normal in this group of patients, since the variation could not be associated with administration of chemotherapy or any nonneoplastic disease process. No patients in this group developed a benign or inflammatory disease. However, in previous studies, transient elevation of CEA has been observed in patients who developed pneumonia, hepatitis, and influenza. False-positive values for calcitonin have been reported in patients with renal failure, gastrointestinal bleeding, and obstructive lung disease (Schwartz et al. 1979).

Figure 2 shows a more serious type of false-positive response of CK-BB that occurred in this patient with nodal metastasis who was NED after response to 5-fluorouracil, Adriamycin, and cyclophosphamide (FAC) and vincristine. This is the one NED patient with the initial CK-BB abnormality that was mentioned earlier. The significantly elevated CK-BB values remained constant for 18 months. Elec-

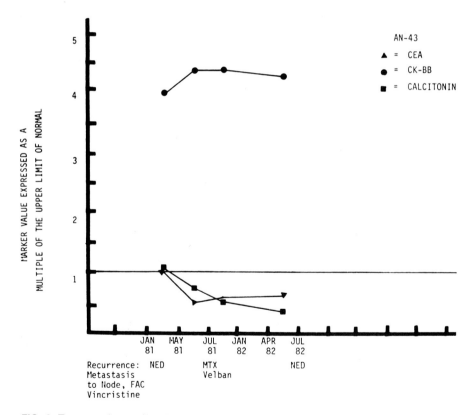

FIG. 2. Tumor-marker profile of a patient with no clinical evidence of disease showing a sustained false-positive response of BB isoenzyme of creatine kinase (CK-BB). (CEA = carcinoembryonic antigen; XRT = irradiation)

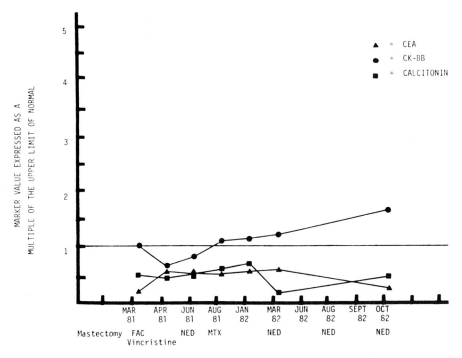

FIG. 3. Tumor-marker profile of a patient with no clinical evidence of disease (NED) showing a slow but progressive false-positive increase of BB isoenzyme of creatine kinase (CK-BB). (CEA = carcinoembryonic enzyme; FAC = 5-fluorouracil, Adriamycin, and methotrexate; MTX = methotrexate)

trophoresis showed this CK activity to be associated with an abnormal migrating isoenzyme, not the BB fraction. Abnormal isoenzymes of this type have been shown to be complexes of immunoglobulin with creatine kinase (Mercer 1980). In any respect, this immunoreactivity is measured as CK-BB by the radioimmunoassay procedure, and, thus, is a true false-positive test result.

Figure 3 shows another type of apparent false-positive response of CK-BB. The slow but steady rise in the CK-BB level might be interpreted as recurrence or progression of disease, but this seems unlikely since this patient has shown no clinical evidence of disease for 16 months. The CK-BB activity for the sample collected in October, 1982, is still too low to be measured by electrophoresis, so we cannot yet determine if this creatine kinase activity is associated with the CK-BB fraction.

Clinically Significant Changes in Marker Values

Our experience with monitoring breast cancer patients in remission gave us the basis for establishing criteria for defining a clinically significant increase in the marker value. For marker values that were initially below the upper limit of normal, we required the marker value to increase above this upper limit and demonstrate a sustained minimum rise of 100%. For initial borderline elevations of the marker, the serial values had to show a minimum 25% increase on each of two serial samples or show a significant increase of at least 50% from the previous value.

Monitoring For Recurrence and Progression

Using this criteria, we then evaluated the response of the markers in those patients at relapse or those who developed progressive disease. Seventeen of the 27 patients in this category showed sequences of marker abnormalities that correlated with disease progression. In nine patients, CEA was the only marker abnormality, and in seven other patients CEA abnormalities occurred along with one of the other markers. Thus, CEA patterns were abnormal in a total of 16 of the 17 patients. The

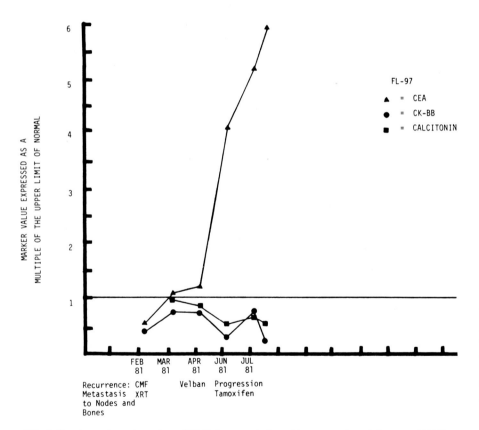

FIG. 4. Carcinoembryonic antigen (CEA) rise correlating with progression of disease. CK-BB = BB isoenzyme of creatine kinase; CMF = cyclophosphamide, methotrexate, and 5-fluorouracil; XRT = irradiation)

CK-BB marker was useful in only one patient in whom the CEA pattern was negative. In all but one patient, the CEA abnormality occurred from 4 months to 1 year before there was clinical evidence of progression. Calcitonin abnormalities only occurred in two patients and in these the serial CEA sequences were also abnormal. Figures 4, 5, and 6 show examples of patients in whom (a) only the CEA pattern was abnormal, (b) both CEA and CK-BB indicated progression, and (c) both CEA and calcitonin abnormalities correlated with progressive disease, respectively.

In the patient shown in Figure 6, the rising CEA levels occurred some 6 months before progression was clinically evident in October of 1981, while the calcitonin rise occurred after the fact. The CK-BB level also began to rise several months after the calcitonin increase, but this change does not meet the criteria for a clinically significant change. The CK-BB showed a rise of 100% and an increase above the upper limit of normal but then dropped back down, suggesting the type of normal variation that was observed with the NED patients.

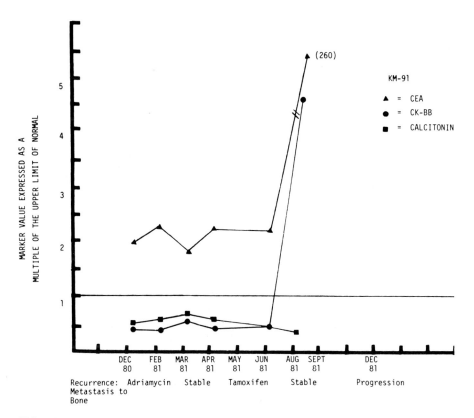

FIG. 5. Disease progression preceded by simultaneous rise of carcinoembryonic antigen (CEA) and BB isoenzyme of creatine kinase (CK-BB).

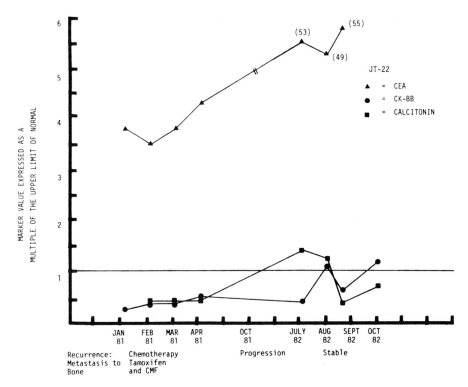

FIG. 6. Tumor-marker profile of a patient with progressive disease. (CEA = carcinoembryonic antigen; CK-BB = BB isoenzyme of creatine kinase; CMF = cyclophosphamide, methotrexate, and 5-fluorouracil)

The profile pattern of the patient with a neck mass, progression, and metastic disease to the lung (Figure 7) suggests that one or more of the markers may eventually demonstrate a clinically significant change, but responses such as these are of limited clinical value.

Monitoring for Response To Therapy

For those five patients who responded to therapy with either a partial or complete remission, the response of CEA and CK-BB correlated well with the clinical course of the patient. Figure 8 shows the marker profile patterns of a patient who demonstrated an immediate response to chemotherapy. The initially elevated CK-BB value obtained before therapy fell to below normal limits in 1 month and remained there. In two other patients, the initially elevated-marker values returned to normal limits when the patients demonstrated only a partial remission.

Figure 9 shows a marker pattern that demonstrated a paradoxical rise of the CEA level in a patient who responded to therapy. This paradoxical rise of CEA is seen in

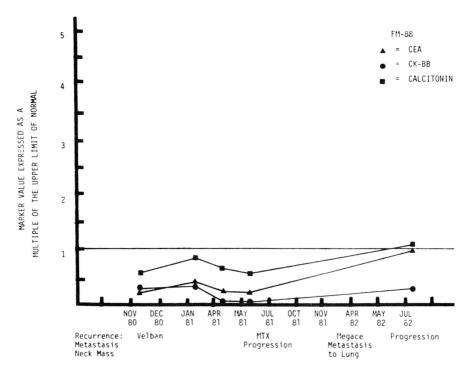

FIG. 7. Clinical evidence of disease progression preceding rise of tumor markers. (CEA = carcinoembryonic antigen; CK-BB = BB isoenzyme of creatine kinase; MTX = methotrexate)

some patients who have either a normal or borderline elevation of CEA before therapy, which may rise to a value of three to six times the initial value while the patient is demonstrating a clinical response to therapy. In these patients, the CEA value usually returns to normal limits within 3 to 6 months after therapy, as is shown by this patient. This type of serum CEA increase may reflect those patients whose tumors produce but do not secrete CEA and then release the CEA into the circulation upon cell death after effective therapy. Paradoxical rises of CK-BB and calcitonin were not observed in our study and have not yet been reported in the literature.

CONCLUSIONS

In summary, our data suggest that the tumor-marker profile consisting of CEA, CK-BB, and calcitonin is of no greater value in monitoring for recurrence of breast cancer than is the CEA test used alone. Calcitonin was of absolutely no value as a tumor marker for breast cancer. This same observation has recently been reported by Fereberger et al. (1982) and by Wahlby and Westman (1979).

While CK-BB abnormalities were observed in 25% of the patients suffering re-

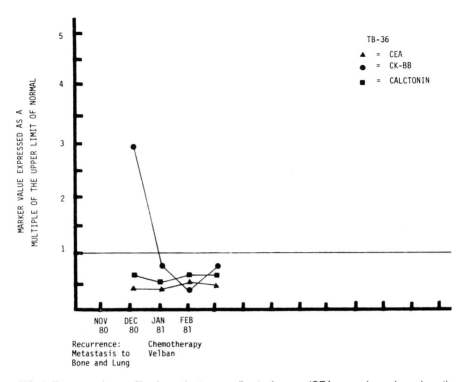

FIG. 8. Tumor-marker profile of a patient responding to therapy. (CEA = carcinoembryonic antigen; CK-BB = BB isoenzyme of creatine kinase)

lapse, serial changes in the marker values were not always consistent with the clinical course of the patient. The tendency of CK-BB to demonstrate both false-positive and false-negative responses severely limits its use as a tumor marker for breast cancer.

We realize that the limited usefulness of CK-BB and calcitonin in the cancer patient population that we observed in this study may be different from that observed in a group of newly diagnosed and previously untreated patients. Therefore, a study of these patients will be required before a final judgment on the usefulness of these markers in breast cancer can be made. Our data emphasizes, again, the value of CEA as a tumor marker and the need for other markers for breast cancer. In that regard, we present this tumor-marker profile approach as a model for the evaluation of new markers as they are defined.

REFERENCES

Bezwoda, W., D. Derman, T. Bothwell, P. MacPhil, J. Levin, and N. DeMoor. 1981. Significance of serum concentrations of carcinoembryonic antigen, ferritin and calcitonin in breast cancer. Cancer 48:1623–1628.

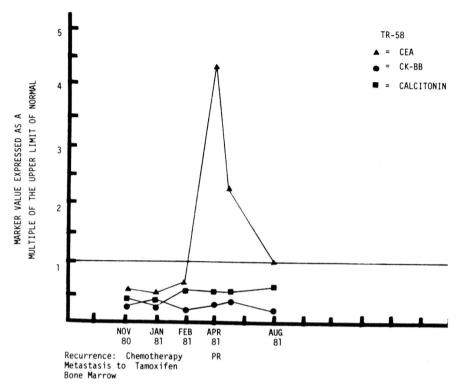

FIG. 9. Paradoxical increase of CEA in a patient responding to therapy. (CEA = carcino-embryonic antigen; CK-BB = BB isoenzyme of creatine kinase; NED = no evidence of disease; FAC = 5-fluorouracil, Adriamycin, cyclophosphamide)

Chatal, J., F. Chupin, G. Ricolleau, and B. Mevel. 1981. Use of serial carcinoembryonic antigen assays in detecting relapses in breast cancer involving high risk of metastasis. Eur. J. Cancer 17:233–238.

Falkson, H., G. Falkson, M. Portugal, J. Van Der Watt, and H. Schoeman. 1982. Carcino-embryonic antigen as a marker in patients with breast cancer receiving postsurgical adjuvant therapy. Cancer 49:1859–1865.

Fereberger, W., G. Leb, A. Pussath, H. Samonigg, and F. Beaufort. 1982. Immunoreactive serum calcitonin in patients with mammary carcinoma. MMW 124:471–472.

Findlay, D., K. Ng, M. Niall, and T. Martin. 1982. Processing of calcitonin and epidermal growth factor after binding to receptors in human breast cancer cells (T-47D). Biochem. J. 206:343–350.

Fritsche, H., C. Tashima, W. Collingsworth, A. Geitner, and J. Van Oort. 1980. A direct com-petitive binding radioimmunoassay for carcinoembryonic antigen. J. Immunol. Methods. 35:115–128.

Fritsche, H., and M. Valdivieso. 1982. Tumor marker testing in oat cell carcinoma of the lung. (Abstract) Proceedings of the 13th International Cancer Congress, Seattle, Sept. 8–15. Seattle, Washington, p. 178.

Lamerz, R., A. Leonhardt, H. Ehrhart, and H. Lieven. 1980. Serial carcinoembryonic anti-gen determinations in the management of metastatic breast cancer. Oncodev. Biol. Med. 1:123–135.

Martin, T., D. Findlay, I. MacIntyre, J. Eisman, V. Michelangeli, J. Moseley, and N. Partridge. 1980. Calcitonin receptors in a cloned human breast cancer cell line (MCF-7). Biochem. Biophys. Res. Commun. 96:150–156.

Mercer, D. 1980. Column chromatographic detection of the atypical creatine kinase isoenzyme in human serum, *in* Progress in Enzymology, D. M. Goldberg and M. Werner, eds. Masson Publishing Co., New York, pp. 59–61.

Mughal, A., G. Hortobagyi, H. Fritsche, A. Buzdar, H. Yap, and G. Blumenschein. 1983. Serial plasma carcinoembryonic antigen measurements during treatment for metastatic breast cancer. JAMA 249:1881–1886.

Schwartz, K., A. Wolfsen, B. Forster, and W. Odell. 1979. Calcitonin in nonthyroidal cancer. J. Clin. Endocrinol. Metab. 49, 438–444.

Wahlby, L. and G. Westman. 1979. Calcitonin and breast cancer. (Abstract) Cancer Treat. Rep. 63, 1184.

Current Controversies in Breast Cancer, edited
by F. C. Ames, G. R. Blumenschein, and E. D. Montague.
University of Texas Press, Austin © 1984.

Potential of Monoclonal Antibody Technology in the Management of Human Mammary Carcinoma

J. Schlom, Ph.D., D. Colcher, Ph.D., P. Horan Hand, Ph.D.,
D. Wunderlich, B.S., M. Nuti, Ph.D., Y. A. Teramoto, Ph.D.,
and D. Kufe, M.D.

*Laboratory of Tumor Immunology and Biology, National Cancer Institute, National
Institutes of Health, Bethesda, Maryland*

Numerous investigators have reported the existence of human mammary tumor-associated antigens (Hollinshead et al. 1974, Avis et al. 1976, Mesa-Tejada et al. 1978, Black et al. 1978, Springer et al. 1979, Leung et al. 1979, Howard and Taylor 1979, Sheikh et al. 1979, Yu et al. 1980). These studies, all conducted with conventional hyperimmune polyclonal sera, however, were hampered with regard to the heterogeneity of the antibody populations employed and the amount of specific immunoglobulin that could be generated. Since the advent of hybridoma technology, monoclonal antibodies of predefined specificity and virtually unlimited quantity can now be generated against a variety of antigenic determinants present on normal or neoplastic cells.

Monoclonal antibodies reactive with human mammary tissues have been generated by a number of laboratories using a variety of immunogens. Several groups have generated monoclonal antibodies against human milk fat globule membranes (Arklie et al. 1981, Taylor-Papadimitriou et al. 1981, Foster et al. 1982a, Foster et al. 1982b). These antibodies react strongly with lactating breast tissues and to a lesser extent with normal resting breast. Monoclonal antibodies have also been generated to estrogen receptors from the MCF-7 human breast tumor cell line (Greene et al. 1980). These antibodies bind to a variety of estrogen receptors, including those purified from monkey endometrium, and can be used to detect estrogen receptor-positive human mammary tumors by immunofluorescence of frozen sections and immunoperoxidase of fixed sections. Human mammary tumor cell lines have been used as immunogens by several laboratories (Krolick et al. 1981, Yuan et al. 1982). The antibody generated against the ZR-75-1 cell line reacts with approximately half of the malignant mammary tumors tested and to more than 80% of the benign mammary tumors tested (Yuan et al. 1982). Monoclonal antibodies have also been generated against human breast fibroblasts, with some reported reactivity to the MCF-7 cell line (Edwards et al. 1980).

Studies previously reported from our laboratory have demonstrated that lympho-

219

cytes obtained from lymph nodes of mastectomy patients may be fused with murine nonimmunoglobulin-secreting myeloma cells to generate human-mouse hybridomas secreting human monoclonal antibodies (Schlom et al. 1980, Wunderlich et al. 1981). One of these monoclonal antibodies (Teramoto et al. 1982) has been shown to be selectively reactive with human breast carcinoma and selected nonbreast carcinoma cells, but is of the IgM isotype. Further attempts to generate human monoclonal antibodies of the IgG isotype are in progress.

A number of laboratories have also generated monoclonal antibodies to a variety of tumors that cross-react with breast tumors. Antibodies prepared using melanomas (Woodbury et al. 1980, Loop et al. 1981, Natali et al. 1982), lung carcinomas (Cuttitta et al. 1981, Mazauric et al. 1982), renal carcinomas (Ueda et al. 1981), and prostate carcinomas (Frankel et al. 1982) as immunogens bind to a variety of breast tumor cell lines or sections of breast tumors. Antibodies to antigens found on normal human cells have shown reactivity with human breast carcinomas (Daar and Fabre 1981).

The rationale of the studies briefly reviewed here was to utilize membrane-enriched extracts of human metastatic mammary tumor cells as immunogens in an attempt to generate and characterize monoclonal antibodies reactive with determinants that would be maintained on metastatic, as well as primary, human mammary carcinoma cells. Multiple assays using tumor cell extracts, tissue sections, and live cells in culture have been employed to reveal the diversity of the monoclonal antibodies generated (Colcher et al. 1981a, Nuti et al. 1982, Nuti et al. 1981, Colcher et al. 1983a, Colcher et al. 1983b, Horan Hand 1983).

RESULTS AND DISCUSSION

Generation of Monoclonal Antibodies

Mice were immunized with membrane-enriched fractions of human metastatic mammary carcinoma cells from either of two involved livers (designated Met 1 and Met 2). Spleens of immunized mice were fused with nonimmunoglobulin secreting NS-1 murine myeloma cells to generate 4,250 primary hybridoma cultures. All hybridoma methodology and assay methods employed have been described previously (Colcher et al. 1981b, Herzenberg et al. 1979). Supernatant fluids from hybridoma cultures were first screened in solid-phase radioimmunoassays (RIA) for the presence of immunoglobulin reactive with extracts of metastatic mammary tumor cells from involved livers and not reactive with extracts of apparently normal human liver. Following passage and double-cloning by endpoint dilution of cultures secreting immunoglobulins demonstrating preferential reactivity with breast carcinoma cells, the monoclonal antibodies from 11 hybridoma cell lines were chosen for further study. The isotypes of all 11 antibodies were determined; 10 were IgG of various subclasses and one was an IgM (Table 1).

The 11 monoclonal antibodies could be divided into three major groups based on their differential reactivity to Met 1 vs. Met 2 in solid-phase RIA (Figure 1). The

Table 1. Reactivity of Monoclonal Antibodies in Solid-Phase Radioimmunoassay (RIA)

Monoclonal Antibody	Isotype	Cell Extracts*			Live Cells†				
		Met 1	Met 2	Liver	Mammary Carcinoma			Melanoma Sarcoma‡	Normal§
					BT-20	MCF-7	ZR-75-1		
B6.2	IgG₁	+++	++	neg	++	+++	++	neg	neg
B14.2	IgG₁	+++	++	neg	++	++	++	neg	neg
B39.1	IgG₁	+++	++	neg	++	++	++	neg	neg
F64.5	IgG₂ₐ	+++	++	neg	++	++	+	neg	neg
F25.2	IgG₁	+++	++	neg	+	+		neg	neg
B84.1	IgG₁	++	+	neg		+	+	neg	neg
B50.4	IgG₁	++	+	neg	neg	+	neg	neg	neg
B50.1	IgG₁	neg	+	neg	neg	+	neg	neg	neg
B25.2	IgM	+++	neg	neg	neg	neg	neg	neg	neg
B72.3	IgG₁	+++	+	neg	neg	+	neg	neg	neg
B38.1	IgG₁	+	+	neg	+++	++	+++	neg	neg
W6/32	IgG₂ₐ	neg	neg	neg	+	+	neg	++	++
B139	IgG₁	+++	++	++	++	++	++	++	++

* Solid-phase RIA: neg, <500; +, 500–2000cpm; ++, 2000–5000cpm; +++, >5000cpm.

† The live-cell immunoassay was performed on human cells: neg, <500cpm; +, 300–1000cpm; ++, 1001–2000cpm; +++, >2000cpm.

‡ Rhabdomyosarcoma (A204), fibrosarcoma (HT-1080), and melanoma (A375, A101D, A875, A3875).

§ Human cell lines were derived from apparently normal breast (HSo584Bst, HSo578Bst), embryonic skin (Detroit 550, 551), fetal lung (WI-38, MRC-5), fetal testis (HSo181Tes), fetal thymus (HSo208Th), fetal bone marrow (HSo074BM), embryonic kidney (FLOW-4,000), fetal spleen (HSo203Sp), and uterus (HSo769Ut).

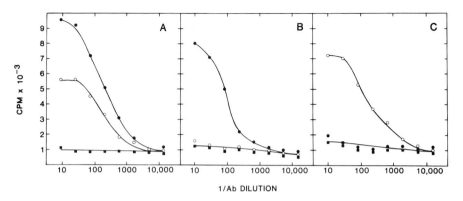

FIG. 1. Reactivity of monoclonal antibodies with extracts of metastatic breast tumors to the liver and normal liver in solid-phase radioimmunoassays. Metastases from patient 1, closed circle; patient 2, open circle; normal liver, square. **A.** monoclonal B6.2; **B.** monoclonal B72.3; **C.** monoclonal B25.2.

immunogen used in the generation of monoclonal B72.3 was Met 1, while the immunogen used for the generation of monoclonal B25.2 was Met 2. All 11 antibodies were negative when tested against similar extracts from normal human liver, a rhabdomyosarcoma cell line, the HBL100 cell line derived from cultures of human milk cells, mouse mammary tumor and fibroblast cell lines, disrupted mouse mammary tumor virus and mouse leukemia virus, purified carcinoembryonic antigen (CEA), and ferritin. Two monoclonal antibodies were used as positive controls in all these studies: (a) W6/32, an antihuman histocompatibility antigen (Barnstable et al. 1978) and (b) B139, which was generated against a human breast tumor metastasis but showed reactivity to all human cells tested (Table 1).

To determine whether the monoclonal antibodies bind cell-surface determinants, each antibody was tested for binding to live cells in culture, i.e., established cell lines of human mammary carcinoma. The nine monoclonal antibodies grouped together on the basis of their binding to both metastatic cell extracts could be further separated into three different groups on the basis of their differential binding to cell-surface determinants (Table 1). Many of the monoclonal antibodies bound to the surfaces of selected nonbreast carcinoma cells. None of the 11 monoclonal antibodies, however, bound to the surfaces of sarcoma or melanoma cells, nor to the surfaces of a variety of cells whose lines were derived from apparently normal human tissues (Table 1). Control monoclonal antibodies W6/32 or B139, however, did bind to all of these cells (Table 1).

Monoclonal antibody B6.2 was further analyzed by Kufe, et al. (1983) for surface binding to a panel of human cell lines using fluorescent-activated cell-sorter analyses. Antibody B6.2 was reactive with five or six breast carcinoma cell lines, but was unreactive with most other carcinomas. Cell lines derived from melanomas, sarcomas, and lymphoid tumors were uniformly unreactive. There was complete agreement in assay results when the same cell lines were tested in live-cell RIA and by cell-sorter analysis. A variety of tissues obtained directly from biopsy specimens were also evaluated via fluorescence-activated cell-sorter analyses. Breast carcinoma cells from patients with malignant pleural effusions were examined. Tumor cells from three of six were positive with B6.2. Single-cell suspensions derived from normal lymphoid tissue, including bone marrow, lymph node, spleen, and tonsil, demonstrated no reactivity.

To further define the specificity and range of reactivity of each of the 11 monoclonal antibodies, the immunoperoxidase technique was employed on tissue sections. All the monoclonal antibodies reacted with mammary carcinoma cells of primary mammary carcinomas, both infiltrating ductal (Figure 2A,B) and lobular (Figure 2D). Formalin-fixed and frozen-section tissue preparations gave comparable results. The percentage of primary mammary tumors that were reactive varied for the different monoclonal antibodies. In many of the positive primary and metastatic mammary carcinomas, not all tumor cells stained. In certain tumor masses, furthermore, heterogeneity of tumor cell staining was observed in different areas of a tumor, and even within a given area, as will be discussed in detail below. A high degree of selective reactivity with mammary tumor cells, and not with apparently normal mammary epithelium, stroma, blood vessels, or lymphocytes of the breast, was also observed (Figure 2A and C). A dark reddish-brown stain (the result of the immunoperoxidase reaction with the diaminobenzidine substrate) was observed only on mammary carcinoma cells, whereas only the light-blue hematoxylin counterstain was observed on adjacent normal mammary epithelium, stroma, and lymphocytes. Occasionally, a few of the apparently normal mammary epithelial cells immediately adjacent to the mammary tumor did stain weakly with the same pattern of staining seen in the tumor cells. The polymorphonuclear leukocytes and histiocytes in the stroma only in the area of mammary tumor also showed positive cytoplasmic staining. This reactivity may be due to antigen shed by the tumor and phagocytized by reactive cells in the immediate proximity.

Experiments were then carried out to determine whether the 11 monoclonal antibodies could detect mammary carcinoma cell populations at distal sites, i.e., in metastases. Since the antibodies were all generated using metastatic mammary carcinoma cells as antigens, it was not unexpected that they all reacted, but with different degrees, to various metastases (Figure 2E, F; Figure 3D). None of the monoclonal antibodies reacted with normal lymphocytes or stroma from any involved or uninvolved nodes. The antibodies were then tested for reactivity to normal and neoplastic nonmammary tissues. Some of the monoclonal antibodies showed reactivity with selected nonbreast carcinomas such as adenocarcinoma of the colon. These observations are currently being extended. Other neoplasms tested, which showed no staining, were sarcomas, lymphomas, glioblastomas, and melanomas. All 11 monoclonal antibodies were negative for cellular reactivity with apparently normal tissues of the following organs: Thyroid, intestine, kidney, liver, bladder, tonsils, and prostate.

A factor in the potential utility of any monoclonal antibody is its selective reactivity. The immunoperoxidase method of staining fixed tissue sections with antibody

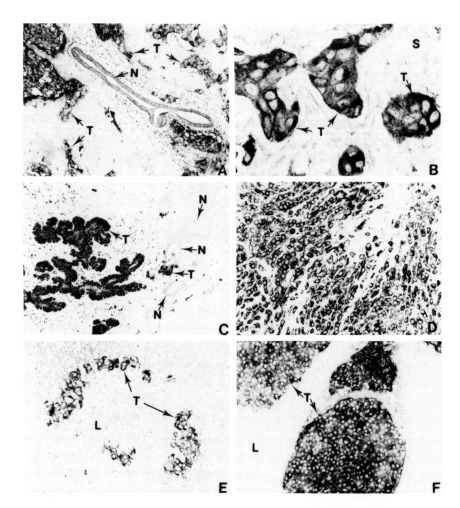

FIG. 2. Immunoperoxidase staining of fixed tissue sections of primary and metastatic mammary carcinomas with monoclonal antibody B6.2. **A.** Infiltrating duct carcinoma. At the center of the field is a negative normal duct (N) surrounded by positive-stained tumor cells (T); 130x. **B.** Higher magnification of tumor cells (T) and stroma (S) from same tissue section shown in panel A; 540x. **C.** Cancerization of a mammary lobule. Note the positive-stained tumor cells (T) and the unstained normal mammary cells (N); 130x. **D.** Infiltrating lobular carcinoma; 220x. **E.** Breast tumor metastasis of the lymph node: tumor cells (T), lymphocytes (L); 220x. **F.** Breast tumor metastasis of the lymph node from another patient: tumor cells (T), lymphocytes (L); 220x.

has the advantage of screening large amounts of tissues in a relatively short time. Moreover, it permits the testing of antibody reactivity with tissues that would otherwise be inaccessible. For example, to date there are no cell lines available from in situ breast carcinoma. A major drawback of using fixed tissue sections in the immunoperoxidase technique, however, is that this procedure makes it extremely difficult

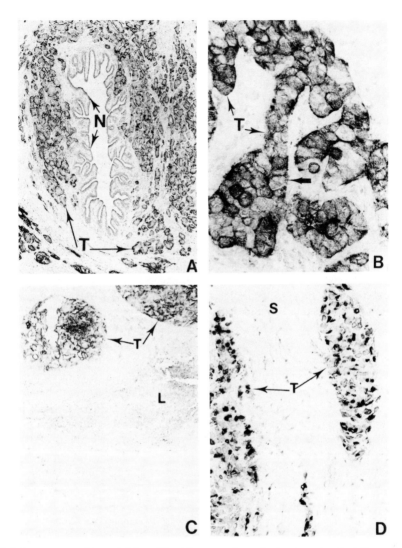

FIG. 3. Immunoperoxidase staining of fixed tissue sections of primary and metastatic mammary carcinomas of four different patients with monoclonal antibody B72.3: **A.** Infiltrating duct carcinoma. At the center of the field is a negative large normal duct (N) surrounded by positively staining infiltrating tumor cells (T); 54x. **B.** Infiltrating duct carcinoma. Note the intense membrane and faint cytoplasmic staining of the tumor cells (T). The broad arrow indicates a negative tumor cell flanked by positive tumor cells; 540x. **C.** In situ element (T) of an infiltrating duct carcinoma. Note the stroma and lymphocytes (L), which are negative; 130x. **D.** Breast tumor metastasis in the pleura. This is an example of the focal pattern of staining. Intense stain is concentrated in the cytoplasm of tumor cells (T). The stroma (S) is negative. 330X.

to define cell-surface reactivities. One must, therefore, also employ techniques using live cells to determine cell-surface binding. These two methods used in tandem represent an excellent way to characterize the differential reactivities of monoclonal antibodies. While monoclonal antibody B6.2 has shown no reactivity to the cell surfaces of any normal human cell lines tested, it has shown some reactivity with subpopulations of polymorphonuclear leukocytes in fixed tissue sections of spleens from some patients using the immunoperoxidase technique. Antibody B6.2 has also shown cell-surface binding reactivity to peripheral blood polymorphonuclear leukocytes but has shown no binding to the cell surfaces of unfixed bone marrow, spleen, lymph node, and tonsil cell preparations from a variety of patients using fluorescent-activated cell-sorter analyses (Kufe et al. submitted for publication). Thus, radiolabeled B6.2 antibody may prove quite useful in detecting mammary carcinoma cells in lymphatics of the axilla and internal mammary chain via intralymphatic inoculation.

Of the 11 monoclonal antibodies described above, B72.3 (an IgG_1) has displayed the most restricted range of reactivity for human mammary tumor versus normal cells. Monoclonal B72.3 was used at various concentrations in immunoperoxidase assays of tissue sections to determine the effect of antibody dose on the staining intensity and the percent of tumor cells stained. Since one cannot titrate antigen in the fixed tissue section, an antibody dilution experiment was performed to give an indication of the relative titer of reactive antigen within a given tissue. A range of antibody concentrations, varying from 0.02 ug to 10 ug of purified immunoglobulin (per 200 ul) per tissue section, was used on each of four mammary carcinomas from different patients. The results (Table 2) demonstrate that (a) different mammary tumors may vary in the amount of the antigen detected by B72.3, (b) a given mammary tumor may contain tumor cell populations that vary in antigen density, and (c) some mammary tumors may score positive or negative depending on the dose of antibody employed.

To further characterize the range of reactivity of B72.3, the immunoperoxidase

Table 2. *Dose of Monoclonal Antibody B72.3 vs. Reactivity of Human Mammary Carcinoma Cells in Immunoperoxidase Assay*

ug B72.3	Tumor Staining Intensity* (% Reactive Tumor Cells)			
	Tumor 1	Tumor 2	Tumor 3	Tumor 4
10	1+(90) 2+(10)	3+(100)	3+(80)	neg
4	1+(5)	2+(100)	3+(80)	neg
2	neg	1+(80)	3+(70)	neg
1	neg	neg	3+(70)	neg
0.2	neg	neg	2+(50)	neg
0.02	neg	neg	2+(30)	neg

*Staining intensity: 1+ weak, 2+ moderate, 3+ strong. 0.02 ug of B72.3 is equivalent to a 1:100,000 dilution of B72.3 produced in mouse ascites fluid.

technique was used to test a variety of malignant, benign, and normal mammary tissues. Using 4 ug of monoclonal antibody per slide, the percent of positive primary breast tumors was 46% (19/41); 62% (13/21) of the metastatic lesions scored positive. Several histologic types of primary mammary tumors scored positive: Infiltrating duct (Figure 3A and B), infiltrating lobular, and comedo carcinomas. Many of the *in situ* elements present in the above lesions also stained (Figure 3C). None of the six medullary carcinomas tested were positive. Approximately two-thirds of the tumors that showed a positive reactivity demonstrated a cell-associated membrane or diffuse cytoplasmic staining (Figure 3B), approximately 5% showed discrete focal staining of the cytoplasm (Figure 3D), and approximately one-fourth of the reactive tumors showed an apical or marginal staining pattern. Metastatic breast carcinoma lesions that were positive were in axillary lymph nodes and at the distal sites of skin, liver, lung, pleura (Figure 3D), and mesentery. Fifteen benign breast lesions were also tested; these included fibrocystic disease, fibroadenomas, and sclerosing adenosis. Two specimens showed positive staining: One case of fibrocystic disease where a few cells in some ducts were faintly positive, and a case of intraductal papillomatosis and sclerosing adenosis with the majority of cells staining strongly. Monoclonal B72.3 was also tested against normal breast tissue and normal lactating breast tissue from patients who did not have cancer and showed no reactivity. A variety of nonbreast cells and tissues were tested and were negative; these included two uteruses, two livers, two spleens, three lungs, two bone marrows, five colons, one stomach, one salivary gland, five lymph nodes, and one kidney.

Differential Binding to Human Mammary and Nonmammary Tumors of Monoclonal Antibodies Reactive with Carcinoembryonic Antigen

The presence of high plasma levels of CEA (Gold and Freedman 1964) has been reported to be an indicator of the possible presence of metastatic disease in patients with cancers of the digestive system, breast, lung, and other sites (Hansen et al. 1974, Krebs et al. 1978, Gold et al. 1979). Using assays based on antibodies to colonic CEA, elevated plasma levels of CEA (above 2.5 ng/ml) have been reported in 38% to 79% of patients with mammary carcinomas (Hansen et al. 1974, Chu and Nemoto 1973, Steward et al. 1974, Menendez-Botet et al. 1976, Lokich et al. 1978, Waalkes et al. 1978, Wilkinson et al. 1980, Chatal et al. 1980). There have been several reports (Vrba et al. 1975, Chism et al. 1977, Pusztaszeri and Mach 1973, Dent et al. 1980, Rogers et al. 1981), however, indicating that CEA is a heterogeneous family of glycoproteins, some of which demonstrate cross-reactivity with each other as well as with so-called "CEA-related" proteins. One issue that has not yet been clearly resolved is the possibility that different tumor cell types may produce, or maintain on their cell surfaces, a CEA that is only partially related to CEAs associated with other malignancies. Monoclonal antibodies should be valuable reagents toward resolving this point. To date, several monoclonal antibodies have been generated and characterized using CEA from colon carcinomas as the immunogen

(Koprowski et al. 1979, Miggiano et al. 1979, Accolla et al. 1980, Mitchell 1980, Kupcik et al. 1981, Rogers et al. 1981). In the studies reported here, monoclonal antibodies were generated to membrane-enriched fractions of human mammary carcinoma metastases and screened for reactivity with purified CEA. The differential binding properties of two of these antibodies (B1.1 and F5.5) to CEA and to breast and nonbreast tumors were investigated. Monoclonal B1.1 is an IgG_{2a}, while F5.5 is an IgG_1.

Both B1.1 and F5.5 precipitated iodinated CEA, resulting in a radiolabeled peak at approximately 180,000 daltons. No precipitation of purified CEA was obtained using monoclonal antibody B6.2 nor with any of the monoclonal antibodies described above. Cross reactivities have been reported (von Kleist and Burtin 1979) between determinants on CEA and an antigen expressed in normal spleens termed

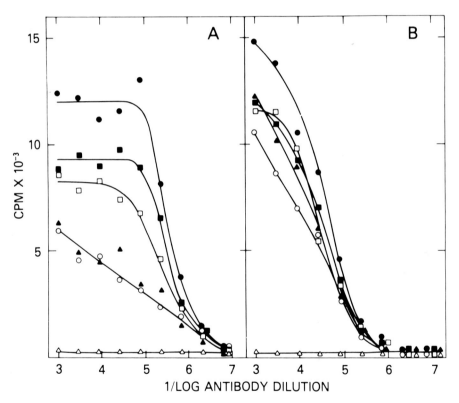

FIG. 4. Titration of monoclonal antibodies B1.1 and F5.5 against five preparations of carcino-embryonic antigen (CEA) from different patients. Thirty nanograms of purified CEA from five different patients were utilized in a solid-phase radioimmunoassay (RIA). CEA DH3B (closed circle); CEA BP160 (open circle); CEA DH2-3 (closed square); CEA HCA3B (open square); CEA JFII (closed triangle); bovine serum albumin (open triangle). Ascitic fluid from mice containing monoclonal antibodies B1.1 (**A**) or F5.5 (**B**) was titered against the different CEA in a solid-phase RIA.

normal cross-reacting antigen (NCA). Monoclonals B1.1 and F5.5 did not react, however, with a normal spleen extract rich in NCA. Purified immunoglobulin preparations of monoclonals B1.1 and F5.5 were then titered for binding to five CEAs purified from five different patients with colon cancer. As can be seen in Figure 4, significant binding was observed with both antibodies to all five CEAs. Monoclonals B1.1 and F5.5 are clearly reactive with different epitopes on the CEA molecule, however, as evidenced by their differential binding to the various CEA preparations. Specifically, monoclonal F5.5 reacted similarly with all five CEA preparations, whereas B1.1 exhibited preferential binding to different CEA preparations. Monoclonal antibodies B1.1 and F5.5 were tested for binding to live cells in culture to further define their range of reactivities and to ascertain whether they bind to antigenic determinants present on the cell surface. As seen in Table 3, both monoclonal antibodies bound to the same three of six established human mammary carcinoma cell lines and to the two colon carcinoma cell lines, but not to the lung carcinoma or vulvular carcinoma cell lines. No surface binding was observed with either antibody to normal breast cell lines nor to a variety of cell lines derived from apparently normal human tissues (Table 3). The two antibodies could be distinguished, however, by their differential reactivity to the surfaces of melanoma cells. B1.1 bound to three of four melanoma cell lines tested, while F5.5 did not bind to any of the four (Table 3). Reactivity with B1.1 was repeatedly observed with late passages (greater than passage 80) of the A204 rhabdomyosarcoma cell line (Table 3). These findings are further substantiated by a comparative titration of B1.1 and F5.5 against breast carcinoma, colon carcinoma, and melanoma cell lines. As seen in Figure 5A, B1.1 binds the melanoma, colon, and breast tumor cell lines comparably. There is a clear preferential binding of monoclonal F5.5, however, with the mammary tumor line as compared to the colon tumor or melanoma cell lines (Figure 5B).

To further identify the range of reactivities of monoclonal antibodies B1.1 and F5.5 with human mammary carcinomas, the immunoperoxidase technique was used on formalin-fixed tumor sections. Positive staining with both B1.1 and F5.5 was observed with three colon carcinomas and three lung carcinomas. Monoclonal antibodies F5.5 and B1.1 reacted positively with 55% and 66%, respectively, of the mammary carcinomas tested. The positive mammary tumors included infiltrating ductal carcinoma, in situ carcinoma, and medullary carcinoma. B1.1 and F5.5 also reacted positively with metastatic mammary tumor cells in lymph nodes and at distal sites.

It is anticipated that studies can now be undertaken to determine whether the presence, intensity, or cellular localization of these reactions, using either or both of these monoclonal antibodies with tissue sections of primary breast lesions, is of any prognostic value. A previous study (Sehested et al. 1981), performed using heterologous antisera and small cell carcinomas of the lung, has indicated that CEA reactivity of tissue sections may have prognostic significance. Since radiolabeled immunoglobulin preparations of heterologous sera to CEA (derived from colon carcinoma) have already been used (DeLand et al. 1979, Goldenberg et al. 1980b) for

Table 3. *Reactivity of Monoclonal Antibodies in Live-Cell RIA**

Cell Type	Cell Line	B1.1	F5.5	B139[†]
Mammary Carcinoma	MCF-7	2,391	2,239	1,343
	ZR-75-1	1,350	1,331	605
	BT-20	1,899	1,563	1,818
	MDA-MB-231	neg	neg	2,800
	ZR-75-31A	neg	neg	3,219
	T47D	neg	neg	2,501
Carcinoma				
Colon	WIDR	1,959	506	2,110
Colon	HT-29	2,683	1,463	2,646
Lung	A549	neg	neg	3,060
Vulva	A431	neg	neg	2,250
Melanoma	A3827	2,840	neg	3,780
	A101D	1,453	neg	4,482
	A875	876	neg	3,747
	A375	neg	neg	4,813
Sarcoma				
Rhabdomyosarcoma	A204,P18-79[‡]	neg	neg	4,456
	P80-90	1,024	neg	4,673
Fibrosarcoma	HT-1080	neg	neg	3,688
Normal				
Breast	HSo584Bst	neg	neg	1,481
Breast	HSo578Bst	neg	neg	1,360
Embryonic skin	D550	neg	neg	2,100
Embryonic skin	D551	neg	neg	2,296
Embryonic kidney	Flow-4,000	neg	neg	2,256
Fetal lung	MRC-5	neg	neg	3,210
Fetal lung	WI-38	neg	neg	2,331
Fetal testis	HSo181Tes	neg	neg	2,298
Fetal thymus	HSo208Th	neg	neg	3,391
Fetal bone marrow	HSo074BM	neg	neg	1,062
Fetal spleen	HSo203Sp	neg	neg	2,500
Fetal kidney	HSo807K	neg	neg	3,682
Uterus	HSo769Ut	neg	neg	1,647

*Live-cell immunoassays were performed as described by Colcher et al. 1981a. Negative (neg) indicates less than 300 cpm above background (approximately 200 cpm).
[†]B139 is a monoclonal antibody that binds to all human cell lines tested.
[‡]At different passage (P) levels within our laboratory, the reactivity with B1.1 was altered. At passage levels below 80, B1.1 was negative; at passage levels above 80, there was significant binding of B1.1.

binding metastatic breast carcinoma lesions in situ, appropriately labeled immuno-globulin or antibody fragment preparations of F5.5 and B1.1 may also eventually prove useful toward this end.

Identification and Purification of Mammary Tumor Associated Antigens

As a first step in the identification of the best source of antigens reactive with the monoclonal antibodies described, monoclonal antibodies were screened by solid-

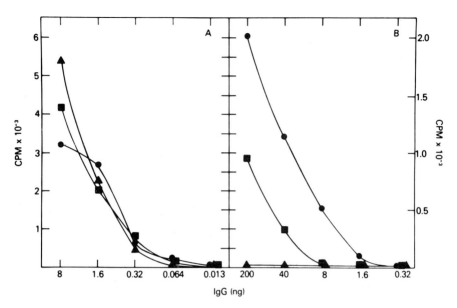

FIG. 5. Reactivity of monoclonal antibodies B1.1 and F5.5 in live-cell radioimmunoassay. Increasing amounts of purified IgG of B1.1 (Panel A) and F5.5 (Panel B) were reacted in a live-cell RIA with 5×10^4 cells of the following established human cell lines: MCF-7, mammary adenocarcinoma (closed circle); HT-29, colon adenocarcinoma (closed square); and A3827, melanoma (closed triangle).

phase RIA for reactivity with a variety of mammary tumor extracts, including primary and metastatic tumors and established cell lines. Monoclonal antibodies B1.1 and B6.2 reacted similarly with tissue extracts and extracts of cell lines. Antibody B72.3, however, showed very strong reactivity with some human tumor extracts, but reacted poorly with mammary tumor cell lines. Two breast tumor metastases to the liver were chosen as the prime sources for antigen identification and purification on the basis of their broad immunoreactivity to all the monoclonal antibodies and the quantity of tumor tissue available.

Immunoprecipitation studies were initiated to determine the molecular weights of the tumor-associated antigens (TAA) reactive with the monoclonal antibodies described. Purified CEA was iodinated and was used as an antigen source for the binding of B1.1 and F5.5. Sodium dodecylsulfate polyacrylamide gel electrophoresis (SDS-PAGE) of the immunoprecipitates showed that the polypeptide precipitated by both monoclonal antibodies is a heterogenous protein with an average molecular weight of 180,000 daltons. An extract of a breast tumor metastasis to the liver was used as the antigen source for the other monoclonal antibodies described. Initial attempts to identify the various reactive antigens in radioiodinated extracts of the metastasis were unsuccessful. The limiting factor appeared to be either an inability to label the desired antigen or an inability to detect an antigen that may constitute a very small percentage of the total tumor mass. To determine which hypothesis was correct, experiments were undertaken to determine whether CEA could be immu-

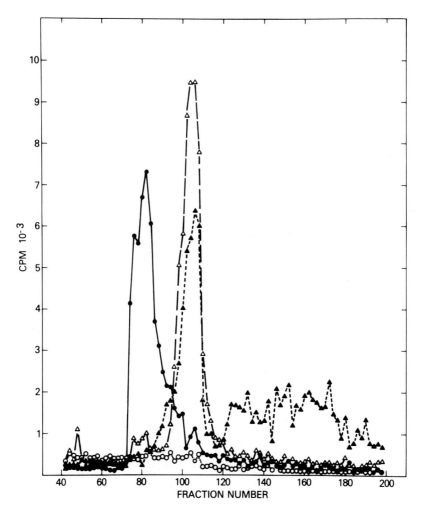

FIG. 6. Gel filtration of an extract of a breast tumor on Ultrogel AcA34. Immunoreactivity of fractions was determined in a solid-phase radioimmunoassay. B72.3 (closed circle); B6.2 (open triangle); B1.1 (closed triangle); phosphate buffered saline (open circle).

noprecipitated in "CEA-spiked" extracts of the mammary tumor metastasis. Purified CEA was iodinated and added to an extract of the breast tumor metastasis at a final concentration of 0.2%; monoclonal antibody B1.1 was able to precipitate the CEA in this extract. However, a similar amount of unlabeled CEA added to the extract prior to labeling was not detected by similar immunoprecipitation procedures. It appeared, therefore, that there was a preferential labeling of proteins other than CEA in this extract. To overcome this problem, experiments were undertaken to increase the relative antigen concentration by partial purification of the extract.

The metastatic liver extract was detergent-disrupted and separated using molecular sieving on Ultrogel AcA34. The column fractions were assayed for reactivity with monoclonals B1.1, B6.2, and B72.3 by solid-phase RIA (Figure 6). The appropriate immunoreactive fractions were then pooled and labeled with ^{125}I. SDS-PAGE analyses of the immunoprecipitates generated are seen in Figure 7. B72.3 immunoprecipitated a complex of four bands with estimated molecular weights of approximately 220,000, 250,000, 285,000, and 340,000 daltons. B1.1 immunoprecipitated a heterogenous component with an average estimated molecular weight of 180,000 daltons. B6.2 immunoprecipitated a 90,000-dalton component, as did several other monoclonal antibodies.

Extracts of a breast tumor metastasis to the liver, normal liver, and the MCF-7 breast tumor cell line, were disrupted and run on SDS-PAGE. The polypeptides were electrophoretically transferred to nitrocellulose filters, and the filters were incubated with IgG from B1.1, B6.2, or B72.3. The filters were washed, and the remaining antibodies were detected with rabbit IgG and ^{125}I-labeled protein A. B72.3 bound to a high molecular weight complex of approximately 220,000–400,000 daltons in the extract from the metastasis. B1.1 bound to a 180,000-dalton polypeptide, and B6.2 bound to a 90,000-dalton polypeptide in extracts of both the breast tumor metastasis and the MCF-7 cell line. These data demonstrate that the

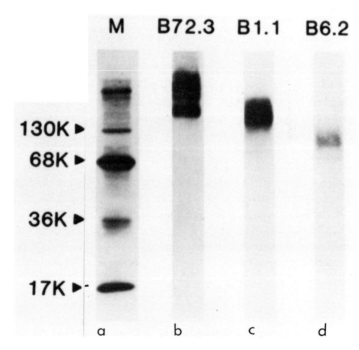

FIG. 7. Immunoprecipitation of ^{125}I-labeled partially purified extract of a human breast tumor. (a) markers (M); (b) immunoprecipitation by monoclonal antibodies B72.3; (c) B1.1; (d) B6.2.

immunoreactivity of the antigenic determinants is not destroyed by SDS and mercaptoethanol, and that molecular weights of the polypeptides in the crude extracts are consistent with those obtained by the immunoprecipitations from semipurified extracts.

Five of the monoclonal antibodies, including B6.2, were reactive with an antigen of approximately 90,000 daltons. To determine whether these antibodies reacted with the same determinants, a competitive binding assay was established. Purified monoclonal antibody B6.2 was labeled with [125]I. Increasing amounts of unlabeled monoclonal antibodies were added to a breast tumor extract followed by the addition of ^{125}I-labeled B6.2 IgG. As little as 10 ng of B6.2 IgG was able to inhibit the binding of the labeled antibody by greater than 90%. Various degrees of competition were also observed with other antibodies (B39.1, B14.2, B50.4, F25.2, B84.1). The ability of some of these monoclonal antibodies to compete for the binding of B6.2 to the breast tumor metastasis extract indicates that these antibodies react to the same antigen. The differences in the slope of the competition curve and the amount of antibody needed to achieve the competition may be due to differences in the affinities of the antibodies to the same epitope. Another possibility may be the existence of spatially close epitopes, which may result in steric inhibition of the binding of ^{125}I-labeled B6.2 to a nearby epitope.

Purification of the 220,000-Dalton High Molecular Weight Complex

Monoclonal antibody B72.3 has been shown to have highly selective reactivity to tumor versus normal tissues. We thus attempted to purify the antigen reactive with B72.3 first, so that further immunological and biochemical characterization could be made. An extract of a breast tumor metastasis to the liver, which contained the highest immunoreactivity with B72.3, was used as the starting material for purification of the 220,000-dalton complex. Following detergent disruption and high-speed centrifugation, the supernatant was subjected to molecular sieving using Ultrogel AcA34. Immunoreactive fractions were then passed through a B72.3 antibody affinity column and eluted with 3M KSCN. Radiolabeled aliquots from the various purification steps were analyzed by SDS-PAGE (Figure 8). Only minimal radioactivity in the high molecular weight range was seen in gel patterns of the AcA34 pool, whereas the affinity column eluant demonstrated the four distinct bands of the 220,000-dalton complex. ^{125}I-labeled B72.3 affinity-purified antigen was tested for immunoreactivity by solid-phase RIA. Approximately 70% of the purified ^{125}I-labeled antigen was bound in B72.3 antibody excess. The identical method of purification was used with a normal human liver extract as the starting tissue, and at no step within the purification scheme was any reactivity with B72.3 detected.

Heterogeneity Among Human Mammary Carcinoma Cell Populations

In 1954, Foulds documented the existence of distinct morphologies in different areas of a single mammary tumor (Foulds 1954). Since then, several investigators

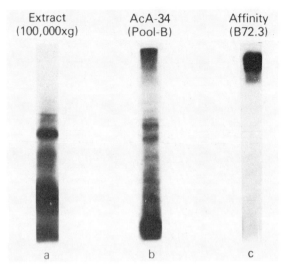

FIG. 8. Purification of mammary tumor-associated antigen reactive with monoclonal B72.3. Sodium dodecyl sulfate and polyacrylamide gel electrophoresis, SDS-PAGE, of ^{125}I-labeled extract from a breast tumor metastasis at various purification steps. An equal amount of each ^{125}I-labeled sample was loaded onto the gel: (a) crude extract; (b) pool of AcA-34 fractions reactive with B72.3; (c) pool of affinity column fractions reactive with B72.3.

have reported the occurrence of heterogeneity in a variety of tumor cell populations (Hart and Fidler 1981, Kerbel 1979). Using a variety of methods and reagents, including heterologous antisera, heterogeneity has also been observed with respect to the antigenic properties of tumor cell populations (Kerbel 1979, Miller and Heppner 1979, Pimm and Baldwin 1977, Poste et al. 1981, Prehn 1970). Consistent with this finding, we have observed antigenic heterogeneity, as defined by the expression of TAA detected by monoclonal antibodies, among and within murine mammary tumor masses (Colcher et al. 1981). The objectives of the studies described below were to use the monoclonal antibodies to: (a) determine the extent of antigenic heterogeneity of specific TAA that exist among human mammary tumors as well as within a given mammary tumor population; (b) determine some of the parameters that mediate the expression of various antigenic phenotypes; and (c) develop model systems in which to study and perhaps eventually control these phenomena.

Formalin-fixed tissue sections of human mammary tumors were examined, using the immunoperoxidase method, in an attempt to determine the range of expression of TAA reactive with monoclonal antibodies (Colcher et al. 1981a). Although some mammary tumors reacted with all monoclonal antibodies tested, other mammary tumors reacted with none. Both fixed and frozen sections gave similar results. Some mammary tumors showed a differential expression of one antigen versus another. As shown in Figure 9, an infiltrating duct mammary carcinoma contains the 90,000 dalton TAA reactive with monoclonal antibody B6.2 (Figure 9a), but not the 220,000 dalton TAA reactive with monoclonal B72.3 (Figure 9b). Conversely, an infiltrating

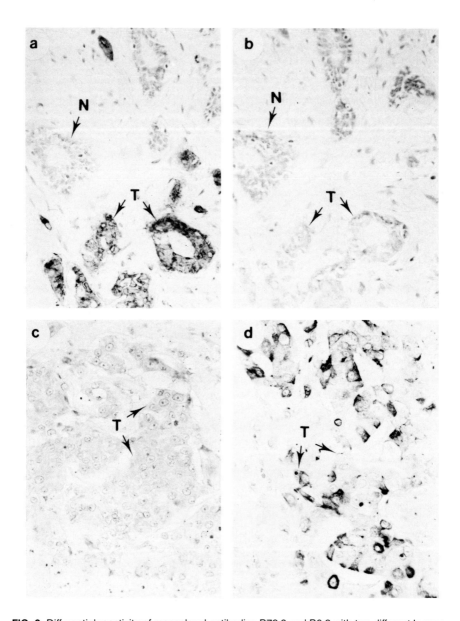

FIG. 9. Differential reactivity of monoclonal antibodies B72.3 and B6.2 with two different human mammary adenocarcinomas using the immunoperoxidase technique. Serial tissue sections in panel A and B are from an infiltrating duct carcinoma; in panel C and D serial sections are from an infiltrating duct carcinoma from another patient. Panel A and C are reacted with monoclonal antibody B6.2. Panel B and D are stained with monoclonal antibody B72.3. Note the stained tumor cells (T) and unstained normal mammary cells (N). (A-C, 220x; D, 330x).

duct mammary carcinoma from another patient expresses the TAA detected only by B72.3 (Figure 9 c–d). To exclude the possibility of variation due to location of tissue within the tumor, several alternate serial sections of the tumors were used in these experiments, and the results were identical.

The immunoperoxidase method was then used to test the reactivity of fixed sections of primary infiltrating duct mammary carcinomas from 45 different patients to a panel of five monoclonal antibodies (Table 4). What emerges is a variety of antigenic phenotypes of the 45 mammary tumors that can be placed into several distinct groups. Reactivity to all five monoclonal antibodies, including B1.1, which is directed against CEA, was demonstrated by the presence of antigens in 6/45 (13.3%) of the mammary tumors, while 9/45 (20.0%) contained none of these TAA (Table 4). The remaining 30 tumors displayed a variety of immunologic phenotypes with the five monoclonal antibodies. What emerges from these studies is a demonstration of the wide range of antigenic phenotypes present in human mammary tumors. Different tumors also differed in their pattern of staining with a given monoclonal antibody. These patterns included focal staining (representing dense foci of TAA in the cytoplasm), diffuse cytoplasmic staining, membrane staining, and apical or luminal staining (representing a concentration of TAA on the luminal borders of cells).

Phenotypic variation was also observed in the expression of TAA within a given mammary tumor. One pattern observed repeatedly was that one area of a mammary tumor contained TAA reactive with a particular monoclonal antibody, while another area of the same tumor was not reactive with the identical antibody (Figure 10a).

Table 4. *Differential Reactivity of Monoclonal Antibodies With Different Human Mammary Tumors**

Tumor Phenotype	No. Patients[†]	Monoclonal Antibody				
		B72.3	B1.1	B6.2	F25.2	B38.1
Group A	6	+	+	+	+	+
Group B	1	+	neg	+	+	+
Group C	2	+	+	+	+	neg
Group D	10	neg	+	+	+	+
Group E	4	neg	+	+	+	neg
Group F	3	+	neg	+	neg	neg
Group G	1	neg	+	neg	+	neg
Group H	2	neg	neg	neg	+	+
Group I	1	neg	+	+	neg	neg
Group J	1	neg	+	neg	neg	neg
Group K	2	neg	neg	+	neg	neg
Group L	3	neg	neg	neg	neg	+
Group M	9	neg	neg	neg	neg	neg
Total:	45					

*Serial sections of formalin-fixed mammary tumors were tested for expression of tumor-associated antigens detected by monoclonal antibodies using the immunoperoxidase method. Tumors were scored positive if antigen was present on 5% or more of carcinoma cells.
†Number of patients with tumor specimens displaying the indicated pattern of reactivity with the monoclonal antibodies.

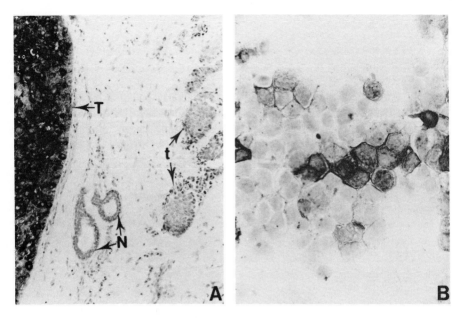

FIG. 10. Heterogeneity of antigenic expression of TAA. **A.** An infiltrating duct mammary carcinoma was reacted with monoclonal antibody B6.2 using the immunoperoxidase technique. Note the stained (T) and unstained (t) tumor cells. Normal mammary cells (N) do not react with the antibody (130x). **B.** Using the cytospin/immunoperoxidase technique as described (32, 36), MCF-7 cells were stained with monoclonal antibody B6.2 (540x).

Another type of antigenic heterogeneity was observed among cells in a given area of a tumor mass. This type of antigenic diversity, termed "patchwork," is demonstrated by the presence of tumor cells expressing a specific TAA directly adjacent to tumor cells negative for the same antigen (Figure 9b). Patterns of reactivity with a specific monoclonal antibody were also observed to vary within a given tumor mass, i.e., antigen was detected in the cytoplasm of cells in one part of the tumor mass and on the luminal edge of differentiated structures in a different part of the same mass.

Heterogeneity of TAA Expression in Human Mammary Tumor Cell Lines

In an attempt to elucidate the phenomenon of variation of antigenic phenotypes in primary human mammary tumors, model systems were examined. Human mammary tumor cell lines, transplanted in athymic mice, demonstrated antigenic heterogeneity. To determine if this phenomenon also exists in human mammary tumor cell lines grown in vitro, MCF-7 cells were tested for the presence of TAA using the cytospin/immunoperoxidase method (Nuti et al. 1982, Horan Hand et al. 1983). As seen in Figure 10B, the MCF-7 cell line contained various subpopulations of cells as defined by variability in expression of TAA reactive with monoclonal antibody B6.2. Positive MCF-7 cells are seen adjacent to cells that scored negative.

Antigenic Drift of Mammary Tumor Cell Populations

Studies were then undertaken to determine if any change in antigenic phenotype occurs during extended passage of cells in culture. The BT-20 cell line, obtained at passage 288, was serially passaged and assayed at each passage level during logarithmic growth. As seen in Table 5, a cell-surface HLA antigen, detected by monoclonal antibody W6/32 (Barnstable et al. 1978), was present at all passage levels, as was the antigen detected by monoclonal antibody B38.1. The antigen detected by monoclonal antibody B6.2 was expressed on the BT-20 cell surface up to passage 319, but was not evident after this passage level. Similarly, monoclonal B14.2 reacted with BT-20 cells only up to passage 317. This phenomenon was repeatedly observed in several separate experiments at approximately the same passage levels. Antigenic drift was also observed with the MCF-7 cell line.

As a result of the phenotypic changes observed after passage in culture, MCF-7 cell lines obtained from four sources were examined for the presence of several cell-surface TAA. Karyotype profiles of the four cell lines were tested and were all identical and characteristic of the MCF-7 cell line. A single LDH band, characteristic of only a few breast tumor cell lines, including MCF-7, was also supportive evidence that these cell lines were indeed MCF-7. Using a live-cell RIA, which detects the reactivity of antigens at the cell surface, antigenic profiles of the four MCF-7 cell lines were determined. Using three monoclonal antibodies (B1.1, B6.2, and B50.4), four different antigenic phenotypes emerged.

To further understand the nature of antigenic heterogeneity of human mammary tumor cell populations, MCF-7 cells were cloned by end-point dilution, and 10 different clones were obtained and assayed for cell-surface TAA. As seen in Figure 11, the parent MCF-7 culture reacts most strongly with monoclonal antibody B1.1 and least with monoclonal B72.3. Clone 6F1 (Figure 11B) exhibits a similar phenotype to that of the parent. At least three additional major phenotypes were observed among the other clones. For example, clone 10B5 is devoid of detectable expression of any of the antigens assayed (Figure 11C), although it does contain

Table 5. *Differential Expression of Tumor-Associated Antigens in BT-20 Cells Upon Passage**

MCL AB	Passage Number					
	316	317	318	319	320	323
W6/32	690[†]	1,620	750	620	700	500
B38.1	2,560	2,280	1,380	1,640	1,550	1,320
B6.2	1,620	2,910	560	710	neg[‡]	neg
B14.2	1,600	1,380	neg	neg	neg	neg

* Monoclonal antibodies (MCL AB) were tested for binding to the surface of BT-20 mammary tumor cells in a live cell radioimmunoassay.
† Values are expressed as cpm above background.
‡ Neg = <200 cpm.

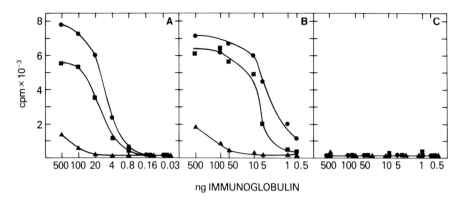

FIG. 11. Reactivity of monoclonal antibodies with the surface of the parent MCF-7 mammary adenocarcinoma cell line and cloned MCF-7 cell populations. Using a live-cell radioimmunoassay, increasing amounts of monoclonal antibodies B1.1 (closed circle), B6.2 (closed square), and B72.3 (closed triangle), were tested for binding to: **A.** the parent MCF-7 cell line; **B.** MCF-7 clone 6F1; **C.** MCF-7 clone 10B5.

HLA and human antigens detected by monoclonal antibodies W6/32 and B139, respectively.

Studies were then undertaken to determine the stability of the cell-surface phenotype of the MCF-7 clones. These cell lines have been monitored through a 4-month period and assayed during log phase at approximately every other passage. A dramatic change in antigenic phenotype was observed in some of the clones, while other MCF-7 clones maintained stable antigenic phenotypes throughout the same observation period.

Antigenic variability of TAA among and within human mammary tumor cell populations presents a potential problem in the development and optimization of immunodiagnostic and therapeutic procedures for breast cancer. Knowledge about the nature of this antigenic heterogeneity may be helpful in the prediction or control of the expression of specific antigenic phenotypes. The studies described have enabled us to demonstrate the extent of specific antigenic variability in vivo among and within human mammary tumor cell populations. Heterogeneity was not only observed within a given mammary tumor cell line, but also among the "same" mammary tumor cell line obtained from four different laboratories. This observation should serve as a caveat to investigators who are utilizing established cell lines in their studies and attempting to correlate their results with those of other laboratories.

In collaboration with Dr. D. Kufe and colleagues (Dana Farber Cancer Institute, Boston, MA), other studies, using fluorescent-activated cell-sorter analyses, have shown that at least two of the monoclonal antibodies developed (B6.2 and B38.1) are most reactive with the surfaces of MCF-7 cells during S phase (Kohler and Milstein 1976). For this reason, all the experiments using cell lines described above were performed with cells in log phase.

Using model systems, including the monoclonal antibodies and the cloned human mammary tumor cell lines described here, determinations of the parameters associated with a distinct change in antigenic phenotype are now feasible. Studies may now be undertaken to examine the relationship between the expression of specific antigenic phenotypes and such variables as morphology, tumorigenicity, drug susceptibility, growth rate, and the presence of specific hormone receptors in cloned mammary tumor cell lines. In view of the widespread variation of antigenic phenotypes among and within human mammary tumors and their implications for the immunodiagnosis and therapy of breast cancer, it would be of importance to determine which potentially clinically useful compounds will enhance the expression of specific TAA on the surface of human mammary tumor cells.

Radiolocalization of Human Mammary Tumors in Athymic Mice by a Monoclonal Antibody

Radioactively labeled antibodies to a variety of TAA have been used to detect the presence of tumors in both experimental animals and humans by gamma scintigraphy. The majority of the antibodies used for clinical trials were constituents of goat or rabbit antisera and were directed against antigens such as CEA (DeLand et al. 1979, Goldenberg et al. 1980b, Mach et al. 1981b) alpha-fetoprotein (Goldenberg et al. 1980a, Goldenberg et al. 1980c, Kim et al. 1980), ferritin (Order et al. 1981), and human chorionic gonadatropin (Goldenberg et al. 1980d, Goldenberg et al. 1981); the studies using anti-CEA demonstrated the localization of malignant breast tumors (DeLand et al. 1979, Goldenberg et al. 1980b). In some of these studies (DeLand et al. 1979, Goldenberg et al. 1980b, Goldenberg et al. 1980d, Goldenberg et al. 1981, Primus and Goldenberg 1980, Mach et al. 1981b) the immunoglobulins have been partially purified using affinity chromotography with an increase in immunoreactivity of the IgG (Primus and Goldenberg 1980). With the development of the hybridoma technology, homogenous populations of monoclonal antibodies (Kohler and Milstein 1975, Kohler and Milstein 1976) to TAA can now be utilized in either lymphangiography, to detect tumors in nodes of the axilla and internal mammary chain, or to detect distal metastases. In the studies described below, monoclonal B6.2, which may be useful in lymphangiography procedures, was utilized. B6.2 IgG was purified and $F(ab')_2$ and Fab' fragments were generated by pepsin digestion. These three forms of the antibody were radiolabeled and used to determine their utility in the radioimmunolocalization of human mammary tumor masses.

Monoclonal antibody B6.2 IgG, obtained from ascitic fluid, was precipitated with ammonium sulfate, dialyzed, and purified by ion exchange chromatography. The IgG was further purified by molecular sieving using an Ultrogel AcA 44 column to remove low molecular weight contaminants. Some of the purified IgG was used to generate $F(ab')_2$ and Fab' fragments. The fragments were purified by molecular sieving and retained all their immunoreactivity to mammary tumor extracts and not normal liver in solid-phase RIA when compared on a molar basis to the intact IgG. The IgG and its fragments were labeled with ^{125}I using the iodogen method, and specific activities of 15–50 uCi/ug of protein were easily obtained. The labeled antibody was shown to bind to the surfaces of live MCF-7 cells and retained the same specificity as the unlabeled antibody. Better than 70% of the antibody remained immunoreactive in sequential saturation solid-phase RIA after labeling.

Athymic mice were implanted with 1–2 mm³ pieces of the transplantable Clouser human mammary tumor. After approximately 10–20 days, the tumors grew to detectable nodules and continued to grow until they obtained diameters of 2.5 cm or more. Some tumors grew rapidly, while others from the same inoculum stopped growing at various times, yielding stable tumors as small as 0.6 cm in diameter. This variation in growth rate and ultimate tumor size, even arising from different aliquots of the same mammary tumor, is important in view of subsequent variations observed among different tumors in the amount of radiolabeled antibody bound per mg of tumor tissue. Athymic mice bearing the Clouser human mammary tumor were injected with 0.1 ug of B6.2 IgG labeled with ^{125}I to a specific activity of approximately 15 uCi/ug. The ratio of radioactivity/mg in the tumor compared to that of various tissues rose over a 4-day period (Figure 12 A–E) and then fell at 7 days. The tumor-to-tissue ratios were 10:1 or greater in the liver, spleen, and kidney at day 4. Ratios of the counts in the tumor to that found in the brain and muscle were greater than 50:1 and as high as 110:1. Lower tumor-to-tissue ratios were obtained when compared to blood and the lungs with their large blood pool. The activity found in the lungs was probably not a consequence of trapping of particulates, as evidenced by the low uptake in the liver and spleen.

When the Clouser mammary tumor-bearing mice were injected with ^{125}I-labeled F(ab')$_2$ fragments of B6.2, higher tumor-to-tissue ratios were obtained (Figure 12 F–J). The tumor-to-tissue ratios in the liver and spleen were 15–20:1 at 96 hours. The tumor-to-tissue ratios were somewhat lower with blood and lungs, but were still higher than those obtained using IgG. This is probably due to the faster clearance of the F(ab')$_2$ fragments as compared to IgG. The tumor-to-kidney ratio was relatively low and was probably due to the more rapid clearance of Fab' fragments, which may have been generated from the F(ab')$_2$ in vivo by the breakage of the cross linking disulfide bonds.

Athymic mice bearing a human melanoma (A375), a tumor that shows no surface reactivity with B6.2 in live-cell RIA, were used as controls for nonspecific binding of the labeled antibody or antibody fragments to tumor tissue. As shown in Figure 12 (open circles), no preferential localization of the monoclonal antibody was observed in the tumor; in fact, the counts per mg in the tumor were lower than those found in many organs, resulting in ratios of less than 1. Similarly, no localization was observed when either normal murine IgG or MOPC-21 IgG$_1$ (the same isotype as B6.2) from a murine myeloma or their F(ab')$_2$ fragments were inoculated into athymic mice bearing Clouser mammary tumors or melanomas, with tumor-to-blood ratios of less than or equal to 0.5:1. Athymic mice bearing human mammary tumors derived from tissue culture cell lines were also injected with labeled B6.2

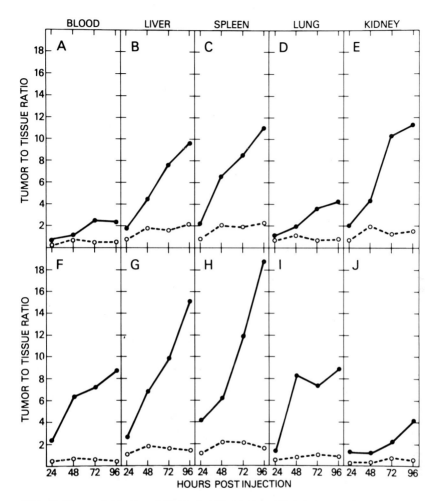

FIG. 12. Tissue distribution of ^{125}I-labeled B6.2 IgG and F(ab')$_2$ in athymic mice bearing human tumor transplants. Athymic mice bearing a transplantable human mammary tumor (Clouser, closed circles) or a human melanoma (A375, open circles) were inoculated with ^{125}I-labeled B6.2. Approximately 1.5 uCi of IgG (Panels A-E) or F(ab')$_2$ (Panels F-J) were injected i.v., and the mice were killed at daily intervals. The radioactivity per milligram of tumor was determined and compared to that of various tissues; the averages of 2–20 mice per group are shown.

antibody and fragments. Tumor-to-spleen and tumor-to-liver ratios of 6–8:1 were obtained using B6.2 F(ab')$_2$ in mice bearing tumors derived from MCF-7 cells and BT-20 cells.

Athymic mice bearing Clouser mammary tumors were also injected with ^{125}I-labeled B6.2 Fab'. The clearance rate of the Fab' fragment was considerably faster than the larger F(ab')$_2$ fragment and the intact IgG. Acceptable tumor-to-tissue ratios were obtained, but the fast clearance rate resulted in a large amount of the labeled Fab' being found in the kidney and bladder, resulting in low tumor-to-kidney ratios. These studies therefore indicate that F(ab')₂ fragments are superior to Fab' or intact IgG in radiolocalization studies of mice with monoclonal antibody B6.2.

Scanning of Athymic Mice Bearing Human Tumors

Studies were undertaken to determine whether the localization of the ^{125}I-labeled antibody and fragments in the tumors was sufficient to detect using a gamma camera. Athymic mice bearing the Clouser mammary tumor or the A375 melanoma were injected i.v. with approximately 30 uCi of ^{125}I-labeled B6.2 IgG. The mice were scanned and then killed at 24-hour intervals. The Clouser tumors were easily detected at 24 hours (Figure 13A) using radiolabeled B6.2 IgG, with a small amount of activity detectable in the blood pool. The tumor remained strongly positive over the 4-day period, with the background activity decreasing to the point where it was barely detectable at 96 hours (Figure 13B). The 0.5-cm diameter tumors localized in Figure 13A and B appear bigger than their actual size; this may be due to the dispersion of rays through the pinhole collimeter. No tumor localization was observed using radiolabeled B6.2 IgG in mice bearing the control human melanoma transplants (Figure 13C).

Mice were also injected with ^{125}I-labeled B6.2 F(ab')₂ fragments. The mice cleared the fragments faster than the intact IgG, and a significant amount of activity was observed in the two kidneys and bladder at 24 hours (Figure 14A), but tumors were clearly positive for localization of the ^{125}I-labeled B6.2 F(ab')₂ fragments. The activity was cleared from the kidneys and bladder by 48 hours, and the tumor-to-

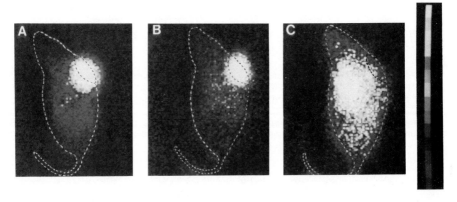

FIG. 13. Gamma camera scanning with B6.2 IgG of athymic mice bearing transplanted human tumors. Athymic mice bearing a transplantable human mammary tumor (Clouser, Panels A and B) or a human melanoma (A375, Panel C) were inoculated with approximately 30 uCi of ^{125}I-labeled B6.2 IgG. The mice were scanned after various time intervals (24 hours, Panel A, C; 96 hours, Panel B) until an equal number of counts were detected in each field. The color bar denotes the relative amounts of activity, with the highest levels at the top of the bar.

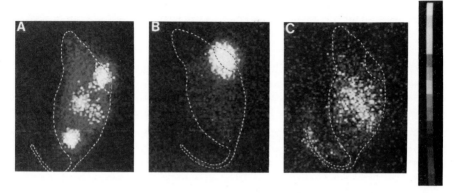

FIG. 14. Gamma camera scanning with B6.2 F(ab')$_2$ of athymic mice bearing transplanted human tumors. Athymic mice bearing a transplantable human mammary tumor (Clouser, Panels A and B) or a human melanoma (A375, Panel C) were inoculated with approximately 30 uCi of ^{125}I-labeled B6.2 F(ab')$_2$. The mice were scanned after various time intervals (24 hours, Panel A; 96 hours, Panels B and C) until an equal number of counts were detected in each field. The color bar denotes the relative amount of activity, with the highest levels at the top of the bar.

background ratio increased over the 4-day period of scanning, with little background and good tumor localization observed at 96 hours (Figure 14B). No localization of activity was observed with the radio-labeled B6.2 F(ab')$_2$ fragments in the athymic mice bearing the A375 melanoma (Figure 14C).

The utility of radiolabeled antibodies for the in vivo localization of tumors in humans has been shown with heterologous polyclonal antibodies to a number of different antigens. Human mammary tumors have been localized using antibodies to CEA (DeLand et al. 1979, Goldenberg et al. 1980b) that have been affinity purified. Murine mammary tumors have been localized using antibodies to murine mammary epithelial antigens generated in rabbits (Wilbanks et al. 1981). These studies required computer-aided background subtraction (employing a second radiolabeled Ig or other protein) and are thus limited in use to institutions with such sophisticated equipment. The use of monoclonal antibodies with defined specificities should eliminate such additional manipulations, and should also thus reduce radiation dose to the patients.

Monoclonal antibodies to murine Thy 1.1 antigens (Houston et al. 1980), Rauscher leukemia virus gp70 (Scheinberg et al. 1982), and to a stage-specific embryonic antigen (Ballou et al. 1979), have been used to show localization of tissues in mice. The study by Houston et al. (1980) using ^{125}I-labeled anti-Thy 1.1 showed selective localization of the antibody to lymphatic tissues in mice containing the antigen. Scheinberg et al. (1982) were able to show the localization of radioactivity in leukemic spleens of mice injected with the Rauscher leukemia virus. This work has been extended with the successful localization of human colon carcinomas in athymic mice and in patients with monoclonal antibodies to CEA (Mach et al. 1981a) and in athymic mice bearing a human germ cell tumor using monoclonal antibodies generated against the tumor (Moshakis et al. 1981). Attempts to localize human tumors in mice with monoclonal antibodies to HLA were unsuccessful (Warenius et al. 1981).

The studies described here demonstrate the ability of radiolabeled monoclonal antibody to detect human breast tumor xenografts in athymic mice. The ^{125}I-labeled antibody and fragments all successfully localized tumors, with the F(ab')$_2$ fragment giving the overall highest tumor-to-tissue ratios. The F(ab')$_2$ fragments may be the best form of the antibody to use because of the potential problem of Fc receptors on a variety of cells binding the labeled IgG and yielding a higher nonspecific distribution of the antibody. The use of an antibody without the Fc portion should also reduce its immunoreactivity in patients and thus minimize an immune response. The smaller fragments also clear the body faster than intact immunoglobulin and should result in a lower whole-body radiation absorbed dose to the host.

Radiolabeled monoclonal antibodies that are reactive with the surface of human mammary carcinoma cells may eventually prove useful in several areas in the management of human breast cancer. The detection of occult metastatic lesions at distal sites via gamma scanning could serve as an adjunct in determining which patients should receive adjuvant therapy, and subsequent scanning may reveal which tumors are responding to therapy. At present, only axillary lymph nodes removed at mastectomy are examined for tumor involvement for use in staging; the extent of nodal tumor involvement in the internal mammary chain is not determined. The use of radiolabeled monoclonal antibodies in lymphangiography of the internal mammary chain may eventually increase the reliability of staging of nodal involvement (both axillary and internal chain) as a prognostic indicator. Along with their potential in the diagnosis and prognosis of breast cancer, monoclonal antibodies coupled with isotopes decaying via high-energy transfer with short range radiation may eventually prove useful as radiotherapeutic agents. This approach, however, is obviously quite complex and would require extensive studies in an experimental model. The system described here, of a radiolabeled monoclonal antibody that is selectively reactive with the surfaces of human mammary tumor cells in vivo may provide an excellent experimental system for such therapy studies.

ACKNOWLEDGMENTS

We wish to thank D. Poole, D. Simpson, J. Howell, J. Collins, J. Crowley, R. Fitzgerald, and A. Sloan for expert technical assistance in these studies. We also thank Dr. D. Stramignoni for many helpful discussions. Some of these studies were supported in part by contract NO1-CP-01018 from the National Cancer Institute, National Institutes of Health, Bethesda, Maryland.

REFERENCES

Accolla, R. S., S. Carrel, and J. P. Mach. 1980. Monoclonal antibodies specific for carcino-embryonic antigen and produced by two hybrid cell lines. Proc. Natl. Acad. Sci. USA 77:563–566.

Arklie, J., J. Taylor-Papadimitriou, W. Bodmer, M. Egan, and R. Millis. 1981. Differentiation antigens expressed by epithelial cells in the lactating breast are also detectable in breast cancers. Int. J. Cancer 28:23–29.

Avis, F., I. Avis, J. F. Newsome, and G. Haughton. 1976. Antigenic cross-reactivity between adenocarcinoma of the breast and fibrocystic disease of the breast. JNCI 56:17–25.

Ballou, B., G. Levine, T. R. Hakala, and D. Solter. 1979. Tumor location detected with radioactively labeled monoclonal antibody and external scintigraphy. Science 206:844–847.

Barnstable, C. J., W. F. Bodmer, G. Brown, G. Galfre, C. Milstein, A. F. Williams, and A. Ziegler. 1978. Production of monoclonal antibodies to group A erthrocytes, HLA and other human cell surface antigens: New tools for genetic analysis. Cell 14:9–20.

Black, M. M., R. E. Zachrau, B. Shore, A. S. Dion, and H. P. Leis. 1978. Cellular immunity to autologous breast cancer and RIII-murine mammary tumor virus preparations. Cancer Res. 38:2068–2078.

Chatal, J. F., F. Chupin, G. Ricolleaua, J. L. Tellier, A. le Mevel, P. Fumoleau, O. Godin, and B. P. le Mevel. 1980. Use of serial carcinoembryonic antigen assays in detecting relapses in breast cancer involving high risk of metastasis. Eur. J. Cancer 17:233–238.

Chism, S. E., L. W. Noel, J. V. Wells, P. Crewther, S. Hung, J. J. Marchalonis, and H. H. Fudenberg. 1977. Evidence for common and distinct determinants of colon carcinoembryonic antigen, colon carcinoma antigen-III, and molecules with carcinoembryonic antigen activity isolated from breast and ovarian cancer. Cancer Res. 37:3100–3108.

Chu, T. M., and T. Nemoto. 1973. Evaluation of carcinoembryonic antigen in human mammary carcinoma. JNCI 51:1119–1122.

Colcher, D., P. Horan Hand, M. Nuti, and J. Schlom. 1981a. A spectrum of monoclonal antibodies reactive with human mammary tumor cells. Proc. Natl. Acad. Sci. USA 73:3199–3203.

Colcher, D., P. Horan Hand, M. Nuti, and J. Schlom. 1983a. Differential binding to human mammary and non-mammary tumors of monoclonal antibodies reactive with carcinoembryonic antigen. Cancer Invest. 1:131–143.

Colcher, D., P. Horan Hand, Y. A. Teramoto, D. Wunderlich, and J. Schlom. 1981b. Monoclonal antibodies define diversity of mammary tumor viral gene products in virions and mammary tumors of the genus *Mus*. Cancer Res. 41:1451–1459.

Colcher, D., M. Zalutsky, W. Kaplan, D. Kufe, F. Austin, and J. Schlom. 1983b. Radiolocalization of human mammary tumors in athymic mice by a monoclonal antibody. Cancer Res. 43:736–742.

Cuttitta, F., S. Rosen, A. F. Gazdar, and J. D. Minna. 1981. Monoclonal antibodies that demonstrate specificity for several types of human lung cancer. Proc. Natl. Acad. Sci. USA 78:4591–4595.

Daar, A. S., and J. W. Fabre. 1981. Demonstration with monoclonal antibodies of an unusual mononuclear cell infiltrate and loss of normal epithelial membrane antigens in human breast carcinomas. Lancet 29:434–438.

DeLand, F. H., E. E. Kim, R. L. Corgan, S. Casper, F. J. Primus, E. Spremulli, N. Estes, and D. M. Goldenberg. 1979. Axillary lymphoscintigraphy by radioimmunodetection of carcinoembryonic antigen in breast cancer. J. Nucl. Med. 20:1243–1250.

Dent, P. B., S. Carrel, and J. P. Mach. 1980. Detection of new cross-reacting carcinoembryonic antigen(s) on cultured tumor cells by mixed hemadsorption assay. JNCI 64:309–316.

Edwards, P. A. W., C. S. Foster, and R. A. J. McIlhinney. 1980. Monoclonal antibodies to teratomas and breast. Transplant. Proc. 12:398–402.

Foster, C. S., E. A. Dinsdale, P. A. W. Edwards, and A. M. Neville. 1982a. Monoclonal antibodies to the human mammary gland: II. Distribution of determinants in breast carcinomas. Virchows Arch. [Pathol. Anat.] 394:295–305.

Foster, C. S., P. A. W. Edwards, E. A. Dinsdale, and A. M. Neville. 1982b. Monoclonal antibodies to the human mammary gland: I. Distribution of determinants in non-neoplastic mammary and extra mammary tissues. Virchows Arch. [Pathol. Anat.] 394:279–293.

Foulds, L. 1954. The experimental study of tumor progression: A review. Cancer Res. 14:327–339.

Frankel, A. E., R. V. Rouse, and L. A. Herzenberg. 1982. Human prostate specific and shared differentiation antigens defined by monoclonal antibodies. Proc. Natl. Acad. Sci. USA 79:903–907.

Gold, P., and S. O. Freedman. 1964. Demonstration of tumor-specific antigens in human colonic carcinomata by immunological tolerance and absorption techniques. J. Exp. Med. 121:439–462.

Gold, P., S. O. Freedman, and J. Shuster. 1979. Carcinoembryonic antigen: Historical perspective, experimental data, in Immunodiagnosis of Cancer, R. B. Herberman and K. R. McIntire, eds. Marcel Dekker, Inc., New York, pp. 147–164.

Goldenberg, D. M., F. H. DeLand, E. E. Kim, and F. J. Primus. 1980a. Xenogeneic antitumor antibodies in cancer radioimmunodetection. Transplant Proc. 12:188–191.

Goldenberg, D. M., E. E. Kim, and F. H. DeLand. 1981. Human chorionic gonadotropin radioantibodies in the radioimmunodetection of cancer and for disclosure of occult metastases. Proc. Natl. Acad. Sci. USA 78:7754–7758.

Goldenberg, D. M., E. E. Kim, F. H. DeLand, S. Bennett, and F. J. Primus. 1980b. Radioimmunodetection of cancer with radioactive antibodies to carcinoembryonic antigen. Cancer Res. 40:2984–2992.

Goldenberg, D. M., E. E. Kim, F. H. DeLand, E. Spremulli, M. O. Nelson, J. P. Gockerman, F. J. Primus, R. L. Corgan, and E. Alpert. 1980c. Clinical studies on the radioimmunodetection of tumors containing alpha-fetoprotein. Cancer 45:2500–2505.

Goldenberg, D. M., E. E. Kim, F. H. DeLand, J. R. vanNagell Jr., and N. Iavadpour. 1980d. Clinical radioimmunodetection of cancer with radioactive antibodies to human chorionic gonadotropin. Science 208:1284–1286.

Greene, G. L., C. Nolan, J. P. Engler, and E. V. Jensen. 1980. Monoclonal antibodies to human estrogen receptor. Proc. Natl. Acad. Sci. USA 77:5115–5119.

Hansen, H. J., J. J. Snyder, E. Miller, J. P. Vandevoorde, O. N. Miller, L. R. Hines, and J. J. Burns. 1974. Carcinoembryonic antigen (CEA) assay. Hum. Pathol. 5:139–147.

Hart, I. R., and I. U. Fidler. 1981. The implications of tumor heterogeneity for studies on the biology and therapy of cancer metastasis. Biochem. Biophys. Acta 651:37–50.

Herzenberg, L. A., L. A. Herzenberg, and C. Milstein. 1979. Cell hybrids of myelomas with antibody forming cells and T lymphocytes with T cells, in Handbook of Experimental Immunology, D. M. Weir, ed. Blackwell Scientific, London, p. 25.1–25.7.

Hollinshead, A. C., W. T. Jaffurs, L. K. Alpert, J. E. Harris, and R. B. Herberman. 1974. Isolation and identification of soluble skin-reactive membrane antigens and normal breast cells. Cancer Res. 34:2961–2968.

Horan Hand, P., M. Nuti, D. Colcher, and J. Scholm. 1983. Monoclonal antibodies to tumor associated antigens define antigenic heterogeneity among human mammary carcinoma cell populations. Cancer Res. 43:728–735.

Houston, L. L., R. C. Nowinski, and I. D. Bernstein. 1980. Specific in vivo localization of monoclonal antibodies directed against the Thy 1.1 antigen. J. Immunol. 125:837–843.

Howard, D. R., and C. R. Taylor. 1979. A method for distinguishing benign from malignant breast lesions utilizing antibody present in normal human sera. Cancer 43:2279–2287.

Kerbel, R. S. 1979. Implications of immunological heterogeneity of tumors. Nature 280:358–360.

Kim, E. E., F. H. DeLand, M. O. Nelson, S. Bennett, G. Simmons, E. Alpert, and D. M. Goldenberg. 1980. Radioimmunodetection of cancer with radiolabeled antibodies to a-fetoprotein. Cancer Res. 40:3008–3012.

Kohler, B., and C. Milstein. 1975. Continuous cultures of fused cells secreting antibody of predefined specificity. Nature 256:494–497.

Kohler, G., and C. Milstein. 1976. Derivation of specific antibody producing tissue culture and tumor lines by cell fusion. Eur. J. Immunol. 6:511–519.

Koprowski, H., Z. Steplewski, K. Mitchell, M. Herlyn, D. Herlyn, and P. Fuhrer. 1979. Colorectal carcinoma antigens detected by hybridoma antibodies. Somatic Cell Genet. 5:957–971.

Krebs, B. P., C. M. Lalanne, and M. Schneider. 1978. Clinical application of carcinoembryonic antigen assay. Proceedings of a Symposium, Nice, France. Excerpta medica, Amsterdam.

Krolick, K. A., D. Yuan, and E. S. Vitetta. 1981. Specific killing of a human breast carcinoma cell line by a monoclonal antibody coupled to the A-chain of ricin. Cancer Immunol. Immunother. 12:39–41.

Kufe, D. W., L. Nadler, L. Sargent, H. Shapiro, P. Horan Hand, F. Austin, D. Colcher, and J. Schlom. 1983. Cell surface binding properties of monoclonal antibodies reactive with human mammary carcinoma cells. Cancer Res. 43:851–857.

Kupcik, H. Z., V. R. Zurawski, Jr., J. G. R. Hurrell, N. Zamcheck, and P. H. Black. 1981. Monoclonal antibodies to carcinoembryonic antigen produced by somatic cell fusion. Cancer Res. 41:3306–3310.

Leung, I. P., G. M. Borden, R. M. Nakamura, D. H. Delteer, and T. S. Edgington. 1979. Frequency of association of mammary tumor glycoprotein antigen and other markers with human breast tumors. Cancer Res. 39:2057–2061.

Lokich, J. J., N. Zamcheck, and M. Lowenstein. 1978. Sequential carcinoembryonic antigen levels in the therapy of metastatic breast cancer: A predictor and monitor of response and relapse. Ann. Intern. Med. 89:902–906.

Loop, S. M., K. Nishiyama, I. Hellstrom, R. G. Woodbury, J. P. Brown, and K. E. Hellstrom. 1981. Two human tumor-associated antigens, p155 and p210, detected by monoclonal antibodies. Int. J. Cancer 27:775–781.

Mach, J. P., F. Buchegger, M. Forni, J. Ritschard, L. Berche, J. D. Lumbroso, M. Schreyer, C. Girardet, R. S. Accolla, and S. Carrel. 1981a. Use of radiolabeled monoclonal anti-CEA antibodies for the detection of human carcinomas by external photoscanning and tomoscintigraphy. Immunology Today:239–249.

Mach, J. P., S. Carrel, M. Forni, J. Ritschard, A. Donath, and P. Alberto. 1981b. Tumor localization of radiolabeled antibodies against carcinoembryonic antigen in patients with carcinoma. N. Engl. J. Med. 303:5–10.

Mazauric, T., K. F. Mitchell, G. J. Letchworth III, H. Koprowski, and Z. Steplewski. 1982. Monoclonal antibody-defined human lung cell surface protein antigens. Cancer Res. 42:150–154.

Menendez-Botet, C. J., J. S. Nisselbaum, M. Fleisher, P. P. Rosen, A. Fracchia, G. Robbins, J. A. Urban, and M. K. Schwartz. 1976. Correlation between estrogen receptor protein and carcinoembryonic antigen in normal and carcinomatous human breast tissue. Clin. Chem. 22:1366–1371.

Mesa-Tejada, R., I. Keydar, M. Ramanarayanan, T. Ohno, C. Feoglio, and S. Speigelman. 1978. Detection in human breast carcinomas of an antigen immunologically related to a group-specific antigen of mouse mammary tumor virus. Proc. Natl. Acad. Sci. USA 75:1529–1533.

Miggiano, V., C. Stahli, P. Haring, J. Schmidt, M. LeDain, B. Glatthaar, and T. Staehelin. 1979. Monoclonal antibodies to three tumor markers: Human chorionic gonadotropin (hCG), prostatic acid phosphatase (PAP) and carcinoembryonic antigen (CEA), in Proceedings of the Twenty-Eighth Colloquium, H. Peeters, ed. Pergamon Press, Oxford, p. 501–504.

Miller, F. R., and G. H. Heppner. 1979. Immunologic heterogeneity of tumor cell subpopulations from a single mouse mammary tumor. JNCI 63:1457–1463.

Mitchell, K. F. 1980. A carcinoembryonic antigen (CEA) specific monoclonal hybridoma antibody that reacts only with high-molecular-weight CEA. Cancer Immunol. Immunother. 10:1.

Moshakis, V., R. A. J. McIlhinney, D. Raghavan, and A. M. Neville. 1981. Localization of human tumor xenografts after i.v. administration of radiolabeled monoclonal antibodies. Br. J. Cancer 44:91–99.

Natali, P. G., B. S. Wilson, K. Imai, A. Bigotti, and S. Ferrone. 1982. Tissue distribution, molecular profile, and shedding of a cytoplasmic antigen identified by the monoclonal antibody 465.125 to human melanoma cells. Cancer Res. 42:583–589.

Nuti, M., D. Colcher, P. Horan Hand, F. Austin, and J. Schlom. 1981. Generation and characterization of monoclonal antibodies reactive with human primary and metastatic mammary tumor cells, in Monoclonal Antibodies and Development in Immunoassay, A. Albertini, and R. Ekins, eds. Elsevier/North Holland Biomedical Press, North Holland, p. 87.

Nuti, M., Y. A. Teramoto, R. Mariani-Costantini, P. Horan Hand, D. Colcher, and J. Schlom.

1982. A monoclonal antibody (B72.3) defines patterns of distribution of a novel tumor associated antigen in human mammary carcinoma cell populations. Int. J. Cancer 29:539–545.

Order, S. E., J. L. Klein, and P. K. Leichner. 1981. Antiferritin IgG antibody for isotopic cancer therapy. Oncology 38:154–160.

Pimm, M. V., and R. W. Baldwin. 1977. Antigenic differences between primary methylcholanthrene-induced rat sarcomas and post-surgical recurrences. Int. J. Cancer 20:37–43.

Poste, G., J. Doll, and I. J. Fidler. 1981. Interactions among clonal subpopulations affect stability of the metastatic phenotype in polyclonal populations of B16 melanoma cells. Proc. Natl. Acad. Sci. USA 78:6226–6230.

Prehn, R. T. 1970. Analysis of antigenic heterogeneity within individual 3-methylcholanthrene-induced mouse sarcomas. JNCI 45:1039–1050.

Primus, F. J., and D. M. Goldenberg. 1980. Immunological considerations in the use of goat antibodies to carcinoembryonic antigen for the radioimmunodetection of cancer. Cancer Res. 40:2979–2983.

Pusztaszeri, G., and J. P. Mach. 1973. Carcinoembryonic antigen (CEA) in non-digestive cancerous and normal tissues. Immunochemistry 10:197–204.

Rogers, G. T., G. A. Rawlins, and K. D. Bagshawe. 1981a. Somatic-cell hybrids producing antibodies against CEA. Br. J. Cancer 43:1–4.

Rogers, G. T., G. A. Rawlins, P. A. Keep, E. H. Cooper, and K. D. Bagshawe. 1981b. Application of monoclonal antibodies to purified CEA in clinical radioimmunoassay of human serum. Br. J. Cancer 44:371–380.

Scheinberg, D. A., M. Strand, and O. Gansow. 1982. Tumor imaging with radioactive metal chelates conjugated to monoclonal antibodies. Science 215:1511–1513.

Schlom, J., D. Wunderlich, and Y. A. Teramoto. 1980. Generation of human monoclonal antibodies reactive with human mammary carcinoma cells. Proc. Natl. Acad. Sci. USA 77:6841–6845.

Sehested, M., F. R. Hirsch, and K. Hou-Hensen. 1981. Immunoperoxidase staining for carcinoembryonic antigen in small cell carcinoma of the lung. Eur. J. Cancer Clin. Oncol. 17:1125–1131.

Sheikh, K. M. A., F. A. Quismorio, G. J. Friou, and Y. Lee. 1979. Ductular carcinoma of the breast. Serum antibodies to tumor-associated antigens. Cancer 44:2083–2089.

Springer, G. F., P. R. Desai, M. S. Murthy, and E. F. Scanlon. 1979. Human carcinoma-associated precursor antigens of the NM blood group system. J. Surg. Oncol. 11:95–106.

Steward, A. M., D. Nixon, N. Zamcheck, and A. Aisenberg. 1974. Carcinoembryonc antigen in breast cancer patients: Serum levels and disease progress. Cancer 33:1246–1252.

Taylor-Papadimitriou, J., J. A. Peterson, J. Arklie, J. Burchell, and R. L. Ceriani. 1981. Monoclonal antibodies to epithelium-specific components of the human milk fat globule membrane: Production and reaction with cells in culture. Int. J. Cancer 28:17–21.

Teramoto, Y. A., R. Mariani, D. Wunderlich, and J. Schlom. 1982. The immunohistochemical reactivity of a human monoclonal antibody with tissue sections of human mammary tumors. Cancer 50:241–249.

Ueda, R., S. Ogata, D. M. Morrissey, C. L. Finstad, J. Szkudlarek, W. F. Whitmore, H. F. Oettgen, K. O. Lloyd, and L. J. Old. 1981. Cell surface antigens of human renal cancer defined by mouse monoclonal antibodies: Identification of tissue-specific kidney glycoproteins. Proc. Natl. Acad. Sci. USA 78:5122–5126.

von Kleist, S., and P. Burtin. 1979. Antigens cross-reacting with CEA, in Immunodiagnosis of Cancer, R. B. Herberman and K. R. McIntire, eds. Marcel-Dekker, Inc, New York, pp. 322–342.

Vrba, R., E. Alpert, and K. J. Isselbacher. 1975. Carcinoembryonic antigen: Evidence for multiple antigenic determinants and isoantigens. Proc. Natl. Acad. Sci. USA 72:4602–4606.

Waalkes, T. P., C. W. Gehrke, D. C. Tormey, K. B. Woo, K. C. Kuo, J. Snyder, and H. Hansen.

1978. Biologic markers in breast carcinoma: IV. Serum fucose-protein ratio, comparisons with carcinoembryonic antigen and human chorionic gonadotrophin. Cancer 41:1871–1882.

Warenius, H. M., G. Galfre, N. M. Bleehen, and C. Milstein. 1981. Attempted targeting of a monoclonal antibody in a human tumor xenograft system. Eur. J. Cancer Clin. Oncol. 17:1009–1015.

Wilbanks, T., J. A. Peterson, S. Miller, L. Kaufman, D. Ortendahl, and R. L. Ceriani. 1981. Localization of mammary tumors in vivo with ^{131}I-labeled Fab fragments of antibodies against mouse mammary epithelial (MME) antigens. Cancer 48:1768–1775.

Wilkinson, E. J., L. L. Hause, E. A. Sasse, R. A. Pattillo, J. R. Milbrath, and J. D. Lewis. 1980. Carcinoembryonic antigen and L-fucose in malignant and benign mammary disease. Am. J. Clin. Pathol. 73:669–675.

Woodbury, R. G., J. P. Brown, M. Y. Yeh, I. Hellstrom, and K. E. Hellstrom. 1980. Identification of a cell surface protein, p97, in human melanomas and certain other neoplasms. Proc. Natl. Acad. Sci. USA 77:2183–2187.

Wunderlich, D., Y. A. Teramoto, C. Alford, and J. Schlom. 1981. The use of lymphocytes from axillary lymph nodes of mastectomy patients to generate human monoclonal antibodies. Eur. J. Cancer Clin. Oncol. 17:719–730.

Yu, G. S. M., A. S. Kadish, A. B. Johnson, and D. M. Marcus. 1980. Breast carcinoma associated antigen: An immunocytochemical study. A brief scientific report. Am. J. Clin. Path. 74:453–457.

Yuan, D., F. J. Hendler, and E. S. Vitetta. 1982. Characterization of a monoclonal antibody reactive with a subset of human breast tumors. JNCI 68:719–728.

STAGE IV DISEASE

Current Controversies in Breast Cancer, edited
by F. C. Ames, G. R. Blumenschein, and E. D. Montague.
University of Texas Press, Austin © 1984.

Clinical Prognostic Factors of Response

Gabriel N. Hortobagyi, M.D.,* Terry L. Smith, B.S.,†
George R. Blumenschein, M.D.,* Sewa S. Legha, M.B., B.S.,‡
Hwee-Yong Yap, M.D.,* and Aman U. Buzdar, M.B., B.S.*

*Departments of *Internal Medicine, †Biomathematics, and ‡Developmental
Therapeutics, The University of Texas M. D. Anderson Hospital and
Tumor Institute at Houston, Houston, Texas*

The number of therapeutic modalities now available for the successful treatment
of breast cancer stimulated us at The University of Texas M. D. Anderson Hospital
and Tumor Institute at Houston to develop methods for determining the probability
of response and survival of individual patients. This goal can be accomplished
effectively for the various hormonal manipulations by means of hormonal receptor
assay (McGuire et al. 1977); however, this test is of no prognostic value when the
patients are treated with combination chemotherapy.

To assess the factors that will predict response to combination chemotherapy, we
performed univariate and multivariate analyses on pretreatment data collected from
546 patients with metastatic breast cancer seen in the Medical Breast Clinic of this
institution. Combination chemotherapy with 5-fluorouracil, Adriamycin, and cyclophosphamide (FAC) induction regimens, and cyclophosphamide, methotrexate, and
5-fluorouracil (CMF) maintenance programs was employed in these patients, all of
whom had clearly measurable lesions.

A complete remission (CR) was defined as disappearance of all clinical and biochemical evidence of active tumor. A partial remission (PR) was defined as a 50% or
greater decrease in the sum of the products of the largest perpendicular diameters of
measurable lesions. Stable disease (SD) represented a steady state with no change
for a minimum of 8 weeks. In all other patients, progressive disease was considered
to be present. Fifty-one pretreatment factors were included in the initial evaluation,
which were related to the host, the tumor, or their interaction (Swenerton et al.
1979). Twenty factors were individually and separately correlated with response to
therapy (CR + PR). Age and menopausal status, which are of prognostic value during endocrine treatment, were conspicuously unrelated to prognosis after chemotherapy. Other factors, such as disease-free interval, correlated with one endpoint
(survival) but not with the other (response). The most prominent host-related and
tumor-related factors of prognostic value for the determination of response are
shown in Table 1. Visual evaluation of these variables suggests that patients who

Table 1. *Prognostic Factors for Response to Therapy: Univariate Analysis*

Factor	Favorable	Unfavorable
Performance status	good	poor
Weight loss	none	> 5%
Skin test response	present	absent
Prior chemotherapy	none	yes
Prior radiotherapy	none	extensive
Extent of disease	minimal	extensive
Number of sites	1–2	≥ 3
Lung metastases	no	yes
Nodal metastases	yes	no
Hemoglobin	> 11 gm/100 ml	< 11
White cell count	> 3,500/μl	< 3,500
Platelet count	> 200,000/μl	< 200,000
Lymphocyte count	> 800/μl	< 800
Albumin	> 4/μl	< 4
Alkaline phosphatase	< 85 U	> 85
Lactic dehydrogenase	< 225 U	> 225

have minimal metastatic disease, good functional status, no prior treatment, and no impairment of vital organ function are much more likely to respond to chemotherapy than those with the opposite characteristics. While this hypothesis is logical, the number of factors to evaluate makes it impractical to predict response based on all the variables.

We performed a stepwise regression analysis including these factors and used a regression equation for calculating the probability of response (Cox 1970): ln (p/(1 − p)) = .6581 − .4045 (weight loss − 1.397) − .3012 (alkaline phosphatase − 2.011) + .6061 (node involvement − .290) + .7582 (hemoglobin − 1.879) − .5535 (prior radiotherapy − 1.183) in which the variables are coded as follows: Weight loss: 1 = < 5%, 2 = 5% to 10%, 3 = > 10%; alkaline phosphatase: 1 = < 85 U, 2 = 86 U to 170 U, 3 = 171 U to 350 U, 4 = > 350 U; nodal involvement: 0 = no, 1 = yes; hemoglobin: 1 = < 11 gm/100 ml, 2 = > 11 gm/100 ml; prior radiotherapy: 1 = none, 2 = 1 to 3 ports irradiated, 3 = > 3 ports irradiated. Table 2 shows the predictive ability of this model when applied to the 546 patients from whom it was derived. The predicted response rates correlated well with the observed response rates in each prognostic subgroup ($P = 0.98$). An even better test of the predictive capability of this model was obtained when this mathematical tool was applied prospectively to another 200 consecutive patients with metastatic breast cancer treated with the same chemotherapeutic regimen (FAC + CMF). Table 3 shows how well the model predicted the outcome in this new patient population ($P = 0.56$) (Hortobagyi, et al. 1983).

The relative importance of each of the factors included in the model varies depending on which ones are considered initially. Therefore, based on findings in the same patient population, several closely related but not identical models can be constructed with identical or similar predictive value.

Table 2. *Comparison of Observed and Expected Response Rates Based on Regression Model**

Predicted Probability of Response	Observed Response Rate	Expected No. of Responders	Observed No. of Responders
< .45	.37	24.2	26
.45–.59	.52	54.8	54
.60–.69	.65	127.5	124
.70–.79	.75	75.5	75
≥ .80	.88	69.2	73

*A retrospective analysis of 546 patients.

Table 3. *Comparison of Observed and Predicted Response Rates Based on Regression Model: A Prospective Analysis of 200 Patients*

Predicted Probability of Response	Observed Response Rate	Expected No. of Responders	Observed No. of Responders
< .45	.44	5.7	8
.45–.59	.57	24.0	25
.60–.69	.70	43.2	45
.70–.79	.67	22.6	20
≥ .80	.80	36.7	35

Prediction of probability of response was only one aspect of the determination of individual prognosis. Our next effort was to apply the same methods to predicting survival after the initiation of chemotherapy. We again applied univariate analysis to the same 51 pretreatment characteristics to assess their predictive capacity for determining survival. The most important factors, as judged by the strength of the statistical correlation, are shown in Table 4 (Swenerton et al. 1979). While many of these factors were found to be important in predicting response, others had no bearing on the response model. A regression model developed by Cox was applied to the analysis, resulting in the following equation (Cox 1972): $\ln(\lambda(t)/\lambda_0(t)) = .370$ (lactic dehydrogenase $- 1.53) + .294$ (performance status $- 1.77) + .474$ (lung $- .26) + .297$ (prior radiotherapy $- 1.89) + .197$ (alkaline phosphatase $- 2.01) + .173$ (extent of disease $- 1.67$) in which the variables are coded as follows: Lactic dehydrogenase: $1 = < 225$ U, $2 = 226$ U to 450 U, $3 = 450$ U; performance status: $1 = 1, 2 = 2, 3 = 3.4$; lung: $1 =$ involved, $0 =$ not involved; prior radiotherapy: $1 =$ none, $2 = 1$ to 3 ports, $3 = > 3$ ports; alkaline phosphatase: $1 = < 85$ U, $2 = 86$ U to 170 U, $3 = 171$ U to 350 U, $4 = > 350$ U; extent of disease (Swenerton et al. 1979): $1 = < 5, 2 = 6$ to 12, $3 = 13$ to 20, $4 = > 20$. The model was fitted in stepwise fashion in the same manner as for the logistic regression model used in predicting response. This model can be fitted to any statistical study of metastatic

Table 4. *Prognostic Factors for Survival in Breast Cancer:*
Univariate Analysis

Factor	Favorable	Unfavorable
Performance status	good	poor
Weight loss	none	> 5%
Skin test response	present	absent
Disease-free interval	long	short
Prior radiotherapy	none	extensive
Hormone responsiveness	yes	no
Bone metastases	yes	no
Extent of disease	minimal	extensive
Number of sites	1–2	≥ 3
Hemoglobin	> 11 gm/100 ml	< 11
White cell count	> 3,500/μl	< 3,500
Platelet count	> 200,000/μl	< 200,000
Lymphocyte count	> 800/μl	< 800
Albumin	> 4 gm/ml	< 4
Calcium	< 11 gm/100 ml	≥ 11
Bilirubin	< 1 mg/ml	> 1
Alkaline phosphatase	< 85 U	> 85
Lactic dehydrogenase	< 225 U	> 225
SGOT*	< 25 U	> 25

*SGOT = serum glutamic oxaloacetic transaminase.

Table 5. *Prediction of Survival by Hazard Ratio**

Hazard Ratio	Median Survival Times in Weeks	
	Model Group (546)	Test Group (200)
< 0.6	149	141
0.6–0.9	108	111
1.0–1.5	80	62
> 1.5	54	52

*Multivariate analysis of prognostic factors for survival. Hazard ratio gives the risk of death per unit of time so that increasing hazard function correlates with decreases in survival time.

breast cancer regardless of whether all patients have died. Complete information about all the variables employed in the equation was available from 536 patients. When the survival model was applied to the population from which it was derived, four distinct prognostic subgroups were identified (Table 5). The clear-cut separation and overall survival rates for the four subgroups shows the excellent predictive capability of the model. Estimated median survival times were defined (or identified) by calculating hazard ratios with the survival model at 137, 114, 62, and 52 weeks for the four subgroups. This same model then was applied to the 200 new patients with metastatic breast cancer treated with FAC + CMF combinations, and again the predictive capability of the equation was confirmed (Table 5).

This model for evaluation of survival does not contain some important prognostic factors since, strictly speaking, they were not pretreatment factors. Thus, the aggressiveness of chemotherapy (dose and frequency) and, most important, the response to treatment were not considered in the analysis (Swenerton et al. 1979). In addition, pretreatment factors of potential value to subgroups of patients, such as disease-free interval and hormonal receptor status, were not included because the information was not available for all patients in the study. Consequently, newer models incorporating these factors need to be devised to more accurately evaluate prognosis.

By employing the prognostic models for determination of response and length of survival described in this paper, one can now predict the prognosis of individual patients who have metastatic breast cancer. The pretreatment factors included in the models for response and survival are simple and easily quantitated during initial history taking or staging evaluation. Whether these models apply equally well to all chemotherapy programs remains to be established. The greatest advantage of this method, in addition to predicting individual prognosis, is that the number of factors needed for prediction of prognosis is limited to three or four, as opposed to the 15 to 20 that otherwise would be needed. Also, the probability of response or survival predicted by the model includes the influence of all the potentially known prognostic factors and, therefore, overrides the influence of individual prognostic variables. Thus, patient subgroups with comparable and uniform prognoses can be selected for planning and evaluation of clinical trials. Another important application of this type of technology is the possibility of individualizing treatment for a patient in the hope of selecting a regimen that will offer the maximum probability of response and survival.

ACKNOWLEDGMENTS

The authors wish to acknowledge the assistance of Mrs. Joan Trammell in the preparation of this manuscript.

REFERENCES

Cox, D. R. 1970. The Analysis of Binary Data. Methuen, London, pp. 87–90.

Cox, D. R. 1972. Regression models and life tables. J. Roy. Statist. Soc. (B) 34:187–220.

Hortobagyi, G. N., T. Smith, S. S. Legha, K. D. Swenerton, E. A. Gehan, H-Y. Yap, A. U. Buzdar, and G. R. Blumenschein, 1983. Multivariate analysis of prognostic factors in metastatic breast cancer. J. Clin. Oncol. (in press).

McGuire, W. L. 1977. Physiological principles underlying endocrine therapy of breast cancer, *in* Breast Cancer: Advances in Research and Treatment: Current Approaches to Therapy, vol. 1, W. L. McGuire, ed. Plenum Medical Book Company, New York, pp. 217–262.

Swenerton, K. D., S. S. Legha, T. L. Smith, G. N. Hortobagyi, E. A. Gehan, H-Y. Yap, J. U. Gutterman, and G. R. Blumenschein. 1979. Prognostic factors in metastatic breast cancer treated with combination chemotherapy. Cancer Res. 39:1552–1562.

Current Controversies in Breast Cancer, edited
by F. C. Ames, G. R. Blumenschein, and E. D. Montague.
University of Texas Press, Austin © 1984.

The Human Tumor Clonogenic Assay:
A Prognostic Factor in Breast Cancer?

Sydney E. Salmon, M.D.

University of Arizona Cancer Center, Tucson, Arizona

INTRODUCTION

In 1977 our group first reported the ability to obtain in vitro soft agar colony formation from a wide variety of human tumors (Hamburger and Salmon 1977). Within the initial group of tumors that we studied there were several metastatic breast cancers from which limited in vitro colony formation was observed; however, we excluded these from our initial publication because, at that time, we lacked sufficient morphologic, cytogenetic, or histochemical data to assure that the observed colonies were composed of breast cancer cells. Subsequently, a number of laboratories have obtained clear evidence that breast cancer cells do form colonies in this assay system, and have documented their origin with morphologic techniques (Salmon 1980a, Von Hoff et al. 1981a, Sandbach et al. 1982, Slocum et al. 1981, Gangi et al. 1981). A typical breast cancer colony is depicted under both low and high magnification in Figure 1. Additional proof of the neoplastic nature of the cells within tumor colonies has been obtained with cytogenetic and nude mouse transplantation studies. In cytogenetic studies (Trent and Thompson 1981), cells within breast tumor colonies were found to have characteristic abnormalities in chromosome 1 that have previously been reported from breast cancer cell lines. An example of a banded karyotype of a breast cancer cell within a tumor colony is depicted in Figure 2, and illustrates abnormality in chromosome 1.

Researchers using colony-transfer techniques have reported breast cancer colonies yielding tumor formation in nude mice in two of three attempts, with histologic confirmation of morphology consistent with breast cancer (Sandbach et al. 1982). The human tumor clonogenic assay (HTCA) has provided an important new focus for studies of cancer biology and developmental therapeutics, because it appears to identify a specific subpopulation of tumor cells capable of repeated cycles of cell division in vitro that are thought to be closely related to tumor stem cells in vivo (Hamburger and Salmon 1977, Salmon 1980b). In fact, growth of tumors in nude mice from in vitro colonies (as has been achieved in human breast cancer) supports the contention that the colonies contain tumor stem cells. Initial studies correlating in vitro chemosensitivity of tumor colony-forming cells (TCFU) from metastatic

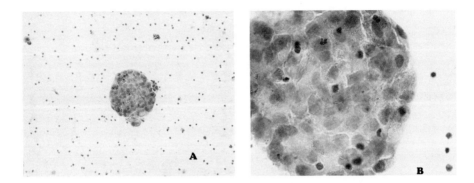

FIG. 1A and B. Human breast cancer colonies grown in soft agar culture prepared with a dried slide technique and stained with the Papanicolau stain (Salmon 1980b). Nonproliferating stromal cells and carcinoma cells are evident in the background around the colony. Colony cells have the typical morphology of adenocarcinoma. (1A) 100X magnification. (1B) 400X magnification.

cancers to clinical response to the same anticancer drugs have suggested a good correlation with response of metastases in patients who have a variety of tumor types (Salmon et al. 1978, Meyskens et al. 1981), including breast cancer (Von Hoff et al. 1981a). Given this background, it would appear that HTCA may prove to have value as a prognostic factor in human breast cancer and aid in understanding aspects of this neoplasm's biology and sensitivity to a wide variety of standard and new therapeutic agents. It has been suggested that HTCA may prove useful in testing the chemosensitivity of breast cancers just as estrogen and progesterone receptor assays are used in hormonal therapy. However, before this goal can be achieved, a number of problems will need to be resolved. In this brief discussion, it is my intent to review selected results obtained to date as well as problems identified in several laboratories involved with cloning human breast cancers in vitro. This topic has also been recently addressed independently by Von Hoff et al. (1981e).

METHODS, RESULTS, AND DISCUSSION

The general methods used for sample collection, preparation, cultivation, and chemosensitivity testing in HTCA are detailed elsewhere (Hamburger and Salmon 1977, Salmon et al. 1978, Salmon 1980b). A general flow diagram for the assay system is depicted in Figure 3.

Breast cancer specimens have been obtained from both primary tumors and solid metastases as well as from malignant effusions or bone marrow aspirates. Several major problems can be identified in relation to in vitro studies of primary breast cancers. These are summarized in Table 1. First, the cloning efficiency in HTCA is quite low, frequently in the range of 0.1% or less, and therefore requires submission of specimens of 1–10 gm to assure the availability of adequate numbers of cells (500,000 nucleated cells per 35-mm agar petri dish). In breast cancer the problem

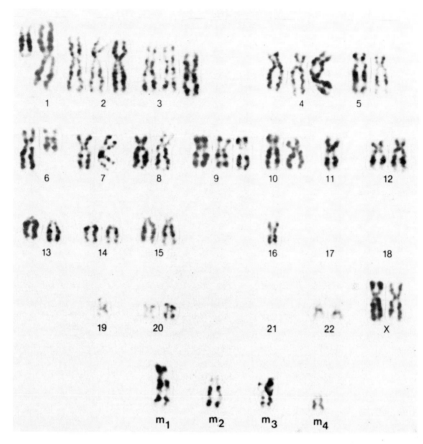

FIG. 2. An example of an abnormal chromosomal complement from breast carcinoma tumor colony-forming units stained with Giemsa banding. The karyotype is described as 45,XX,-1, +1q-, +2, +3, +4, -6, +6q-, +9, -11, -16, -17, -17, -18, -18, -19, -21, -21, +M_{1-4}. Among these many abnormalities is the deletion of the short arms of one of the first chromosomes. Four unidentified marker chromosomes were also noted. (Figure kindly provided by J. Trent and F. Thompson.)

of obtaining adequate cell numbers for HTCA is compounded by other diagnostic needs and logistic difficulties. A major requirement in dealing with primary tumors is assuring that adequate tissue is available for standard histopathology and for hormone-receptor testing. The receptor assays generally require submission of up to 1 gm of tumor tissue. With T1 and many T2 tumors, there is little if any tissue remaining for baseline colony growth studies and far too little for significant chemosensitivity testing. This problem is not likely to be resolved until immunohistochemical techniques become available for estrogen- and progesterone-receptor testing and until higher cloning efficiencies are attainable for breast cancer. Thus, most of the primary breast cancers submitted to our laboratory are from patients who have

TUMOR STEM CELL ASSAY

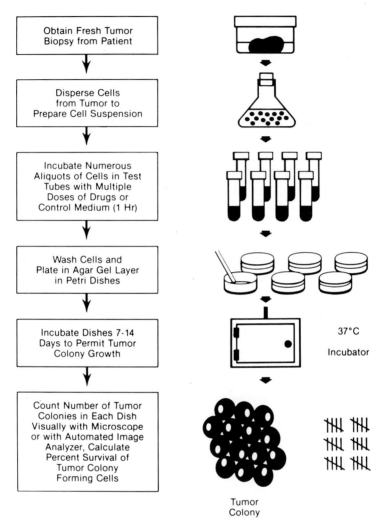

FIG. 3. Flow diagram of steps in drug-sensitivity assay. (Reproduced from Salmon 1980b, with permission of Alan R. Liss, Inc.)

high-risk tumors (e.g., T3-T4), and their test results may not be representative of smaller primaries. A second significant problem results from the density and tight adhesion of breast cancer cells that frequently diffusely invade the stromal connective tissue, making it difficult to obtain adequate numbers of cells using simple mechanical disaggregation techniques. We had negligible success in obtaining adequate numbers of breast cancer cells, even from larger primary tumors, with stan-

Table 1. *Problems Encountered in Attempting to Carry Out Clonogenic Assays in Human Breast Cancer*

Inadequate biopsy specimen size in T_1 and some T_2 primaries.
Tissue requirements for histopathology and estrogen-receptor testing.
Difficult to obtain tumor from many metastatic sites (e.g., bone, intradermal).
Difficult to disaggregate tumor cells from stroma.
Low cloning efficiency.
Evidence of heterogeneity of growth and drug sensitivity between primary tumors and metastases.
Correlations difficult to make with multiagent therapy.
Metastatic tumor often submitted from "end stage" patients.

dard mechanical disaggregation techniques (Salmon 1980b). However, using a reported enzymatic disaggregation technique incorporating a combination of DNAse and collagenase (Slocum et al. 1981), we have obtained adequate numbers of tumor cells for culture in about 80% of adequate size primary or metastatic breast cancer specimens submitted to our laboratory. However, cell numbers are still rather limited in T1 and some T2 tumors. Problems are also encountered in dealing with the question of tumor procurement from metastatic sites, e.g., many patients have inaccessible tumor present in bone, and it has been extremely difficult to disaggregate intradermal metastases. The latter problem has also been noted by others (Sandbach et al. 1982). Overall, our current success rate at obtaining adequate baseline colony growth (>30 colonies/plate) is only in the range of 50%. Thus, only 40% of submitted primary breast cancer specimens yield both enough tumor cells for culture and exhibit adequate colony growth in vitro. Similar results have recently been reported from other laboratories (Sandbach et al. 1982).

As of October 1982, adequate in vitro growth (>30 colonies/plate) of breast cancer cells has occurred in 66 specimens submitted for chemosensitivity testing. The mean number of drugs tested per specimen (generally at two concentrations in triplicate plus six controls) was 6.9 and was identical to that attained in other tumor types. Figure 4 depicts a survival-concentration curve for breast tumor colony-forming units (TCFU) exposed to a series of anticancer drugs and the antiestrogen tamoxifen. Heterogeneity in response was observed to the different agents.

Both estrogen receptor-positive and estrogen receptor-negative tumors grow in similar fashion in HTCA (Sandbach et al. 1982, Von Hoff et al. 1981e). We have carried out testing of the antiestrogen tamoxifen by continuous exposure in agar against specimens from 20 patients with breast cancer. In general, we observed minor or moderate sensitivity in some specimens, but in no instance was growth reduced to $<35\%$ of control. In these initial studies the fetal calf serum may have contained some estrogen, and additional studies are now underway in charcoal-stripped serum. With respect to a number of cytotoxic drugs tested at standard laboratory concentrations, the percent reduction in survival observed was not as great as observed in other tumor types (e.g., ovarian cancer). The standard agents doxorubicin, cyclophosphamide, fluorouracil, methotrexate, vinblastine, mitomycin, and the investigational agent recombinant leukocyte interferon A, have all been

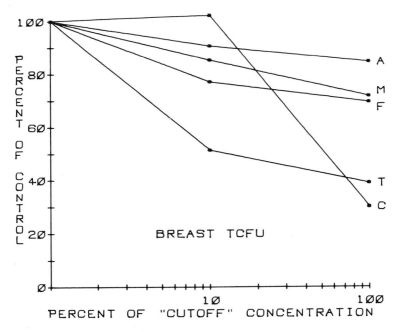

FIG. 4. In vitro sensitivity response of tumor colony-forming units (TCFU) from a patient with metastatic breast cancer to a series of anticancer drugs. The upper "cutoff concentrations" (μg/ml) indicated in the figure were as follows: A (Adriamycin or doxorubicin, 0.1); M (methotrexate, 10); F (fluorouracil, 5); C (cyclophosphamide, 10); T (tamoxifen, 5×10^{-5}M). Tamoxifen was tested by continuous exposure in the agar while the other agents were exposed to the cells for 1 hour prior to plating. The active product of cyclophosphamide, 4-hydroperoxycyclophosphamide, was used for testing purposes.

tested against at least 20 breast cancers grown in HTCA in our laboratory. The results of these studies are summarized in Figure 5. The results differ somewhat from those we have observed in some other "clinically sensitive" tumor types. Specifically, it was not unusual to see survival reduced to 50% of control or less, but rather uncommon for it to be reduced to less than 30% of control. The relative ranking of agents with respect to activity was also somewhat unexpected, specifically the somewhat reduced activity of doxorubicin. However, the exact rank for any given agent depends on the in vitro cutoff concentration selected, and this is subject to change based on clinical correlations in specific tumor types. A related phenomenon has been reported from Von Hoff's laboratory (Sandbach et al. 1982). They also found limited sensitivity (<30% of control) in breast cancer, but indicated that positive clinical correlations in breast cancer were observed in patients whose TCFU showed reduction to between 30% and 50% of control. Based on such observations, they suggested that reduction in survival of TCFU to 50% of control or less (at appropriate drug dosage) may be an adequate definition of in vitro sensitivity for breast cancer. However, it is troublesome that the in vitro response rates observed with some conventional agents, such as doxorubicin, are not as high as those ob-

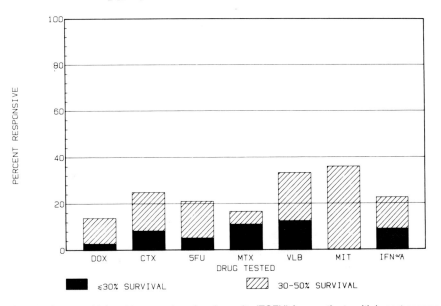

FIG. 5. In vitro sensitivity of tumor colony-forming units (TCFU) from patients with breast cancer to standard cytotoxic agents and to recombinant leukocyte interferon A (IFN-αA). The proportion of patients whose cells exhibited marked (solid bar) or intermediate (hatched bar) sensitivity is depicted. All drugs (μg/ml) were tested for 1 hour prior to plating except for IFN-αA, which was tested by continuous exposure. The summaries based on the highest concentration tested are: DOX = doxorubicin (0.1); CTX = cyclophosphamide (10); 5FU = 5-fluorouracil (5); MTX = mitomycin C (0.1); IFN = αA (0.004); VLB = vinblastine (.01). Each drug was tested against at least 20 breast cancers grown in the human tumor clonogenic assay.

served in the clinic. In our experience, the frequency of in vitro sensitivity to doxorubicin (50% of control at 0.1 μg-hours of exposure) was only 13.9%; in the report of Sandbach et al. (1982), it was 18%. The rate of clinical response in this group of patients would be projected to be closer to 30%. One possible explanation relates to heterogeneity in growth and sensitivity of TCFU in the primary tumor and its metastases. This circumstance has recently been reported by Schlag and Schreml (1982). While it is difficult to obtain primary tumors and metastases simultaneously (and have both exhibit adequate in vitro growth), this was accomplished by Schlag and his co-workers for several breast cancers and a variety of other tumor types (Schlag and Schreml 1982). They noted that, in general, the gross cloning efficiency (percentage of colonies formed/500,000 nucleated cells plated) was significantly lower in breast cancer primary tumors than in the same patient's lymph node metastases. Additionally, for the limited number of solid tumors they studied for chemosensitivity, they did not find a correlation between the sensitivity of the primary tumor and its metastases. However, the cellular compositions of a primary tumor and its metastases vary considerably, and it must be recognized that metasta-

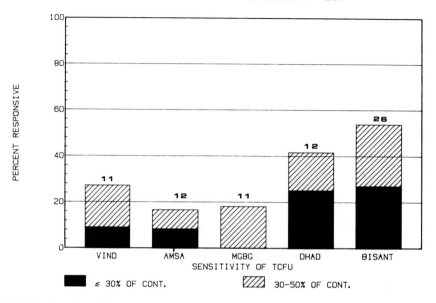

FIG. 6. In vitro phase II sensitivity studies of tumor colony-forming units from patients with breast cancer tested against five investigational agents. All drugs (μg/ml) were tested for 1 hour prior to plating. The summaries are based on the highest concentration tested. (VIND = vindesine; AMSA = 4′-(-acridinylamino-methansulfon-anisidide); MGBG = methyglyoxalbisguanethyl hydrazone; DHAD = dihydroxyanthracenedione (mitoxantrone); BISANT = bisantrene).

ses likely represent subclones from the primary tumor and may exhibit growth and drug sensitivity heterogeneity in relation to the primary tumor. These observations suggest that drug sensitivity results obtained during tests of primary tumors will have to be interpreted with caution and may not be applicable to treatment of metastases. Clinical correlations reported to date with HTCA in both our laboratory (Salmon et al. 1978, Alberts et al. 1980, Meyskens et al. 1981) and Von Hoff's (1981a,c) have been limited to testing of metastatic disease with correlations to the response of metastases. It therefore remains quite uncertain whether in vitro chemosensitivity testing will have relevance to the results of adjuvant chemotherapy in breast cancer. This question is likely only to be answered by prospective correlative trials (Salmon 1980c), wherein patients who are selected to receive a specified adjuvant chemotherapy regimen have their primary tumors tested in vitro against the treatment they will receive. Under these circumstances, the assay results would be independent of the treatment plan for the patient, and correlations could be sought between assay results and relapse-free and overall survival.

Beyond such applications for evaluating individualized "tailoring" of treatment of patients, HTCA has been increasingly applied to the area of new drug development for both preclinical new drug screening and for "in vitro phase II trials." Considerable progress has already occurred in the application of HTCA for in vitro phase II trials. In such studies, new drugs that are being considered for clinical trial are tested in vitro against a variety of tumor types in HTCA. In vitro phase II trials have clearly identified single-agent activity for the current new drugs mitoxantrone (Von Hoff et al. 1981b) and bisantrene (Alberts et al. 1982, Von Hoff et al. 1981c), and helped to target these drugs for clinical trials in breast cancer. Both agents recently have been found to induce remissions in advanced breast cancer, providing a good correlation with predictions from HTCA studies. Results of in vitro phase II trials with mitoxantrone, bisantrene, and several other agents are depicted in Figure 6. Using such in vitro phase II trials, we recently also identified significant activity in a new doxorubicin analog (4'deoxydoxorubicin), which is more potent than its parent compound and appears to lack cardiac toxicity in mice (Salmon et al. 1981, Salmon and Durie 1982, Casazza et al. 1981). This agent has significant activity against breast cancer in this assay system (Figure 7), and the drug has recently been slated for clinical trial. An approach such as this one has particular importance in relation to identifying potential new agents that have activity against a substantial proportion of previously untreated breast cancers (in vitro). In breast cancer, new agents would be unlikely to be tested in other than heavily pretreated patients who have relapsed after receiving multiple combinations of standard anticancer drugs.

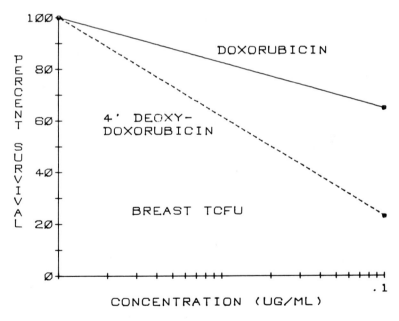

FIG. 7. Comparative sensitivity of tumor colony-forming units (TCFU) to doxorubicin (Adriamycin) and its semisynthetic congener 4'deoxydoxorubicin in a patient with breast cancer. The 4'deoxy derivative has recently entered clinical trial. As evidenced by in vitro studies such as this, the antitumor potency of 4'deoxydoxorubicin is significantly greater than that of the parent compound.

A phase II clinical trial in such advanced patients is undesirable, as it often markedly underestimates the activity of a new agent. HTCA is now also being tested systematically by the National Cancer Institute (NCI) to determine whether it can play a role in primary drug screening for new agents tested in vitro against tumors from patients who have received no prior chemotherapy (Shoemaker et al. 1982). In the NCI studies breast cancer is one of the signal tumors being tested by HTCA. It will be of interest to see whether the NCI study identifies any novel structures for breast cancer that were missed by standard in vivo immune screening systems.

Improvements in the in vitro culture system for breast cancer and development of a better understanding of the biological problem of tumor heterogeneity may increase the applicability of HTCA for human breast cancer.

ACKNOWLEDGMENTS

The author thanks his colleagues for their participation in many of the studies cited from his laboratory: Laurie Young and Joyce Lebowitz for technical assistance, Jerry Isaman for computer graphics, and Toni Meinke for preparation of the manuscript.

These studies were supported in part by grants CA-21839, CA-17094, and CA-23074 from the National Cancer Institute, U.S. Department of Health and Human Services.

REFERENCES

Alberts, D. S., C. Mackel, R. Pocelinko, and S. E. Salmon. 1982. Phase I clinical investigation of 9,10-anthracenedicarboxaldehyde bis ((4,5-dihydro-1H-imidazol-2-yl)hydrazone) dihydrochloride with correlative in vitro human tumor clonogenic assay. Cancer Res. 42:1170–1175.

Alberts, D. S., S. E. Salmon, H. S. G. Chen, E. A. Surwit, B. Soehnlen, L. Young, and T. Moon. 1980. In vitro clonogenic assay for predicting response of ovarian cancer to chemotherapy. Lancet 2:340–342.

Casazza, A. M., O. Bellini, G. Savi, and A. DiMarco. 1981. Antitumor activity and cardiac toxicity of 4'deoxydoxorubicin (4'deoxydx) in mice. (Abstract) Proc. Amer. Assoc. Cancer Res. 22:267.

Gangi, D., N. Legros, B. Heule-Vanden, W. Mattheiem, and J. C. Heuson. 1981. Stem cell assay in solid breast carcinoma. (Abstract) Proc. Amer. Assoc. Cancer Res. 22:156.

Hamburger, A. W., and S. E. Salmon. 1977. Primary bioassay of human tumor stem cells. Science 197:461–463.

Meyskens, F. L., T. E. Moon, B. Dana, E. Gilmartin, W. J. Casey, H. S. G. Chen, D. H. Franks, L. Young, and S. E. Salmon. 1981. Quantitation of drug sensitivity by human metastatic melanoma colony forming units. Br. J. Cancer 44:787–797.

Salmon, S. E. 1980a. Background and overview, in Cloning of Human Tumor Stem Cells, S. E. Salmon, ed. Alan R. Liss, Inc., New York, pp. 3–14.

Salmon, S. E., ed. 1980b. Cloning of Human Tumor Stem Cells. Alan R. Liss, Inc., New York.

Salmon, S. E. 1980c. Perspectives on future directions, in Cloning of Human Tumor Stem Cells, S. E. Salmon, ed. Alan R. Liss, Inc., New York, pp. 315–330.

Salmon, S. E., and B. G. M. Durie. 1982. In vitro phase II trial of 4'deoxydoxorubicin (4'deoxydx) with comparisons to doxorubicin (dx). (Abstract) Proc. Am. Soc. Clin. Oncol. 23:9.

Salmon, S. E., A. W. Hamburger, B. Soehnlen, B. G. M. Durie, D. S. Alberts, and T. E. Moon.

1978. Quantitation of differential sensitivity of human tumor stem cells to anticancer drugs. N. Engl. J. Med. 298:1321–1327.

Salmon, S. E., R. M. Liu, and A. M. Casazza. 1981. Evaluation of new anthracycline analogs with the human tumor stem cell assay. Cancer Chemother. Pharmacol. 6:103–109.

Sandbach, J., D. D. Von Hoff, G. Clark, A. B. Cruz, M. Obrien, and The South Central Texas Human Tumor Cloning Group. 1982. Direct cloning of human breast cancer in soft agar culture. Cancer 50:1315–1321.

Schlag, P., and W. Schreml. 1982. Heterogeneity in growth pattern and drug sensitivity of primary tumor and metastases in the human tumor colony forming assay. Cancer Res. 42:4086–4089.

Shoemaker, R. H., M. K. Wolpert-DeFilippes, R. W. Makuch, and J. M. Venditti. 1982. The National Cancer Institute program for new drug screening with the human tumor clonogenic assay. (Abstract) Proceedings of the 13th International Cancer Congress, Seattle, Washington, p. 569.

Slocum, H. K., Z. P. Pavelic, Y. M. Rustum, P. J. Creaven, C. Karakousis, H. Takita, and W. R. Greco. 1981. Characterization of cells obtained by mechanical and enzymatic means from human melanoma, sarcoma, and lung tumors. Cancer Res. 41:1428–1434.

Trent, J. M., and F. H. Thompson. 1982. Cytogenetic analysis of tumor colony forming cells from human breast cancer: Evidence for clonal karyotypic heterogeneity. Breast Cancer Research and Treatment 3:292.

Von Hoff, D. D., J. Casper, E. Bradley, J. Sandbach, D. Jones, and R. Makuch. 1981a. Association between human tumor colony forming assay results and response of an individual patient's tumor to chemotherapy. Am. J. Med. 70:1027–1032.

Von Hoff, D. D., C. A. Coltman, Jr., and B. Forseth. 1981b. Activity of mitoxantrone in a human tumor cloning system. Cancer Res. 41:1853–1855.

Von Hoff, D. D., C. A. Coltman, Jr., and B. Forseth. 1981c. Activity 9-10anthracenedicarboxaldehyde bis ((4,5-dihydro-1H-imidazol-2yl)hydrazone) dihydrochloride (CL-216,942) in a human tumor cloning system. Cancer Chemother. Pharmacol. 6:141–144.

Von Hoff, D. D., C. Page, G. Harris, G. Clark, J. Cowan, C. A. Coltman, and The South Central Texas Human Tumor Cloning Group. 1981d. Prospective clinical trial of a human tumor cloning system. Proc. Amer. Assoc. Cancer Res. 22:154.

Von Hoff, D. D., J. Sandbach, C. K. Osborne, C. Metelmann, G. H. Clark, and M. Obrien. 1981e. Potential and problems with the growth of breast cancer in a human tumor cloning system. Breast Cancer Research and Treatment 2:141–148.

Current Controversies in Breast Cancer, edited
by F. C. Ames, G. R. Blumenschein, and E. D. Montague.
University of Texas Press, Austin © 1984.

Aggressive Systemic Therapy for Metastatic Breast Cancer

Douglass C. Tormey, M.D., Ph.D., Joyce C. Kline, M.D., Dori
Kalish-Black, M.S., Thomas E. Davis, M.D., Richard R. Love,
M.D., and Paul P. Carbone, M.D.

Department of Human Oncology, University of Wisconsin, Madison, Wisconsin

Since the introduction of modern combination chemotherapy for metastatic breast cancer in 1969 (Cooper 1969), response rates for initial chemotherapy regimens have varied from 50% with cyclophosphamide (Cytoxan) (CYT), methotrexate (MTX), and 5-fluorouracil (5-FU) based regimens to over 70% with Adriamycin (ADR), CYT, 5-FU and dibromodulcitol (DBD), ADR, vincristine (VCR) based regimens. Complete response rates ranged from 8% to 22% in these same trials. Regimens associated with higher response rates in these trials also tended to be associated with longer median times of disease control and survival (Table 1).

Because of the apparent plateau in the complete remission (CR) rate in these trials, we attempted to ascertain if exposure to a high drug density could enhance the CR rate to >50%. To assess the durability of the remission, the patients were to be taken off chemotherapy shortly after obtaining CR. In addition, postsystemic therapy consolidation radiotherapy was introduced into the trial to attempt to reduce the high relapse rate observed in early patients at identical prestudy sites of gross disease.

MATERIALS AND METHODS

Patient Population

Women patients eligible for the protocol had metastatic breast cancer with an ECOG performance status of 0, 1, 2, or 3 (Oken et al. 1982), at least one bidimensionally measurable disease component, age ≤65 years, no prior exposure to DBD, VCR, or ADR, and no prior chemotherapy for metastatic disease (prior hormone therapy or interferon therapy was allowed; also, patients failing adjuvant therapy >6 months after its completion were eligible). All patients signed informed consent forms. Patients with creatinine levels >1.5 mg/100ml, SGOT >600 IU/ml, or bilirubin levels >5.0 mg/100ml were not eligible.

Table 1. Historical Data from Selected Randomized Trials*

| Regimen | No. of Patients | %CR+PR | %CR | Median Time to Failure (Months) | | Median Survival (Months) | | Study Reference[†] |
				All Patients	CR	All Patients	CR	
CMF	40	62	8	6.2	NS	17.0	NS	1
CAF	38	82	18	10.0	NS	27.2	NS	
CAF	46	63	13	11.4	10.7+	20.0+	NS	2
DAV/CMF	48	71	10					
CMFVP-C	86	50	9	5.0		16.0		3
CMFVP-I	109	50	11	5.0	16.0	13.0	32.0	
CAFVP	107	71	15	7.0		19.0		
AV	166	56	12	5.7	11.9	13.7	19.4	4
CMF	79	57	15	5.3	14.3	14.5	25.0	
CMFP	86	63	16	9.1	15.0	16.4	36.0	
CMF	26	55	17	5.6		12.5		5
CMFP	33	70	21	7.0		18.0		
CMF/AV	29	58	22	10.9	16.2	17.8	30.0	
CMFP/AV	102	58	14	10.4		16.3		
CMFP	80	59	14	8.9		19.4		

*Abbreviations are as follows: CR = complete response; PR = partial response; CMF = cyclophosphamide (CYT) + methotrexate (MTX) + 5-fluorouracil (5FU); CAF = CYT + Adriamycin (ADR) + 5FU; DAV = dibromodulicitol (DBD) + ADR + vincristine (VCR); CMFVP-C = CMF + VCR + prednisone (PRED) given weekly; CMFVP-I = CMFVP given intermittently; CAFVP = CYT + ADR + 5FU + VCR + PRED; AV = ADR + VCR; CMFP = CMF + PRED; DAV/CMF = three cycles of DAV rotating with three cyles of CMF; CMF/AV = two cycles of CMF rotating with two cycles of AV; CMFP/AV = two cycles of CMFP rotating with two cycles of AV; NS = data not stated.
[†] (1) Bull et al. 1978; (2) Tormey et al. 1979; (3) Tormey et al. 1981; (4) Tormey et al. 1982a; (5) Tormey et al. 1983.

Treatment Plan

Patients were scheduled to be treated with six 28-day cycles of systemic therapy or to be treated until they achieved CR followed by three additional cycles, whichever was longer. Consolidation radiotherapy was delivered to the prestudy sites of disease involvement when the 11th patient entry had completed her systemic therapy. Each 28-day systemic therapy cycle consisted of the drug regimen at doses shown in Figure 1. After the 17th entry, bleomycin (BLEO) was dropped from the regimen because of its pulmonary toxicity (see RESULTS). Treatment delays of up to 2 weeks were allowed between cycles to allow recovery of white blood cell (WBC) counts; in this instance, the Day 22 prednisone (PRED) dosage was repeated. No dose modifications were made during a treatment cycle for low blood counts except for DBD, which was discontinued after Day 7 for WBC counts <3000/mm³ or platelet (PLT) counts <75,000/mm³. Infections or febrile states were not considered reasons to modify therapy. Selection of the full drug doses to be delivered for each subsequent cycle was based on nadir blood counts and delays as shown in Table 2. If on Day 1 of treatment, despite a 1- to 2-week delay, the WBC counts were still <4000/mm³ or the PLT counts were <100,000/mm³, the ADR and DBD doses were further reduced as shown in Table 3. The MTX and leucovorin (LF) doses were modified for renal function and MTX serum levels as shown in Table 4. Vincristine toxicities led to dose reductions of up to 75% for severe paresthesias or if the patient had difficulty walking on her heels or walking up stairs without using her hands; the drug was never omitted. Dose-reduction criteria for hepatic, cardiac, and gastrointestinal abnormalities were available but were utilized in only one patient.

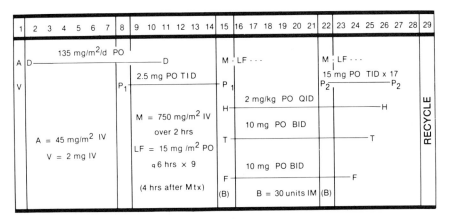

FIG. 1. Drug doses and scheduling for each 28-day systemic therapy cycle. (D = dibromodulcitol; A = Adriamycin; V = vincristine; P = prednisone; M = methotrexate; T = tamoxifen; H = hexamethylmelamine; F = fluoxymesterone; B = bleomycin; LF = leucovorin; PO = orally; TID = three times a day; IV = intravenously; QID = four times a day; BID = two times a day; IM = intramuscularly)

Table 2. *Guidelines for Selection of Full Drug Doses for Each Ensuing Cycle**

Nadir WBC[†]	ADR	DBD	All Others	Nadir PLT
>1,600	100%	100%	100%	>40,000
≤1,600	75%	50%[‡]	100%	≤40,000
Cycle Delay	DBD	d 22 MTX	All Others	
≤1 week	100%	100%	100%	
>1 week	50%[‡]	75%	100%	

*The lowest doses commensurate with either of these tables were used, i.e., the tables were not additive.
[†]Abbreviations are as follows: WBC = white blood cells; ADR = Adriamycin; DBD = dibromodulcitol; PLT = platelets; MTX = methotrexate.
[‡]DBD dose reductions were in days of therapy. If following a dose modification these guidelines required no further reductions, the doses in the next cycle were increased by 25% of the 100% dose in an attempt to return to 100% dosing.

Table 3. *Dose Reductions Employed on the Day of Initiation of Each Cycle of Therapy**

WBC[†]	ADR	DBD	or	PLT	ADR	DBD	All Other
<4,000	75%	75%[‡]		<100,000	75%	50%[‡]	100%
<2,500	50%	50%[‡]		< 75,000	50%	25%[‡]	100%

*These reductions were superimposed upon any reductions required by Table 2.
[†]Abbreviations are as follows: WBC = white blood cells; ADR = Adriamycin; DBD = dibromodulcitol; PLT = platelet.
[‡]DBD dose reductions were in days of therapy.

Patient Evaluations

Pretreatment and posttreatment evaluations consisted of history and physical examination, measurements of all lesions, complete blood count (CBC), urinalysis, liver and renal function chemistries, bone scan (and, if abnormal, x-rays), liver and brain scans, mammography (if indicated), chest x-rays, computerized axial tomography of lesions (where indicated), cardiac evaluation, and staging conferences between the medical oncologist and radiotherapist.

During therapy, CBCs were obtained weekly. All tumor measurement studies and chemistries were performed at 2- to 4-week intervals, renal, cardiac, and pulmonary function studies at 1- to 3-month intervals, and creatinine and MTX levels following Days 15 and 22 of MTX therapy.

The response criteria were those used by the Eastern Cooperative Oncology Group (Oken et al. 1982). Briefly, a CR required the total disappearance of all reversible evidence of disease for at least 4 weeks; a partial response (PR) consisted of no lesions progressing (vide infra) and at least a 50% reduction in the area of all measurable tumor in at least 50% of the involved organ sites for at least 4 weeks;

Table 4. Guidelines for Methotrexate (MTX) and Leucovorin (LF) Dosing Based on Renal Function and MTX Levels*

Day 14 or 21 Pre-MTX Creatinine	% MTX	Initial LF Dose	24-Hour Creatinine Level†	Change LF Dose to	24-Hour MTX Level†	48-Hour MTX Level‡	LF to Give
≤1.00	100	15 mg/m²x 9	≤1.0	15 mg/m² x 9	$<10^{-6}$M	$<10^{-7}$M	15 mg/m²x 9
1.01–1.59	50	30 mg/m²x 12	>1.0 and ↑ >25%	30 mg/m² to total of 12 LF doses	$>10^{-6}$M	$>10^{-7}$M	Increase to 100 mg/m² to total of 15 LF doses
1.6–2.0	25	100 mg/m²x 15	>1.0 or ↑ >50%	100 mg/m² to total of 15 doses	$>10^{-5}$M	$>10^{-6}$M	Increase to 100 mg/m², obtain every 24-hour follow-up levels and continue LF until level $<10^{-9}$M
>2.0	0	—	—	—	—	—	—

*Patients with third-space fluid accumulations were monitored with MTX levels at 24-hour intervals until the level decreased below 10^{-9}M. The MTX dosing was designed to provide 2- to 4-hour levels of $>10^{-4}$M; if this did not occur the MTX dose was escalated 25% in the subsequent cycle.
†Creatinine levels were used as initial guidelines and were overridden by MTX levels.
‡The 48-hour level overrode the 24-hour level.

progressive disease (PD) was assigned with the development of any new lesions or a ≥25% increase in the area of any existing lesion within 4 weeks. Relapse was defined as PD following PR or CR, using the minimal measurements obtained as the baseline for calculations. Time to treatment failure (TTF) and survival were measured, respectively, from the onset of therapy to PD, relapse, or death.

RESULTS

Response Rates

There were 18 CR (78%, 95% confidence interval = .61, .95) among the 23 patient entries. Three patients (13%) achieved PR and two (9%) had PD. Two additional recent entries are in PR in cycle 1. Complete responses were observed across each of the patient characteristics of age, disease-free interval after mastectomy, menopausal status, estrogen-receptor status, dominant disease (12/17 visceral, 6/6 soft tissue), number of sites of involvement (14/15, 1–2; 4/8, ≥3), performance status (16/19, 0–1; 2/4, 2–3), and prior therapy. One of the three patients with PR had achieved a CR in pleura, breast, and skin but died of pulmonary fibrosis with a PR in osseous disease and nonevaluable liver disease. A second patient with a PR achieved a CR in skin and nodes and a PR in lung and bone. The third patient with a PR achieved a CR in liver, nodes, and skin but a PR in bone. Only performance status and number of involved pretreatment organ sites were prognostic for response ($P \leq .05$).

The median time to PR was 27 days (range 7–99) and to CR was 61 days (range 14–215). The number of cycles delivered in CR in the 17 patients completing therapy was 0 in one patient, 1.0–1.9 in two, 2.0–2.9 in two, 3.0–3.9 in five, 4.0–4.9 in three, and ≥5 in four. The median duration of systemic therapy in these patients was 6.4 months, with a range of 5.1 to 10.5 months.

Time to Treatment Failure (TTF) and Survival

The TTF (17/23 failures) and survival (12/23 failures) are, respectively, 11.6 and 19.2 months for all patients and 13.5 and 25.4 months for all patients with CR. Censoring the two BLEO-related deaths increases the overall TTF and survival to 12.2 and 22.2 months, respectively, and of CR to 14.2 and 30.8 months. The median time off all systemic therapy for the patients with CR was 7.8 months. The only pretreatment factor that was prognostic for TTF was performance status ($P < .05$).

Effect of Radiotherapy

The effect of radiotherapy was analyzed with respect to failure patterns within individual involved sites. This analysis deleted the patients with PD or drug-related PR, those with early deaths due to pulmonary fibrosis, and one patient who had just completed radiotherapy. Among the 15 evaluable patients, there were 62 individual sites of prestudy disease involvement. Relapses occurred at 21/32 (66%) individual sites not receiving radiotherapy compared to 5/30 (17%) sites receiving radiotherapy ($P < .001$).

Side Effects

The most life-threatening side effects were leukopenia and thrombocytopenia (Table 5). Overall, leukopenia $<1000/mm^3$ occurred in 12 patients, and thrombocytopenia $<25,000/mm^3$ occurred in 10. Septic states occurred with leukopenia in six patients; five of these were bacteriologically sterile. The sixth patient died from rapidly progressive lymphangitic pulmonary disease in the presence of leukopenia and documented sepsis. Nine of the 17 patients receiving BLEO experienced clinical and/or laboratory evidence of pulmonary toxicity despite a maximum protocol dose of 180 units. Two patients died of documented progressive pulmonary fibrosis at total BLEO doses of 120 and 180 units. An additional three patients experienced dyspnea, and four more had clinical, chest x-ray, and/or diffusion changes. It was for this reason that BLEO was dropped from the protocol with the 18th patient (the CR rate before and after this decision was 13/17 and 5/6). In addition, almost all patients experienced alopecia, mild depression, and malaise. Oropharyngeal erythema or pain related to MTX was reported by five patients, and ulceration was observed in one additional patient. One patient developed a lower extremity thrombophlebitis. Other side effects observed with the systemic therapy are included in Table 5.

Side effects relating to consolidation radiotherapy were primarily pulmonary. Three patients experienced radiation pneumonitis, two of whom required tempo-

Table 5. *Major Side Effects Encountered During Chemotherapy**

Side Effect	N	Side Effect	N
WBC <2,000	8	nausea (mild)	3
<1,000	12	with emesis (transient)	10
PLT <50,000	7	poorly controlled	4
<25,000	10	VCR-mild paresthesias	4
Septic state-clinically	5	+ requiring dose reduction	12
proved	1	+ reversible weakness	2
Pulmonary dyspnea	5	steroid effects-peripheral (mild)	10
+ severe fibrosis	2	central nervous system (mild)	11
		visual complaints (transient)	8

*Abbreviations are as follows: WBC = white blood cells; PLT = platelet; VCR = vincristine.

rary inpatient and outpatient medical support. The latter two received, respectively, doses of 5,000–5,400 rad to the chest wall, axilla, internal mammary nodes, and supraclavicular fossa, and 1,200 rad to the total lung with boosts to 4,800 rad in the left mediastinum and portions of the left lower lobe and left upper lobe.

Postrelapse Therapy

Seven patients were reinduced with the original protocol and three with a CYT substitute for DBD. In this group one patient achieved CR and four achieved PR. Five additional patients were treated with various combinations without effect. Survival from relapse after the original protocol was a median of 5.8 months overall and 7.2 months for the original CR patients. Among the 10 patients reentering the induction program after relapse, the median survival from the start of reinduction was 9.6 months (range 0.9–31.3, 9/10 failures).

DISCUSSION

This pilot study was initiated to ascertain whether a continuous exposure to pulses of active agents delivered over a short time could increase the cell kill, as judged by a high CR rate. That the concept that exposure to a high drug density is effective is strongly supported by the CR rate of 78%. The durability of the CR (13.5 months TTF) was similar to that in trials in which continuing maintenance therapy was utilized.

The CR rate appeared to be higher than that in historical trials (Bull et al. 1978, Tormey et al. 1979, 1981, 1982a, 1983) across all pretreatment characteristics analyzed. Inverse response relationships were present with respect to performance status and number of organ sites involved. Both of these measures are generally thought to be crude indirect measures of tumor burden. Thus, it would appear that at CR rates in excess of 50% the most important predictor for response is tumor burden.

The overall TTF and survival appeared to be higher than observed in the historical trials (Bull et al. 1978, Tormey et al. 1979, 1981, 1982a, 1983, Tormey and Gelman 1981); however, these parameters among those with CR were similar to those of the patients with CR in historical trials. This latter result occurred in the absence of continuing maintenance therapy. Similar results have been observed in two previous trials (Canellos et al. 1974, Smalley et al. 1976) and predicted from an analysis of two others (Tormey and Gelman 1981).

The observation that relapses tended to occur in the unirradiated pretreatment disease sites suggests an inability to eliminate residual disease at those sites by systemic therapy. Although it is possible that more prolonged therapy would eliminate this residual disease, it is our view, based on kinetic modeling, that the failure is due to 1) initially resistant cells, i.e., "naked resistance" (Goldie and Coldman 1979), 2) decreasing drug dosage leading to decreasing cell kill, or 3) the development of a "temporary G_1," protected state. The "naked resistance" argument clearly applies to kinetic modeling and is clinically suggested in the 5/10 patients that failed to achieve second CR. The decreased drug dosing hypothesis again is compatible with modeling approaches. Of special interest was the second CR along with the effect of radiotherapy upon relapses at prestudy disease sites. These data suggest that residual small cohorts of cells may be placed into a relatively refractory G_1 or G_0

state. One explanation for this occurrence would be an insufficient vascular supply due to drug-related destruction of the tumor periphery along with its vascular supply.

Finally, the effect of radiotherapy in this trial, while supporting the above hypothesis, also suggests a role for the introduction of combined modality therapy as a consolidation approach in the treatment of metastatic breast cancer. Such therapy may be effective either by eliminating the reproductive and metastatic capacity of cell niduses or by simply delaying the expression of these properties.

The side effects from this treatment program were significant. The observations with BLEO suggested a drug synergy with respect to pulmonary fibrosis and led to discontinuation of the drug. Significant hematologic suppression was observed, but it is not clear how much more occurred over other reported studies since blood counts were always recorded weekly in our trial. It would appear that the Day 1 counts, cycle delays encountered, and drug-dose decreases encountered were similar to our previous experience with a DBD, ADR, VCR regimen (Tormey et al. 1979). Considerable physician support was required for most patients due to malaise coupled with a mild depression, which appeared to be related to the intensity of frequent visits and testing during the period of therapy.

In summary, this pilot trial has suggested that exposure to a high drug density is capable of raising the CR rate in metastatic breast carcinoma to over 50% and that localized postsystemic therapy radiation therapy is capable of preventing relapse at previous sites of disease. The relative importance of each of the drugs used and their relative timing in our trial can only be assessed by larger studies. It is our view that the results obtained and the concepts developed concerning the duration of therapy and its intensity and the role and timing of radiotherapy deserve further testing to evaluate their biological and clinical effects.

ACKNOWLEDGMENTS

This investigation was supported by Grant Numbers CA 20432 and CA 14520 awarded by the National Cancer Institute, U.S. Department of Health and Human Services.

REFERENCES

Bull, J. M., D. C. Tormey, S. H. Li, P. P. Carbone, G. Falkson, J. Blom, E. Perlin, and R. Simon. 1978. A randomized comparative trial of Adriamycin versus methotrexate in combination drug therapy. Cancer 41:1649–1657.

Canellos, G. P., V. T. DeVita, G. L. Gold, B. A. Chabner, P. S. Schein, and R. C. Young. 1974. Cyclical combination chemotherapy for advanced breast carcinoma. Brit. Med. J. 1:218–220.

Cooper, R. G. 1969. Combination chemotherapy in hormone resistant breast cancer. (Abstract) Proc. Am. Assoc. Cancer Res. 10:15.

Goldie, J. H., and A. J. Coldman. 1979. A mathematic model for relating the drug sensitivity of tumors to their spontaneous mutation rate. Cancer Treat. Rep. 63:1727–1733.

Oken, M. M., R. H. Creech, D. C. Tormey, J. Horton, T. E. Davis, E. T. McFadden, and P. P.

Carbone. 1982. Toxicity and response criteria of the Eastern Cooperative Oncology Group. Cancer Clin. Trials 5:649–655.

Smalley, R. V., S. Murphy, C. M. Huguley, Jr., and A. A. Bartolucci. 1976. Combination versus sequential five-drug chemotherapy in metastatic carcinoma of the breast. Cancer Res. 36:3911–3916.

Tormey, D. C., G. Falkson, R. M. Simon, J. Blom, J. M. Bull, M. E. Lippman, S-H. Li, J. G. Cassidy, and H. C. Falkson. 1979. A randomized comparison of two sequentially administered combination regimens to a single regimen in metastatic breast cancer. Cancer Clin. Trials 2:247–256.

Tormey, D. C., and R. S. Gelman. 1981. Relationship between time to treatment failure and survival and between time to response and response duration in metastatic breast cancer: Implications for treatment. Cancer Clin. Trials 4:355–362.

Tormey, D. C., R. Gelman, P. R. Band, M. Sears, S. N. Rosenthal, W. DeWys, C. Perlia, and M. A. Rice. 1982a. Comparison of induction chemotherapies for metastatic breast cancer: An Eastern Cooperative Oncology Group Trial. Cancer 50:1235–1244.

Tormey, D. C., R. Gelman, and G. Falkson. 1983. Prospective evaluation of rotating chemotherapy in advanced breast cancer: An Eastern Cooperative Oncology Group Trial. Cancer Clin. Trials 6:1–18.

Tormey, D. C., L. Leone, M. Perloff, and C. Bloomfield. 1981. Evaluation of intermittent vs continuous and of Adriamycin vs methotrexate 5-drug chemotherapy regimens for breast cancer. (Abstract) Proc. Am. Soc. Clin. Oncol. 19:320.

Current Controversies in Breast Cancer, edited
by F. C. Ames, G. R. Blumenschein, and E. D. Montague.
University of Texas Press, Austin © 1984.

Promising New Agents for Metastatic Breast Cancer

Hwee-Yong Yap, M.D.,* Aman U. Buzdar, M.D.,*
Gabriel Hortobagyi, M.D.,* George R. Blumenschein, M.D.,*
and Gerald Bodey, M.D.†

*Departments of *Internal Medicine and †Developmental Therapeutics, The University of
Texas M. D. Anderson Hospital and Tumor Institute at Houston, Houston, Texas*

In recent years, in spite of intensive efforts and numerous innovative therapeutic approaches in the management of patients with advanced metastatic breast cancer, the achievement of durable complete remission (CR) remains an ellusive goal (Legha et al. 1979). Further progress in the therapy of patients with breast cancer will require our continuing efforts toward the evaluation of new drugs and the development of alternative therapies. Although it has been increasingly difficult to evaluate new agents in breast cancer because of extensive prior treatments, a wide variety of agents of differing mechanisms of action, nevertheless, have been found to be effective in refractory metastatic breast cancer. Since this review cannot be comprehensive, I will only concentrate on a few of these promising agents in three broad areas: Hormonal therapy, biologic therapy or immunotherapy, and finally chemotherapy.

HORMONAL THERAPY

Adrenalectomy, a historical standard surgical procedure for the management of patients with advanced breast cancer by hormonal manipulation, has been variously reported to induce objective remissions in 25–50% of patients with response durations of 9–12 months. Unfortunately, this ablative surgical procedure carries a definite risk of morbidity and mortality, especially in debilitated patients. Aminoglutethimide, an aramatase inhibitor, was first developed as an anticonvulsant approximately 20 years ago. It has recently been shown in several series to be an effective form of endocrine therapy in advanced breast cancer. Aminoglutethimide decreases adrenal steroid synthesis, but its principal method of action is thought to be inhibition and conversion of adrenal androgens to estrogen in the peripheral tissues. Various dose schedules of aminoglutethimide (Table I) have been employed with comparable results. In general, the escalating dose schedule appears to be better tolerated. The most common side effects have been drowsiness, skin rash, lethargy, depression, and nausea. In the majority of patients, these side effects have

Table 1. *Aminoglutethimide Dose Schedule*

A) Aminoglutethimide
1. 250 mg p.o.* four times daily
2. 250 mg p.o. twice daily for 1–2 weeks
   subsequent escalation to 250 mg four times daily
3. 250 mg p.o. three times daily for 2 weeks
   subsequent escalation to 250 mg four times daily

B) Replacement Therapy
1. Cortisone acetate 37.5 to 50 mg/day with or without
   fludrocortisone 0.1 mg daily
2. Hydrocortisone 30 to 80 mg/day with or without fludrocortisone
3. Dexamethasone 0.75 to 3 mg/day

*p.o. = by mouth.

Table 2. *Aminoglutethimide*

	No. Pts.	No. Responded
A) After Tamoxifen Therapy		
1. UT M. D. Anderson Hospital tamoxifen responders	44	18 (43%)
2. Cancer Institute*		
tamoxifen responders	41	22 (53.6%)
tamoxifen nonresponders	50	16 (32%)
3. Ludwig Institute[†]		
tamoxifen responders	10	4 (40%)
tamoxifen nonresponders	21	4 (19%)
4. Mayo Clinic		
tamoxifen responders	4	1 (25%)
tamoxifen nonresponders	7	0
B) ER[‡]-Positive Pts. or Hormonal Responders		
1. University of Miami	44	19 (43%)
C) Phase II Trials		
1. Royal Marsden Hospital[§]	190	53 (27%)
2. Upstate Medical Center	91	30 (33%)

*Melbourne, Australia.
[†]Sidney, Australia.
[‡]ER = estrogen receptor.
[§]London, England.

been transient, of 1–2 weeks duration from start of therapy. Cessation of therapy due to poor tolerance has occurred in less than 5% of patients in most reported literature series.

Our trial with aminoglutethimide, conducted at The University of Texas M. D. Anderson Hospital and Tumor Institute at Houston, was given to patients, mostly responders to tamoxifen, after prior standard endocrine therapy. Table II compares results of our study to others reported in the literature (Murray 1982, Kaye 1982, Ingl 1982) in which aminoglutethimide was also given to patients previously treated with tamoxifen. Our response rate of 39% in patients with prior response to tamoxifen was comparable to that achieved by other centers. Of interest were response rates of 19–32% reported in patients who had not previously responded to tamoxifen. Lower response rates of less than 35% were observed when aminoglutethimide was given to patients regardless of prior hormonal response or estrogen receptor (ER) status (Table II). Thus, pooling of worldwide data would suggest that aminoglutethimide has the same order of activity as tamoxifen. This has since been confirmed by many prospective randomized studies of tamoxifen and aminoglutethimide (Smith et al. 1981; Lipton et al. 1982).

BIOLOGIC THERAPY OR IMMUNOTHERAPY

This is an area of research that has recently generated a great deal of excitement. Interferon is a naturally occurring protein that has potent antiviral, antiproliferative, and immunomodulating properties. Interferons have been shown to inhibit tumor growth and prolong survival in experimental tumor models. A phase II study was initiated here at UT M. D. Anderson Hospital in 1978 with leukocyte interferon. In this study, leukocyte interferon was given at two induction dose schedules of 5 million or 9 million antiviral units daily, intramuscularly, for 4–26 weeks. Responding patients were maintained on a schedule of 3 million units three times weekly (Gutterman et al. 1980). Seventeen patients with recurrent metastatic breast cancer were entered in the study. All of these patients had failed conventional treatments with surgery, radiotherapy, hormonal therapy, and, in most cases, chemotherapy. Partial responses (PR) were seen in four of 11 patients treated with 3 million units and in two of six patients treated with 9 million units. Responses were seen predominantly in soft tissue sites and in patients who had prior response to systemic chemotherapy or hormonal therapy. A subsequent multiinstitutional trial with leukocyte-derived interferon was conducted by the American Cancer Society (Borden et al. 1982). In this study, leukocyte interferon was given initially daily for 28 days at 3 million units; subsequently, responding or stable patients were randomized to receive interferon for 2 additional weeks, either at the initial dose of 3 million units or at an escalated dose of 9 million units. Following these additional weeks of therapy, responding patients were further randomized to discontinue maintenance therapy or receive maintenance therapy at the low dose of 3 million units for a period equal to the time to PR. Of the 26 patients entered in the study, 23 were considered evaluable, and there were five PR and four minor responses. Patients who were randomized to receive maintenance therapy had longer durations of response compared with those who were randomized to discontinue interferon. The sites of response included the lymph nodes, chest wall, pleura, and bladder, in which involvement had been proven by biopsy. None of the patients entered in the study had received prior systemic chemotherapy for recurrent metastatic breast cancer.

Recent advances in recombinant DNA technology have provided a method of producing a large quantity of interferon using bacterial cells. A recent phase I study was conducted by a group of investigators at Stanford University with recombinant leukocyte A interferon in eight patients with advanced cancer (Horning et al. 1982).

Their preliminary observations suggest evidence of antitumor activities in breast cancer, lymphoma, and chronic myelogenous leukemia. Thus, the eventual role of interferon in the treatment of patients with breast cancer remains to be defined. The increasing availability of interferon will, hopefully, facilitate the ultimate establishment of the efficacy of interferon in the treatment of breast cancer patients in the near future.

CHEMOTHERAPY

A number of interesting novel chemotherapeutic compounds have recently entered clinical trials, both in this country and in Europe:

1. Anthracene derivatives:

Both mitoxantrone and bisantrene are anthracene derivatives that were synthesized and developed in an effort to identify a DNA-reactive cytotoxic agent similar to doxorubicin with a broad spectrum of antitumor activity, but devoid of cardiotoxicity (Johnson et al. 1979). The drug mitoxantrone was the first to be clinically evaluated and has since been found to be well tolerated without significant toxicity, except for mild nausea and vomiting. Myelosuppression was dose limiting. Unfortunately, our data suggest its potential for cardiotoxicity in patients previously treated with 350 mg/m^2 or more of Adriamycin (Schell et al. 1982). Cardiotoxicity has not been reported in patients not previously treated with Adriamycin. Bisantrene has not, to date, demonstrated any evidence of cardiotoxicity, and, except for phlebitis, the drug is generally well tolerated. Significant alopecia has not been seen with either drug.

Immediately following completion of our phase I study with mitoxantrone, we initiated a phase II study in refractory metastatic breast cancer employing a 5-day intermittent dose schedule. There were one CR and five PR among 27 evaluable patients, giving an overall response rate of 22% in a group of heavily pretreated patients (Yap et al. 1982). The majority of these patients had had at least three prior chemotherapeutic regimens. These results suggest that mitoxantrone probably has the same order of activity as doxorubicin for the treatment of breast cancer patients.

Subsequent phase II studies (Table III) employing a single schedule of 10–14 mg/m^2 intravenously (I.V.) every 3–4 weeks were undertaken by investigators at the Royal Marsden Hospital (Stuart-Harris and Smith 1982), the clinical screening group of the European Organization on Research and Treatment of Cancer (EORTC) (Jager et al. 1982) and the Southwest Oncology Group (SWOG) (Knight et al. 1982). Analysis of these results suggests a dose-response phenomenon. Aside from the study conducted by the SWOG, most investigators have reported antitumor activities with mitoxantrone in metastatic breast cancer.

Bisantrene (Table IV) has been evaluated both at our institution (Yap et al. 1982) as well as by investigators at The University of Texas Health Science Center at San Antonio (Osborne et al. 1982) with comparable results. Our study was initiated at the recommended phase-II dose of 250 mg/m^2 given as a single dose I.V. every 3

Table 3. *Mitoxantrone: Phase II Studies*

A) Royal Marsden Hospital*		
No. treated	29	
Complete response	0	
Partial response	8	
Mixed response	2	
B) E.O.R.T.C.[†]		
No. evaluable	53	
Partial response	10	
C) S.W.O.G.[‡]	Good Risk	Poor Risk
No. entered	25	67
No. evaluable	20	53
Partial response	0	3 (4%)
Stable disease	5	7
Progressive disease	15	43

*London, England.
[†]European Organization on Research and Treatment of Cancer, Brussels, Belgium.
[‡]Southwest Oncology Group, Houston, Texas.

Table 4. *Bisantrene*

A) UT M. D. Anderson Hospital	
Treatment plan: 250 mg/m^2 IV every 3 weeks	
Results: no. entered	44
no. evaluable	40
partial response	9 (22%)
stable disease	13
progressive disease	21
B) UT Health Science Center at San Antonio	
Treatment plan: 260 mg/m^2 IV every 3 weeks	
Results: no. entered	30
no. evaluable	30
complete response	2
partial response	4
stable disease	10
progressive disease	14
response rate	20%

weeks. Subsequently, because of the lack of myelosuppression, the starting dose was escalated in most patients to 300 mg/m^2. Most of our patients treated with bisantrene had had extensive prior chemotherapeutic regimens, and all had failed prior therapy with doxorubicin-containing combinations. It does appear that both bisantrene and mitoxantrone are effective new agents.

2. Elliptinium acetate

Elliptinium acetate (Juret et al. 1982) is a synthetic derivative of ellipticine, a naturally occurring plant alkaloid. It has a high DNA affinity and a very favorable chemotherapeutic index in L1210 leukemias. In addition, it has been found to be

Table 5. *Elliptinium Acetate: Phase II Studies in Breast Cancer*

A) Institute of Gustave-Roussy, Villejuif, France

No. of patients	57
Complete response	2
Partial response	8
Stable disease	12
Response rate	17.5%

B) Centre Francois Baclesse, Caen, France

Prior Treatment	No. Patients	Responded* (%)
Conventional, including		
doxorubicin	56	16 (29)
Endocrine therapy only	40	15 (37)

C) EORTC,[†] Brussels, Belgium

No. of patients	36
Partial response	7 (19%)
Stable disease	13 (36%)
Progressive disease	16
Duration of response	2 to 8 months

*Duration of response: 3 to 17 weeks.
[†]European Organization on Research and Treatment of Cancer.

less toxic than ellipticine. Elliptinium acetate first entered clinical trials in Europe in 1977, and several phase I–II studies have since been completed. Elliptinium acetate has now entered phase I evaluations in this country. Promising clinical data have already been generated in three phase II studies conducted in Europe in patients with metastatic breast cancer as shown in Table V. Employing a weekly I.V. dose of 100 mg/m^2, investigators in both Belgium and France have reported significant activity in patients with refractory breast cancer. A response rate in excess of 25% was seen among patients previously exposed to extensive chemotherapy, whereas patients who have had no prior systemic chemotherapy had a higher response rate of 37%. A subsequent multiinstitutional study undertaken by the EORTC utilizing the same weekly dose schedule of 100 mg/m^2 revealed comparable results. As with earlier studies, the lack of significant myelosuppression was the predominant finding. No hepatic toxicity or cardiotoxicity was observed, and the drug did not cause alopecia. Dryness of the mouth was the most frequent toxicity and occurred in two-thirds of the patients. Other side effects were less frequent, including nausea, vomiting, phlebitis, and occasional cases of hemolysis, neuropsychiatric symptoms, and renal failure. In view of significant activities in refractory breast cancer reported by most European investigators and the lack of myelosuppression, elliptinium acetate deserves further study and may have an important role in combination chemotherapy for the treatment of breast cancer.

DISCUSSION

The last decade has seen tremendous progress in the management of patients with metastatic breast cancer who have failed primary cytotoxic therapy. Our intensive research efforts have led to the identification of an increasing number of new agents that possess not only significant antitumor activity but also fewer side effects. New hormonal agents that can inhibit the conversion of androgenic precursors to estrogenic compounds are on the horizon. The tremendous advances in recombinant DNA technology will also provide investigators with an easy availability of a large quantity of interferons for the conduct of clinical trials. Many biologic response modifiers have also recently entered phase I–II evaluations. In the field of chemotherapy, in addition to the few novel compounds presented earlier, analog research has produced a large number of anthracycline and cisplatin analogs that have recently entered clinical evaluations in this country and in Europe. It seems more than likely that the 1980's will be an exciting era for all clinicians who are committed to improving the care of cancer patients.

REFERENCES

Borden, E. C., J. F. Holland, and T. L. Dao. 1982. Leukocyte-derived interferon (Alpha) in human breast cancer. Ann. Int. Med. 79:1–6.

Gutterman, J. U., G. Blumenschein, and R. Alexanian. 1980. Leukocyte interferon-induced tumor regression in human metastatic breast cancer, multiple myeloma, and malignant lymphoma. Ann. Int. Med. 93:399–406.

Horning, S. J., J. F. Leving, and R. N. Miller. 1982. Clinical and immunologic effects of recombinant leukocyte A interferon in eight patients with advanced cancer. JAMA 247:1718–1722.

Jager, R., P. Cappelaere, and H. Earl. 1982. Phase II clinical trial of mitoxantrone: 1, 4-dihydroxy-5-8-bis(((2-((2-hydroxyethyl)amino)ethyl)amino))9,10 anthracenedione dihydrochloride in solid tumors and lymphomas. (Abstract) Proc. Am. Soc. Clin. Oncol. 1:89.

Johnson, R. K., R. K. Y. Zee-Cheng, and W. W. Lee. 1979. Experimental antitumor activity of aminoanthraquinones. Cancer Treat. Rep. 63:425–439.

Juret, P., J. F. Heron, J. E. Couette, T. Delozier, and J. Y. Le Talaer. 1982. Hydroxy-9-methyl-2-ellipticinium for osseous metastases from breast cancer: A 5-years experience. Cancer Treat. Rep. 66:1909–1916.

Ingl, J. N., S. J. Green, D. L. Ahmann, J. H. Edmondson, W. C. Nichols, S. F. Frytak, and J. Rubin. 1982. Progress report on two clinical trials in women with advanced breast cancer. Trial I: Tamoxifen versus tamoxifen plus aminoglutethimide; Trial II: Aminoglutethimide in patients with prior tamoxifen exposure. Cancer Res. (suppl.) 42:3461s–3467s.

Kaye, S. B., R. L. Woods, R. M. Fox, A. S. Coates, and M. H. N. Tatersall. 1982. Use of aminoglutethimide as second-line endocrine therapy in metastatic breast cancer. Cancer Res. (suppl.) 42:3445–3447.

Knight, W. A., III, D. D. Von Hoff, B. Tranum, and R. O'Bryan. 1982. Phase II trial of dihydroxyanthracenedione (DHAD, mitoxantrone) in breast cancer. Proc. Am. Soc. Clin. Oncol. 1:87.

Legha, S. S., A. U. Buzdar, and T. L. Smith. 1979. Complete remissions in metastatic breast cancer treated with combination drug therapy. Ann. Int. Med. 91:847–852.

Lipton, A., H. A. Harvey, and R. J. Santen. 1982. Randomized trial of aminoglutethimide versus tamoxifen in metastatic breast cancer. Cancer Res. 42:3434s–3436s.

Murray, R. M., and P. Pitt. 1982. Use of Aminoglutethimide in tamoxifen-resistant patients: The Melbourne experience. Cancer Res. (suppl.) 42:3437–3441.

Osborn, C. K., D. D. Von Hoff, and J. Sandback. 1982. Activity of bisantrene in a phase II study in advanced breast cancer. Proc. Am. Soc. Clin. Oncol. 1:87.

Schell, F. C., H. Y. Yap, G. R. Blumenschein, M. Valdivieso, and G. P. Bodey. 1982. Potential cardiotoxicity with mitoxantrone. Cancer Treat. Rep. 66:1641–1643.

Smith, I. E., A. L. Harris, and M. Morgan. 1981. Tamoxifen versus aminoglutethimide in advanced breast carcinoma. A randomized cross-over trial. Br. Med. J. 283:1432–1434.

Stuart-Harris, R. C., and I. E. Smith. 1982. Mitoxantrone: A phase II study in the treatment of patients with advanced breast carcinoma and other solid tumors. Cancer Chemother. Pharmacol. 8:179–182.

Yap, H-Y., G. R. Blumenschein, F. Schell, A. Buzdar, M. Valdivieso, and G. Bodey. 1981. Dihydroxyanthracenedione: A promising new drug in the treatment of metastatic breast cancer. Ann. Intern. Med. 95:694–697.

Yap, H-Y., B. S. Yap, and G. R. Blumenschein. 1982. Bisantrene, an active new drug in the treatment of metastatic breast cancer. Cancer Res. (in press).

Current Controversies in Breast Cancer, edited
by F. C. Ames, G. R. Blumenschein, and E. D. Montague.
University of Texas Press, Austin © 1984.

Chemohormonal Therapy in Metastatic Breast Cancer

Frederick R. Ahmann, M.D., and Stephen E. Jones, M.D.

Department of Internal Medicine, University of Arizona Cancer Center, Tucson, Arizona

The therapy of recurrent or metastatic breast cancer has evolved significantly over the past 25 years. Endocrine therapy, until the 1970s, was the primary palliative treatment of this disease, dating from 1894 when oophorectomy was demonstrated to result in breast cancer regression (Beaston 1896). However, endocrine therapies are limited by several factors. Overall, only one in three unselected cases of metastatic breast cancer can be expected to respond to hormonal therapy (Stoll 1972), and survival has averaged only 1 year when endocrine therapy is the only treatment given (Cutler et al. 1969). If patients have involvement of either liver or lung, survivals of even shorter duration are found (Cutler et al. 1969).

The introduction of cytotoxic chemotherapy carried with it a high expectation of altering these limitations. Aggressive combination chemotherapy regimens have led to improved response rates approaching 75% and have additionally led to median survivals of over 2 years in unselected patients (Jones 1980). However, cures of metastatic breast cancer are rare, improvements in response rates and survival appear to have plateaued, and the toxicity of cytotoxic chemotherapy is a significant limiting factor.

Interest has more recently focused on a therapeutic approach combining endocrine and cytotoxic therapy. A major rationale is that endocrine maneuvers and cytotoxic chemotherapy may exert their anticancer effects through different modes of action (Stoll 1979). Consequently, a combination of the two could theoretically result in either additive or synergistic anticancer effects. The key to discussing the results of published clinical trials utilizing combined chemohormonal therapy in metastatic breast cancer is a recognition that many prognostic variables influence outcome and make interpretation of studies difficult (Nash et al. 1980). Chemotherapy and endocrine therapy can be administered concurrently or sequentially in either order. Patient populations to be studied may have very different characteristics, especially those predicting a response to hormonal therapy. Because estrogen-receptor (ER) and progesterone-receptor (PR) protein studies provide a high predictive index of response to endocrine maneuvers (Lippman and Allegra 1978), a knowledge of the presence of these particular characteristics in patients would be ideal but is seldom available. Similarly, groups of patients who have previously received hormonal or cytotoxic therapy before entering on a combined modality study will have a different prognosis than previously untreated patients. Additional complicating factors in interpreting these trials are the choices of chemotherapy that can vary by agent or agents, drug doses, and schedule, as well as the choices of hormonal therapy. Gland ablation and estrogens, progesterones, androgens, and anti-estrogens are all recognized effective hormonal maneuvers of different efficacy that can be utilized in combined modality studies (Stoll 1972). Thus, analysis of studies considering all of these factors and others is difficult. Accordingly, we will divide chemohormonal trials into five categories and discuss each separately.

OOPHORECTOMY AND CHEMOTHERAPY IN
PREMENOPAUSAL PATIENTS

Six studies have utilized a therapeutic approach of oophorectomy with or without chemotherapy in premenopausal women with metastatic breast cancer (Table 1). Study design was similar in most studies. In 1973, the Cancer and Leukemia Group B (CALGB) conducted a study based on a previous report from South Africa of combined chemohormonal therapy as well as their own success with combination chemotherapy utilizing cyclophosphamide, methotrexate, and 5-fluorouracil (5-FU) (CMF) plus vincristine and prednisone (CMFVP) (Falkson et al. 1979). The CALGB study randomized 145 previously untreated premenopausal women to be treated with oophorectomy plus CMFVP, oophorectomy plus cyclophosphamide, or oophorectomy followed by CMFVP at the time of relapse. Estrogen-receptor studies were unavailable at the time this study was initiated. Response rates in the combined therapy groups were 72% and 65%, respectively, and were significantly greater than the 18% response rate noted in patients treated initially with oophorectomy alone. However, there was no statistical difference in overall survival between any of the treatment groups.

The Swiss Group for Clinical Cancer Research (SAKK) has performed two trials of combined chemohormonal therapy in premenopausal patients. In the initial study, SAKK randomized 42 previously untreated premenopausal patients to receive either oophorectomy plus CMFVP or CMFVP chemotherapy alone (Brunner et al. 1977). The 19 patients who received the combined modality therapy had a significantly higher response rate and median survival when compared to those who received chemotherapy alone. The second Swiss study, which is still ongoing, is more complicated. In a preliminary report, 80 premenopausal women had been randomized to undergo oophorectomy followed by chemotherapy or followed by chemotherapy upon relapse (Jungi et al. 1980). Three different chemotherapy regimens were employed with a separate randomization. Hence, six different treatment groups were created. An interim analysis that evaluated concurrent versus delayed chemotherapy revealed a higher response rate for the concurrent combined therapy group but no significant difference in median survival (Jungi et al. 1980).

At the Mayo Clinic, a similar study was performed. Seventy-three evaluable, untreated, premenopausal patients with metastatic breast cancer all underwent oopho-

Table 1. *Oophorectomy Plus Chemotherapy in Previously Untreated Premenopausal ER-Unknown Patients*

Institution* (Reference)	Treatment Groups[†]	Number Evaluable	CR + PR[‡] Response Rate (%)	Median (Months) RFS[§]	Survival
CALGB	oophorectomy + CMFVP vs	53	72	17	26
	oophorectomy + C vs	54	65	16	23
	oophorectomy → CMFVP[‖]	38	18+50[#]	5+8	30
SAKK	oophorectomy +CMFVP vs	19	74	9.5	19.9
	CMFVP	23	43	7.8	13.2
SAKK	oophorectomy +CMFP, CMFVP, CMFAP vs	42	57	NA[¶]	20.5
	oophorectomy → CMFP, CMFVP, CMFAP on relapse	38	19+26	NA	20.4
Mayo Clinic	oophorectomy +ChFP vs	36	38	8.2	30.3
	oophorectomy → ChFP	37	27+21[#]	3.9	20.3
ECOG	oophorectomy +CMF	20	NA	17.5	41.3
	oophorectomy → chemotherapy	14	NA	6.1	40.4

* Abbreviations are as follows: CALGB = Cancer and Leukemia Group B; SAKK = Swiss Group for Clinical Cancer Research; ECOG = Eastern Cooperative Oncology Group.
[†] Abbreviations are as follows: C = cyclophosphamide; M = methotrexate, V = vincristine, P = prednisone, F = 5-fluorouracil, A = Adriamycin, Ch = chlorambucil.
[‡] CR = complete response, PR = partial response.
[§] RFS = relapse-free survival.
[‖] Given sequentially upon relapse.
[#] Induction and sequential therapy response rates.
[¶] NA = not available.

rectomy and were then randomized to receive immediate chemotherapy with chlorambucil, 5-FU, plus prednisone (ChFP) or identical ChFP upon relapse (Ahmann et al. 1977). Although this study included patients with nonmeasurable disease (making any assessment of accurate response rates difficult), there was a significant increase in relapse-free survival and overall survival, favoring the use of immediate combined chemohormonal therapy over hormonal therapy.

In the most recent study published in this area, the Eastern Cooperative Oncology Group (ECOG) entered 106 previously untreated premenopausal patients who underwent oophorectomy. Those who achieved either stable disease or a response were then randomized to receive CMF chemotherapy either immediately or upon relapse (Rossof et al. 1982). This study design was important in that it assured that the patients who were randomized to receive either immediate or delayed chemotherapy had demonstrated some response to endocrine therapy and would therefore theoretically benefit from a combined therapy approach. However, only 34 of the 106 patients achieved tumor regression with ovarian ablation and hence were eligible for randomization. Of the 20 patients who received immediate chemotherapy with CMF, the relapse-free survival was 17.5 months versus only 6.1 months for the group receiving delayed chemotherapy. However, overall survival in both treatment groups did not differ significantly: 41.3 versus 40.4 months (Rossof et al. 1982).

In summary, six clinical trials of oophorectomy plus chemotherapy have been performed in a relatively homogeneous population of previously untreated premenopausal women. A higher response rate appears to be obtainable with combined chemohormonal therapy, but no clear overall survival impact can be deduced. However, no clinical trial involving even a moderate number of patients has provided information about ER protein, which would allow an assessment of treatment effects in important subgroups of patients.

ESTROGEN (DIETHYLSTILBESTROL) PLUS CHEMOTHERAPY

Until recently, Diethylstilbestrol (DES) was one of the commonest additive hormonal therapies for postmenopausal women with metastatic breast cancer. Overall, 30% to 35% of unselected postmenopausal patients respond to DES therapy (Council on Drugs 1960). Not surprisingly, several groups have studied the effects of combined chemotherapy plus DES therapy (Table 2).

The first reported trial of combined chemohormonal therapy with DES was conducted in the late 1960s at a Queens Hospital center affiliation in Jamaica, New York (Firat and Olshin 1968). Thirty-two evaluable postmenopausal patients were randomized to receive either combined DES plus cyclophosphamide or the same treatment given sequentially. This study was limited by the small number of patients treated. There was no difference in response rates, and no survival information was published.

The Swiss Group for Clinical Cancer Research published the results of a trial in which 96 postmenopausal patients were treated with either DES plus a CMFVP regimen of combination chemotherapy or with the same chemotherapy alone (Brunner et al. 1977). The combined modality therapy group, when analyzed, had fewer patients with bony metastases. The higher response rate reported for this treatment group must be interpreted with this knowledge, though the difference in response rate was not statistically significant. Overall median survival, however, was prolonged with combined chemohormonal therapy compared to chemotherapy.

One of the few studies in this field using ER data was carried out at the University of Wisconsin (Kiang et al. 1981). There, 87 evaluable, previously untreated postmenopausal women were stratified as ER positive, ER negative, or ER unknown. Patients who were ER positive or unknown were randomized to receive either DES and then cyclophosphamide plus 5-FU given at relapse or to receive this same treatment given concurrently. Estrogen-receptor negative patients were ran-

Table 2. DES Plus Chemotherapy in Previously Untreated Postmenopausal Patients

Institution (Reference)	Treatment†	Number Evaluable	ER Status‡			CR + PR§ Response Rate (%)	RFS‖ (Median Months)	Survival
			+	−	unk.			
SAKK*	DES + CMFVP vs	48	0	0	48	63	8.4	26.7
	CMFVP	48	0	0	48	54	10.6	19.2
Queens Hospital New York	DES + C vs	18	0	0	18	28	NA#	NA
	DES → C	14	0	0	14	29	NA	NA
University of Wisconsin	CF	11	0	11	0	18	NA	NA
	DES → CF¶ vs	28	15	0	13	44	NA	NA
	DES + CF	48	15	11	22	67	NA	NA

* SAKK = Swiss Group for Clinical Cancer Research.
† DES = diethylstilbestrol; C = cyclophosphamide; M = methotrexate; F = 5-fluorouracil; V = vincristine; P = prednisone.
‡ ER = estrogen receptor; (+) positive; (−) negative.
§ CR = complete response; PR = partial response.
‖ RFS = relapse-free survival.
¶ Given sequentially on relapse.
# NA = not available.

domized to receive either chemotherapy with cyclophosphamide plus 5-FU or to receive combined chemohormonal therapy with DES plus cyclophosphamide and 5-FU. The concurrent combined therapy groups showed higher response rates when compared with those receiving either chemotherapy alone or sequential therapy. Additionally, a superior median survival was found in both the ER-positive and the ER-unknown groups with combined chemohormonal therapy.

In summary, two moderately large studies combining chemohormonal therapy with DES have been reported. In both, combined chemohormonal therapy appears to be associated with higher response rates and improved survival when compared to the use of chemotherapy alone or to sequential use of these modalities.

TAMOXIFEN PLUS CHEMOTHERAPY

Because serum estrogen levels may not fall to zero after oophorectomy or adrenalectomy, an alternative therapeutic strategy has been to block estrogen effects. Drugs that bind to ER or block the action of estrogens are termed antiestrogens and have demonstrated to have activity in the treatment of metastatic breast cancer in both pre- and postmenopausal patients (Legha et al. 1978). At present, the first widely available antiestrogen, tamoxifen, has largely replaced DES as the first-line hormonal agent in patients with metastatic breast cancer. Thus, several studies have examined the effect of combining chemotherapy with tamoxifen (Table 3).

In 1976, the European Organization for Research on the Treatment of Cancer (EORTC) published a preliminary report of a pilot study of tamoxifen plus chemotherapy consisting of courses of Adriamycin and vincristine alternating with cyclophosphamide, methotrexate, and 5-FU (Heuson 1976). Fifty-five postmenopausal patients were treated. A response rate of 73% was reported, but no survival data were given.

More recently, another group in Italy investigated the effects of therapy with CMF plus tamoxifen versus CMF followed by tamoxifen at relapse (Cocconi et al. 1982). One hundred thirty-three postmenopausal patients were randomized; approximately 40% had previously been treated with another endocrine therapy. Estrogen-receptor protein studies were available for approximately 50% of the patients, and a majority were ER positive. The response rate to combined chemohormonal therapy was superior, with a trend towards improved relapse-free survival. However, overall survival was similar as was the response rate. Survival of ER-positive and ER-negative patients was not compared, probably due to inadequate numbers of patients.

In a preliminary report from The University of Texas M. D. Anderson Hospital and Tumor Institute at Houston, improved survival for patients who had initially responded to tamoxifen therapy and were then given combination chemotherapy with 5-FU, Adriamycin, and cyclophosphamide (FAC) was noted when compared to survival of patients who suffered progressive disease on initial tamoxifen and were then treated with FAC chemotherapy (Legha et al. 1982). This treatment approach was used in 85 women, of whom 69 were postmenopausal. A small sub-

Table 3. Tamoxifen Plus Chemotherapy

Institution* (Reference)	Treatment†	Number Evaluable	Prior Hormonal Therapy	Prior Chemotherapy	ER Status‡ +	−	Unk.	Number Premenopausal	Number Postmenopausal	CR + PR§ Response Rate (%)	Median (Months) RFS||	From Treatment
EROTC	T + alt. AV-CMF	55	NA#	NA	0	0	55	0	55	73	NA	NA
Parma, Italy	CMF→T' vs CMF + T	71	30	0	13	7	21	0	71	51	10.9	25.6
		62	26	0	15	4	17	0	62	74	11.8	18
UT M. D. Anderson Hospital	T + FAC vs T + FACT vs FACT	36	0	0	0	0	36	0			13	20
		40	0	0	0	0	40	16	69	81	23.5	39
		9	0	0	0	0	40				23.5	39
NCI	CAMF vs CAMF + T + premarin	90	NA	some			90	NA	NA	62	13	17
			NA	some				NA	NA	60	17	39
SAKK	T + CMFP, LMFVP LMFAP vs T→ LMF, LMFVP LMFAP	74	0	0	0	0	74	0	74	44	NA	17.8
		75	0	0	0	0	75	0	75	40**	19.4	25.6
U. of A.	TAC	63	15	0	12	12	39	6	57	82	18.5	27.3

*Abbreviations are as follows: EROTC = European Organization for Research on the Treatment of Cancer; NCI = National Cancer Institute; SAKK = Swiss Group for Clinical Cancer Research; U. of A. = University of Arizona.
†Abbreviations are as follows: T = tamoxifen; A = Adriamycin; V = vincristine; C = cyclophosphamide; M = methotrexate; F = 5-fluorouracil; P = prednisone; L = chlorambucil (Leukeran).
‡ER = estrogen receptor; (+) positive; (−) negative.
§CR = complete response; PR = partial response.
||RFS = relapse-free survival.
#NA = not available.
'Given sequentially upon relapse.
**Includes chemotherapy responses upon tamoxifen relapse.

group of nine patients received combined chemohormonal therapy with FAC and tamoxifen initially because of life-threatening disease. The overall response rate was 81%, and relapse-free survival was longer in tamoxifen responders (23.5 months) than in the tamoxifen-insensitive patients (13 months). Overall median survival was almost doubled in the tamoxifen responders (39 months).

In another recent trial, 90 patients were randomized to receive combination chemotherapy with cyclophosphamide, Adriamycin, methotrexate, and 5-FU (CAMF) or the same chemotherapy plus tamoxifen and premarin (Lippman et al. 1982). Although the response rate in the combined chemohormonal therapy group was not improved, there was a significant benefit in both relapse-free survival and overall survival for the combined therapy group.

Utilizing a study design similar to their oophorectomy with or without chemotherapy trial, the SAKK has published early results from a study of postmenopausal patients involving tamoxifen (Jungi et al. 1980). All patients were initially treated with tamoxifen, and half were randomized to receive additionally one of three combination chemotherapy regimens. The group that initially received tamoxifen alone was treated at relapse with the same chemotherapy. At interim evaluation, the response rate for the combined chemohormonal therapy group was no higher than the response rate of those receiving initial hormonal therapy plus chemotherapy at first relapse. Thus far no overall survival advantage has been indicated for initial combined therapy either. However, this study involves six different treatment groups and must accrue more patients with longer follow-up before potential differences can be detected.

At the University of Arizona, we have carried out a pilot study with almost 2 years of median follow-up. Sixty-three consecutive patients previously untreated with chemotherapy have been treated with tamoxifen plus Adriamycin and cyclophosphamide (TAC) (Ahmann et al. 1981). An 82% response rate was observed with a median relapse-free survival of 80 weeks and a median overall survival of 118 weeks. Estrogen-receptor protein data was available on 24 of the 63 patients, and in that small group ER status was not of apparent prognostic significance for overall survival ($P = 0.56$); however, most patients were postmenopausal. Indeed an initial time to first recurrence of more than 2 years was a significant prognostic factor in survival, suggesting that presumed ER positivity might be important.

These results with TAC were compared to a similar population of patients with metastatic breast cancer treated with Adriamycin plus cyclophosphamide alone (AC) (Jones et al. 1975). The overall response rate and complete response rate for TAC was virtually identical to that observed with AC (82% vs. 78% with about 20% of patients achieving a CR). However, survival associated with TAC was significantly better than with AC. With further analyses of prognostic factors between these two groups, it now appears that differences in these factors might account for the differences observed in survival.

Of particular interest in light of our results with TAC is a clinical trial under way by the Australian-New Zealand group. In this trial, which has not yet been formally reported, patients with previously untreated metastatic breast cancer were randomized to receive tamoxifen alone, AC chemotherapy alone, or TAC chemohormonal therapy with appropriate crossover at relapse (J. Forbes, personal communication 1982). The final results of this trial are awaited with interest; the trial appears to be a definitive evaluation of sequential versus combined modality therapy.

In summary, combined chemohormonal therapy with tamoxifen has been the best-studied therapeutic schema. These studies have in general encompassed aggressive combination chemotherapy regimens and have largely been utilized in postmenopausal patients. What is most clear from these studies is that a high response rate can be achieved. While some studies have reported survival benefit, there is no clear overall trend to the concurrent combined therapy approach. However, there is certainly no therapeutic disadvantage to this approach in terms of response rate and survival.

ANDROGENS PLUS CHEMOTHERAPY

Androgens were one of the first hormonal therapies to be combined with chemotherapy. This occurred for two reasons: Not only were androgens a recognized second-line hormonal therapy inducing an overall response rate approximately half that of estrogens in postmenopausal patients, but androgens were known to be nonspecific bone marrow stimulants (Council on Drugs 1960). Because myelosuppression is a dose-limiting toxicity of cytotoxic chemotherapy, much speculation exists as to whether the addition of androgens to chemotherapy might induce a higher response rate not only by having direct antitumor effects but by allowing a higher dose of cytotoxic chemotherapy to be delivered (Table 4).

In 1973 a report from Manchester Hospital in England summarized a study of 78 postmenopausal patients who were randomized to receive one of three treatments: Daily cyclophosphamide, nandrolone, or a combination of these two drugs (Cole et al. 1973). There were no responses noted in the 26 patients who received androgen therapy alone, and only 1 of 22 patients treated with both agents responded. Seven patients who received cyclophosphamide alone achieved a response, and this group had a significantly prolonged survival. The results of the study are difficult to interpret as it is unlikely that concurrent androgen use would detract from therapeutic results.

A similar study was conducted in the United States comparing the use of single-agent 5-FU, testolactone, or a combination of these two drugs (Goldberg et al. 1975). The use of 5-FU resulted in tumor regressions in only two of 35 patients, while testolactone therapy produced eight responses in 40 patients. The combined therapy group had five responses among 36 patients treated.

The Mayo Clinic has also published results of a study utilizing androgens and chemotherapy in postmenopausal patients with advanced breast cancer (Eagan et al. 1975). Forty-nine patients were randomized to receive three different treatment arms: Chemotherapy with methotrexate, Adriamycin, and vincristine; chemotherapy with CFP; and combined therapy with CFP plus calusterone. Only 12 pa-

Table 4. Androgens Plus Chemotherapy in ER-Unknown Patients

Institution* (Reference)	Treatment†	Number Evaluable	Prior Hormonal Therapy	Prior Chemotherapy	Number Premenopausal	Number Post-menopausal	CR + PR‡ Response Rate (%)	RFS§ (Median Months)	Survival (Median Months)
U. of A.	AC + calusterone vs AC	20	NA‖	0	20	18	65	21.5	23.5
Mayo Clinic	MAV vs CFP	36	some		11	25	53	11.5	11.5
		23	some	0	0	23	48	7.4	NA
	CFP vs CFP + calusterone	14	some	0		14	57	5.8	NA
		12	some	0	0	12	50	8.1	NA
ECOG	CMF	73	most	0	11	62	NA	6.7	19.8
	CMF + fluoxymesterone	67	most	0	13	54	NA	9.5	23.3
Cooperative Breast Cancer Group	F vs testolactone	35	NA	NA	13	22	6	NA	NA
		40	NA	NA	13	27	20	NA	NA
	F + testolactone	36	NA	NA	16	20	14	NA	NA
Manchester Hospital	C vs nandrolone	30	some	NA	0	30	23	6.2	17
		26	some	NA	0	26	0		10
	C + nandrolone	22	some	NA	0	22	5	8	10

(ECOG treatment note: RESPONSE — CMF, CMFP, AV with arrows pointing to CMF and CMF + fluoxymesterone)

* Abbreviations are as follows: U. of A. = University of Arizona; ECOG = Eastern Cooperative Oncology Group.
† Abbreviations are as follows: A = Adriamycin; C = cyclophosphamide; M = methotrexate; V = vincristine; F = 5-fluorouracil; P = prednisone.
‡ CR = complete response; PR = partial response.
§ RFS = relapse-free survival.
‖ NA = not available.

tients in the study received combined therapy. No statistical difference was detected in response rate or relapse-free survival among all patients, but the small number of patients limits the analysis.

In a much larger trial, ECOG evaluated the use of androgens in maintenance after patients achieved remission with chemotherapy (Tormey et al. 1981). This study randomized 481 patients to be placed in one of several remission-induction groups utilizing combination chemotherapy. The 140 patients who achieved a response lasting 6 months were then rerandomized to receive maintenance therapy with either CMF or CMF plus fluoxymesterone. There was no statistical difference in the re-mission induction rate of the therapies utilized. However, those patients who received CMF plus androgen maintenance had an increase in relapse-free and overall survival. In this study, the androgen-treated patients appeared to have had better bone marrow tolerance to cytotoxic chemotherapy (Tormey et al. 1981).

A small study that utilized combination chemotherapy with or without androgens for remission induction was carried out at the University of Arizona (Lloyd et al. 1979). Twelve patients who had received prior androgen therapy were treated with AC, and 44 other patients who had not previously been treated with androgens were randomized to receive AC alone or AC plus calusterone. The combined chemo-hormonal therapy arm included more postmenopausal patients and produced a higher response rate and statistically significant longer relapse-free survival and overall survival than AC alone.

In summary, the studies of combined chemohormonal therapy with androgens in advanced breast cancer have been of interest. Results suggest that there may be a modest benefit in some treatment groups for combined therapy similar to that seen in studies of chemotherapy plus tamoxifen.

PROGESTATIONAL AGENTS PLUS CHEMOTHERAPY

Progestational agents in metastatic breast cancer are clearly active, even in pa-tients who have failed initial hormonal therapy with tamoxifen (Ross et al. 1982). Moreover, these agents are widely used in Europe and have been combined with chemotherapy in at least three studies (Table 5).

The Swiss Group for Clinical Cancer Research has reported a study of 75 postmenopausal patients who had failed previous hormonal therapy (Brunner et al. 1977). Patients were randomized to receive therapy with CMFVP with or without medroxyprogesterone. Each therapy group showed a response rate exceeding 50%, but there was no statistical difference in response rates, relapse-free survival, or overall survival.

A similar study was carried out in London (Rubens et al. 1978). Sixty-nine evalu-able patients who had previously received endocrine therapy were randomized to receive Adriamycin and vincristine with or without norethisterone acetate. The re-sponse rates were not significantly different between treatments, and there was no difference in relapse-free survival.

Recently a preliminary report detailed findings in 256 postmenopausal patients

Table 5. Progestational Agents Plus Chemotherapy in Postmenopausal ER-Unknown Patients

Institution (Reference)	Treatment*	Number Evaluable	Prior Hormonal Therapy	Prior Chemotherapy	CR + PR[†] Response Rate (%)	RFS[‡]	Median (Months) Survival
Italy (28)	VAC + MPA vs VAC	{ 179	NA[§] NA	NA NA	50 48.2	16 9	NA NA
Guy's Hospital, London (31)	AV vs AV + norethisterone acetate	33 36	33 36	0 0	61 53	8.8 8.8	15 8
SAKK[ǁ] (4)	CMFVP + medroxyprogesterone vs CMFVP	38 37	38 37	0 0	53 63	8.9 10	18.1 22.8

*Abbreviations are as follows: V = vincristine; A = Adriamycin; C = cyclophosphamide; M = methotrexate; P = prednisone; F = fluorouracil.
[†]CR = complete response; PR = partial response.
[‡]RFS = relapse-free survival.
[§]NA = not available.
[ǁ]SAKK = Swiss Group for Clinical Cancer Research.

who received therapy with vincristine, Adriamycin, plus cyclophosphamide (VAC) with or without medroxyprogesterone (Pellegrini et al. 1982). There was no difference in the response rates of the two therapies. However, with a median follow-up of 12 months, there was a significant survival benefit for the combined chemohormonal therapy group.

Except for recent preliminary reports, combined chemohormonal therapy with progestational agents has been employed for patients previously treated with other hormonal therapies. This approach must still be regarded as experimental until more definitive trials are carried out.

SUMMARY

Combined chemohormonal therapy continues to be of great interest to physicians who treat patients with metastatic breast cancer. These therapies theoretically accomplish their anticancer effects via different mechanisms of action and could be combined with little danger of increased toxicity. A basic difficulty in studying this concept is the large number of potential prognostic variables that are known to influence outcome, including menopausal status, ER protein levels, previous treatment, multiple endocrine therapy options, multiple chemotherapeutic possibilities, and the apparent observation that endocrine effects are modest in comparison to the effects of combination chemotherapy. Therefore, definitive clinical trials require large numbers of patients (e.g., 150 per treatment group) to detect small differences in response rates or survival.

Until recently, the best patient population to test a combined chemohormonal treatment has been untreated premenopausal patients. In this group, the standard hormonal therapy is oophorectomy (tamoxifen is also commonly used). However, hormonal receptor data is unavailable from any published study in this group of patients. Response rates all favor combined chemohormonal therapies, but a significant positive effect on survival is less clear. The clinical trial that needs to be undertaken should study premenopausal patients at first relapse, focusing on those with ER-positive tumors and randomizing between effective combination chemotherapy (e.g., CMF, CMFVP, AC, VAC, FAC) with or without oophorectomy (or tamoxifen). Patients treated with chemotherapy should receive the appropriate hormonal therapy at relapse. Until this type of trial is completed, there will not be a definitive answer about immediate chemohormonal therapy versus the sequential use of both modalities.

Studies encompassing endocrine treatment modalities other than tamoxifen have also produced variable results. No definite conclusions are possible concerning therapy with progestational agents when combined with chemotherapy, other than that no deleterious effects appear to occur when the therapies are combined. Studies including DES and androgens are encouraging enough to support additional work in this area.

Tamoxifen plus chemotherapy has been evaluated more than any other endocrine modality in combination with chemotherapy. However, ER data are available in only two of the six studies reported to date. High response rates are reported from these studies, largely consisting of postmenopausal patients, but in one randomized study there was no clear survival benefit for patients receiving combined therapy when compared to survival in those receiving sequential therapy. Many of the questions regarding combined chemotherapy with tamoxifen may be answered by a large clinical trial currently ongoing in Australia in which patients are randomized to receive sequential hormonal chemotherapy, sequential chemohormonal therapy, or combined chemohormonal therapy with Adriamycin, cyclophosphamide, and tamoxifen (J. Forbes, personal communication 1982). Once again, the definitive clinical trial should focus on ER-positive tumors at first relapse and evaluate effective chemotherapy with or without tamoxifen (or possibly progestational agents). Without this trial, it will be impossible to define any advantage for combined initial therapy over sequential therapies. At this time, it is clear that combined chemohormonal therapy does not cause inferior results and may be used with some success in patients with life-threatening disease who might not otherwise tolerate a 2- to 3-month trial of endocrine therapy alone. However, there is also no clear evidence of a marked therapeutic advantage of combined chemohormonal therapy, and in unselected patients the combination effects appear, overall, to be less than additive.

ACKNOWLEDGMENTS

This investigation was supported in part by Stuart Pharmaceuticals and by Grant Number CA-17094 awarded by the National Cancer Institute, U.S. Department of Health and Human Services.

REFERENCES

Ahmann, F. R., S. E. Jones, T. E. Moon, S. L. Davis, and S. E. Salmon. 1981. Improved survival of patients with advanced breast cancer treated with Adriamycin-cyclophosphamide plus tamoxifen. (Abstract) Proc. Am. Amer. Assoc. Cancer Res. 22:148.

Ahmann, D. L., M. J. O'Connell, R. G. Hahan, H. F. Bisel, R. A. Lee, and J. H. Edmonson. 1977. An elevation of early or delayed adjuvant chemotherapy in pre-menopausal patients with advanced breast cancer undergoing oophorectomy. N. Engl. J. Med. 297:356–360.

Beaston, G. T. 1896. On the treatment of inoperable cases of carcinoma of the mamma: Suggestions for a new method of treatment with illustrated cases. Lancet 2:104.

Brunner, K. Q., R. W. Sonntag, P. Albert, H. H. Senn, G. Martz, P. Orbecht, and P. Maurice. 1977. Combined chemo- and hormonal therapy in advanced breast cancer. Cancer 39:2923–2933.

Cocconi, G., V. De Lisi, C. Boni, and P. Mori. 1982. CMF vs. CMF plus tamoxifen (T) in postmenopausal metastatic breast cancer. (Abstract) Proc. Am. Soc. Clin. Oncol. 1:75.

Cole, M. P., L. D. H. Tod, and P. M. Wilkinson. 1973. Cyclophosphamide and nandrolone decanoate in the treatment of advanced carcinoma of the breast: Results of a comparative controlled trial of the agents used singly and in combination. Br. J. Cancer. 27:396–399.

Council on Drugs: Report to the Council. 1960. Androgens & estrogens in treatment of disseminated mammary carcinoma: Retrospective study of 1944 patients. JAMA 172:1271–1283.

Cutler, S. J., H. L. Davis, and S. G. Taylor. 1969. Classification of patients with disseminated cancer of the breast. Cancer 24:861–879.

Eagan, R. T., D. L. Ahmann, J. H. Edmonson, R. G. Hahn, and H. F. Bisel. 1975. Controlled evaluation of the combination of Adriamycin (NSC-123123), vincristine (NSC-67574), and methotrexate (NSC-740) in patients with disseminated breast cancer. Cancer Chemotherapy Reports 6:339–342.

Falkson, G., H. D. Falkson, O. Glidewell, V. Weinberg, L. Leone, and J. F. Holland. 1979. Improved remission rates and remission duration in young women with metastatic breast cancer following combined oophorectomy and chemotherapy. Cancer 36:308–310.

Firat, D., and S. Olshin. 1968. Treatment of metastatic carcinoma of the female breast with combination of hormones and other chemotherapy. Cancer Chemotherapy Reports 52:743–750.

Goldberg, I. S., N. Sedransk, H. Volk, A. Segaloff, R. M. Kelley, and C. R. Haines. 1975. Combined androgen and antimetabolite therapy of advanced female breast cancer. Cancer 36:308–310.

Heuson, J. C. 1976. Current overview of EORTC clinical trials with tamoxifen. Cancer Treat. Rep. 60 (7):857–865.

Jones, E. E. 1982. Breast Cancer, in Current Concepts in the Use of Doxorubicin Chemotherapy, S. E. Jones, ed. Grafiche Milani, Milan, Italy, pp. 23–36.

Jones, S. E., B. G. M. Durie, and S. E. Salmon. 1975. Combination chemotherapy with Adriamycin and cyclophosphamide for advanced breast cancer. Cancer 36:90–97.

Jungi, W. F., K. W. Brunner, and F. Cavalli. 1980. Sequential or combined hormono-chemotherapy in disseminated breast cancer. Reviews on Endocrine Related Cancer 5 (Suppl.): 29–42.

Kiang, D. T., D. H. Frenning, J. Gay, A. I. Goldman, and B. J. Kennedy. 1981. Combination therapy of the hormone and cytotoxic agents in advanced breast cancer. Cancer 47:452–456.

Legha, S., G. Blumenschein, G. Hortobagyi, A Buzdar, H. Yap, and G. Bodey. 1982. Treatment of metastatic breast carcinoma using a combination of 5-fluorouracil (F), Adriamycin (A), Cyclophosphamide (C), and Tamoxifen (T). Proc. Am. Soc. Clin. Oncol. 1:C–299.

Legha, D. D., H. L. Davis, and F. M. Muggia. 1978. Hormonal therapy of breast cancer: New approaches and concepts. Ann. Intern. Med. 88:69–77.

Lippman, M. D., and J. C. Allegra. 1978. Receptors in breast cancer. N. Engl. J. Med. 299: 930–933.

Lippman, M. E., J. Cassidy, M. Wesley, and R. C. Young. 1982. A randomized attempt to increase the efficacy of cytotoxic chemotherapy in metastatic breast cancer by hormonal synchronization. (Abstract) Proc. Am. Soc. Clin. Oncol. 1:79.

Lloyd, R. E., S. E. Jones, and S. E. Salmon. 1979. Comparative trial of low-dose Adriamycin plus cyclophosphamide with or without additive hormonal therapy in advanced breast cancer. Cancer 43:60–65.

MacDonald, I. 1962. Endocrine ablation in disseminated mammary carcinomas. Surg. Gynecol. Obstet. 115:215–222.

Nash, C. H., S. E. Jones, T. E. Moon, S. L. Davis, and S. E. Salmon. 1980. Prediction of outcome in metastatic breast cancer treated with Adriamycin combination chemotherapy. Cancer 46:2380–2388.

Nemoto, T., J. Horton, T. Cunningham, R. Sponzo, D. Rosner, R. Diaz, and T. Cao. 1975. Update report: Comparison of combination chemotherapy (FCP) vs. Adriamycin (ADM) vs. adrenalectomy (ADX) in breast cancer. (Abstract) Proc. Am. Assoc. Cancer Res. 16:46.

Oberfield, R. A., R. Caddy, A. G. Pazianos, and F. A. Salzman. 1979. Adrenalectomy-oophorectomy and combined chemotherapy for carcinoma of the breast with metastases. Surg. Gynecol. Obstet. 148:881–886.

Osteen, R. T., J. T. Chaffey, F. D. Moore, and R. E. Wilson. 1978. An aggressive multimodality approach to locally advanced carcinoma of the breast. Surg. Gynecol. Obstet. 147:75–78.

Pellegrini, A., G. Robustelli, R. Esteveg, A. Luchina, J. B. DeSilvaneto, V. L. Puerto, H. Cortes-Funes, and J. Arrazotoa. 1982. Vincristine, Adriamycin, cyclophosphamide (VAC) versus vincristine, Adriamycin, cyclophosphamide plus high dose medroxyprogesterone acetate

(VAC + HD-MPA): A randomized multi national clinical trial in metastatic breast cancer. (Abstract no. 1629) Proceedings of the 13th International Cancer Congress, Florence, Italy.

Ross, M. B., A. U. Buzdar, and G. R. Blumenschein. 1982. Treatment of advanced breast cancer with megestrol acetate after therapy with tamoxifen. Cancer 49:413–417.

Rossof, A. H., R. Gelman, and R. H. Creech. 1982. Randomized evaluation of combination chemotherapy vs. observation alone following response or stabilization after oophorectomy for metastatic breast cancer in pre-menopausal women. Am. J. Clin. Oncol. 5:253–259.

Rubens, R. D., R. H. J. Began, R. K. Knight, S. A. Sexton, and J. L. Hayward. 1978. Combined cytotoxic and progestogen therapy for advanced breast cancer. Cancer 42:1680–1686.

Stoll, B. A. 1979. Prospects for combined endocrine-cytoxic treatment in breast cancer. Reviews on Endocrine Related Cancer 5:29–37.

Stoll, B. A. 1981. Breast cancer: Rationale for endocrine therapy, *in* Hormonal Management of Endocrine-Related Cancer, B. A. Stoll, ed. Lloyd-Luke, Ltd., London, pp. 77–91.

Tormey, D. C., R. Gelman, P. R. Band, M. Sears, M. Bauer, J. C. Arseneau, and G. Falkson. 1981. A prospective evaluation of chemohormonal therapy remission maintenance in advanced breast cancer. Breast Cancer Res. Treat. 1:111–119.

Current Controversies in Breast Cancer, edited
by F. C. Ames, G. R. Blumenschein, and E. D. Montague.
University of Texas Press, Austin © 1984.

Potential for Cure of Metastatic Breast Cancer by Combined Modality Therapy

George R. Blumenschein, M.D., and Kavitha Pinnamaneni, M.D.

*Department of Internal Medicine, The University of Texas M. D. Anderson Hospital and
Tumor Institute at Houston, Houston, Texas*

Combined modality therapy of breast cancer is a treatment that includes both regional therapy (surgery or irradiation) and systemic therapy (chemotherapy or hormonal therapy). Such combination treatment is considered when complete clinical eradication of measurable cancer cannot be achieved by regional or systemic treatment alone.

Response to chemotherapy is in part related to tumor volume. Bulky disease responds less well to chemotherapy than does a smaller tumor burden (Swenerton et al. 1979). When small nodal metastases or small single metastases at other sites are treated with 5-fluorouracil, doxorubicin, and cyclophosphamide (FAC), the complete·remission (CR) rate approaches 40% and the duration of these remissions exceeds a median of 18 months. While chemotherapy is capable of dealing with a microscopic tumor burden, as evidenced by multiple reports of its success in prolonging relapse-free survival when given postoperatively to patients who have stage II breast cancer (Buzdar et al. 1979a, Bonadonna et al. 1977, Holland 1977), patients who have metastatic breast cancer and enter complete remission as a result of chemotherapy usually relapse in the site or sites of initial metastatic involvement (Legha et al. 1979). This suggests that even in circumstances where breast cancer is sensitive to drugs, the number of tumor cells is too great for chemotherapeutic elimination of every cancer cell.

The type of chemotherapy and the doses of drugs administered appear to have a significant effect on breast cancer response in both measurable metastatic disease and microscopic metastatic breast cancer (Swenerton et al. 1979, Buzdar et al. 1981, Bonadonna and Valagussa 1981). Doxorubicin in combination with cyclophosphamide and 5-fluorouracil have been compared to other drug combinations not containing doxorubicin in both metastatic breast cancer and adjuvant trials. In the metastatic disease trials, doxorubicin combination therapy achieved higher complete and partial remissions and was associated with longer remission durations (Bull et al. 1978, Smalley et al. 1977). These results were predicted from review of earlier reports of nondoxorubicin combinations used for therapy of stage IV breast cancer (Canellos et al. 1976, Smalley et al. 1976, Brambilla et al. 1976) and those

307

Table 1. *Response Rates of Doxorubicin Combinations Versus CMF Combinations in Patients with Metastatic Breast Cancer**

| | % CR + PR | |
| | Doxorubicin | CMF |
Trial	Combination	Combination
Smalley et al.	61	42
Bull et al.	82	62

*Abbreviations are as follows: CMF = cyclophosphamide, methotrexate, and 5-fluorouracil; CR = complete remission; PR = partial remission.

Table 2. *Five-Year Relapse-Free Survival of Stage II Breast Cancer Patients Receiving Adjuvant Chemotherapy*

Chemotherapy Program*	% Patients Relapse-Free at 5 Years
L-PAM + 5-FU	57
CMF	61
FAC	75
No chemotherapy	45

*Abbreviations are as follows: L-PAM = L-phenylalanine mustard; 5-FU = 5-fluorouracil; CMF = cyclophosphamide, methotrexate, 5-fluorouracil; FAC = 5-fluorouracil, doxorubicin, cyclophosphamide.

utilizing doxorubicin (Jones et al. 1975, Hortobagyi et al. 1979). A summary of comparative trials of cyclophosphamide, methotrexate, and 5-fluorouracil (CMF) to doxorubicin combinations is shown in Table 1.

Adjuvant trial comparisons of doxorubicin combination chemotherapy to non-doxorubicin combinations are few in number, but they also show improved relapse-free survival to be associated with doxorubicin combination therapy (Jones et al. 1982, Misset et al. 1982). The 5-year relapse-free (RF) survival of patients with stage II breast cancer treated by the most commonly utilized adjuvant programs is shown in Table 2. Again, a modest benefit exists for patients treated with doxorubicin combination as compared to alkeran, 5-fluorouracil, and CMF. It should be noted, however, that adjuvant CMF with vincristine and prednisone, given aggressively and with attendant significant toxicity, can achieve the same results as doxorubicin combination therapy in stage II patients with greater than three positive axillary nodes (Bonadonna et al. 1977).

The efficacy of CMF and doxorubicin combinations is related to dose. This has been reported for 5-fluorouracil, doxorubicin, and cyclophosphamide (FAC) in metastatic disease (Swenerton et al. 1979, Jones et al. 1975, Lloyd et al. 1979) and stage II disease (Buzdar et al. 1981). Similarly, CMF has been shown to be very sensitive to dose reduction (Bonadonna and Valagussa 1981).

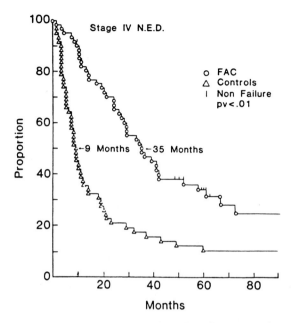

FIG. 1. Relapse-free survival curves for patients with solitary first metastasis treated at UT M. D. Anderson Hospital 1967–1973 (controls), with surgery and/or irradiation, and with regional therapy plus 5-fluorouracil, doxorubicin, cyclophosphamide (FAC) 1974–1977. Median follow-up for FAC is 80 months. (NED = no evidence of disease)

The surgical excision or irradiation for cure of solitary or confined breast cancer metastases has been a long-standing practice (Chu et al. 1976, Tapley 1976). A review of patients so treated at The University of Texas M. D. Anderson Hospital and Tumor Institute at Houston between 1967 and 1973 showed them to have a 9-month median duration of relapse-free survival following regional treatment of initial metastases (Blumenschein et al. 1977) (Figure 1). Patients with chest wall recurrence on the side of the primary breast cancer or regional lymph node recurrences had an improved opportunity for relapse-free survival over patients with recurrences at sites distant to the region of the initial breast cancer. The site of initial metastasis predicted for the duration of relapse-free survival is shown in Table 3.

Regional therapy of small single metastatic breast cancers provided complete clinical remissions for 100% of these patients. The durations of these remissions, however, are relatively short. Half of patients so treated showed evidence of recurrent metastases by 9 months. While only 40% of similar patients achieved complete remission when chemotherapy alone was used, the duration of these remissions was twice as long (Legha et al. 1979).

In 1974, UT M. D. Anderson Hospital initiated a combined regional systemic therapeutic program for treatment of solitary breast cancer metastasis in patients who had received no prior chemotherapy (Buzdar et al. 1979b). Metastatic disease was usually resected, but certain sites were treated with irradiation alone (e.g.,

Table 3. *Percent Patients Relapse Free at 5 Years Following Excision or Irradiation of Initial Single Metastasis in Stage IV Breast Cancer Patients By Site of Recurrence*

Site	Total Patients	No. Relapse Free	% Relapse Free
Regional lymph node	10	2	20
Chest wall	40	2	5
Lung, skin (distant from site of mastectomy)	6	1	16
Bone	6	0	–

single-bone metastasis) and some received both surgical treatment and regional radiotherapy. Patients were then restaged to be certain they were free of other systemic metastases and were started on FAC chemotherapy with nonspecific bacille Calmette Guerin (BCG) immunotherapy. Since BCG therapy was shown in later studies to add no therapeutic benefit, it will not be considered further here (Buzdar et al. 1982a). 5-Fluorouracil was administered in a dose of 400 mg/m^2 IV on days 1 and 8, doxorubicin was administered in a dose of 40 mg/m^2 IV on day 1, and cyclophosphamide was given in a dose of 400 mg/m^2 on day 1. The program was repeated every 28 days until a total cumulative dose of 450 mg/m^2 doxorubicin was achieved. At that point, methotrexate (30 mg/m^2) was substituted for doxorubicin, and chemotherapy was continued until a total elapsed time of 24 months of systemic therapy had been administered.

The median duration of relapse-free survival for the group of 62 patients entered on the study between 1974 and 1977 was 35 months. Analysis of this group at 7 years median follow-up showed 24% disease free (Figure 1). By achieving complete remission with debulking regional therapy and following with systemic therapy for stage IV breast cancer, the median relapse-free survival (RFS) was nearly twice that achieved by CR from systemic therapy alone and nearly quadruple that achieved by regional therapy alone (Table 4). There is a suggestion that the more aggressive the regional treatment, e.g., combination irradiation and surgery, the more durable the

Table 4. *Complete Response and Remission Duration in Months by Regional Therapy (Surgery or Irradiation) or Chemotherapy (FAC)* in Stage IV Breast Cancer Patients with Single Metastasis or Minimal Tumor Burden*

Treatment	% CR[†]	Median Duration of Remission
Regional therapy	100	9
Chemotherapy (FAC)	38	18

*FAC = 5-fluorouracil, doxorubicin, cyclophosphamide.
[†]CR = complete remission.

Table 5. *Relapse-Free Survival of Patients with Minimal Metastatic Breast Cancer by Regional Therapy, Chemotherapy, and Combination Regional and Chemotherapy*

Treatment	Median Duration of CR* in Months
Regional	9
Chemotherapy	18
Combination regional and chemotherapy	35

*CR = complete response.

Table 6. *Patients Relapse-Free at 5 and 7 Years Following Regional Treatment and Chemotherapy for Single Sites of Metastasis by Site*

Site	Total	5 Yrs.	(%)	7 Yrs.	(%)
Regional lymph node	17	7	(41)	7	(41)
Chest wall	19	9	(31)	9	(31)
Visceral (skin, lung, brain, ovary)	7	2	(28)	1	(14)
Bone	9	2	(22)	1	(11)

remission duration (Blumenschein et al. 1979). The site of initial solitary recurrence is predictive for remission duration. Patients with regional nodal recurrence or chest wall recurrence enjoy longer disease-free survival than do patients with bone or visceral sites of recurrence (Table 6).

Many clinical situations arise during the management of breast cancer that afford the physician an opportunity to consider the use of combined regional and systemic therapy. This combination is well established for stage II and III breast cancer and is coming into increasing use in T_4 and inflammatory breast cancer (Nervi et al. 1979a,b, Buzdar et al. 1982b).

Important questions remain to be explored when combining regional and systemic therapy. The advantage of combining hormonal treatment with chemotherapy and the timing of regional treatment and systemic treatment are but a few. It is hoped that studies in progress will provide additional information in these areas.

Given the limitations of today's most efficacious systemic treatment programs and the long-recognized limitation of regional treatment, it seems appropriate to combine these two modalities whenever possible to provide breast cancer patients with the best opportunity for prolonged complete remissions and the small chance for very prolonged complete remissions.

REFERENCES

Blumenschein, G. R., A. U. Buzdar, G. N. Hortobagyi, and C. K. Tashima. 1979. Adjuvant chemoimmunotherapy following regional therapy for initial solitary metastases of breast cancer (stage IV NED), *in* Adjuvant Therapy of Cancer II, S. E. Jones, and S. E. Salmon, eds. Grune and Stratton, New York, pp. 303–310.

Blumenschein, G. R., A. U. Buzdar, G. N. Hortobagyi, and H-Y. Yap. 1981. Adjuvant chemo-immunotherapy of regionally treated stage IV breast cancer patients: A 5-year follow-up, *in* Adjuvant Therapy of Cancer III, S. E. Salmon and S. E. Jones, eds. Grune and Stratton, New York, pp. 427–434.

Blumenschein, G. R., A. U. Buzdar, C. K. Tashima, G. N. Hortobagyi, and J. U. Gutterman. 1977. Adjuvant chemoimmunotherapy of stage IV (NED) breast cancer, *in* Adjuvant Therapy of Cancer, S. E. Salmon and S. E. Jones, eds. North Holland Publishing Company, Amsterdam, pp. 139–146.

Bonadonna, G., A. Rossi, P. Valagussa, A. Banfi, and V. Veronesi. 1977. The CMF program for operable breast cancer with positive axillary nodes: Updated analysis on the disease-free interval, site of relapse, and drug tolerance. Cancer 39:2904–2915.

Bonadonna, G., and P. Valagussa. 1981. Dose-response effect of adjuvant chemotherapy in breast cancer. N. Engl. J. Med. 305:1–6.

Bonadonna, G., P. Valagussa, A. Rossi, G. Tancini, C. Brambilla, S. Marchini, and U. Veronesi. 1981. Multimodal therapy with CMF in resectable breast cancer with positive axillary nodes: The Milan Institute experience, *in* Adjuvant Therapy of Cancer III, S. E. Salmon and S. E. Jones, eds. Grune and Stratton, New York, pp. 435–444.

Brambilla, C., M. DeLena, A. Rossi, P. Valagussa, and G. Bonadonna. 1976. Response and survival in advanced breast cancer after two non-cross-resistant combinations. Br. Med. J. 1:801–804.

Bull, J. M., D. C. Tormey, S. H. Li, P. P. Carbone, G. Falkson, J. Blom, E. Perlin, and R. Simon. 1978. A randomized comparative trial of Adriamycin versus methotrexate in combination drug therapy. Cancer 41:1649–1657.

Buzdar, A. U., G. R. Blumenschein, J. U. Gutterman, C. K. Tashima, G. N. Hortobagyi, T. L. Smith, L. T. Campos, W. L. Wheeler, E. M. Hersh, E. J. Freireich, and E. A. Gehan. 1979a. Postoperative adjuvant chemotherapy with fluorouracil, doxorubicin, cyclophosphamide, and BCG vaccine: A follow-up report. JAMA 242:1509–1513.

Buzdar, A. U., G. R. Blumenschein, G. N. Hortobagyi, S. S. Legha, H-Y. Yap, L. T. Campos, and E. M. Hersh. 1982a. Adjuvant chemotherapy with 5-fluorouracil, doxorubicin (Adriamycin) and cyclophosphamide, with or without BCG immunotherapy in stage II or III breast cancer, *in* Immunotherapy of Human Cancer, W. D. Terry and S. A. Rosenberg, eds. Elsevier/North Holland, New York, pp. 175–181.

Buzdar, A. U., G. R. Blumenschein, T. L. Smith, C. K. Tashima, G. N. Hortobagyi, H-Y. Yap, J. U. Gutterman, E. M. Hersh, and E. A. Gehan. 1979b. Adjuvant chemoimmunotherapy following regional therapy for isolated recurrences of breast cancer (stage IV NED). J. Surg. Oncol. 12:27–40.

Buzdar, A. U., E. D. Montague, J. L. Barker, G. N. Hortobagyi, and G. R. Blumenschein. 1982b. Management of inflammatory carcinoma of breast with combined modality approach: An update. Cancer 47:2537–2542.

Buzdar, A. U., T. L. Smith, G. R. Blumenschein, G. N. Hortobagyi, E. M. Hersh, and E. A. Gehan. 1981. Adjuvant chemotherapy with fluorouracil, doxorubicin, and cyclophosphamide (FAC) for stage II or III breast cancer: 5-year results, *in* Adjuvant Therapy of Cancer III, S. E. Salmon and S. E. Jones, eds. Grune and Stratton, New York, pp. 419–426.

Canellos, G., S. J. Pocock, S. G. Taylor, M. E. Sears, D. J. Klaasen, and P. R. Band. 1976. Combination chemotherapy for metastatic breast carcinoma. Cancer 38:1882.

Chu, F. C. H., F. Lin, J. H. Kim, S. H. Huh, and C. J. Gormatis. 1976. Locally recurrent carcinoma of the breast: Results of radiation therapy. Cancer 37:2677.

Fisher, B., C. Redmond, N. Wolmark, and participating NSABP investigators. 1981. Breast cancer studies of the NSABP: An editorialized overview, *in* Adjuvant Therapy of Cancer III, S. E. Salmon and S. E. Jones, eds. Grune and Stratton, New York, pp. 419–426.

Holland, J. F. 1977. Therapy of primary breast cancer. Israeli J. Med. Sci. 13:829–836.

Hortobagyi, G. N., J. U. Gutterman, G. R. Blumenschein, C. K. Tashima, M. A. Burgess, L. Einhorn, A. U. Buzdar, S. P. Richman, and E. M. Hersh. 1979. Combination chemoimmunotherapy of metastatic breast cancer with 5-fluorouracil, Adriamycin, cyclophosphamide, and BCG. Cancer 44:1955–1962.

Jones, S. E., B. G. M. Durie, and S. E. Salmon. 1975. Combination chemotherapy with Adriamycin and cyclophosphamide for advanced breast cancer. Cancer 36:90–97.

Jones, S. E., T. E. Moon, G. Bonadonna, P. Valagussa, S. Rivkin, and T. Powles. 1982. Computer-based comparative analysis of the Milan, Arizona and Southwest Oncology Group (SWOG) adjuvant trials. (Abstract) Proceedings of the International Conferences on Advances in the Adjuvant Therapy of Cancer, London, England.

Legha, S. S., A. U. Buzdar, T. L. Smith, G. N. Hortobagyi, K. D. Swenerton, G. R. Blumenschein, E. A. Gehan, G. P. Bodey, and E. J. Freireich. 1979. Complete remission in metastatic breast cancer treated with combination drug therapy. Ann. Intern. Med. 91:847–852.

Lloyd, R. E., S. E. Jones, and S. E. Salmon. 1979. Comparative trial of low-dose Adriamycin plus cyclophosphamide with or without additive hormonal therapy in advanced breast cancer. Cancer 43:60–65.

Misset, J. L., M. Delgado, R. Plagne, D. Belpamme, J. Gurrin, P. Fumoleau, R. Metz, and G. Mathe. 1982. Three-year results of a randomized trial comparing CMF to Adriamycin (ADM), vincristine (VCR), cyclophosphamide (CPM), and 5-fluorouracil (5-FU) (AVCF) as adjuvant therapy for operated breast cancer: A "group inter-France" trial. (Abstract) Proceedings of the International Conferences on Advances in the Adjuvant Therapy of Cancer, London, England.

Nervi, C., G. Arcangeli, F. Concolino, and M. Cortese. 1979a. Improved survival with combined modality treatment for stage IV breast cancer. Int. J. Radiat. Oncol. Biol. Phys. 5:1317–1321.

Nervi, C., G. Arcangeli, F. Concolino, and M. Cortese. 1979b. Prolonged survival with postirradiation adjuvant chemotherapy in stage IV breast cancer, *in* Adjuvant Therapy of Cancer II, S. E. Jones and S. E. Salmon, eds. Grune and Stratton, New York, pp. 311–317.

Smalley, R. V., J. Carpenter, A. Bartolucci, C. Vogel, and S. Krauss. 1977. A comparison of cyclophosphamide, Adriamycin, 5-fluorouracil (CAF) and cyclophosphamide, methotrexate, 5-fluorouracil, vincristine, prednisone (CMFVP) in patients with metastatic breast cancer. Cancer 40:625–632.

Smalley, R. V., S. Murphy, C. M. Huguley, and A. A. Bartolucci. 1976. Combination versus sequential five-drug chemotherapy in metastatic carcinoma of the breast. Cancer Res. 36:3911.

Swenerton, K. D., S. S. Legha, T. L. Smith, G. N. Hortobagyi, E. A. Gehan, H-Y. Yap, J. U. Gutterman, and G. R. Blumenschein. 1979. Prognostic factors in metastatic breast cancer treated with combination chemotherapy. Cancer Res. 39:1552–1562.

Tapley, N. D. 1976. Clinical Applications of the Electron Beam. J. Wiley and Sons, New York, p. 220.

NEWER SURGICAL ASPECTS OF
BREAST ONCOLOGY

Current Controversies in Breast Cancer, edited
by F. C. Ames, G. R. Blumenschein, and E. D. Montague.
University of Texas Press, Austin © 1984.

Cystosarcoma Phylloides:
The Military Experience

Richard M. Briggs, M.D., Michael Walters, M.D.,
and Daniel Rosenthal, M.D.

General Surgery Service, Brooke Army Medical Center, Fort Sam Houston, Texas

Cystosarcoma phylloides is a rare breast tumor representing 0.5% to 2.5% of all breast malignancies (Lester and Stout 1954, Treves and Sunderland 1951). Although impressive by virture of its frequent large size, it is a poorly understood tumor. Though its name would indicate otherwise, it is rarely cystic, only occasionally leafy, and seldom sarcomatous in behavior. Many attempts have been made in the literature to predict the biological behavior of cystosarcoma on the basis of its histologic appearance and to tailor the magnitude of surgery accordingly. Several problems, however, have complicated these attempts. First, no institution has had enough cases to perform a randomized study. Second, reports emanating from tertiary-care cancer centers with complex cases tend to skew statistics concerning the course of the disease following various surgical therapies. Third, cystosarcoma is a biologically fickle tumor. These histologically benign lesions do recur, and such tumors classified as malignant frequently are cured with local excision. Finally, age appears to be a major factor in how these tumors behave. Adolescent women rarely develop recurrent disease or metastasis regardless of the histologic classification of the tumor or surgical procedure performed.

Part of the confusion regarding the true nature of cystosarcoma phylloides is derived from early case reports and descriptions of the tumor. The prominent Berlin pathologist Johannes Mueller (1838) first described the lesion and coined the term cystosarcoma phylloides. He emphasized its benign nature and lack of malignant potential. For the next century, authors applied numerous descriptive terms in reports on the same tumor. McDonald and Harrington (1950), in reviewing the literature, identified 28 terms for the same lesion and recommended a 29th name of their own.

The malignant potential of cystosarcoma phylloides was not appreciated until 1931 when Lee and Pack (1931) summarized the literature as a collective study of 105 cases, including an additional four cases of their own. In the group of 91 patients for whom follow-up was mentioned, there were six recurrences, and one patient eventually died of pulmonary metastasis.

In the early 1950s, two landmark studies were published, one by Treves and Sunderland (1951) from Memorial Hospital and the other by Lester and Stout (1954) from Presbyterian Hospital, both in New York. In these studies, clinical behavior of cystosarcoma was correlated with pathologic features. These two studies are of interest in that one reports the experience of a referral cancer hospital and the other of a busy general hospital. The conclusions drawn from the Memorial study proposed that the metastasic potential of cystosarcoma could be predicted from histologic characteristics. On the other hand, the Presbyterian group found that only two of five metastasic lesions could be classified malignant using the Memorial criteria. In addition, two patients with lesions classified as benign developed distant metastasis.

Cognizant of these problems, Norris and Taylor (1967) proposed more specific criteria for the classification of cystosarcoma based on the degree of stromal cellular atypism, the number of mitotic figures per high power field, and infiltrative versus pushing tumor margins. Utilizing the above criteria as well as tumor size, they were able to further identify those lesions likely to recur or metastasize. Nevertheless, they conceded that a clear-cut separation of benign from malignant tumors could not be made by histologic appearance alone.

With these problems in mind, we decided to review the military experience with cystosarcoma phylloides and try to formulate a more rational approach to treatment for women with this disease.

MATERIALS AND METHODS

This study was comprised of 38 cases of cystosarcoma phylloides collected from the tumor registries of 10 military medical centers during the 26-year period between 1954 and 1980. The records of each patient were examined for clinical features, operative treatment, histologic classification, and long-term follow-up. All histologic specimens were reexamined at the Armed Forces Institute of Pathology, Washington D.C., and histologically classified benign, borderline, and malignant according to the criteria proposed by Norris and Taylor. Patients with the diagnosis of giant fibroadenoma or true sarcoma of the breast were excluded from the study. Also excluded were patients in whom follow-up through 1980 was unavailable.

RESULTS

Cystosarcoma phylloides appeared in all age groups, though the largest number occurred during the fifth decade of life. The average age was 38 years. Ethnically, the lesion appeared in 28 Caucasians, five Blacks, two Hispanics, one Filipino, one Japanese, and one Samoan. No patient developed a contralateral cystosarcoma, nor was any familial tendency noted. The chief complaint in 29 patients was the recent onset of a rapidly growing nontender breast mass. Twenty-five women had noticed the mass less than 6 months prior to seeking medical attention; however, in three the lesion had been present greater than 1 year. Two lesions were found on routine physical examination.

On physical examination, the lesion was described as firm and freely movable in essentially all cases. In no instance was skin dimpling or nipple retraction reported.

The average size was 5.2 cm, but larger tumors were not uncommon. The largest tumor in the series measured 18 cm in diameter.

Although axillary adenopathy was palpable in seven patients, no specimen contained nodes positive for tumor.

Xeromammography

Twelve patients underwent preoperative xeromammography. In nine of the twelve patients, the lesion was felt to represent a benign fibroadenoma. In only three patients did the xeromammograms indicate possible malignancies on the basis of indistinct tumor margins. In no instance was the lesion correctly identified as a cystosarcoma phylloides.

Histologic Classification

Histologically, the lesions were differentiated from benign fibroadenomas, on the basis of stromal cellularity and the presence of mitotic nuclei, and from the true sarcomas of the breast, by both epithelial and stromal elements contained within the tumor. Utilizing this criteria for classification of cystosarcoma, 22 lesions were classified as benign, 14 malignant, and two borderline.

Associated Neoplasms

Four patients developed six other malignancies subsequent to the successful surgical treatment of their cystosarcoma (Table 1). A fifth patient, a 14-year-old Samoan girl, developed a malignant cystosarcoma following a prior left lower extremity amputation for osteosarcoma and radical abdominal surgery for advanced ovarian carcinoma. She died as a result of the ovarian carcinoma with no evidence of recurrent cystosarcoma. Although one patient died of an infiltrating ductal carcinoma of the contralateral breast, no other association with ductal breast carcinoma was identified.

On the other hand, 10 women each had excision of at least one fibroadenoma. Six fibroadenomas occurred in the opposite breast and four in the ipsilateral breast.

Table 1. *Associated Cancers in Five Patients with Cystosarcoma Phylloides*

Type	Result
Endometrioid carcinoma of ovary	died 3 years later
Infiltrating ductal carcinoma of breast	death from metastasis
Colon carcinoma	death from metastasis
Osteosarcoma left femur,	death
Cystadenocarcinoma of ovary	
Melanoma of retina, Cervical	alive and well
carcinoma	

Table 2. *Treatment in 37 Patients with Cystosarcoma Phylloides*

	Tumor Excision	Simple Mastectomy	Radical Mastectomy	Subcutaneous Mastectomy
Benign	11 (52.3%)	6 (28.6%)	–	4 (19.0%)
Malignant	4 (28.6%)	4 (28.6%)	6 (42.8%)	–
Borderline	1 (50%)	(50%)	–	–

Treatment and Results

As seen in Table 2, nearly one-half of the patients underwent excision as the only treatment method. Simple mastectomy was the next most common procedure. Other patients underwent either standard radical, modified radical, or subcutaneous mastectomy.

When the study was terminated in January 1982, all living patients had been contacted by mail or telephone. Death summaries or autopsy reports were available on all patients dying from unrelated causes. No patients died as a result of cystosarcoma phylloides, but two patients did develop local recurrences. One tumor recurred in a 50-year-old lady 6 months following the excision of a 2-cm benign cystosarcoma. She was subsequently treated with a quadrantectomy and remained disease free 19 years later. The second recurrence followed the simple excision of a 3-cm malignant lesion in a 62-year-old white female. The patient then underwent a standard radical mastectomy and had negative axillary nodes. Although she remains disease free 16 years later, she suffers significant lymphedema of the extremity.

DISCUSSION

Over the years, the treatment of patients with cystosarcoma phylloides has remained controversial primarily due to the relatively rare incidence of the tumor and conflicting reports regarding its recurrence rate and metastatic potential based on histologic appearance. As seen from Table 3, the recurrence rate in benign cystosarcomas varied from 25% in the study of Pietruszka and Barnes (1978) from Pittsburgh to 3.5% reported by Lester and Stout (1954) from Presbyterian. Likewise, the recurrence rate for malignant cystosarcomas ranged from 5.8% to 50%. Thus, the poor correlation between biologic behavior and histologic appearance noted in the two patients in this study with recurrent disease is in agreement with the findings of others.

An explanation for this poor correlation may rest in the manner in which cystosarcoma phylloides is classified. Not uncommonly, stromal differentiation in the same malignant cystosarcoma will vary from a totally benign to frankly anaplastic appearance, the final designation being based on the most malignant-appearing areas of the tumor. Consequently, some metastasizing cystosarcomas classified as benign may in fact have had small malignant foci that more meticulous examination would have uncovered.

Table 3. *Number of Recurrences of Cystosarcoma*
Phylloides by Histology in Five Studies

	Benign	Malignant	Borderline
Mayo Clinic	3/23	1/6	—
Pittsburgh	4/16	1/17	1/3
Memorial	4/41	9/18	9/18
Presbyterian	1/28	2/20	2/10
Military	1/22	1/14	0/2
Total	13/130 (10%)	14/75 (18%)	12/33 (36%)

Equally controversial is the preferred surgical treatment of cystosarcoma phylloides. Treves and Sunderland (1951) recommended radical mastectomy after observing metastasis in one-half of their patients with microscopically malignant tumors. A later report from the same institution noted no recurrence in 13 patients undergoing various procedures (McDivit, Urban, and Farrow 1967). Based on their report, they remarked: "Had Treves and Sunderland's recommendation of radical mastectomy been followed, we might now attribute the 100% cure rate to the therapeutic effectiveness of radical mastectomy." Nevertheless, they concede part of the high success rate to the earlier detection and treatment of the tumor.

In reviewing the data from our military series and other large series in the literature, one arrives at several conclusions that should be considered when planning therapy. First, lymphatic spread to axillary nodes rarely occurs. In a collective review of five large series with a total of 244 patients, including patients in this series, axillary lymph node involvement was found in only one case, and this followed the recurrence of a 15-cm tumor in the upper outer quadrant (Treves and Sunderland 1951, Lester and Stout 1954, Pietruszka and Barnes 1978, and West et al. 1971). The authors felt that direct tumor invasion of the lymph nodes was a possibility. Therefore, standard radical mastectomy or modified radical mastectomy should play essentially no role in the surgical treatment of patients with this disease.

Another consideration is that local excision is accompanied by a higher incidence of recurrence than is simple mastectomy. In a compiled series of 119 patients treated with simple excision, 26 (21.8%) developed recurrent lesions. By comparison, in 83 patients from the same institutions undergoing simple mastectomy, only 6 (7.2%) required further surgery for recurrent lesions. Consequently, simple mastectomy is the standard procedure to which any lesser operation must be compared. For the majority of women with cystosarcoma phylloides, simple mastectomy offers the best therapy regardless of histologic type.

An alternative procedure, especially in younger women in whom cosmesis may be an important consideration, is subcutaneous mastectomy with immediate reconstruction. Theoretically subcutaneous mastectomy offers the same advantages as simple mastectomy in patients in whom total excision of the tumor with adequate margins would be curative. Unlike other breast carcinomas, multicentricity and involvement of the subareolar ductal tissue are not characteristic. Therefore, complete excision of the tumor along with most of the breast tissue should provide a high expectation of cure and excellent conditions for reconstruction.

Four patients in our series underwent subcutaneous mastectomy as their primary form of treatment. Their ages ranged from 29 to 43 years; tumor diameters ranged from 2 cm to 4 cm. All lesions showed histologically benign pathology. No patient developed recurrent disease, and all expressed satisfaction with the cosmetic result.

On the basis of this limited clinical experience, subcutaneous mastectomy appears to be an acceptable alternative if certain criteria are met: 1) The patient must express a desire for nipple preservation and breast reconstruction; 2) due to the higher recurrence rate in older patients, only women less than 50 years of age should be considered candidates for the procedure; 3) the tumor needs to be histologically benign; 4) the procedure should be limited to lesions less than 4 cm in diameter.

The optimal therapy in adolescent patients is likewise controversial due to the small number of these patients in any series. The management of cystosarcoma phylloides in teenagers was first examined by Amerson (1970). In his review of 355 cases of cystosarcoma from the American literature, he found 20 patients under the age of 20 with the diagnosis of cystosarcoma phylloides. There were two recurrences in this group but no instances of death or distant metastasis.

Andersson and Bergdahl (1978) studied the Swedish experience with cystosarcoma in young women and found three cases in adolescents. All three were treated with simple excision and sustained no recurrent lesions.

In the reports from the Mayo Clinic (West et al. 1971) and Pittsburgh (Pietruszka and Barnes 1978), two adolescents in each series were identified as having benign cystosarcomas. The four patients received local excision as the primary form of treatment with no recurrent tumors.

The only known case of metastatic disease in an adolescent patient was reported from the National Institutes of Health in a 14-year-old Romanian female (Hoover et al. 1975). This virulent and eventually fatal tumor involved the chest wall, back, and lungs in spite of vigorous surgical, radiation, and chemotherapeutic management.

The military experience with cystosarcoma in adolescents is similar to the findings of others except that patients in this age group make up a larger percentage than seen in other series. As seen in Table 4, the lesions ranged from 1.5 cm to 13 cm and averaged 6 cm in diameter. Eight of nine lesions were excised and of these no tumors recurred. One 12-year-old child received a radical mastectomy for a 13-cm malignant lesion and sustained no recurrence at follow-up 14 years later.

It therefore appears reasonable that simple excision is sufficient therapy in adolescents. Furthermore, if a cystosarcoma is enucleated under the clinical impression of a fibroadenoma, the patient can be safely observed provided the pathologist is assured of its benignity.

The final problem to be broached is that of recurrence after primary treatment. Although some authors feel recurrent lesions tend to degenerate histologically, in general, benign lesions recur as benign lesions and malignant recur as malignant.

Table 4. *Adolescents with Cystosarcoma Phylloides*

Age	Tumor Size	Pathology	Treatment	Result
12	13 cm	malignant	radical mastectomy	well 14 years
14	6 cm	benign	excision	well 13 years
19	1.5 cm	borderline	excision	well 2 years
16	10 cm	benign	excision	well 5 years
17	5 cm	benign	excision	well 7 years
19	5 cm	benign	excision	well 21 years
19	5 cm	benign	excision	well 2 years
14	6 cm	malignant	excision	died 6 months ovarian cancer
16	3 cm	benign	excision	well 2 years

Furthermore, recurrent malignant tumors usually contain only the stromal elements, whereas recurrent benign lesions contain both stromal and epithelial components suggesting unrecognized amputation of bosselations at the initial excision. Also, a local recurrence does not portend progressive disease or an ominous prognosis. Most patients are rendered disease free by complete removal of the recurrent lesion.

For adolescents and young women with a small benign recurrence, wide excision or quadrantectomy should be sufficient therapy. For older women or women with larger lesions, the recurrence should be treated with simple mastectomy. In patients treated previously with a simple mastectomy, wide excision is recommended.

Although no patients in this series developed distant metastasis, cystosarcoma phylloides does spread by the hematogenous route; the lungs and bone are the most common sites of metastatic disease. Even though clinical trials are few, radiation and chemotherapy apparently have little effect on the clinical course of metastatic disease, and death usually ensues within 2 years of diagnosis.

RECOMMENDATIONS

The successful management of cystosarcoma phylloides, like that of many cancers, requires early diagnosis of the tumor and adequate surgical treatment. Unfortunately, the usual scenario involves an unsuspecting surgeon, who enucleates the lesion, considering it to be a benign fibroadenoma, and later discovers that he has excised a cystosarcoma phylloides. He is then faced with the dilemma of whether to advise reoperation or close observation, knowing that a recurrence rate of 20–30% is expected.

If the patient is an adolescent, observation is entirely acceptable because the recurrence rate is low in adolescents. If reoperation is elected, the procedure should be limited to a quandratectomy of the area involved. For the older patient, wide excision offers a much lower rate of cure and should only be selectively used. Subcutaneous mastectomy or simple mastectomy is the recommended procedure depending on the patient's desires, tumor size, and tumor histologic category.

The obvious way to avoid the situation of reoperation is to request frozen sections on all tumors removed from the breast. Although in the past this appeared to be a waste of resources in the majority of cases, in the era of estrogen receptors for ductal breast carcinoma it is practically mandatory. Then with a knowledge of tumor histology, small benign lesions can be excised with a margin of normal tissue and with a high expectation of cure. For larger or malignant lesions, simple mastectomy could be performed at the initial procedure or at a later date.

CONCLUSIONS

Although it is apparent in reviewing this series and the literature that no single series satisfies the statistical requirements to reach sound conclusions, the guidelines in this paper propose that tumor size, histology, and patient age should all be considered prior to proceeding with surgery. As always, treatment needs to be individualized, and surgical judgment must take precedence in formulating therapeutic decisions.

REFERENCES

Al-Jurf, A., W. A. Hawk, and G. Crile. 1978. Cystosarcoma phylloides. Surg. Gynecol. Obstet. 146:358–364.

Amerson, J. R. 1970. Cystosarcoma phylloides in adolescent females: A report of seven patients. Ann. Surg. 171:849–858.

Andersson, A., and L. Bergdahl. 1978. Cystosarcoma phylloides in young women. Arch. Surg. 113:742–744.

Blichert-Toft, M., J. P. Hansen, O. Hansen, and T. Schiodt. 1975. Clinical course of cystosarcoma phylloides related to histologic appearance. Surg. Gynecol. Obstet. 140:929–932.

Browder, W., J. T. McQuitty, and J. C. McDonald. 1978. Malignant cystosarcoma phylloides. Am. J. Surg. 136:239–241.

Hoover, H. C., A. Trestioreanu, and A. S. Ketcham. 1975. Metastatic cystosarcoma phylloides in an adolescent girl: An unusually malignant tumor. Ann. Surg. 181:279–282.

Lee, B. J., and G. T. Pack. 1931. Giant intracanalicular fibroadenomyxoma of the breast: The so-called cystosarcoma phylloides mammae of Johannes Mueller. Am. J. Cancer 15:2583–2609.

Lester, J., and A. P. Stout. 1954. Cystosarcoma phylloides. Cancer 7:335–353.

McDivit, R. W., J. A. Urban, and J. H. Farrow. 1967. Cystosarcoma phylloides. Johns Hopkins Med. J. 120:33–45.

McDonald, J. R., and S. Harrington. 1950. Giant fibroadenoma of the breast "Cystosarcoma Phylloides." Ann. Surg. 131:243–251.

Mueller, J. 1838. Ueber den feinern Bau und die Formen der krankhaften Geschwulste. G. Reimer, Berlin, pp. 54–60.

Norris, H. J., and H. B. Taylor. 1967. Relationship of histologic appearance to behavior of cystosarcoma phylloides: Analysis of ninety-four cases. Cancer 20:2090–2099.

Pietruszka, M., and L. Barnes. 1978. Cystosarcoma phylloides: A Clinicopathologic analysis of forty-two cases. Cancer 41:1974–1983.

Treves, N., and D. A. Sunderland. 1951. Cystosarcoma phylloides of the breast: A benign and malignant tumor. Cancer 4:1286–1332.

West, T. L., L. H. Weiland, and O. T. Clagett. Cystosarcoma phylloides. Ann. Surg. 173: 520–528.

Current Controversies in Breast Cancer, edited
by F. C. Ames, G. R. Blumenschein, and E. D. Montague.
University of Texas Press, Austin © 1984.

Chest Wall Resection and Reconstruction in Breast Cancer Patients

David L. Larson, M.D.,* and Marion J. McMurtrey, M.D.†

*Departments of *Head and Neck Surgery and †Thoracic Surgery, The University of Texas
M. D. Anderson Hospital and Tumor Institute at Houston, Houston, Texas*

Until recently, the only role of the plastic surgeon in the treatment of the breast cancer patient has been to reconstruct the breast after mastectomy. Yet, the cosmetic result of reconstruction was usually unsatisfactory to the patient after multistaged procedures. The recent availability of the musculocutaneous (MC) flap has added a new dimension to the treatment of patients with primary or locally recurrent breast cancer. This flap consists of a muscle and its overlying skin, taken as a unit and rotated on a single, vascular pedicle, so that a large mass of tissue can be safely introduced into a significant defect in a single-stage procedure. Not only can the plastic surgeon provide a satisfactory reconstruction of an amputated breast (Figures 1,2), but he may, with the help of the oncologic surgeon, assist the clinical oncologist in the primary care of the breast cancer patient.

The experience in chest wall reconstruction associated with the treatment of breast cancer at The University of Texas M. D. Anderson Hospital and Tumor Institute at Houston was reviewed. From September 1979 to September 1982, 28 patients have undergone chest wall resection and immediate reconstruction. All patients had either primary breast cancer, locally recurrent disease, or a complication related to previous treatment of breast cancer. The average defect measured 170 cm and usually included a portion of the underlying ribs or sternum or both.

Perhaps the most effective demonstration of the use of these flaps can be seen by the following illustrative cases.

Case 1: (Figures 3–6) A 55-year-old patient presented with a large, necrotic tumor of the right breast. The patient failed to respond to full course irradiation and multiple courses of chemotherapy. Local hyperthermia yielded a bleeding tumor mass that threatened the patient's life. At surgery, the tumor mass of the chest wall was removed, and immediate reconstruction performed with a rectus abdominus MC flap.

In this situation, patient salvage from sepsis was aided by aggressive resection and appropriate reconstruction.

Case 2: (Figures 7–8) A young female ignored a massive breast cancer, resulting in infection of chest wall skin not involved with tumor. Resection and reconstruction

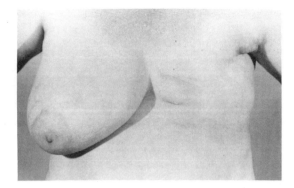

FIG. 1. Patient after modified radical mastectomy.

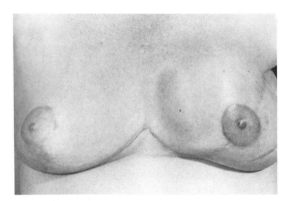

FIG. 2. Result of right reduction mammoplasty and left breast reconstruction with latissimus dorsi musculocutaneous flap. Medial thigh skin used for areola and nipple reconstruction.

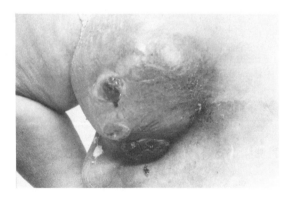

FIG. 3. Persistent disease after radiation therapy and chemotherapy.

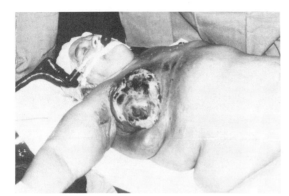

FIG. 4. Necrotic bleeding mass of chest wall after local hyperthermia.

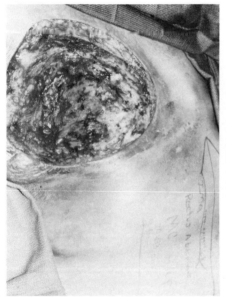

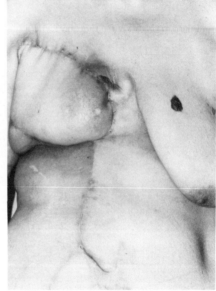

FIG. 5. Defect after chest wall resection. Note outline of rectus abdominus musculocutaneous flap, which will be rotated 180° from abdomen to cover chest wall.

FIG. 6. Result at 2 weeks; adjunctive therapy can be initiated. Note primary closure of donor site aides in decreasing tissue morbidity.

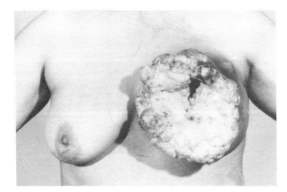

FIG. 7. Previously untreated breast cancer.

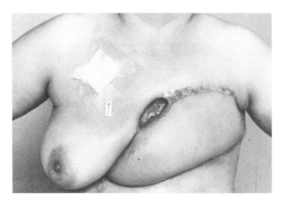

FIG. 8. Result at 4 weeks using rectus abdominus musculocutaneous flap. Clean wound at superior margin of flap will heal secondarily and does not compromise immediate use of chemotherapy.

resulted in a superficial infection that responded to antibiotics and drainage; healing progressed so that she could start chemotherapy within 4 weeks after mastectomy.

By decreasing the tumor burden in a large open wound that was chronically infected, the MC flap produced a clean wound that allowed additional adjunctive treatment without fear of tissue breakdown.

Case 3: (Figures 9–10) Following definitive surgery, radiation, and chemotherapy, this patient had residual breast cancer of the chest wall. After resection of two ribs and part of the sternum, the chest was reconstructed using a latissimus dorsi MC flap.

Again, by decreasing tumor burden and acting in concert with the ablative surgeons, the reconstructive surgeon was able to provide safe, simultaneous coverage of the wound.

Case 4: (Figures 11–13) This middle-aged patient presented with pus in the depths of a sternal wound after mastectomy and radiation therapy. At surgery, a pericardial abscess was found.

In this circumstance, the thoracic surgeon and the plastic and reconstructive surgeon combined their efforts to remove the radionecrotic ulcer and cover the area

Latissimus Dorsi
Musculocutaneous Flap

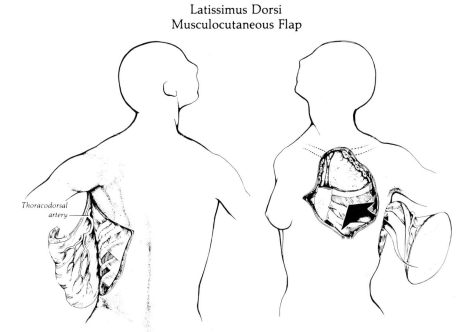

Thoracodorsal artery

FIG. 9. Latissimus dorsi musculocutaneous flap and arc of rotation from back to anterior chest wall. This is the same flap used in Figure 2 for breast reconstruction. (Reproduced from Larson et al. 1982, with permission of J. P. Lippincott.)

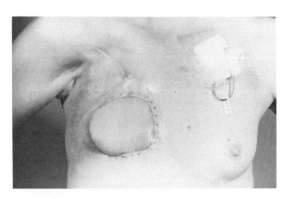

FIG. 10. After radiation therapy, local recurrence was resected and the breast reconstructed using the latissimus dorsi musculocutaneous flap.

with an available MC flap. This patient's problem was compounded by the pericardial abscess, which would certainly have resulted in death had immunosuppression followed additional chemotherapy. Now that the patient has sufficient coverage, more definitive systemic treatment can be given.

Case 5: (Figure 14–16) This 55-year-old patient with stage IV breast cancer was treated initially with high-dose radiation and chemotherapy, resulting in a complete

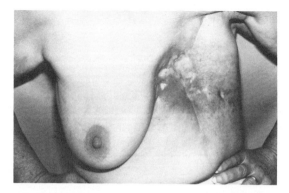

FIG. 11. Radionecrotic ulcer following radical mastectomy; tumor was also present at wound margins.

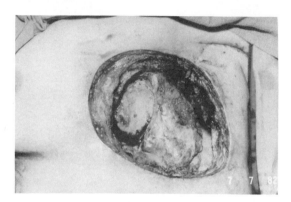

FIG. 12. Defect after removal of three ribs, half of sternum, and overlying skin. An unsuspected pericardial abscess was also drained.

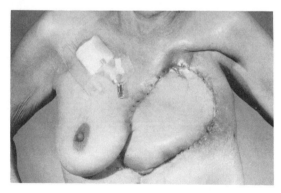

FIG. 13. Result at 3 weeks shows patient ready to undergo chemotherapy.

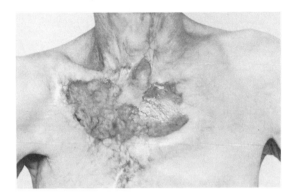

FIG. 14. Patient sustained full-thickness loss of tissue secondarily to thermal injury in previously irradiated chest wall skin. (Reproduced from Larson et al. 1982, with permission of J. P. Lippincott.)

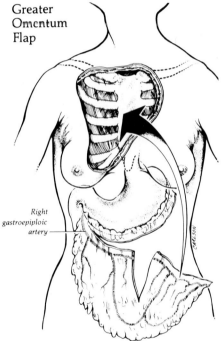

Greater
Omentum
Flap

*Right
gastroepiploic
artery*

FIG. 15. Arc of rotation of omental flap used with skin graft to resurface damaged skin of anterior chest wall. (Reproduced from Larson et al. 1982, with permission of J. P. Lippincott.)

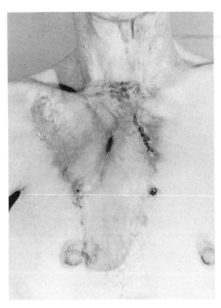

FIG. 16. Result at 3 months. (Reproduced from Larson et al. 1982, with permission of J. P. Lippincott.)

response. Two years later, she accidentially caught her blouse on fire and sustained a full-thickness thermal loss of irradiated skin. This resulted in a chronic, painful wound of the chest wall. Reconstruction of this soft tissue defect was accomplished by the use of an omental flap and skin graft.

Treatment of breast cancer by surgery, radiation, or chemotherapy results in tissue morbidity. When more than one modality is used, additional tissue morbidity usually ensues. By awareness of the additional capabilities of surgery over and above mastectomy and lymphadenectomy, the oncologist can provide his patient with more effective methods of dealing with breast cancer and the related complications.

REFERENCES

Larson, D. L., M. J. McMurtrey, E. Irish, and H. J. Howe. 1982. Major chest wall reconstruction after chest wall irradiation. Cancer 49:1286–1293.

McCraw, J. B., D. G. Dibbell, and J. H. Carraway. 1977a. Experimental definition of independent myocutaneous vascular territories. Plast. Reconstr. Surg. 60:212–220.

McCraw, J. B., D. G. Dibbell, and J. H. Carraway. 1977b. Clinical definition of independent myocutaneous vascular territories. Plast. Reconstr. Surg. 60:341–352.

Current Controversies in Breast Cancer, edited
by F. C. Ames, G. R. Blumenschein, and E. D. Montague.
University of Texas Press, Austin © 1984.

Immediate Reconstruction in the Treatment of Carcinoma of the Breast

Thomas G. Frazier, M.D., F.A.C.S.,*† and
R. Barrett Noone, M.D., F.A.C.S.‡

*Departments of *Surgery and †Plastic Surgery, The Bryn Mawr Hospital, Bryn Mawr,
Pennsylvania, and ‡The Bryn Mawr Tumor Institute, Haverford, Pennsylvania*

Probably no other ablative procedure in surgery carries the devastating psychological impact of amputation of the breast for carcinoma. The abrupt change in body image and alteration of female form in a society that places such great emphasis on physical appearance has often been suggested as a reason for the failure of self-detection programs as well as obvious patient delay in diagnosis. Too often, as cancer surgeons in pursuit of cure of the disease, we neglect to consider the quality of the life we are preserving. Our goal and, in fact, the goal of all cancer therapy should be to optimize the quality of survival as well as the quantity. With this in mind, it is worthwhile to review some of the historical perspectives that have evolved to our present consideration of immediate reconstruction as an adjunct to the treatment of primary breast cancer.

In 1970, Hueston and McKenzie first described immediate breast reconstruction after radical mastectomy. A number of authors, both in this country and abroad, have continued to improve on this approach, and as the technique of reconstruction evolved, interest moved from a delayed approach (Cronin et al. 1977, Dowden et al. 1979) to consideration of an immediate approach (Georgiade et al. 1981, Horton et al. 1979).

Our own experience with immediate reconstruction began with the development of a protocol in 1977 to see if, in fact, immediate reconstruction was a practical and rational alternative in the treatment of carcinoma of the breast. The advantages to immediate reconstruction seemed quite obvious. The disadvantages seemed to center primarily around concern regarding interference with healing and perhaps adverse effects on adjuvant therapy, survival, and the detection of recurrent disease. In addition, we also had concerns about patient acceptance of immediate reconstruction following mastectomy. A number of authors, particularly plastic surgeons, had expressed concerns that patients may not appreciate less-than-perfect reconstructions unless they have had time to live with the inconvenience of a deformity and an external prosthesis. In May of 1981 (Noone et al. 1982), we evaluated our own patients' acceptance with a series of in-depth interviews and found an overwhelming patient acceptance of this particular procedure. We have now adopted this as a valuable option in the treatment of selected patients who have primary carcinoma of the breast.

In reviewing the various technical advantages that have helped us, we have developed a protocol we think is extremely important to the success we have had with this procedure. Our decision to go ahead with immediate reconstruction began almost simultaneously with the use of the submuscular prosthesis and the use of fluorescein to evaluate the viability of skin flaps. With these factors having made the application of immediate reconstruction a technical possibility, we then began to evaluate which patients would be good candidates for immediate reconstruction. The experience of others in dealing with minimal breast cancer (Frazier et al. 1977) led us to believe that the survivals with this group and perhaps with patients who had slightly larger tumors (as great as 1.0 cm in diameter) would be adequate for immediate reconstruction attempts. Subsequent work communicated personally by Larson and Copeland at The University of Texas M. D. Anderson Hospital and Tumor Institute at Houston has convinced us that with stage I carcinoma of the breast the recurrence is very rarely submuscular and, therefore, these patients would be at a very low risk of developing an occult recurrence after immediate reconstruction.

There are at least three or four options that can be exercised in immediate reconstruction of the breast. Some authors have thought a "delayed" immediate reconstruction is best, in which the reconstruction takes place on day 3 or 4 after the final pathological report is in and there has been additional time to evaluate the viability of the skin flaps. While we took this approach for several patients early in our experience, we found this technique to be of no advantage, since even patients who had lymph node involvement had no delay in their future chemotherapy or radiation therapy. In addition, this technique had the added disadvantage of requiring a second anesthetic for the reconstruction procedure. We have also performed one immediate breast reconstruction operation using the rectus abdominus muscle flap in a patient who wanted immediate reconstruction without an artificial prosthesis. While this gave a very satisfactory cosmetic result, the surgical time required, in excess of 3.5 hours for the combined procedure, makes this an unacceptable alternative. We have also discontinued the use of latissimus dorsi flaps as an additional method for obtaining muscle and skin coverage in immediate reconstruction for this same reason.

We now take a two-team approach to immediate reconstruction, utilizing one anesthetic and two teams of surgeons. This is in contrast to the recommendations of others (Wilkinson et al. 1982), but we believe the two-team approach is extremely important in the preservation of an adequate cancer ablative procedure without introducing any bias on the part of the oncologic surgeon.

MATERIALS AND METHODS—PATIENT SELECTION

At present, we offer immediate reconstruction to those patients who have stage I carcinoma of the breast and whose tumor size is 1.0 cm or less anywhere in the breast or up to 2.5 cm or less in the lateral aspect of the breast. All patients must have clinically negative axillary lymph nodes and staging studies negative for disseminated disease. All patients have had their diagnoses by an outpatient biopsy procedure. The histology and size of the primary tumor are evaluated. All patients have an excisional biopsy that includes a small margin of normal surrounding tissue. The usual studies for estrogen and progesterone receptors are also performed. Staging studies are then carried out. The oncologic surgeon discusses the options for the treatment of primary carcinoma of the breast. Prior to their surgery, they discuss immediate reconstruction with the oncologic surgeon and then consult with the plastic surgeon. At this time, photos of previous patients who have undergone reconstruction are shown to these patients. Opportunities for counseling with previous patients who have undergone immediate reconstruction are available. Those patients electing to undergo mastectomy have a complete axillary dissection of all three levels of lymph nodes. After the modified radical mastectomy has been completed, the plastic surgeon enters the room, the patient is again prepared for surgery and redraped, and the surgical defect is evaluated to determine whether the patient is a satisfactory candidate for an immediate reconstructive procedure. Over 90% of our patients who wish to be considered for immediate reconstruction do have satisfactory surgical defects; those who do not have satisfactory defects usually undergo reconstruction within 6 months.

Using the Madden mastectomy technique, we are able to preserve the pectoralis major and minor muscles and the medial and lateral anterior thoracic nerve supply so that submuscular reconstruction may be performed. The pectoralis major is detached from the sixth rib origin, and a pocket is created to the sternal border. The serratus anterior is raised along the sixth rib in an inferolateral direction and is dissected to the anterior axillary line to provide lateral and inferior muscle coverage for the prosthesis. The flap of rectus abdominus fascia is developed 3.0 cm to the corresponding contralateral intramammary fold. A gel-inflatable prosthesis is inserted to approximate the weight of the removed mastectomy specimen. Total submuscular closure around the prosthesis and hemostasis beneath the skin flap and axilla are achieved with 2-0 and 3-0 vicryl suture material. Suction catheter drains are used, and both intraoperative and postoperative antibiotic coverage with a cepholasporin is continued. Patients considered for immediate reconstruction are given one dose of preoperative antibiotics as well. Dressings are usually removed in 48 hours, and a bra-supported soft dressing is used for the remainder of the patient's hospital stay. Postoperatively, both the oncologic surgeon and the reconstructive surgeon examine the patient at regular intervals for the potential development of metastases.

RESULTS

Forty-five consecutive patients who underwent immediate reconstruction for primary breast carcinoma ranged in age from 35 to 63 years (mean 46.2 years). All patients have been followed from 6 to 60 months (mean 31.4 months; median 26.3 months). No patient has been lost to follow-up.

Table 1. *Pathologic Node Involvement*

Result	Patients	%
Negative nodes	34	75.6
Positive nodes	11	24.4
Number of involved nodes		
1–3	8	
4+	3	

Table 2. *Complications and Morbidity*

Hematoma and implant loss*	2
Significant cellulitis	1
Superficial flap necrosis	2
Total	5 (11.1%)

*Subsequently replaced at 6 months.

Thirty-nine patients had tumors 1.0 cm or less in diameter (86.7%), and six patients had lateral tumors 1.0 to 2.5 cm in diameter (13.3%). All patients had clinically negative axillae and had clinical stage I disease.

Thirty-four patients (75.6%) subsequently had pathologically confirmed negative axillary lymph nodes, and 11 patients (24.4%) had positive nodes (Table 1).

Only two patients (4.9%) had loss of the implant, and one patient had the implant replaced 6 months later with satisfactory results. Other minor complications included significant cellulitis and superficial flap necrosis (Table 2).

Of the 11 patients who had positive lymph nodes, all were offered adjuvant chemotherapy. Seven accepted, three refused, and one accepted x-ray therapy only. All patients began adjuvant therapy within 4 weeks of surgery.

Three patients had recurrences, but no patient had local recurrence. Of the patients who had distant recurrences, two died at 36 and 38 months, respectively, and one is alive with supraclavicular nodal disease.

Three other patients are dead, one at 6 months of an unrelated cause and two of metastatic disease (4.9%).

Of our first 30 patients, 28 were interviewed for patient acceptance of cosmetic result. Of those, 92.8% thought reconstruction had achieved their desired goals, and 96.4% recommended reconstruction at the time of mastectomy.

DISCUSSION

Because of the results we have had with this approach, we are comfortable in offering it as a routine part of our treatment for primary carcinoma of the breast in selected patients. While this seems to put a fair amount of emphasis on the quality of life, we feel strongly that immediate reconstruction is still not for everyone and that our real goal in offering immediate reconstruction is to make the best of a bad situation. As long as immediate reconstruction can be performed without any compromise of the patient's cure or cancer treatment, we believe it should be offered. We believe that most of our success in utilizing this procedure has been based on the two-step biopsy technique. This gives the patient a period of time to adjust to the fact that she has breast cancer and to participate in the actual treatment she is to receive. In addition, we have a very sophisticated patient population from a university-affiliated community hospital in a high socioeconomic suburban setting. Patients are informed, educated persons, and the opportunity they have to participate in decisions regarding their reconstructions may, in fact, have contributed to their overall happiness with the reconstruction effort. The only disadvantage we have encountered in immediate reconstruction has been a slightly delayed return of shoulder motion because of stiffness in the pectoralis muscle. Two patients did require physical therapy. The increased operating time was not considered to be a significant problem for us, although coordinating numerous consultations on relatively short notice did occasionally present scheduling problems. Again, we must emphasize that proper selection of the patient for this procedure requires consideration of patient and tumor factors. Such considerations are essential if the results desired by the physician and patient are to be achieved.

REFERENCES

Cronin, T. D., J. Upton, and J. M. McDonough. 1977. Reconstruction of the breast after mastectomy. Plast. Reconstr. Surg. 59:1–14.

Dowden, R. V., C. E. Horton, F. E. Rosato, and J. B. McCraw. 1979. Reconstruction of the breast after mastectomy for cancer. Surg. Gynecol. Obstet. 149:190.

Frazier, T. G., E. M. Copeland, H. S. Gallager, D. D. Paulus, Jr., and E. C. White. 1977. Prognosis and treatment in minimal breast cancer. Am. J. Surg. 133:697–701.

Georgiade, G. S., N. G. Georgiade, K. S. McCarty, Jr., B. J. Ferguson, and H. F. Siegler. 1981. Modified radical mastectomy with immediate reconstruction for carcinoma of the breast. Ann. Surg. 193:565–573.

Horton, C. E., F. E. Rosato, J. B. McCraw, and R. V. Dowden. 1979. Immediate reconstruction following mastectomy for cancer. Clinics Plast. Surg. 6:37.

Hueston, J., and G. McKenzie. 1970. Breast reconstruction after radical mastectomy. Aust. N.Z. J. Surg. 39:367–370.

Noone, R. B., T. G. Frazier, C. Z. Hayward, and M. S. Skiles. 1982. Patient acceptance of immediate reconstruction following mastectomy. Plast. Reconstr. Surg. 69:632–638.

Wilkinson, L. H., O. A. Peloso, and W. G. Dail, Jr. 1982. Modified radical mastectomy with immediate breast reconstruction. Arch. Surg. 117:579–582.

Current Controversies in Breast Cancer, edited
by F. C. Ames, G. R. Blumenschein, and E. D. Montague.
University of Texas Press, Austin © 1984.

Analysis of the Prognosis of Minimal and Occult Breast Cancers

Gary W. Unzeitig, M.D.,* Gloria Frankl, M.D.,† Mona Ackerman,
R.N.,† and Theodore X. O'Connell, M.D.*

*Departments of *Surgery and †Radiology, Southern California Kaiser-Permanente
Medical Center, Los Angeles, California*

In the 10-year period between 1971 and 1981, 32,814 women were examined by xeromammography at the Los Angeles Kaiser-Permanente Medical Center. Of the patients examined, 1,135 breast cancers were demonstrated, of which 26% (296) were occult, that is, not palpable on clinical examination. Of these patients with occult lesions, 247 underwent subsequent treatment at our institution (Table 1) and follow-up is complete to date. Patients with occult cancers were referred by their primary physicians for routine mammography, for breast complaints other than a mass, or for follow-up of previous breast disease. All patients with xerographic abnormalities suggestive of cancer were referred for surgical consultation.

RESULTS

The patients are divided into two groups, occult/minimal and occult/nonminimal, on the basis of the pathologist's description of the primary lesion. As defined by Gallager (1971), minimal breast cancer is lobular carcinoma in situ, intraductal carcinoma, or invasive carcinoma less than or equal to 0.5 cm in diameter.

Eighty patients, or 32%, had occult/minimal breast cancers. There were 51 intraductal and 29 infiltrating ductal carcinomas less than or equal to 0.5 cm. There were no lobular carcinomas in situ detected by xeromammography. Twenty-five patients (31%) were premenopausal, and 55 patients (69%) were postmenopausal. Only one patient was less than 35 years old.

Sixty-nine patients (86%) with occult/minimal breast cancer underwent modified radical mastectomies four had simple mastectomies, four had radiation alone, two had biopsy alone, and one had radiation and axillary dissection.

Seventy patients underwent axillary dissections as part of their treatment, and in no cases were axillary metastases found. The follow-up has ranged from 1 to 10 years, and there have been no recurrences or cancer-related deaths in these 80 patients.

One hundred sixty-seven patients had occult/nonminimal lesions, that is, infil-

Table 1. *Occult Breast Cancers in 247 Patients*

| | | Type | | Menopausal Status | |
No. Patients	Intraductal	Infiltrating Ductal	Lobular in situ	Pre	Post
80 Minimal	51	29	0	25 (31%)	55 (69%)
167 Nonminimal	0	167	0	42 (25%)	125 (75%)

trating ductal carcinomas greater than 0.5 cm. Forty-two patients (25%) were pre-menopausal, and 125 patients (75%) were postmenopausal.

One hundred fifty-four patients (92%) underwent modified radical mastectomies, and 13 patients had lesser procedures because of metastatic disease already present or other serious illness.

Of the 154 patients undergoing axillary dissection, 114 patients (74%) had negative axillary lymph nodes while 40 patients (26%) had axillary metastases. Follow-up ranged from 1 to 10 years.

Of the 167 patients with nonminimal tumors, there were 23 deaths: 19 from breast cancer and 4 from unrelated disease. In addition, there were nine recurrences in patients who are still alive and undergoing treatment. Of the cancer-related deaths, three occurred in patients with negative axillary lymph nodes (2.6%), nine in patients with positive lymph nodes (22.5%), and seven in patients who did not undergo axillary dissection. This is an overall recurrence rate of 13% and a mortality rate from breast cancer of 11.6%.

These results for the occult/nonminimal group are more favorable than those reported in a 1980 regional survey of all breast cancers treated within the Kaiser-Permanente Medical Care Program (unpublished report). All breast cancers treated initially between 1973 and 1978 were reviewed, including both occult and palpable lesions. Of 2,620 cases, 1,510 (58%) had negative lymph nodes, and 1,110 (42%) had positive lymph nodes. They had 16% and 42% mortality rates, respectively, at 5 years. The overall mortality of all breast cancers seen at 5 years was 31% (Table 2).

DISCUSSION

Most of the studies to date that have addressed the issue of minimal breast cancer have used the terms occult, early, or minimal cancers synonymously. Gallager (1971) was the first to define minimal breast cancer. Since that time there have been

Table 2. *Nodal Status and Follow-up*

No. Patients	Negative Nodes	Positive Nodes	Recurrences	Deaths From Cancer
80 Minimal	70 (100%)	0	0	0
167 Nonminimal	114 (74%)	40 (26%)	21 (13%)	19 (11.6%)
2,620 All Kaiser (Palpable + occult)	1,510 (58%)	1,110 (42%)		(31%)

Table 3. *All Tumors Intraductal, Lobular in situ, Infiltrating Ductal Less Than or Equal To 0.5 cm*

Author	No. Patients	Negative Nodes	Positive Nodes
Bedwani (1981)	204	77% (157)	23% (47)
Moskowitz (1976)	32	100% (32)	0
Rosen (1980)*	129	99%	1%
Unzeitig	70	100% (70)	0

*Intraductal and lobular in situ carcinoma only.

few studies that have looked specifically at the nodal status and survival of a large group of patients with these minimal lesions.

A study by Bedwani et al. (1981) reviewed data from the American College of Surgeons long-term breast cancer survey and reported axillary metastases in 23% of patients with invasive carcinomas less than 0.5 cm. They reported no difference in survival of patients with tumors 0.5 cm or less when compared with survival of patients with tumors measuring 0.6 to 1 cm. Other articles by Rosen (1980) and by Letton (1980) report axillary metastases in 1% and 2.5% of the preinvasive lesions, respectively. Moskowitz et al. (1976) reported no axillary metastases in their group of 32 patients with minimal breast cancers. These researchers' data are compared with ours in Table 3.

In our group, there were no axillary metastases in patients with tumors measuring 0.5 cm or less. These differences may reflect better techniques in early detection of minimal cancers with xeromammography or more accurate or consistent pathologic staging.

Some confusion exists as to the difference between occult and minimal breast cancer. We believe it is extremely important to differentiate between occult/minimal and occult/nonminimal breast cancer. Minimal breast cancers, as defined by Gallagher, are intraductal, lobular in situ, or invasive cancers less than or equal to 0.5 cm in diameter, while occult tumors are not palpable but may be of any size. We reviewed all of our occult cancers detected by xeromammography and found that 80 (32%) were minimal cancers by the above definition. No patients in this group had axillary metastases, and there were no recurrences with a follow-up to 10 years. This contrasts significantly with patients who had occult tumors greater than 0.5 cm in diameter. This group had an axillary nodal involvement rate of 26%, a recurrence rate of 13%, and a mortality rate of 11.6%. Menopausal status was similar in both groups as was treatment, with 86% in the occult/minimal group and 92% in the occult/nonminimal group undergoing modified radical mastectomies. All our patients with breast cancer (occult and palpable combined) have a 42% incidence of axillary nodal involvement and an overall mortality of 31% at 5 years. Although the results in the occult/nonminimal group are significantly better than those of all breast cancer patients in our medical center, they in no way compare to the results in the occult/minimal group.

Occult breast cancers differ significantly between minimal and nonminimal tumors as regards both treatment and prognosis. The nonminimal cancers should be treated as any palpable carcinoma. Although patient survival is better than that of patients with palpable breast cancers, the incidence of recurrence and death in the nonminimal group, even among those patients with negative lymph nodes, is significant. More conservative treatment approaches, however, could be considered for the minimal breast cancer group, but prospective controlled studies should be done to determine the long-term risks of developing invasive carcinoma and recurrences in patients so treated.

SUMMARY

Among 32,814 women examined by xeromammography at the Los Angeles Kaiser-Permanente Medical Center in the last 10 years, 1,135 breast cancers were demonstrated. Twenty-six percent of these cancers (296) were occult, that is, not palpable on clinical examination. These cancers are divided into occult/minimal (80 patients) and occult/nonminimal (167 patients). Minimal cancers as defined by Gallager (1971) are intraductal, lobular in situ, or invasive cancers less than or equal to 0.5 cm in diameter. In the occult/minimal group, none had positive axillary lymph nodes, and there were no recurrences with a follow-up to 10 years. In the occult/nonminimal group, 26% had axillary nodal involvement, and there was a recurrence rate of 13% and a mortality of 11.6%. Occult breast cancers differ significantly between minimal and nonminimal tumors as regards both treatment and prognosis. The nonminimal cancers should be treated as any palpable carcinoma. More conservative treatment approaches, however, could be considered for the minimal group, but prospective controlled studies should be done to determine the long-term risks of developing invasive carcinoma and recurrences in patients so treated.

REFERENCES

Bedwani, R., J. Vana, D. Rosner, R. Schmitz, and G. Murphy. 1981. Management and survival of female patients with "minimal" breast cancer. Cancer 47:2769–2778.

Gallager, H. S., J. H. Farrow, and M. Galante. 1971. Early breast cancer. What is it? South. Med. Bull. 59:10–12.

Gallager, H. S., and J. E. Martin. 1971. An orientation to the concept of minimal breast cancer. Cancer 28:1505–1507.

Letton, A. H., and E. M. Mason. 1980. The treatment of nonpalpable carcinoma of the breast. Cancer 46:980–982.

Moskowitz, M., S. Pemmaraju, J. Fidler, D. Sutorius, P. Russell, P. Scheinok, and J. Holle. 1976. On the diagnosis of minimal breast cancer in a screenee population. Cancer 37:2543–2552.

Rosen, P. P., D. W. Braun, and D. E. Kinne. 1980. The clinical significance of pre-invasive breast carcinoma. Cancer 46:919–925.

Current Controversies in Breast Cancer, edited
by F. C. Ames, G. R. Blumenschein, and E. D. Montague.
University of Texas Press, Austin © 1984.

Localization of Occult Breast Lesions

J. L. Hoehn, M. D., J. M. Hardacre, M.D., M. K. Swanson, M.D.,
M. E. Kuehner, M.D., and G. H. Williams, M.D.

*Department of Surgery, Marshfield Clinic, and Marshfield
Medical Foundation, Marshfield, Wisconsin*

With the increased emphasis on early detection of breast cancer, more asymptomatic women are being subjected to mammography. Consequently, an increased number of nonpalpable lesions are being described, and the patient is referred to the surgeon for removal of the area of mammographic concern. Blind procedures, especially quadrant resections of the breast, are often quite deforming and still risk missing the area of mammographic concern. Five to 8% of the patients who underwent a blind procedure required a subsequent operation to find the area of mammographic abnormality (Rosen and Snyder 1977, Solmer et al. 1980).

Many refinements have been offered in the literature to help the surgeon find the area of mammographic concern. Injection techniques involve injecting a mixture of vital dye and radiopaque substance into the breast in the area of mammographic abnormality (Simon et al. 1972). These substances, however, tend to diffuse into the fat of the breast, particularly if there is any delay in the time between injection and biopsy. Additionally, the added radiopaque substance may obscure the microcalcifications that must be seen on specimen radiography to assure removal of the area of concern.

The use of skin markers and grids have been advocated by Malone et al. (1975). However, with any surface marker there may be considerable shift between the skin surface relative to a deeply situated, nonpalpable lesion, especially in large and pendulous breasts. Single or multiple hypodermic needles taped to the skin of the breast have been advocated (Dodd et al. 1966). These tend to dislodge during filming, transport from x-ray to surgery, skin preparation in surgery, as well as during the operative procedure itself. Additionally, such skin markers may cause false assumptions to be made. With compression of the breast during filming, the needle may be driven more deeply into the substance of the breast. With the patient in the lateral position, the needle may fall away from the area of concern.

The barbed wire was first reported by Funderburk and Flax (1976). Frank et al. (1976) reported their experience with a commercially available device (Frank Breast Biopsy Guide, Randall Faichney Corp. [Ranfac], Avon Industrial Park, Avon, Mass. 02327). We have reported our series using this same device illustrating its efficacy in finding the lesion with rapidity and conservation of breast substance (Hoehn et al. 1982). This communication updates our first 4 years experience at the Marshfield Clinic.

RESULTS

From May 1978 through April 1982, 128 patients underwent 137 needle localization procedures for nonpalpable breast lesions. The age of the patients ranged from 28–82 with a mean of 56.9 years. Fifty-four of the lesions contained microcalcifications (Figure 1), and the tissues were additionally subjected to specimen radiography. Eighty-three lesions did not contain microcalcifications (Figure 2). The histology of the lesions is as depicted in Table 1. There were 24 occult carcinomas discovered, and none were lobular carcinoma in situ (Table 2). All patients were treated by modified radical mastectomy, and only one patient (4.2%) had metastatic disease in the lymph nodes.

To assure accuracy in the removal of the area of mammographic concern in the 112 lesions that were not removed by mastectomy, follow-up mammograms confirmed removal for 94 lesions and specimen radiography for six lesions. Follow-up films are still pending for nine lesions. One patient's lesion was altered in configuration after biopsy and has remained stable for over 3 years. One patient refused follow-up mammograms. One lesion was missed, and a secondary procedure was

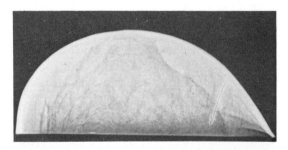

FIG. 1. Adjacent to the course of the localizing wire, microcalcifications are noted. This was a 3-mm intraductal carcinoma in a 55-year-old patient.

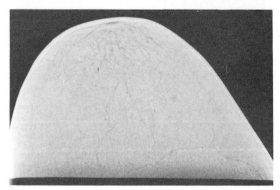

FIG. 2. A 6-mm infiltrating duct carcinoma in a 63-year-old female.

Table 1. *Histology*

Fibrocystic disease	52
Fibroadenoma	31
Carcinoma	24
Fibrous breast	13
Lymph node	9
Benign breast	3
Papilloma	2
Hibernoma	1
Fat necrosis	1
Hemangioma	1

Table 2. *Occult Carcinomas**

Histology	No.	Size	Microcalcifications
Intraductal	11	microscopic to 5 mm	9
Infiltrating duct	10	6–24 mm (mean 13 mm)	1
Tubular	2	1.0 & 1.5[†]	0
Mucinous	1	7 mm	0

*Range in size from microscopic to 24 mm.
[†]Only patient with axillary metastasis (4.2%).

required for removal. This was a fibroadenoma. Of the 24 patients with carcinoma of the breast, 23 are alive and free of disease. One patient has died of metastatic ovarian carcinoma.

COMPLICATIONS

In addition to the lesion that was missed as noted above, one patient developed a wound infection. Two patients had migration of the wire into the breast substance because of breast manipulation. This resulted in a prolonged operation to find the wire and remove both the wire and the area of mammographic concern. Migration can be easily prevented by bending the free end of the wire guide in excess of 90° and by not manipulating the breast once the wire is placed, especially in very large and mobile breasts.

COMMENT

No matter which technique for localization is used, it is absolutely necessary that the area of mammographic concern be seen on both the medial to lateral projection as well as the cephalocaudad projection with absolute certainty. We have not utilized this technique for lesions that lie immediately below the nipple and areola because this area can be conveniently sampled by a central duct resection. Additionally, it is important not to premedicate the patient prior to the wire placement because the patient will need to cooperate with the technician in radiology.

In our setting the placement of the device is done in the radiology suite. The site on the breast for insertion is chosen by a two-plane plot technique from the original mammograms. After cleansing the breast, a small amount of local anesthetic is injected into the skin overlying the area of mammographic concern. To facilitate introduction of the needle and wire guide, a stab wound is made with a no. 11 blade. The needle is introduced to the approximate depth as noted in the original mammograms and is then withdrawn leaving the wire guide in place. The patient is subjected to the same two mammographic views as she had originally and is brought to the operating room for the biopsy. Although close proximity of the wire guide to the lesion is helpful, the guide functions merely as a reference point at the time of surgery. Multiple needle placements and x-ray exposures are not necessary. Approximately one-third of these patients have been outpatients.

We have delayed definitive operation in those patients with either very small or microscopic lesions. In those patients who have adequate tumor volume and have consented to mastectomy, we have proceeded with a modified radical mastectomy upon frozen section results.

The incidence of metastasis to the axillary lymph nodes was 4.2% in our series but varies in the literature from 0–32% (Solmer et al. 1980 and Malone et al. 1975). A node sampling procedure is imperative to identify the patients at high risk for future failure so that they may be offered adjunctive chemotherapy.

Confirming removal of the area of mammographic concern is especially important when discrete lesions were not found at the time of biopsy. By 3–6 months after the operation, the surgical residual is minimal, and the mammographic appearance of the breast has usually returned to baseline. In only one of our patients has there been a question about persistence of the lesion. The appearance of the lesion was altered by the biopsy and has remained stable for over 3 years.

CONCLUSION

This technique provides the surgeon with a simple and reliable method to find nonpalpable areas of mammographic concern. In doing so, carcinoma of the breast is diagnosed at an early stage with minimal lymph node involvement.

ACKNOWLEDGMENTS

The authors wish to thank Donna Van Meter, RTR, Joan Riedel, RTR, and Patricia Schaub, RTR, for their willing cooperation with the needle placements and Ray Wade, RTR, for his invaluable assistance with specimen radiography, and Loretta Keding for her patience and secretarial skills.

REFERENCES

Dodd, G. D., K. Fry, and W. Delany. 1966. Preoperative Localization of Occult Carcinoma of the Breast in Management of the Patient with Cancer. W. B. Saunders, Philadelphia, p. 88.

Frank, H. A., F. M. Hall, and N. L. Steer. 1976. Preoperative localization of nonpalpable breast lesions demonstrated by mammography. N. Engl. J. Med. 295:259–260.

Funderburk, W. W., and R. L. Flax. 1976. Localization of nonpalpable carcinoma of the breast utilizing mammography: Technique A. Breast 2:28–29.

Hoehn, J. L., J. M. Hardacre, M. K. Swanson, and G. H. Williams. 1982. Localization of occult breast lesions. Cancer 49:1142–1144.

Malone, L. J., G. Frankl, R. A. Dorazio, and J. H. Winkley. 1975. Occult breast carcinomas detected by xeroradiography: Clinical Considerations. Ann. Surg. 181:133–136.

Rosen, P. P., and R. E. Snyder. 1977. Nonpalpable breast lesions detected by mammography and confirmed by specimen radiography: Recent experience. Breast 3:13–16.

Simon, N., G. J. Lesnick, W. N. Lerer, and A. L. Bachman. 1972. Roentgenographic localization of small lesions of the breast by the spot method. Surg. Gynecol. Obstet. 134:572–574.

Solmer, R., J. Goodstein, and C. Agliozzo. 1980. Nonpalpable breast lesions discovered by mammography. Arch. Surg. 115:1067–1069.

Current Controversies in Breast Cancer, edited
by F. C. Ames, G. R. Blumenschein, and E. D. Montague.
University of Texas Press, Austin © 1984.

Choice of Anesthesia for Breast Biopsy

Gordon F. Schwartz, M.D.,* Maryalice Cheney, M.D.,* Juan J.
Noguera, M.D.,* Mary Frances Boyle, M.D.,* and
Stephen A. Feig, M.D.†

*Departments of *Surgery and †Radiology, Jefferson Medical College,
Philadelphia, Pennsylvania*

How comforting it would be to our patients if we could precisely define which of the patients who present with breast complaints have significant disease, so that the vast majority who do not could be reassured without subjecting them to breast biopsy. Not only is the prospect of breast biopsy a formidable and enervating experience to endure because of the possible diagnosis of cancer, but, even when it is over and the results are benign, it is an operation that may have to be repeated again within the patient's lifetime. Unlike appendicitis, which is a one-time procedure, a woman may face an additional biopsy for another, perhaps more significant, reason at a later time. Therefore, it is incumbent upon those of us who perform breast biopsy to make this procedure as palatable as we can to those women who must undergo it.

Most practicing surgeons have been trained to perform breast biopsy in the hospital, using general anesthesia under inpatient circumstances. Only in the past few years has this practice been criticized as much for fiscal as for humanitarian reasons. As the costs of medical care have escalated, patients, surgeons, and third-party insurers have sought ways of keeping costs as low as possible, without jeopardizing quality of care. Thus, outpatient breast biopsy using local anesthesia has become advocated as an alternative to inpatient biopsy under general anesthesia (Klamer and Fry 1980).

Almost simultaneously, the anachronistic physician-patient attitude of "do as I say" has been supplanted by a shared responsibility for health care, in which the patient demands the privilege of making her own decisions with the help of her caring and concerned physician. In this context, the traditional approach of one-step biopsy, frozen section, and "whatever else might be necessary" has been challenged by patients as well as physicians.

This study was undertaken to answer several questions: 1) Is breast biopsy using local anesthesia an acceptable or preferable alternative to the conventional practice of inpatient breast biopsy using general anesthesia? 2) Is breast biopsy using local anesthesia cost effective? 3) Is the separation of biopsy and definitive treatment for breast cancer a reasonable alternative to the traditional one-step procedure, involving biopsy, frozen section, and mastectomy, under the same anesthesia?

MATERIALS AND METHODS

Between January 1977 and June 30, 1982, 2,643 new private patients sought evaluation by the senior author (G.F.S.) for a perceived breast problem. Of this total number of new patients, 817 (30.9%) underwent breast biopsy, 36 bilateral, so that the total number of biopsies was 853. All biopsies were performed in the same operating room suite at Thomas Jefferson University Hospital in Philadelphia using either general or local anesthesia.

Choice of general or local anesthesia was suggested at the time the biopsy recommendation was made. Occasionally, patients expressed strong preference for or against one type of anesthesia, and, when not contraindicated for medical reasons, the patient's preference was respected. In general, biopsies for clinically occult lesions were performed using general anesthesia through the course of this study.

Patients for whom general anesthesia was used were almost always admitted to the hospital the evening before surgery, undergoing physical examination and laboratory studies. They were discharged from the hospital either on the evening of surgery if they had recovered from the anesthesia or the next morning after the dressing was changed. Patients undergoing biopsy under local anesthesia came to the operating room immediately prior to the scheduled procedure and were discharged from the hospital immediately upon completion of the procedure.

Technique of biopsy was the same for both groups of patients. Whenever possible, a circumareolar incision was used, especially in young women and almost always if the preoperative likelihood of malignancy was deemed small or the lesion was located in the upper inner quadrant of the breast. When the lesion was judged too far from the areolar margin for a circumareolar incision, a curvilinear incision parallel to the areolar margin was made in the skin lines directly over the lesion. When the preoperative diagnosis was cancer, the incision was usually parallel to the areolar margin, but directly over the lesion. When a presumed benign lesion was encountered, it was usually excised in its entirety with a tiny rim of contiguous normal breast. If the lesion appeared malignant on inspection at the time of biopsy, an incisional biopsy was performed, in which only enough tissue was removed to secure the diagnosis without equivocation and to determine the presence of estrogen and progesterone receptors. If the lesion was small, so that excisional versus incisional biopsy was merely an exercise in semantics, then it was usually removed in its entirety. No sutures were ever placed within the substance of the breast to close "dead space" because of our concern with subsequent deformity of the breast contour. Instead, a sliver of Penrose drain was placed in the depths of the wound and brought out through the incision. The areolar muscle or dermis was closed with interrupted sutures of 5-0 Dexon or Vicril, and the skin was reapproximated with interrupted 6-0 Nylon sutures. Fluff gauzes were placed over the wound, and the chest was wrapped circumferentially with elastic bandages fixed in place with adhesive tape and safety pins. The next morning, either at home or before discharge, the dressing was changed and the drain removed. The only subsequent dressing was the patients own bra with a small square of gauze between the incision and the bra. No adhesive tape was ever used on the skin of the breast.

For lesions that were not palpable, i.e., clinically occult, and for which biopsy had been recommended on the basis of a suspicious mammogram, needle-guided biopsy was employed (Schwartz et al. 1978). Once the needle had been inserted into the breast and taped in place by the radiologists, the patient was brought to the operating room, and the biopsy was performed using general anesthesia. General anesthesia was preferred because of the need to dissect through the breast looking for the "needle in the haystack" and, at the same time, trying to avoid the excision of needless volumes of breast tissue. This often required considerable manipulation of breast tissue often causing more discomfort than biopsy of a palpable lesion. Moreover, some of the radiographic findings were so minimal that concern was raised that infiltration of local anesthesia into the area might distort the architecture of the breast enough to interfere with the excision of the suspicious lesion and with interpretation of the specimen radiograph. Proof that the entire suspicious area was removed was verified by specimen radiography. These patients were also discharged according to the same time schedule as patients undergoing biopsy for palpable lesions.

The diagnosis was given to the patient in all cases as soon as it became available. If frozen section had been performed, the diagnosis was shared with the patient as soon as she was awake if general anesthesia had been used; if local anesthesia was employed, the patient was informed before she left the operating room suite. In general, the diagnosis was not immediately available for lesions that were clinically occult, since frozen sections were rarely requested for these lesions. We have preferred to submit all of this tissue for paraffin sections and not risk losing what might be the most significant portion of the specimen in the cryostat. When cancer was disclosed, the patient was informed of the diagnosis, metastatic workup was initiated, and the patient was scheduled for what we call a conference appointment to discuss the options of therapy. These biopsy techniques offer patients superior cosmetic results, with an inconspicuous scar and no loss of breast contour. The procedure is made palatable enough so that if another biopsy is required subsequently, it will not be avoided because of the unpleasant memory or the visible reminder of a previous formidable experience.

RESULTS

Table 1 shows the breakdown of all breast biopsies performed using local and general anesthesia from 1977 to 1982. Table 2 shows the breakdown of unilateral breast biopsies performed using local and general anesthesia for the same time period. Of note is the reversal in practice that has occurred.

In 1977, 19.4% of all breast biopsies were performed using local anesthesia, while 80.6% were performed using general anesthesia. These figures include uni-

Table 1. *Anesthesia for Breast Biopsy, 1977–1982*

	Year					
	77	78	79	80	81	82
Local						
Unilateral	20	40	89	130	151	91
Bilateral	–	2	4	8	8	3
Needle-guided	–	–	1	2	–	7
Total	20	44	98	148	167	104
%	19.4	45.8	75.9	80.9	79.1	79.4
General						
Unilateral	64	37	18	11	12	4
Bilateral	3	2	–	4	1	–
Needle-guided	13	11	13	16	30	23
Total	83	52	31	35	44	27
%	80.6	54.2	24.1	19.1	20.9	20.6

Table 2. *Unilateral Breast Biopsies, 1977–1982*

	Year					
	77	78	79	80	81	82
Local	20	40	89	130	151	91
General	64	37	18	11	12	4
Total	84	77	107	141	163	95
% Local	23.8	51.9	83.2	92.2	92.6	95.8
% General	76.2	48.1	16.8	7.8	7.4	4.2

lateral, bilateral, and needle-guided biopsies as well. If unilateral biopsies alone are considered, in 1977, 23.8% were performed using local anesthesia, and 76.2% were performed using general anesthesia. In 1978, although 54.2% and 45.8% of all biopsies were performed using general and local anesthesia, respectively, if unilateral biopsies are considered separately, the ratio of general versus local begins to reverse (48.1% general, 51.9% local). The reversal is complete by 1979 when 75.9% of all biopsies were performed using local anesthesia and 24.1% using general anesthesia. Considering unilateral biopsies only, patient and physician preference for local anesthesia began in 1978 and was overwhelming by the end of the study period. Currently (1982) less than 5% of biopsies are performed using general anesthesia.

Of the 853 biopsies performed, approximately one out of four (26.7%) proved to be malignant (Table 3).

Only two of the 817 patients in this series preferred biopsy with frozen section, using general anesthesia, with immediate treatment if the diagnosis proved to be malignant. All of the others, when offered the alternative, preferred to separate biopsy from treatment if the lesion proved to be malignant.

Table 3. *Distribution of Diagnoses*

| | Year | | | | | | | |
	77	78	79	80	81	82	Total	%
Benign	88	78	106	124	139	90	625	73.3
Malignant	15	18	23	59	72	41	228	26.7
Total	103	96	129	183	211	131	853	

Table 4. *Complications in 853 Breast Biopsies*

Complication	Number	Anesthesia
Wound Infection	2	1 local, 1 general
Hematoma	2	2 local
Total	4	
%	0.46	

Approximate current hospital charges for breast biopsies using local anesthesia are $500 versus $2,500 for general anesthesia. These figures do not include the professional fees for the surgeon, or surgeon and anesthesiologist.

Of the total group of 853 biopsies, there were four complications, two hematomas, and two wound infections (Table 4). The hematomas both occurred in patients undergoing biopsy with local anesthesia. The wound infections occurred in one patient who received local anesthesia and in one patient given general anesthesia. All complications were managed on an outpatient basis.

DISCUSSION

This study demonstrates an increasing utilization of local anesthesia for breast biopsy between the years 1977 and 1982, paralleling changes in physician and patient preference. Up until 1977, the only indications for local anesthesia for breast biopsy were patient demand or significant intercurrent illness that contraindicated general anesthesia. Local anesthesia was generally looked upon with disfavor, the only reasons cited being the possibility of missing the lesion and an increased likelihood of hematoma or infection. Similarly, the separation of biopsy from definitive treatment for breast cancer had been unnecessary, since all patients underwent radical mastectomy once the diagnosis of cancer was secure. An occasional patient might insist upon separate biopsy because of concern about the accuracy of the diagnosis, preferring to await the paraffin sections rather than chancing the loss of her breast on the basis of frozen section results alone. Occasionally, the nature of the diagnosis on frozen section was obscure, so that waiting for the paraffin sections was deemed medically appropriate. For example, intraductal papilloma and papillary carcinomas are difficult to distinguish on frozen section, so that we have never asked for frozen section when dealing with lesions producing nipple discharge. As the treatment for breast cancer became more selective in nature, in that the treatment recommendation depended upon the individual patient circumstances and options of therapy were offered when appropriate for the patient's own considerations, the advantage of separating the biopsy from the subsequent treatment became obvious. No longer is it necessary to consider all of the "what if's" at the time of the preoperative discussion, and no longer is it necessary to make patients undergo extensive preoperative laboratory examinations, such as liver function studies, chest x-ray, or bone scans, when the diagnosis proves to be benign. Patients with cancer can be addressed individually, each woman feeling that her treatment will be custom tailored to her own situation. Fears about a mistaken diagnosis are now assuaged. Concerns about tumor dissemination when biopsy and treatment are separated are unproven. Data from the Mayo Clinic indicate that a short delay between biopsy and treatment is not harmful (Pierce et al. 1956), and we have not observed any increased incidence of wound complications, local or distant recurrence, or other complications in the 5 years of this study. Admittedly, it will be at least another 5 years before 10-year data are available for analysis in enough patients to make substantive statements in this regard. Haagensen's data with respect to incisional biopsy (Haagensen, 1981) indicate a preference for this technique over excisional biopsy in terms of dissemination of cancer.

The low incidence of complications following breast biopsy is probably the bare minimum to be expected with any surgically "clean" procedure. There was no difference between complications after local and those after general anesthesia. Thus, avoidance of hematoma or infection is not a valid reason for choosing general over local anesthesia. Almost without exception, when questioned after the procedure, the majority of women, even those most reluctant to undergo biopsy under local anesthesia, have been delighted with the outcome. No patient undergoing biopsy under local anesthesia has remarked that she would choose general anesthesia if there were a "next time." Cosmetic results have been equal and excellent in all patients regardless of anesthesia chosen.

Those women diagnosed with breast cancer after having undergone biopsy have expressed the most gratitude for not being intimidated into an immediate decision about what comes next, even when the subsequent treatment was mastectomy nonetheless. All of these women felt that they were being treated as individuals, their own concerns and fears being addressed, and not merely being plugged into an operating schedule and receiving the same treatment as all patients. It is not germane to this discussion to consider the various options for therapy, i.e., radiation therapy versus mastectomy, etc., but discussion of these options followed by a final recommendation based upon individual considerations has been most appreciated by all patients.

Finally, the difference in cost between biopsy using local anesthesia and using general anesthesia is staggering, a factor of about five. Assuming the surgeon's fees to be the same, this fivefold increase in cost is even greater when one considers the professional fees of the anesthesiologist, who need not be involved at all if the biopsy is performed using local anesthesia. Those who cite the cheaper costs for the one-step procedure in patients with cancer forget that the majority of breast biopsies are performed for what proves to be benign disease.

The original questions that were posed have been answered, we believe, in favor of local anesthesia for most breast biopsies. We do still prefer general anesthesia for needle-guided biopsies for nonpalpable calcifications and also for selected patients who require bilateral biopsies. Even in this latter category, although the procedure is extended in time, most women are still willing to undergo biopsy under local anesthesia, which we encourage for bilateral breast biopsy.

No firm statements may be made with respect to the long-term outlook for patients with breast cancer who have undergone biopsy and have then been treated separately at a later date. There is no question that this separation of biopsy from treatment has found considerable favor with patients. Until there is proof that this so-called two-stage procedure is harmful, we shall continue to advocate it as the most comfortable, courteous, and concerned approach for the patient who may have breast cancer.

REFERENCES

Haagensen, C. D., C. Bodian, and D. E. Haagensen. 1981. Biopsy, *in* Breast Carcinoma: Risk and Detection, C. D. Haagensen, C. Bodian, and D. E. Haagensen, eds. W. B. Saunders Company, Philadelphia, pp. 516–525.

Klamer, T. W., and D. E. Fry. 1980. The merits of breast biopsy under local anesthesia. Cur. Surg. 37:126–128.

Pierce, E. H., O. T. Clagett, J. R. McDonald, and R. P. Gage. 1956. Biopsy of the breast followed by radical mastectomy. Surg. Gynecol. Obstet. 103:559–564.

Schwartz, G. F., S. A. Feig, and A. S. Patchefsky. 1978. Clinicopathologic correlations and significance of clinically occult mammary lesions. Cancer 41:1147–1153.

Current Controversies in Breast Cancer, edited
by F. C. Ames, G. R. Blumenschein, and E. D. Montague.
University of Texas Press, Austin © 1984.

The Use of the Latissimus Dorsi Myocutaneous Flap in the Reconstruction of the Breast after Mastectomy

Thomas M. Biggs, M.D., F.A.C.S.

Department of Plastic Surgery, St. Joseph Hospital, Houston, Texas

In the reconstruction of a breast that has been removed due to malignancy, the goal is to create a mound or a mass of tissue that, in shape and consistency, resembles a natural breast. The Silastic gel prosthesis has provided the surgeon with mass (T. Cronin and Gerow 1964) and, in patients with ample muscle and skin remaining after the mastectomy, this prosthesis may be placed beneath these tissues for breast reconstruction (Cronin and Cronin 1979, Snyderman and Guthrie 1971). Our own experience (Cronin and Biggs 1980), as well as that of others (Bostwick 1979), has shown that simple prosthesis placement is adequate for some breast reconstructions (Figure 1a and b). If adequate tissue is not present or if a desire for larger breasts exists, it may be necessary to bring in additional tissue to satisfy these needs (Wolf and Biggs 1979).

Our initial effort at bringing in additional tissue involved local transposition or rotational flaps (Cronin et al. 1977) (Figure 2a and b). Although we frequently produced good reconstructions using this technique, consistency of excellence was lacking, and in radical mastectomy patients the amount of tissue necessary to cover the ribs was of such magnitude that we were unable to accomplish as complete a reconstruction as we wished.

The introduction of the latissimus dorsi myocutaneous flap for breast reconstruction was a great step forward (Bostwick et al. 1978). The latissimus dorsi gets most of its blood supply from the thoracodorsal artery, which also acts as a carrier for the blood supply to the overlying skin. For these reasons the entire muscle can be dissected away from its origin on the fascia of the paraspinal muscles and over the ribs distally and, with an ellipse of overlying skin attached to the muscle, rotated and passed subcutaneously to the anterior chest (Figures 3, 4a and b, 5a,b, and c). The muscle and skin can then be fashioned over a gel prosthesis to create a natural shape for the reconstruction (Figure 6). The technical aspects of the design of the flap and placement of the muscle vary, and each case must be approached individually.

This reconstruction can be performed after mastectomy as soon as the wounds are healed (Figure 7a and b). The patient remains in the hospital 3 to 4 days, and all sutures are removed by 8 days. Occasionally, however, sutures are left in the donor site on the back longer if the wound has been closed under excess tension. When

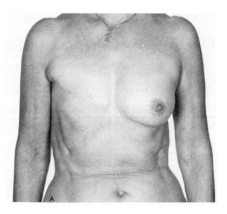
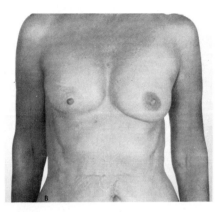

FIG. 1A. Preoperative photograph of a patient with small breasts who had undergone modified radical mastectomy. **B.** Postoperative view of the same patient with a Silastic gel prosthesis placed beneath the remaining muscle and skin. The nipple has been reconstructed. The shape is akin to the opposite breast but is little more than a mound with very little projection.

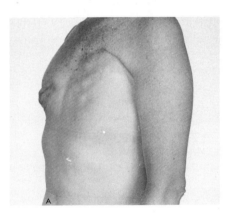
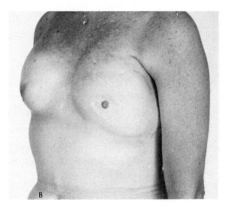

FIG. 2A. Patient who underwent a left modified radical mastectomy of the left breast and a simple mastectomy of the right breast. **B.** One year after reconstruction of the left breast with a rotational flap from the abdomen and a Silastic gel prosthesis placed beneath. A gel prosthesis was placed beneath the available tissues of the right breast, and a nipple was reconstructed. The procedure is adequate, but the breast is a mound and does not have a globular shape. There is a deficiency of tissue near the axilla.

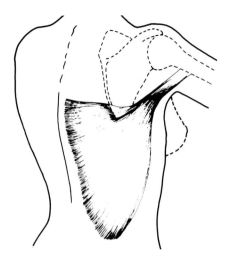

FIG. 3. The location of the latissimus dorsi muscle in the back. The thoracodorsal artery supplies the blood for this muscle and its overlying skin and enters the muscle high in the axilla; thus, when the muscle is freed it can be rotated to the anterior chest along with the overlying skin.

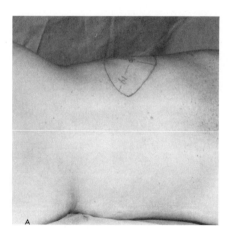
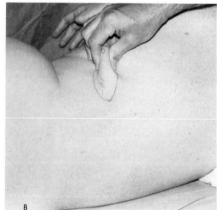

FIG. 4A. The location of the skin flap is directly over the latissimus dorsi muscle. **B.** The patient is placed in the extended position for the dissection but is moved to the flexed position so the wound can be closed.

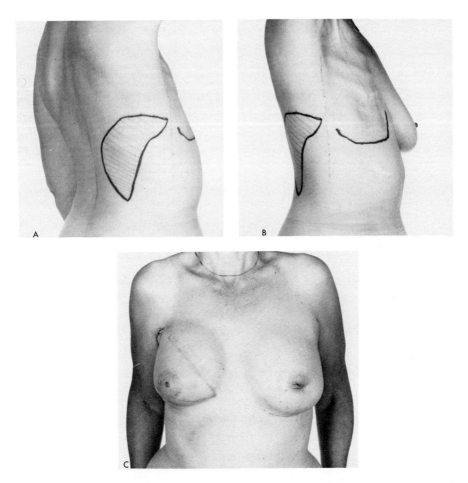

FIG. 5A. The design of a flap so that the most lateral portion of the flap will rotate anteriorly and not extend into the axilla. **B.** The dissection of the anterior chest and the elevation of the flap onto the posterior chest create two large spaces. It is imperative to leave a bridge of intact tissue between these two spaces and pass the flap through a small tunnel as high in the axilla as possible. **C.** The location of the flap on the anterior chest with the lateral portion going anteriorly and not into the axilla. This patient has also had a subcutaneous mastectomy with reconstruction.

radiotherapy is instituted we prefer to reconstruct the breast as soon as possible after completion of therapy as long as erythema does not persist. We believe the well-vascularized muscle beneath the irradiated skin may prevent or preclude some of the changes often seen after radiotherapy.

Bilateral reconstruction can be performed in one stage (Figure 8a and b). While we use the recumbent position for unilateral cases, the prone position is preferred for raising bilateral flaps. After the flaps are raised, they are placed into the axilla

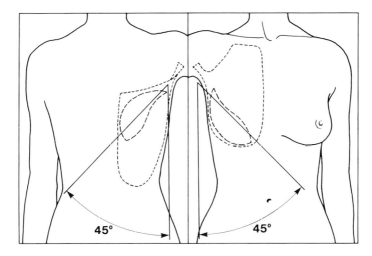

FIG. 6. The rotation of the myocutaneous flap transposes an arc of 90° as it goes from the back to the front. The muscle for resection can be determined on the back and can be moved to the anterior chest in the appropriate fashion. Likewise, the location of the skin island can be determined so that it will fit properly on the anterior chest.

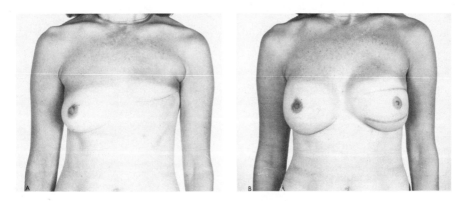

FIG. 7A. Patient 1 month after modified radical mastectomy. **B.** Four months after latissimus dorsi myocutaneous flap reconstruction of the left breast and nipple reconstruction. On the right she has had a subcutaneous mastectomy with reconstruction. The flap has been placed in the position where it would be most effective in creating the desired shape. The old scar was ignored.

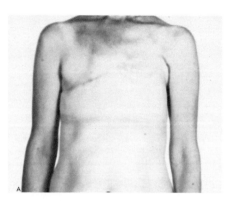
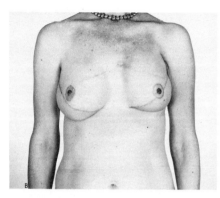

FIG. 8A. Patient 4 years following bilateral modified radical mastectomy. **B.** One year following bilateral latissimus dorsi myocutaneous flap reconstruction with bilateral nipple reconstruction. This patient had inadequate tissue on the left side, necessitating additional tissue to achieve a full breast with adequate shape.

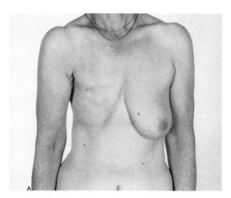
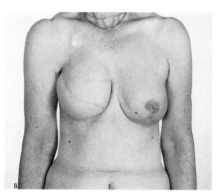

FIG. 9A. Two years following radical mastectomy. **B.** The patient 6 months following latissimus dorsi myocutaneous flap reconstruction of the right breast. The left breast had a subcutaneous mastectomy with a mastopexy. A variety of options are available for the remaining breast, and each case should be determined individually.

for storage while the donor wounds are closed. The patient is then rotated onto her back, and the flaps brought forward onto the chest.

The opposite breast and the nipple can be dealt with at the time of reconstruction or later (Figures 9a and b, 10a and b). A subcutaneous mastectomy, mastopexy, reduction mammoplasty, or augmentation mammoplasty can be adequately performed at the time of reconstruction. Nipple reconstruction, if desired by the patient, is somewhat more precise after healing has taken place.

Other sites for distal tissue include free flaps with microvascular anastamosis (Fugino et al. 1976) or rectus abdominus myocutaneous flaps (Scheflan and Dinner

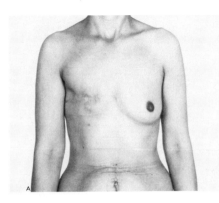 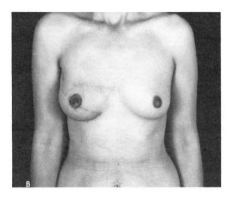

FIG. 10A. Patient 6 months following modified radical mastectomy who desired reconstruction of the new breast to match the size and shape of the opposite breast as much as possible. **B.** Six months following latissimus dorsi reconstruction. The reconstructed breast is similar in size and shape to the opposite breast. It was necessary to abandon the old mastectomy scar, and the skin flap was placed to create the desired shape.

1983). The latter may be preferable if the latissimus dorsi is absent or if there is an excessive subclavicular hollow. The former is preferred only when all other sources are unavailable.

REFERENCES

Bostwick, J. 1979. Breast reconstruction and comprehensive approach. Clin. Plast. Surg. 6:143.

Bostwick, J., L. Vasconez, and M. Jurkiewicz. 1978. Breast reconstruction after a radical mastectomy. Plast. Reconstr. Surg. 61:682.

Cronin, T., and T. Biggs. 1980. Breast reconstruction following mastectomy, *in* International Advances in Surgical Oncology, G. Murphy, ed. Alan R. Liss, New York, pp. 29–48.

Cronin, T., and E. Cronin, 1979. Reconstruction of the breast without additional skin or muscle flaps. Clin. Plast. Surg. 6:1.

Cronin, T., and F. Gerow. 1964. Augmentation mammaplasty: A new "natural feel" prosthesis (Transactions of the Third International Congress of Plastic Surgery, Washington, D.C.) Exerpta Medica, Amsterdam, pp. 41–49.

Cronin, T., J. Upton, and J. McDonough. 1977. Reconstruction of the breast after mastectomy. Plast. Reconstr. Surg. 59:1–14.

Fugino, T., T. Harashina, and K. Enomoto. 1976. Primary breast reconstruction after a standard radical mastectomy by a free flap transfer: A case report. Plast. Reconstr. Surg. 58:372.

Scheflan, M., and M. Dinner. 1983. The transverse abdominal island flap: Part I. Indications, contraindications, results and complications. Ann. Plast. Surg. 10:24–35.

Snyderman, R., and R. Guthrie. 1971. Reconstruction of the female breast following radical mastectomy. Plast. Reconstr. Surg. 46:565.

Wolf, L., and T. Biggs. 1979. Breast reconstruction following mastectomy. Am. J. Surg. 138:777.

RADIATION ONCOLOGY AND BREAST CANCER

Current Controversies in Breast Cancer, edited
by F. C. Ames, G. R. Blumenschein, and E. D. Montague.
University of Texas Press, Austin © 1984.

Treatment Results, Cosmesis, and Complications in Stages I and II Breast Cancer Patients Treated by Excisional Biopsy and Irradiation

Alvaro A. Martinez, M.D.,*† and Daniel Clarke, M.D.*

Department of Radiology, Stanford University School of Medicine, Stanford, California, and †Department of Oncology, Mayo Clinic, Rochester, Minnesota

While considerable controversy remains concerning the best treatment modality for patients with early breast cancer, modern radiation therapy has become in some centers an acceptable alternative to radical surgery in the primary management of early-stage breast carcinoma, and locoregional control rates in excess of 90% are being achieved (Bedwinek 1981, Hellman et al. 1980, Martinez and Goffinet 1981, Montague et al. 1979, Pierquin et al. 1980). Recognition of factors that can modify cosmesis is important because breast preservation is a major concern to patients who refuse mastectomy. Since there have been few analyses of treatment sequelae (Clarke et al. 1982, Clarke et al. 1983, Harris et al. 1979), this study was undertaken to identify variables that influence both cosmetic results and treatment complications in these patients. Also, the treatment results of this prospective clinical trial are presented.

MATERIALS AND METHODS

Between May 1973 and December 1980, 77 patients with stage I or stage II adenocarcinoma of the breast were treated by primary radiotherapy at Stanford University Medical Center. Seventy-nine breasts were treated; two patients presented with bilateral cancers. Table 1 correlates stage and menopausal status.

Radiation Therapy Policies

A complete description of our treatment technique has been reported previously (Martinez and Goffinet 1981, Martinez and Clarke 1983) (Table 2). Since radiation doses and fractionation schedules were modified during the treatment period, we were able to correlate these changes with treatment results. Early in this series, five patients were treated with 250-rad fractions four times per week, with total doses ranging from 5,000 to 5,500 rad. Ten patients received 5,000 rad using 200-rad

Table 1. *Stanford University Patient Population
(May 1973–Dec 1980)**

Patients		Clinical Stage	
		I	II
Premenopausal	45	22	23
Postmenopausal	34	13	21
Total	79	35	44

*Median follow-up 40 months.

Table 2. *Treatment Policy (1973–1980)*

Daily Dose	Fractions/ Week	Total Dose*	Breasts Treated
250 rad	4/week	5,000–5,500 rad	5
200 rad	5/week	5,000 rad	10
180 rad	5/week	4,500–5,000 rad	64

*1,800–2,500 rad by ^{192}Ir implant = 64 breasts; 1,500–2,500 rad by electron beam = 10 breasts.

fractions five times per week. Our current policy is to deliver 4,500 to 5,000 rad at 180 rad per fraction five times per week. Sixty-four patients have been treated in this fashion. All fields were treated daily in all patients in this series. Two to four weeks following completion of external-beam radiation, preplanned ^{192}Ir implants delivering 1,800 to 3,000 rad to the tumor volume and tumor margins were performed in 64 breasts. The implant volume ranged from 20 cc to 170 cc. Fifteen patients did not undergo ^{192}Ir breast implants. Of these, 10 received electron boosts to the tumor volume, three had supervoltage boosts, and two had no additional treatment.

Computerized dosimetry at multiple levels was obtained in all patients. Inhomogeneity of ± 5% across the irradiated breast was accepted. Compensators were frequently utilized to correct for variation in dose. Patients with extremely large breasts had from 8 to 12% inhomogeneity throughout the irradiated volume.

Surgical Techniques

All patients were advised to have excisional biopsies of their tumors, and gross excision was performed in 76 instances. Two patients had incisional biopsies, and one patient had a needle biopsy. Careful pathologic examination of tumor margins was not done in most patients.

Our policy has been to recommend an axillary dissection for patients who are candidates for adjuvant chemotherapy. Thirty-eight patients had axillary dissections, 12 had axillary samplings, and 29 patients had no axillary staging. Table 3 compares the mean and the range of number of nodes removed during each surgical

Table 3. *Axillary Staging Procedure*

Procedure	Cases	Nodes Mean	Range
Dissection	38	18	8–36
Sampling	12	3	1–6
None	29	0	0

procedure. Eighteen nodes was the mean value for patients who had dissected axillary nodes compared to three nodes for those who had axillary sampling. We strongly recommend that removal of the primary tumor and the axillary contents be done through two separate incisions, to avoid contamination of the axillary area if all nodes are negative.

Follow-Up and Evaluation

All patients in this study have been examined by the two authors. Ninety-one percent of the patients were examined during the 6 months immediately preceding the closing date of the study, while 90% were seen within the last year. At each examination, the following complications, if present, were carefully documented: 1) breast edema, 2) skin discoloration, 3) breast fibrosis, 4) arm edema, 5) impairment of arm mobility or function, and 6) rib fractures. If present, each was scored as mild, moderate, or severe. Other complications, such as axillary hematoma or seroma, basilic vein thrombosis, axillary or breast infection, radiation pneumonitis, and myositis, were recorded if present. Whether the excisional biopsy affected cosmesis was also reported. The overall cosmetic result was scored as excellent, satisfactory, or unsatisfactory. The criteria were:

Excellent—Appearance of the breast almost identical in size and configuration to the opposite breast; no breast deformity either from fibrosis or biopsy; no readily apparent permanent skin changes, such as telangiectasia or atrophy.

Satisfactory—Mild to moderate breast asymmetry, with no more than ⅓ volume loss secondary to biopsy or retraction from fibrosis; any readily apparent treatment sequelae such as breast retraction from the biopsy scar or telangiectasia over the implanted site.

Unsatisfactory—Marked breast asymmetry; severe fibrosis; greater than ⅓ volume loss secondary to biopsy or retraction from fibrosis.

When there was disagreement regarding a complication or the cosmetic result, the complication was marked as present and the lower of the two cosmetic results was scored. Currently, our patients are being interviewed to determine their own evaluation of cosmesis.

Multiple patient characteristics were recorded and evaluated for their correlation with various complications and the cosmetic results. Breast size was determined as A, B, C, or D for each patient, with breast size approximating the breast cup size.

All patients with D cup or greater were scored as D. In addition, patient age, menopausal status, and tumor size were analyzed.

Contingency tables were prepared relating patient characteristics with outcome (complication or cosmetic result). The significance of the correlation between the characteristic and outcome was assessed by means of the chi-square test.

RESULTS

Locoregional control was achieved in 74 of 79 breasts (94%), with a median follow-up of 40 months. Table 4 shows the correlation of locoregional control with "T" stage. Two patients, whose failures occurred at 7 months and at 35 months after irradiation, underwent salvage surgery and postoperative chemotherapy. Since their cosmetic results are now unsatisfactory due to the salvage surgery, the cosmetic result scored at their last follow-up prior to relapse was used for this analysis. The other three patients with local failure presented concomitantly with widespread disease. Mastectomies were not performed in these patients.

Eight patients developed discrete masses in the treated breasts. Excisional biopsy of these masses revealed fat necrosis in four patients, which were clinically indistinguishable from recurrent cancer. A complete description of the clinical features of fat necrosis simulating carcinoma was previously reported (Clarke et al. 1983).

Complications Related to Surgery

Surgical complications resulted primarily from the axillary dissection and are summarized in Table 5. Lymphedema of the breast, a commonly observed reaction

Table 4. *Locoregional Control of T_1–T_2, N_0–N+ Lesions.**

T-Stage	No. patients	Locoregional Failure
T1	43	1 (2%)
T2	36	4 (11%)
Total	79	5 (6%)

*Minimal follow-up 24 months, median follow-up 40 months; 94% or 74/79 pts. with locoregional control.

Table 5. *Complications Associated with Axillary Dissection (38 Patients)*

Breast edema	87%
Axillary seroma or hematoma	31.6%
Arm edema	26%
Basilic vein thrombosis	20%
Axillary abscess	7.9%
Impaired arm mobility (transient)	5%

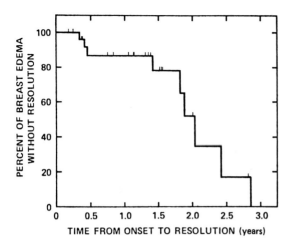

FIG. 1. Time to complete resolution of breast edema in 33 patients with early onset of lymphedema of the breast following axillary dissection.

that has been previously reported (Clarke et al. 1982), was observed in 51% of the patients and was directly related to the extent of the axillary staging procedure. Of the 38 patients receiving axillary dissections, breast edema occurred in 33 (87%). Twenty-five percent of patients undergoing axillary sampling, and only 7% of patients with no axillary surgery, developed breast edema (Clarke et al. 1982). Lymphedema of the breast is transient, with resolution of all cases observed by 3 years (Figure 1).

Axillary seroma or hematoma formation was seen in 12 patients or 32%. All of these patients have had axillary dissections and developed their complications prior to the initiation of radiotherapy. Multiple needle aspirations of the accumulated fluid were required in these patients. Four out of the 12 patients during the first year of follow-up developed an axillary mass that was round, smooth, very hard, and fixed to the chest wall. Excisional biopsy was performed in all four cases; no tumor was found, only a cystic capsule with organized hematoma and fibrosis. Of interest is that only one of these patients had received irradiation to the axilla.

Arm edema has been observed in 11 patients (14%). Ten of these complications occurred acutely as a result of axillary dissection, for an incidence of 26% in the dissected population; one patient developed edema after a high axillary radiation dose (6,500 rad), and another developed transient arm edema in association with an axillary tumor recurrence. Breast edema was present in all 10 patients who developed arm edema following axillary dissection. Two patients had mild functional arm impairment; however, there has been good improvement in both patients after physical therapy.

Eleven patients, or 14% of the entire group, had a reduction in cosmetic score, mostly from excellent to satisfactory due to either an excessively large biopsy (quadrentectomy or partial mastectomy) or a poorly placed incisional scar.

Less common complications included basilic vein thrombosis in eight patients or 10% of the population. Seven of the eight with thrombosis followed axillary dissection, and one occurred in conjunction with axillary recurrence of carcinoma. Postirradiation axillary abscesses occurred in three patients, all of whom had axillary dissections. Two of the abscesses developed 6 months after treatment and their cause is not clear.

Complications Related to Radiation Therapy

Radiation therapy complications are summarized in Table 6. Breast fibrosis has been observed in 18 patients (22.7%): 13 mild, 2 moderate, and 3 severe. Mild fibrosis was a finding that was appreciated on breast palpation but not recognized on inspection in the upright position.

Four of five patients treated with 250-rad fractions developed fibrosis and two of the three severe cases were in this group (Table 7). Severe fibrosis was noted in a patient who received 5,500 rad in 250-rad fractions to the entire breast in 1973. No field size reductions were made. The second patient received 5,500 rad in 250-rad fractions and a high-dose, large-volume ^{192}Ir implant in 1975. The third case of severe fibrosis was seen in a patient treated in 1976 with 5,000 rad in 200-rad fractions followed by a large-volume high-dose implant (2,595 rad to 170 cc volume at 30 rad per hour). No statistically significant difference in the degree of breast fibrosis was found between patients who received 200 rad per fraction and those who received 180 rad per fraction; however, the trend indicates a lesser degree of breast fibrosis in the latter group. When breast fibrosis was correlated with breast cup size, there was a trend towards increased fibrosis with larger breasts, but this correlation was not statistically significant ($P=0.11$) (Table 8). Both patients who were treated

Table 6. *Complications Associated with Radiation Therapy*
(79 Breasts)

Breast fibrosis (mild)	16%
Breast fibrosis (moderate)	3%
Breast fibrosis (severe)	4%
Painful myositis	5%
Telangiectasia	5%
Pneumonitis (mild)	3%
Asymptomatic rib fractures	3%
Postimplant bleeding	1%
Arm edema	1%

Table 7. *Correlation of Breast Fibrosis and Dose per Fraction*

Fibrosis		Dose Per Fraction 250 × 4	200 × 5	180 × 5
None	62	20%	60%	85%
Mild	12	40%	20%	13%
Moderate	2	0%	10%	2%
Severe	3	40%	10%	0%
Total	79	5	10	64

Table 8. *Correlation of Fibrosis and Breast Size*

			Breast Size		
Fibrosis		A	B	C	D*
Present	17	0%	22%	22%	33%
Absent	62	100%	78%	78%	67%
Total	79	8	32	27	12

*Patients with D-cup or greater breast size were scored as D.

with 250-rad fractions and developed severe fibrosis had D-size breasts. Of the patients who were treated with 250-rad fractions and did not develop severe fibrosis, two had B and one had a C breast size.

There was no correlation between fibrosis and the implanted volume or the implanted dose. The combined effect of implanted volume and implanted dose was also investigated, and no correlation was found.

Since only three patients in this series received greater than 5,000 rad to the entire breast, the influence of high external-beam radiation dose could not be evaluated.

No match-line effect has been observed in our patients as reported by other authors (Harris et al. 1979). This may be due to differences in our immobilization techniques or differences in our radiation fields, as discussed previously (Martinez and Goffinet 1981, Martinez and Clarke 1983).

Transient hyperpigmentation in the irradiated field was seen in all patients. It was particularly marked in those areas that received radiation boost doses with electrons; however, this problem resolved over a period of months. One patient had prominent telangiectasia over the implanted site. In patients treated with 250-rad fractions and who went on to develop severe fibrosis, telangiectasia and skin atrophy were present.

Mild radiation pneumonitis was seen in two patients; neither required hospitalization, steroids, or antibiotics. Asymptomatic rib fractures have developed in two patients, and one patient had postimplant bleeding, which was controlled with pressure. As discussed previously, one patient developed arm edema after 6,500 rad to the axilla.

Painful myositis occurred in four patients and was secondary to the ^{192}Ir implant in close proximity to or superficially into the pectoralis muscle.

All surgical- and radiation therapy-related complications were studied for their correlation with patients' age, weight, menopausal status, and tumor size; no significant correlations were found.

Cosmetic Results

Overall cosmetic result was analyzed and scored as excellent in 62 patients (78%), satisfactory in 14 patients (18%), and unsatisfactory in three patients (4%). Figure 2 illustrates a patient with excellent cosmetic results at 52 months after com-

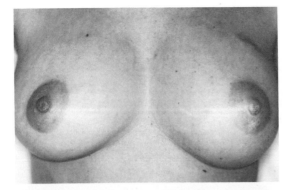

FIG. 2. Thirty-two-year-old pre-menopausal female with $T_2 N_0$ carcinoma of left breast 52 months after completion of therapy. She had received excisional biopsy, axillary dissection, 4500-rad external beam and 2000-rad ^{192}Ir boost. Excellent cosmetic result. result.

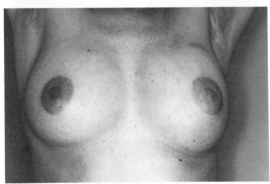

FIG. 3. The same patient of Figure 2 with her arms up. Symmetrical upward displacement of breasts and nipples. No limitation in shoulder movement.

pletion of external beam irradiation and ^{192}Ir implant. Figure 3 shows the same patient with her arms up, documenting the symmetrical upward displacement of both breasts and nipples. Currently patients are being interviewed to determine their own evaluation of cosmesis, and to date 82% of patients have been sampled (Table 9). Patients have tended to give a higher score to their cosmetic results than have physicians. In addition, there were no patients who scored their cosmetic results lower than did their physicians. Most patients who were scored as satisfactory by the physicians scored their own results as excellent. One patient with severe fibrosis who was scored as unsatisfactory, was happy with her result and gave it a score of satisfactory.

Breast size was a major determinant of the cosmetic result (Table 10); excellent results were achieved in patients with small breasts, while those with very large breasts fared less well. All patients with A-cup size had excellent results, while only 50% of patients with D-cup or greater were scored as excellent.

The patients' body weight also had a direct correlation with cosmesis. Ninety percent of the patients who weighed less than 120 pounds had excellent cosmetic results, while only 46% of patients in the group weighing more than 161 pounds had excellent results (Table 11).

Table 9. *Physician-Patient Cosmetic Result Scoring*

Cosmetic Result	Physician	Patient
Excellent	78%	91%
Satisfactory	18%	7%
Unsatisfactory	4%	2%
Total patients	79	65

Table 10. *Correlation of Cosmetic Result and Breast Size**

Cosmetic Result		Breast Size			
		A	B	C	D
Excellent	62	100%	84%	78%	50%
Satisfactory	14	0%	13%	22%	33%
Unsatisfactory	3	0%	3%	0%	17%
Total	79	8	32	27	12

*Probability = .02.

Table 11. *Correlation of Body Weight and Cosmetic Result**

Cosmesis		Body Weight (lbs.)		
		<120	121–160	>161
Excellent	62	90%	81%	46%
Satisfactory	14	5%	19%	36%
Unsatisfactory	3	5%	0%	18%
Total	79	21	47	11

*Probability = 0.001.

Table 12. *Correlation of Cosmetic Result and Tumor Size*

Cosmetic Result		Tumor Size (cm)		
		0–2.0	2.1–3.9	4.0–5.0
Excellent	62	85%	86%	47%
Satisfactory	14	10%	14%	47%
Unsatisfactory	3	5%	–	6%
Total	79	42	22	15

Tumor size was also a factor that affected the cosmetic result (Table 12). When the tumor was 4.0 cm or greater, an excellent cosmetic result was achieved in only 7/15 (47%). In breasts with tumors less than 4.0 cm, an excellent result was noted in 86%. There was no difference in cosmetic results between T_2 lesions that ranged 2.0 to 3.9 cm and T_1 tumors. However, it is important to note that only one breast with a

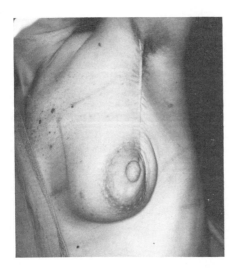

FIG. 4. Sixty-year-old postmenopausal female with T_1N_0 carcinoma of the left breast. Excisional biopsy and low axillary sampling through the same incision. Notice the significant breast retraction and deformity. Photograph was taken the day external beam irradiation began. The cosmetic result was decreased to satisfactory due to moderate breast asymmetry and retraction of tissues.

tumor 4.0 cm or greater achieved an unsatisfactory result, and this was secondary to poor radiation therapy technique.

Surgical technique also had a significant influence on cosmesis. Eleven patients had a reduction in cosmesis secondary either to a large biopsy (quadrantectomy or partial mastectomy), as documented in Figure 4, or to an excisional biopsy scar that was not parallel to skin lines, resulting in subsequent breast retraction. Four occurred in patients with tumors 4.0 cm or greater.

The type of boost therapy delivered to the tumor bed (^{192}Ir implantation or electron-beam therapy) did not influence the cosmetic result. Additionally, there was no correlation between patient age or menopausal status and the cosmetic result.

DISCUSSION

Many patients find radical surgery unacceptable as a treatment modality in the management of breast carcinoma. Primary radiation therapy appears to be a treatment alternative in the management of early stage breast carcinoma, since local control rates in excess of 90% have been obtained. While breast preservation is a major advantage of primary radiotherapy, it is also important to maximize the functional and cosmetic result to minimize the physical and psychological sequelae of treatment. This study has attempted to identify surgical factors, radiation treatment variables, and patient characteristics that alter cosmesis.

Surgical Factors

The first step in the treatment of a patient with early stage breast cancer is an excisional biopsy. In our patients, 11 of 79 (14%) had a reduction in their cosmetic result secondary to excisional biopsy. Often this resulted from a poorly planned or very large excision that did not run parallel to skin lines and resulted in breast retraction. In a few patients, an excessive biopsy resulted in significant loss of breast tissue. When possible, we recommend a circumareolar incision. If the lesion is located more peripherally and is in the upper half of the breast, a circumferential incision in the direction of Langer's lines is advised. If the tumor is in the lower half of the breast, a radial incision is recommended.

When the use of adjuvant chemotherapy is considered, axillary staging is important in planning treatment. We strongly recommend the use of two separate incisions, one for the removal of the primary tumor and a second one for the axillary staging procedure. Breast edema occurred after axillary dissection in 87% of patients, but gradually resolved over a 3-year period. Axillary seroma or hematoma developed in 12 patients or 31.6% of the dissected axillae. Four of these 12 patients developed an axillary mass with the clinical characteristics of a regional recurrence during the first year of follow-up. However, after excisional biopsy of the palpable mass no tumor was found in any of the specimens. Twenty-five percent of patients developed mild arm edema after axillary dissection. In two cases there was mild arm function impairment. Twenty percent of the patients developed basilic vein thrombosis prior to initiation of radiotherapy. Additionally, three patients developed abscesses in the tail of the breast and axilla following axillary dissection and irradiation. The cause was not clear, but the combined staging procedure and subsequent irradiation are implicated.

Twenty-five percent of patients developed breast edema as a result of axillary sampling, but no cases of arm edema were observed. There is clearly a much lower incidence of complications following axillary sampling than after a thorough axillary dissection. The incidence of skip metastases to the apex of the axilla that would be detected with a dissection but missed with a sampling is 0% to 10% (Haagensen 1971, Smith et al. 1977). Potential gains and risks must be considered individually when axillary staging is planned.

Radiation Therapy Factors

Daily fractionation was found to be an important treatment factor; 250 rad per day was unacceptable, resulting in a high incidence of fibrosis. Four of five patients treated in this fashion developed fibrosis. There was little variation in total dose in this series, and the influence of dose could not be evaluated. Excisional biopsy, followed by minimum tumor dose of 4,500 to 5,000 rad in 180- to 200-rad fractions, with all fields treated daily, appears optimal for achieving local control with excellent cosmesis.

The type of boost therapy given to the tumor bed (^{192}Ir implantation or electron-beam therapy) did not influence the cosmetic result, although most patients in this series received ^{192}Ir implants. The dose and volume of the implant did not affect fibrosis or cosmesis.

Patient Characteristics

Patient characteristics that influenced cosmesis were identified. Patients with breasts of D size (D-cup or larger) achieved poorer cosmesis than patients with smaller breasts. This may be secondary to: a) an increased fat content in the larger breasts, making them particularly sensitive to high-dose-per-fraction irradiation, and b) to the dose inhomogeneity due to the large separation between the two tangential fields. Eighty percent of patients with D-size breasts treated at 180 rad per fraction achieved excellent results. Thus, careful attention to treatment technique is especially important in patients with large breasts.

Tumor size was found to correlate with the cosmetic result, with excellent results obtained in 86% of patients with tumors less than 4 cm; only 47% of breasts with cancers greater than 4 cm had excellent cosmetic results. However, a satisfactory result was obtained in another 47% of breasts with large tumors, resulting in an excellent or satisfactory score in 94% of T_2 lesions 4 cm or greater. These results would support the use of primary radiotherapy for 4- to 5-cm lesions, since acceptable postirradiation cosmesis can be obtained in most of these patients.

To obtain the best local control and cosmetic results, careful attention not only to the excisional biopsy and radiation therapy techniques but also to the individual patient's characteristics is important. This entails a joint effort by both surgeons and radiation oncologists. With a median follow-up of 40 months, the locoregional control rate of 94% and the excellent to satisfactory cosmetic result in 96% of patients supports primary radiotherapy as a treatment alternative to radical surgery in stages I and II breast carcinoma.

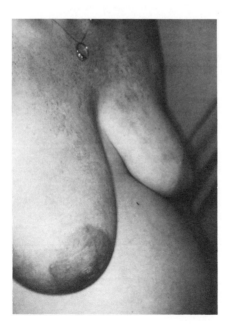

FIG. 5. Twenty-nine-year-old female with T_2N_0 carcinoma of the left breast, 38 months after completion of irradiation. The patient is 8 months pregnant. Notice moderate skin discoloration of the irradiated breast, as well as the small degree of breast engorgement.

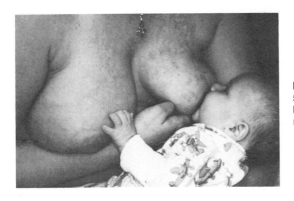

FIG. 6. The same patient of Figure 5, four months later, breastfeeding her 3-month-old baby from the irradiated breast.

Postmenopausal patients having undergone irradiation can experience pregnancy, as shown in Figure 5, and can not only deliver normal babies but provide the newborn with the gratifying experience of breast feeding from both mammary glands (Figure 6).

REFERENCES

Bedwinek, J. 1981. Treatment of stage I and II adenocarcinoma of the breast by tumor excision and irradiation. Int. J. Radiat. Oncol. Biol. Phys. 7:1553–1559.

Clarke, D., A. Martinez, R. Cox, and D. Goffinet. 1982. Breast edema following staging axillary node dissection in patients with breast carcinoma treated by radical radiotherapy. Cancer 49: 2295–2299.

Clarke, D., J. Curtis, A. A. Martinez, L. Fajardo, and D. Goffinet. 1983. Fat necrosis of the breast simulating recurrent carcinoma after primary radiotherapy in the management of early stage breast carcinoma. Cancer 52:442–445.

Haagensen, C. D. 1971. Lymphatics of the Breast, 2nd ed. W. B. Saunders Co., Philadelphia, p. 346.

Harris, J. R., M. B. Levene, G. Sevensson, and S. Hellman. 1979. Analysis of cosmetic results following primary radiation therapy for stages I and II carcinoma of the breast. Int. J. Radiat. Oncol. Biol. Phys. 5:257–261.

Hellman, S., J. R. Harris, and M. G. Levene. 1980. Radiation therapy of early carcinoma of the breast without mastectomy. Cancer 46:988–994.

Martinez, A., and D. R. Goffinet. 1981. Irradiation with external beam and interstitial radioactive implant as primary treatment for early carcinoma of the breast. Surg. Gynecol. Obstet. 152: 285–290.

Martinez, A. A., and D. Clarke. 1983. Medical practice and the California law: Is radiation an alternative to mastectomy for patients with early breast cancer? West. J. Med. 138:676–680.

Montague, E. D., A. E. Gutierrez, J. L. Barker, N. Tapley, and G. Fletcher. 1979. Conservation surgery and irradiation for the treatment of favorable breast cancer. Cancer 43:1058–1061.

Pierquin, B., R. Owen, C. Maylin, Y. Olmezquine, M. Raynal, W. Mueller, and S. Honnoun. 1980. Radical radiation therapy of breast cancer. Int. J. Radiat. Oncol. Biol. Phys. 6:17–24.

Smith, J., J. Gamez-Araujo, H. Gallager, E. White, and C. McBride. 1977. Carcinoma of the breast. Analysis of total lymph node involvement versus level of metastasis. Cancer 39:527–532.

Current Controversies in Breast Cancer, edited
by F. C. Ames, G. R. Blumenschein, and E. D. Montague.
University of Texas Press, Austin © 1984.

Irradiation of Hepatic Metastases in Breast Cancer

Albert S. Braverman, M.D.,* Inder Bhutiani, M.D.,†
Chul Sohn, M.D.,† Diodato Villamena, M.D.,*
Marvin Rotman, M.D.,† and Jose Marti, M.D.‡

*Departments of *Medicine, †Radiation Oncology, and ‡Surgery, Downstate Medical
Center, State University of New York, Brooklyn, New York*

Hepatic metastases (HM) occur in as many as 50% of metastatic breast cancer (MBC) patients (Phillips et al. 1954). Since these metastases often become massive, they may constitute one of the largest tumor deposits in the body. Their presence has been shown to be a poor prognostic factor for response to endocrine therapy or chemotherapy (Nemoto and Dao 1966, George and Hoogstraten 1978, Nash et al. 1980). In this study, HM in 18 breast cancer patients were irradiated as soon as detected, with or without concomitant systemic therapy. The results suggest that hepatic irradiation (HRT) may contribute to the prolongation of life in patients who have MBC.

MATERIALS AND METHODS

Patients

Hepatic metastases were irradiated as soon as discovered in all patients with MBC at the Downstate and Kings County Hospital Medical Centers between 1977 and 1982. Of the 18 patients treated, two died of metastases at other sites within a month, one refused to complete treatment, one had irradiation of the porta hepatis only, and one, who was profoundly icteric when HRT was begun, died of hepatic failure before completion of treatment. Thirteen patients were evaluable (Table 1).

The criterion for HM was that at least two focal areas of decreased isotope uptake appeared on technitium sulfur colloid liver scanning. However, in most cases HM were first detected because of gross hepatomegaly (Figure 1).

In nine patients, HM were among the first metastases to be detected and were irradiated as part of the first therapy for MBC the patients received. Six patients had minimal or no extrahepatic metastases at the time they were irradiated.

Therapy

Five patients had no treatment prior to HRT except for mastectomy. Three had had adjuvant therapy only, and five had had systemic therapy with multiple chemo-

Table 1. *Patient Data*

Pt.	Age	Prior XRT*	Other Metastases	Concomitant XRT	Subsequent XRT	Post-HRT Survival (months)	Outcome
DD	50	none	skin, bone	CMF	ADR, VBN	18+	in remission, with ascites
FG	58	none	bone	CMF	ADR, VBN	40	no relapse of hepatic metastases
DG	73	CMF, ADR, TAM	bone, skin	5-FU	VBN, AG	11	hepatic metastases
RH	52	adjuvant CMF	none	ADR	none	2+	in remission
LH	67	CMF, CA, TAM, AG	bone, CNS	none	M-C, VBN	12	no relapse of hepatic metastases
DL	57	TAM	breast, bone pleura	CAF	CAF	15+	lost to follow-up
EM	34	none	bone	CMF	ADR, VBN	11	relapsed with ascites, increasing SGOT, pleural effusions
IM	63	CAF	bone, lung	CAF	CAF	7+	no subsequent systemic XRT
MM	45	adjuvant CMF	none	none	ADR, VBN	12+	lost to follow-up, in remission
GM	54	adjuvant CMF	supraclavicular nodes	none	ADR, VBN	5	relapse of hepatic metastases
GP	63	CMF, ADR	axillary nodes, breast	ADR	none	4	relapse of hepatic metastases
RS	53	none	breast, bone lung	CAF	CAF	5	no relapse of hepatic metastases
NW	60	adjuvant L-PAM CMF	bone	none	ADR, VBN	11	no relapse of hepatic metastases

*Abbreviations are as follows: XRT = irradiation; HRT = hepatic irradiation; CMF = cyclophosphamide, methotrexate, 5-fluorouracil; ADR = Adriamycin; VBN = vinblastine; TAM = tamoxifen; 5-FU = 5-fluorouracil; CNS = central nervous system; M-C = mitomycin-C; AG = aminoglutethimide; CA = cyclophosphamide and Adriamycin; CAF = cyclophosphamide, Adriamycin, 5-fluorouracil; L-PAM = L-phenylalanine mustard.

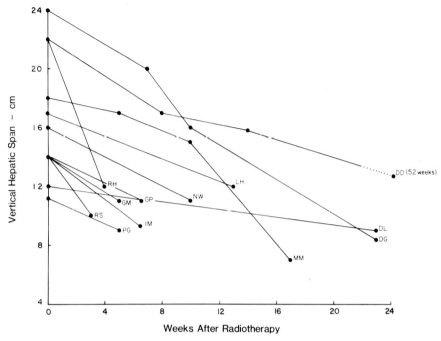

FIG. 1. Decrease in vertical hepatic span following hepatic irradiation.

therapeutic and endocrine modalities (Table 1). The whole liver was irradiated in all patients. Eight patients received 3,000 to 3,500 rad, four received 2,500 rad, and one received 2,000 rad. In most cases, HRT was delivered 3 to 5 days per week in 150- to 250-rad fractions. Seven patients received chemotherapy and HRT simultaneously, and all received systemic chemotherapy or endocrine therapy following the completion of HRT.

RESULTS

Regression of hepatomegaly, as determined by measurement of the vertical hepatic span, occurred in all patients, and was greater than 50% in all patients who had massive hepatomegaly (Figure 1). Scans confirmed the decrease in hepatic size, but focal areas of decreased uptake persisted, even in long-term survivors. Pain and tenderness were eliminated in all. Marked improvement in abnormal liver chemistry occurred in all patients who had such symptoms prior to HRT (Table 2).

The relative roles of systemic chemotherapy and HRT in achieving objective regression of HM were difficult to evaluate accurately. Extrahepatic metastases progressed during HRT in four of the seven patients who received concomitant chemotherapy, indicating failure of systemic therapy. However, regression of HM was usually not complete until 4 to 8 weeks following completion of HRT, when all patients were already receiving systemic therapy.

Table 2. *Liver Chemistries Before (B) and After (A) Hepatic Irradiation*

Patient	Bilirubin		Alkaline Phosphatase		SGOT*		LDH[†]	
	B	A	B	A	B	A	B	A
DD	0.7	0.3	350	350	170	55	600	250
DG	0.6	0.3	410	217	114	29	482	267
DL	0.7	0.2	500	250	400	36	380	320
EM	7.6	0.9	374	245	245	55	642	460
IM	0.3	0.3	166	88	33	32	675	207
GP	0.5	0.3	159	91	57	24	300	113
RS	4.4	0.5	656	96	293	53	351	112

*SGOT = serum glutomic oxaloacitic transaminase.
[†]LDH = lactic dehydrogenase.

The median survival of the patients was 11.5 months following HRT (Figure 2). Three patients suffered relapse with recurrent hepatomegaly and hepatic failure 11, 5, and 4 months, respectively, following HRT. Three are alive without evidence of relapse of HM 17, 8, and 1 month following HRT, while two were lost to follow-up while still in remission at 15 and 12 months. Four patients died of extrahepatic metastases at 40, 12, 11, and 5 months, respectively, following HRT.

Toxicity

Mild nausea, with little vomiting, occurred in most patients, and transient dysphagia occurred in two patients. There was no evidence of acute hepatotoxicity. Ascites developed terminally in association with overt recurrence of hepatic metastases in three patients. In another, ascites occurred terminally without jaundice, but with recurrent serum glutamic oxaloacetic transaminase (SGOT) and lactic dehydrogenase (LDH) elevations. In a fourth patient, ascites developed without liver failure (see below).

No cutaneous inflammation occurred in the irradiated areas in patients who received Adriamycin (ADR). Initial ADR doses were adjusted downward by 25%, as is usual in all patients with liver disease, but it was ultimately possible to deliver full doses to all patients without unusual toxicity.

Illustrative Cases

Possible Delayed Hepatotoxicity—Patient DD

This patient presented with cachexia, massive hepatomegaly, and no other evidence of metastases. Hepatic irradiation and combination chemotherapy with cyclophosphamide, methotrexate, and 5-fluorouracil (CMF) were initiated, bringing about slow regression of hepatomegaly and improvement in liver chemistry. Four months later, cutaneous and bone metastases were found; treatment with ADR was

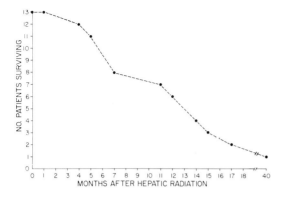

FIG. 2. Survival following hepatic irradiation.

initiated. Three months afterwards (7 months after HRT), massive ascites developed without hepatic failure. Ascites have been controlled for the past 10 months with a LeVeen shunt without relapse at any site.

Prolonged Survival Following HRT—Patient FG

This patient presented with a painful lytic lesion of the right femur, an otherwise negative bone scan, and minimal hepatomegaly. Scan findings were equivocal, but liver biopsy confirmed metastases. Hepatic irradiation and CMF were initiated, resulting in improvement of bone pain and regression of hepatomegaly. After 30 months of clinical remission, bone metastases occurred. The patient responded transiently to treatment with ADR but died at 40 months without evidence of hepatic relapse.

HRT and Endocrine Therapy—Patient DG

After 4 years of CMF, tamoxifen (TAM), and ADR therapy for extensive bone metastases, this patient presented with massive hepatomegaly, bone pain, severe anemia, thrombocytopenia, and skin nodules. Hepatic irradiation with 5-fluorouracil infusion, followed by vinblastine infusion (VBN), produced striking regression of hepatomegaly without affecting her other metastases. Treatment with aminoglutethimide (AG) was then initiated with complete remission of bone pain, cytopenia, and skin nodules. She suffered a relapse after 10 months with evidence of hypoadrenalism and rapidly progressive hepatomegaly, resulting in hepatic failure.

DISCUSSION

There are no published studies of HRT in MBC, but 45 of 183 patients in four major studies of HRT for HM had MBC (Phillips et al. 1954, Turek-Maischeider and Kazem 1975, Borgelt et al. 1981, Leibel et al. 1981). Their results were not categorized for HM site of origin, but, like ourselves, these authors noted little toxicity with HRT and generally good responses, including improvement of liver function and regression of hepatomegaly. The survival times of their patients were short, averaging 11 to 18 weeks, but the treatment was administered primarily for pain palliation in terminal patients, most of whom had metastases from gastrointestinal primary tumors unresponsive to chemotherapy.

Four hundred thirty-six of 1,629 patients reported in 16 recent studies (Jones et al. 1975, Canellos et al. 1976, Smalley et al. 1977, Presant et al. 1977, Lokich et al. 1977, Russell et al. 1978, Tranum et al. 1978, Kennealey et al. 1978, Muss et al. 1978, Creech et al. 1979, Rainey et al. 1979, Hortobagyi et al. 1979a, Yap et al. 1979, Henderson et al. 1981, Yap et al. 1981, Tormey et al. 1982) of chemotherapy for MBC, in which site-specific data were given, had HM. The incidence was 50% in an earlier postmortem study (Phillips 1954), perhaps because of subclinical liver involvement.

Hepatic metastases have been reported (Nemoto and Dao 1966) to presage a poor response to endocrine therapy, and they appear to respond less well to endocrine therapy than metastases to other sites (Kiang and Kennedy 1977, Harvey et al. 1979, Santen et al. 1982). Their presence also predicts a poor response of MBC to chemotherapy, including treatment with ADR (George and Hoogstraten 1978, Nash et al. 1980).

The reason for these findings may be that a correlation exists between the presence of HM and a more advanced stage of disease. Alternatively, HM may be specifically less responsive to these modalities, perhaps because in breast cancer patients they arise from other metastases rather than from the primary tumor. We have observed two patients in whom HM were progressing rapidly while pulmonary metastases were responding objectively to chemotherapy. The 11.5-month median survival time of our patients, therefore, seems encouraging, especially considering how advanced the HM in many of our patients were. Hepatic irradition may, therefore, be a valuable adjunct to effective modern therapies for MBC, not only for palliation of local symptoms but as a means of prolonging life.

Hepatic irradiation is most likely to have this effect if it is applied when HM are at their earliest detectable stage. Moreover, although we and others have irradiated jaundiced patients without ill effects, the treatment is probably more hazardous in the presence of hepatic failure. Because of breast cancer patients' potentially long survival, the possibility of delayed radiation toxicity must be taken into account, especially considering the radiomimetic agents these patients usually receive. The major histopathologic lesion of the human liver caused by irradiation at these doses occurs from damage to sinusoidal vessels with relative sparing of hepatocytes (Ogata et al. 1963, Ingold et al. 1968, Reed and Cox 1966, Rubin and Casarett 1968).

Although collaterals form, the late development of clinically significant presinusoidal or postsinusoidal block cannot be ruled out. The appearance of ascites in one of our patients without evidence of relapse of HM may have been due to a radiation-induced postsinusoidal block. Conversely, five patients followed from 11 to 40 months did not develop ascites.

The usefulness and long-term toxicity of HRT in MBC can only be determined by a randomized study in which systematic efforts are made to detect patients who have HM as early as possible. Once they are found, their random assignment to appropriate systemic therapy, with or without HRT, should provide the information necessary to evaluate this therapeutic modality.

ACKNOWLEDGMENTS

We gratefully acknowledge the assistance of Dr. C. Julian Rosenthal in providing information concerning two of the patients, and of Dr. Nathan Solomon in interpreting hepatic scans.

REFERENCES

Borgelt, B. B., R. Gelber, L. W. Brady, T. Griffin, and F. R. Hendrickson. 1981. The palliation of hepatic metastases: Results of the radiation therapy oncology group pilot study. Int. J. Radiat. Oncol. Biol. Phys. 7:587–591.

Canellos, G. P., V. T. DeVita, G. L. Gold, B. A. Chabner, P. S. Schein, and R. C. Young. 1976a. Combination chemotherapy for advanced breast cancer: Response and effect on survival. Ann. Intern. Med. 84:389–392.

Canellos, G. P., S. J. Pocock, S. G. Taylor, III, M. E. Sears, D. J. Klaasen, and P. R. Band. 1976b. Combination chemotherapy for metastatic breast carcinoma. Cancer 38:1882–1886.

Creech, R. H., R. B. Catalano, D. T. Harris, P. F. Engstrom, and P. J. Grotzinger. 1979. Low-dose chemotherapy of metastatic breast cancer with cyclophosphamide, Adriamycin, methotrexate, 5-fluorouracil (CAMF) versus sequential cyclophosphamide, methotrexate, 5-fluorouracil (CMF) and Adriamycin. Cancer 43:51–59.

George, S. L., and B. Hoogstraten. 1978. Prognostic factors in initial response to therapy in patients with advanced breast cancer. JNCI 60:731–736.

Harvey, H. A., R. J. Santen, J. Osterman, E. Samojlik, D. S. White, and A. Lipton. 1979. A comparative trial of transsphenodial hypophysectomy and estrogen suppression with aminoglutethimide in advanced breast cancer. Cancer 43:2207–2214.

Henderson, I. C., R. Gelman, G. P. Canellos, and E. Frei III. 1981. Prolonged disease-free survival in advanced breast cancer treated with "super-CMF" Adriamycin: An alternating regimen employing high-dose methotrexate with citrovorum factor rescue. Cancer Treat. Rep. 65 (Suppl. 1):67–75.

Hortobagyi, G. N., J. U. Gutterman, G. R. Blumenschein, C. K. Tashima, M. A. Burgess, L. Einhorn, A. U. Buzdar, S. P. Richman, and E. M. Hersh. 1979a. Combination chemoimmunotherapy of metastatic breast cancer with 5-fluorouracil, Adriamycin, cyclophosphamide and BCG. Cancer 43:1225–1233.

Hortobagyi, G. N., J. U. Gutterman, G. R. Blumenschein, C. K. Tashima, M. A. Burgess, L. Einhorn, A. U. Buzdar, S. P. Richman, and E. M. Hersh. 1979b. Combination chemoimmunotherapy of metastatic breast cancer with 5-fluorouracil, Adriamycin, cyclophosphamide and BCG. Cancer 44:1955–1962.

Ingold, J. A., G. B. Reed, M. S. Kaplan, and M. A. Bagshaw. 1968. Radiation hepatitis. Am. J. Roentgenol. 93:200–208.

Jones, S. E., B. G. Durie, and S. E. Salmon. 1975. Combination chemotherapy with Adriamycin and cyclophosphamide for advanced breast cancer. Cancer 36:90–97.

Kennealey, G. T., B. Boston, M. S. Mitchell, M. K. Knobf, S. N. Bobrow, J. F. Pezzimenti, R. Lawerence, and J. R. Bertino. 1978. Combination chemotherapy for advanced breast cancer. Cancer 42:27–33.

Kiang, D. T., and B. J. Kennedy. 1977. Tamoxifen (antiestrogen) therapy in advanced breast cancer. Ann. Intern. Med. 87:687–690.

Leibel, S. A., S. E. Order, C. J. Rominger, and S. O. Asbell. 1981. Palliation of liver metastases with combined hepatic irradiation and misonidazole. Cancer Clin. Trials 4:285–293.

Lokich, J. J., A. T. Skarin, R. J. Mayer, I. C. Henderson, R. H. Blum, and E. Frei, III. 1977. Adriamycin plus alkylating agents in the treatment of metastatic breast cancer. Cancer 40:2801–2805.

Muss, H. B., D. R. White, F. Richards, II, M. R. Cooper, J. J. Stuart, D. V. Jackson, L. Rhyne, and C. L. Spurr. 1978. Adriamycin versus methotrexate in five-drug combination chemotherapy of advanced breast cancer. Cancer 42:2141–2148.

Nash, C. H., S. E. Jones, T. E. Moon, S. L. Davis, and S. E. Salmon. 1980. Prediction of outcome in metastatic breast cancer treated with Adriamycin combination chemotherapy. Cancer 46:2380–2388.

Nemoto, T., and T. L. Dao. 1966. Significance of liver metastasis in women with disseminated breast cancer undergoing endocrine ablative surgery. Cancer 19:421–427.

Ogata, K., J. Mizawaki, and M. Yoshida. 1963. Hepatic injury following radiation therapy. J. Exp. Med. 9:240–251.

Phillips, R., D. A. Karnofsky, L. D. Hamilton, and J. J. Nickson. 1954. Roentgen therapy of hepatic metastases. Am. J. Roentgenol. 71:825–834.

Presant, C. A., A. V. Amburg, III, and C. Klahr. 1977. Adriamycin, 1-3 bis (2-chloroethyl)-1-nitrosourea (BCNU, NSC 409962) and cyclophosphamide therapy of drug-resistant metastatic breast carcinoma. Cancer 40:987–993.

Rainey, J. M., S. E. Jones, and S. E. Salmon. 1979. Combination chemotherapy for advanced breast cancer utilizing vincristine, Adriamycin, and cyclophosphamide (VAC). Cancer 43:66–71.

Reed, G. B., and J. A. Cox, Jr. 1966. The human liver after radiation injury. Am. J. Pathol. 48:597–611.

Rubin, P., and G. W. Casarett. 1968. Clinical Radiation Pathology, vol. 1. W. B. Saunders, Philadelphia, pp. 270–284.

Russell, J. A., J. W. Baker, P. J. Dady, H. T. Ford, J. C. Gazet, J. A. Mckinna, A. G. Nash, and T. J. Powles. 1978. Combination chemotherapy of metastatic breast cancer with vincristine, Adriamycin and prednisolone. Cancer 41:396–399.

Santen, R. J., T. J. Worgul, A. Lipton, H. Harvey, A. Boucher, E. Samojlik, and S. Wells. 1982. Aminoglutethimide as treatment of postmenopausal women with advanced breast carcinoma. Ann. Intern. Med. 96:94–101.

Smalley, R. V., J. Carpenter, A. Bartolucci, C. Vogel, and S. Krauss. 1977. A comparison of cyclophosphamide, Adriamycin, 5-fluorouracil (CAF) and cyclophosphamide, methotrexate, 5-fluorouracil, vincristine, prednisone (CMFVP) in patients with metastatic breast cancer. Cancer 40:625–632.

Tormey, D. C., R. Gelman, P. R. Band, M. Sears, S. N. Rosenthal, W. DeWys, C. Perlia, and M. A. Rice. 1982. Comparison of induction chemotherapies for metastatic breast cancer. Cancer 50:1235–1244.

Tranum, R., B. Hoogstraten, A. Kennedy, C. B. Vaughn, B. Samal, T. Thigpen, S. Rivkin, F. Smith, R. L. Palmer, J. Costanzi, W. G. Tucker, H. Wilson, and T. R. Maloney. 1978. Adriamycin in combination for the treatment of breast cancer. Cancer 41:2078–2083.

Turek-Maischeider, M. T., and I. Kazem. 1975. Palliative irradiation of liver metastases. JAMA 232:625–628.

Yap, H-Y:, G. R. Blumenschein, C. K. Tashim, G. N. Hortobagyi, A. U. Buzdar, and C. L. Wiseman. 1979. Combination chemotherapy with vincristine and methotrexate for advanced refractory breast cancer. Cancer 44:34–43.

Yap, H-Y., G. R. Blumenschein, G. P. Bodey, G. N. Hortobagyi, A. U. Buzdar, and A. DiStefano. 1981. Vindesine in the treatment of refractory breast cancer: Improvement in therapeutic index with continuous 5-day infusion. Cancer Treat. Rep. 65:775–779.

Current Controversies in Breast Cancer, edited
by F. C. Ames, G. R. Blumenschein, and E. D. Montague.
University of Texas Press, Austin © 1984.

The Clinical Application of CT Scanning in the Treatment of Primary Breast Cancer

Barbara F. Danoff, M.D., James M. Galvin, D.Sc., Elizabeth
Cheng, B.S., Robert K. Brookland, M.D., William D. Powlis, M.D.,
and Robert L. Goodman, M.D.

*Department of Radiation Therapy, University of Pennsylvania School of Medicine,
Philadelphia, Pennsylvania*

Excisional biopsy and definitive radiotherapy have been employed with increasing frequency in the treatment of patients with stages I and II breast cancer. Results comparable to those achieved with mastectomy in terms of local-regional control and survival have been reported (Amalric et al. 1982, Bedwinek et al. 1980, Chu et al. 1980, Hellman et al. 1980, Pierquin et al. 1980, Veronesi et al. 1981). Recent studies (Bonadonna et al. 1976, Bonadonna and Valagussa 1981, Fisher et al. 1981) have also suggested a survival benefit for patients with histologically positive axillary nodes who receive adjuvant chemotherapy. Current treatment regimens, therefore, combine primary radiotherapy and adjuvant chemotherapy in patients with histologically positive nodes.

Complications following primary radiotherapy for breast cancer have been well documented (Bedwinek et al. 1980, Chu et al. 1980, Hellman et al. 1980, Pierquin et al. 1980) and include arm edema, pneumonitis, brachial plexus injury, pericarditis, pleural effusion, rib fracture, fibrosis, and necrosis. However, the effect of adjuvant chemotherapy on the frequency and severity of these complications remains to be determined. Enhancement of the effects of radiation on normal tissues may occur with various chemotherapy agents employed in the treatment of breast cancer (Phillips and Fu 1976, Phillips and Fu 1977, Phillips and Fu 1978). An enhanced radiation response in the lung has been noted with Adriamycin, cyclophosphamide, and vincristine and in the heart with Adriamycin (Phillips and Fu 1976, Phillips and Fu 1977). Preliminary studies (Botnick et al. 1982, Danoff et al. 1983, Lichter 1983) have noted an increased incidence of symptomatic pneumonitis, arm edema, and rib fractures in patients receiving concomitant or sequential chemotherapy and primary radiotherapy. The selection and sequencing of agents as well as refinements in radiotherapy technique may ultimately alter the nature of the complications observed as well as their incidence.

In an attempt to quantitate the amount of lung and heart currently included in the standard radiation fields for the definitive treatment of breast cancer, a specially modified computed tomographic (CT) scanner was employed (Galvin et al. 1982). This report presents the clinical findings to date and recommendations for treatment modifications that may minimize complications related to the heart and lung.

MATERIALS AND METHODS

Between March and August 1982, 22 patients undergoing primary radiotherapy for stages I and II breast cancer had CT scans performed as part of their treatment planning. The CT scanner employed is a modified version of the second generation Pfizer 0200 scanner with a scan time of 30 seconds and a scan aperture of 56 cm.

The radiotherapy technique consisted of opposed tangential fields to the breast. The superior border of the field was the sternoclavicular joint. The lateral and inferior borders were 1–2 cm beyond the palpable breast tissue. The medial border was 3 cm across the midline when the internal mammary nodes were included within the tangential fields; the medial border was midline when these nodes were not irradiated. Both fields were treated per day with compensating wedge filters. No bolus was used. The apical axillary and supraclavicular nodes were treated with a separate anterior field angled 12° to avoid divergence through the spinal cord and vertebral bodies. The inferior border of this field was matched to the tangents, and the superior border was at the level of the cricothyroid groove. The medial border was midline, and the lateral border was at the humeral head.

Radiation was directed to the breast only in 13 patients, to the breast and internal mammary nodes in four patients, and to the breast and apical axillary-supraclavicular nodes in five patients. The internal mammary nodes were treated in two of these last five patients. Twelve patients had right-sided primary lesions, and 10 had left-sided lesions.

After simulation and delineation of the tangential and supraclavicular fields, CT scans were obtained to visualize the treatment fields and anatomy in cross section. The patients were scanned in the treatment position and an immobilization cast and an angle board were used. In order to adapt to the size of the tunnel, the patients were scanned and treated in a one-arm-up position rather than the usual two-arms-up position.

Radiopaque catheters were placed on the patient's skin to indicate the entrance points for the tangential and supraclavicular fields. The selected treatment fields were then scanned in cross section at intervals of 2 cm. The exact position of each cross-sectional image was indicated on a scout view. This view is a computer-produced digital image that was generated by rectilinear scanning of the patient both in the anterior and tangential projection. The representation of the treatment field on the patient's contour and cross-sectional anatomy was then plotted. The area of ipsilateral lung or heart included within the treatment field was electronically traced and then calculated by computer software. This area, integrated over the appropriate CT slices, represented the volume. The total ipsilateral lung and heart volumes were obtained in a similar fashion by integrating the area over all the CT slices.

As no patient was treated with tangent and hockey-stick field arrangement, information regarding the amount of ipsilateral lung and heart included within these fields was obtained by electronically tracing them on the digital radiograph. The medial border of the hockey stick was drawn at midline with the lateral border 5 cm to the ipsilateral side. The medial border of the tangents was drawn to overlap the hockey stick .5 cm. Lung and heart volumes were again determined by tracing the area included within the fields and integrating this over the appropriate CT slices.

The amount of lung in centimeters visualized within the tangential fields, at the center of the field on the simulator films, was recorded for each patient and compared to the volume obtained from the CT scan. For left-sided lesions, the maximum amount of heart in centimeters visualized within the tangential simulator films was also recorded.

Dose distributions then generated and displayed as an overlay on the anatomical information provided by the CT slice.

RESULTS

Tables 1 and 2 compare the volume of lung obtained from the CT scan with the amount of lung visualized on the simulator tangential fields. While there is a trend to increasing lung volumes with an increasing amount of lung seen on the simulator

Table 1. *Volume of Lung* Versus Centimeter of Lung Visualized on Simulator Tangential Fields—Tangents Only*

Lung on Simulator Film	No. Pts.	Lung Volume (%)	Median Lung Volume (%)
2.0–2.5 cm	4	13,14,17,33	15.5
2.6–3.0 cm	5	16,19,19,22,33	19
3.1–3.5 cm	7	16,18,20,24,24, 29,34	24

*Determined by computed tomographic scan.

Table 2. *Volume of Lung* Versus Centimeter of Lung Visualized on Simulator Tangential Fields—Tangents and IMN†*

Lung on Simulator Film	No. Pts.	Lung Volume (%)	Median Lung Volume (%)
2.6–3.0 cm	4	23,25,25,28	25
3.1–3.5 cm	2	30,33	31.5

*Determined by computed tomographic scan.
†Internal mammary nodes.

Table 3. *Volume of Lung* [*] *Tangents Versus Tangents and IMN* [†]

	2.6–3.0 cm[‡]	3.1–3.5 cm[‡]
Tangential field		
Range	16–33%	16–34%
Median	19%	24%
Tangential field and IMN		
Range	23–28%	30–33%
Median	25%	31.5%

[*] Determined by computed tomographic scan.
[†] Internal mammary nodes.
[‡] Measurement of lung on simulator film.

Table 4. *Volume of Lung* [*] *Tangents Versus Tangents and Supraclavicular Field Versus Tangents and Hockey Stick*

	Volume of Lung (%)	
Tangential Field	Tangential and Supraclavicular Fields	Tangential and Hockey-Stick Fields
16	25	35 (22[†])
19	24	41 (25)
23	40	43 (26)
24	31	39 (34)
30	36	47 (30)

[*] Determined by computed tomographic scan.
[†] ( ) Volume of lung receiving $\geq$ 50% of dose.

films, there is significant anatomic variation. It can also be seen that tangential breast irradiation includes approximately 20 to 25% of the ipsilateral lung volume. Bringing the medial border of the tangential field 3 cm across midline to include the internal mammary nodes increased this volume 25 to 30% (Table 3).

There was no significant difference in the lung volume included within the tangential fields for right- versus left-sided lesions.

The addition of the supraclavicular field to the tangential fields increased the ipsilateral lung volume within the treated fields by 5 to 17% in the five patients so treated (Table 4). In comparing tangential and supraclavicular irradiation with the simulated tangents and hockey-stick field arrangement, it can be seen that the latter increased the volume of ipsilateral lung irradiated by an additional 3 to 17%. However, if only the volume of lung that received $\geq$ 50% of the dose when the hockey-stick and tangential fields were used is considered, the results are similar to those with tangential and supraclavicular field irradiation (Table 5).

Tables 5 and 6 depict the volume of heart included in the tangential breast fields. For left-sided lesions, the average volume is 12%. There was significant anatomic

Table 5. *Volume of Heart* Versus Centimeter of Heart Visualized on Simulator Tangential Fields (Left-Sided Primary)*

Heart on Simulator Film	No. Pts.	Heart Volume (%)	Median Volume (%)
.5−1.0 cm	2	6,9	7.5
1.5−2.0 cm	6	5,6,10,12,15,17	11
2.1−2.5 cm	2	12,28	20

*Determined by computed tomographic scan.

Table 6. *Volume of Heart* Tangents Versus Tangents and Hockey Stick*

	Heart Volume (%)	
	Tangential Field	Tangential and Hockey-Stick Fields
Left-sided primary	6	69
	9	40
	17	53
Right-sided primary		17
		22
		24

*Determined by computed tomographic scan.

variation and little correlation with the amount of heart seen on the simulator films (Table 6). The addition of the hockey stick to the tangential fields significantly increased the volume of heart included within the treatment fields both for right- and left-sided lesions (Table 6).

DISCUSSION

With the increasing use of primary radiotherapy and adjuvant chemotherapy in the treatment of patients with early breast cancer, attention has been drawn to the nature and incidence of complications resulting from the combined treatment. The present study provides data regarding the volume of lung and heart included within the standard treatment fields as obtained from a specially modified CT scanner. The advantages of the scanner used include the ability to scan the patient in the treatment position with an immobilization cast and an angle board, the ability to generate dose distributions for the volume of interest, and the ability to make field changes and variations in the absence of the patient by electronically tracing them on a digital radiograph.

Tangential breast irradiation results in inclusion of 20 to 25% of the ipsilateral lung volume in the treatment field. Displacement of the medial border 3 cm across midline does not significantly increase the volume. There is, however, significant anatomic variation that accounts for the poor correlation between the amount of lung or heart seen on the simulator film and the volume determined by the CT scan. If one considers only the amount of lung receiving $\geq$ 50% of the dose, there may be no advantage of the tangential-supraclavicular field arrangement over the tangential and hockey-stick fields in terms of volume of lung irradiated. However, the use of the hockey-stick field markedly increased the volume of heart irradiated, and, therefore, should not be used in patients receiving chemotherapy regimens containing Adriamycin. The addition of the supraclavicular field to the tangential field may significantly increase the volume of lung irradiated. In such patients, consideration may be given to the omission of this field. A recent study (Sarrazin et al. 1982) has shown no additional benefit to regional node irradiation in patients with histologically positive nodes who receive adjuvant chemotherapy.

The use of the CT scanner in the treatment planning of breast cancer may ultimately result in optimization of treatment fields and in refinement of techniques that will minimize complications. Decisions to include more or less lung or heart can be based on actual measurements. A current use also involves the selection of an optimum electron beam energy and beam angulation for boost treatment. The margins of surgical bed are clipped at the time of excisional biopsy. The depth, position, and volume encompassed by the clips are outlined by the scan. This information is then used to select the optimum electron-beam energy, field size, and beam angulation to minimize radiation dose to the underlying lung.

BIBLIOGRAPHY

Amalric, R., F. Santamaria, F. Robert, J. Seigle, C. Altschuler, J. M. Kurtz, J. M. Spitalier, H. Brandore, Y. Ayme, J. F. Pollet, R. Burmeister, and R. Abed. 1982. Radiation therapy with or without primary limited surgery for operable breast cancer. A 20-year experience at the Marseilles Cancer Institute. Cancer 49:30–34.

Bedwinek, J. M., C. A. Perez, S. Kramer, L. Brady, R. Goodman, and G. Grundy. 1980. Irradiation as the primary management of stage I and II adenocarcinoma of the breast. Cancer Clin. Trials 3:11–18.

Bonadonna, G., E. Brusamolino, P. Valagussa, L. Brugnatelli, A. Rossi, C. Brambilla, M. De-Lena, G. Tancini, E. Bajetta, and U. Veronesi. 1976. Combination chemotherapy as an adjuvant treatment in operable breast cancer. N. Engl. J. Med. 294:405–410.

Bonadonna, G., and P. Valagussa. 1981. Dose response effect of adjuvant chemotherapy in breast cancer. N. Engl. J. Med. 304:10–15.

Botnick, L. E., S. Come, C. Rose, M. Goldstein, R. Lange, S. Tishler, and L. Schnipper. 1982. Primary breast irradiation and concomitant adjuvant chemotherapy (CMF), in Conservative Management of Breast Cancer, J. R. Harris, S. Hellman, and W. Silen, eds. J. B. Lippincott Co., Philadelphia, pp. 321–328.

Chu, A. M., O. Cope, R. Russo, C. C. Wange, M. D. Schultz, C. Wang, and G. Rodkey. 1980. Treatment of early stage breast cancer by limited surgery and radical irradiation. Int. J. Radiat. Oncol. Biol. Phys. 6:25–30.

Danoff, B. F., R. L. Goodman, J. H. Glick, D. G. Haller, and T. F. Pajak. 1983. The effect of adjuvant chemotherapy on cosmesis and complications in patients with breast cancer treated by definitive irradiation. Int. J. Radiat. Oncol. Biol. Phys. (in press).

Fisher, B., C. Redmond, and N. Wolmark. 1981. Breast Cancer Studies of the NSABP: An editorialized overview, *in* Adjuvant Therapy of Cancer III, S. Salmon and S. Jones, eds. Grune and Stratton, New York, pp. 359–369.

Galvin, J. M., E. Cheng, P. Bloch, and R. L. Goodman. 1982. CT-simulation: A modified computerized tomographic scanner for use in radiation therapy. (Abstract) Proceedings of the American Society of Therapeutic Radiologists 24th Annual Meeting. Int. J. Radiat. Oncol. Biol. Phys. 8:82.

Hellman, S., J. R. Harris, and M. B. Levine. 1980. Radiation therapy of early carcinoma of the breast without mastectomy. Cancer 46:988–994.

Lichter, A. S., M. E. Lippman, C. R. Gorrell, T. M. d'Angelo, B. K. Edwards, and E. V. deMoss. 1983. Adjuvant chemotherapy in patients treated primarily with irradiation for localized breast cancer, *in* Conservative Management of Breast Cancer, J. R. Harris, S. Hellman, and W. Silen, eds. J. B. Lippincott Co., Philadelphia, pp. 299–310.

Phillips, T. L., and K. K. Fu. 1976. Quantification of combined radiation therapy and chemotherapy effects on critical normal tissues. Cancer 37:1186–1200.

Phillips, T. L., and K. K. Fu. 1977. Acute and late effects of multimodal therapy on normal tissues. Cancer 40:489–494.

Phillips, T. L., and K. K. Fu. 1978. The interaction of drug and radiation effects on normal tissues. Int. J. Radiat. Oncol. Biol. Phys. 4:59–64.

Pierquin, B., R. Owen, C. Maylin, Y. Otmezguine, M. Raynal, W. Mueller, and S. Hanneun. 1980. Radical radiation therapy of breast cancer. Int. J. Radiat. Oncol. Biol. Phys. 6:17–24.

Sarrazin, D., M. Le, F. Fontaine, and R. Arriajada. 1982. Conservative treatment versus mastectomy T_1 or small T_2 breast cancer: The experience of the Institute Gustave-Roussy, *in* Conservative Management of Breast Cancer, J. R. Harris, S. Hellman, and W. Silen, eds. J. B. Lippincott Co., Philadelphia, pp. 299–310.

Veronesi, U., R. Saccozzi, M. DelVecchio, A. Banfi, C. Clemente, M. DeLena, G. Gallus, M. Greco, A. Luini, E. Maruloini, G. Muscolino, F. Rilke, G. Salvadori, A. Zecchini, and F. Zucali. 1981. Comparing radical mastectomy with quadrantectomy, axillary dissection and radiotherapy in patients with small cancers of the breast. N. Engl. J. Med. 305:6–11.

Current Controversies in Breast Cancer, edited
by F. C. Ames, G. R. Blumenschein, and E. D. Montague.
University of Texas Press, Austin © 1984.

New Information on Breast Carcinoma and the Eye

Linda Mewis, M.D., Sue Ellen Young, M.D., and
Rosa A. Tang, M.D.

*Department of Ophthalmology, The University of Texas Medical School at Houston,
Houston, Texas*

Only in the past decade has it been recognized that metastatic carcinoma is the most common intraocular malignancy. The numbers of Americans affected each year are phenomenal; estimates range from 1,150 to 25,300 in one report (Ferry and Font 1974) and 15,000 in another (Nelson et al. 1982). Among this group, metastatic breast carcinoma accounts for about half in most large series (Ferry and Font 1974, Stephens and Shields 1979). Both the oncologist and the ophthalmologist underestimate the magnitude of the problem.

Because the course of breast cancer spans decades, and its prevalence as a cause of ocular disease is high, a retrospective study of 250 patients treated for breast primaries at The University of Texas M. D. Anderson Hospital and Tumor Institute at Houston between 1973 and 1980 was conducted. Only metastases to the choroid, the most frequently involved site, were studied. Ferry and Font (1974, 1975, Font and Ferry 1976) studied 227 patients with metastases to the eye and orbit. In these studies, metastases to the choroid were most common, followed by metastases to the orbit and anterior segment in order of frequency. In our series, four areas in which information was limited were addressed. First, changes in vision in the involved eyes receiving medical therapy alone or plus irradiation were documented. Second, a large number of cancer patients were examined during life for evidence of ocular metastasis. Other recent data on metastatic involvement was obtained from autopsy studies of eyes of cancer patients (Bloch and Gartner 1971) or surgical specimens (Ferry and Font 1974). Clinical examination of groups of cancer patients has been rarely performed (Albert et al. 1967). This fact relates to the scarcity of ophthalmic care at tumor centers and the presence of eye involvement in patients with advanced disease who are sometimes gravely ill.

A third area addressed by this study is unique. It has been assumed in the past that hematogenous seeding of the tumor accounts for at least some metastases to distant sites. If this is true, metastatic pulmonary disease should precede eye and central nervous system (CNS) spread. This assumption was investigated clinically in the 67 patients with choroidal metastases. Finally, an attempt was made to document possible ocular side effects of treatment for choroidal deposits, i.e. irradiation. Other parameters previously reported for such patients including survival, interval from diagnosis of primary to ocular disease, right-versus-left eye involvement, and age at diagnosis were verified.

MATERIALS AND METHODS

Two hundred fifty female patients with known breast carcinoma primaries underwent complete ophthalmic examinations between 1973 and 1980 at UT M. D. Anderson Hospital. Sixty-seven patients with choroidal metastases were identified (94 eyes). A clinical diagnosis of choroidal metastatic disease was made rather than a surgical diagnosis because of risk to the eye. However, all the patients had proven breast primaries, typical choroidal involvement, and spread of the disease to other sites at some time during their course. As of November 1981, 60 of the patients were known dead, three lost to follow up, and four alive.

RESULTS

Of the 67 patients with choroidal disease, the age at diagnosis ranged from 28 to 71 years, with a median age of 51 (Figure 1). The interval from diagnosis of the primary to ocular disease ranged from 6 months to 14 years 3 months with a median of 3 years. Survival after diagnosis of choroidal involvement varied from 5 days to 50 months, with a median of 9 months. These findings are similar to those of other authors (Ferry and Font 1974, Stephens and Shields 1979, Maor et al. 1977).

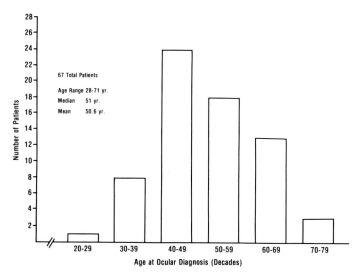

FIG. 1. Age at diagnosis of ocular disease by decades (reproduced from Mewis and Young 1982, with permission of Lippincott/Harper).

Ophthalmic texts (Hogan and Zimmerman 1962) and some series (Stephens and Shields 1979) state that metastatic involvement of the left eye is more common than that of the right. The rationale for this is the anatomic arrangement of the carotid arterial system. The tumor cells en route to the right common carotid must pursue a more tortuous course via the innominate artery. The left common carotid branches directly off the aorta, a straighter path to the left eye. Other authors (Ferry and Font 1974) have found no left-sided predominance. In this series of 67 patients, the right eye was affected in 18 patients (26.9%) and the left in 22 patients (32.8%). Both eyes were affected at the first evaluation in 21 patients, and in six patients involve ment of the second eye followed the first within 9 months. Bilateral disease oc curred, therefore, in 27 patients, or 40.3%. In addition, multiple metastatic foci were common as suggested by Stephens and Shields (1979). Thirty-two patients had three to 16 deposits, eight had one in each eye, and 35 had only one deposit. Most metastases occur in the posterior pole, not in the periphery.

Most patients presented because of a decrease in vision (44 of 67). Nine patients, whose cases will be discussed later, had no eye complaints. Four patients had noted visual field abnormalities. Three patients were referred because of an eye abnor mality noted by the oncologist (e.g. papilledema). Seven patients had diverse com plaints including metamorphopsia (distortion), diplopia, photophobia, or ptosis.

Vision and Treatment

Changes in vision over time were evaluated in 45 patients for whom follow-up exams were available. The patients on whom no follow-up was available either died within 3 months of ocular diagnosis or lived far from this center. We have no reason to believe these patients represent treatment failures. Of the 45 patients, 66 eyes were affected. Irradiation was advised for metastases that had caused or were threat ening to cause a decrease in vision, had associated retinal detachments, or were definitely enlarging on medical therapy. All patients with choroidal metastases were treated medically with chemotherapy or hormonal therapy. Irradiation treatment consisted of 2,500 to 3,000 rad of ^{60}Co delivered through a lateral portal usually in 10 fractions (Maor et al. 1977). Such treatment minimizes ocular side effects such as loss of lashes, corneal changes, and cataract. If the choroidal lesion was only an incidental finding and did not threaten vision, the eye was observed on medical therapy. A 1-mm change in size was readily visible in most cases.

The results of treatment were generally favorable (Table 1). Among 52 irradiated eyes, 35 had stabilization of vision, 14 had an improvement of two lines or more in vision on a standard visual acuity chart. Two eyes lost two or more lines of acuity, one due to optic nerve disease, and another had a drop in acuity from 20/15 to 20/30 over the month after diagnosis for unknown reasons. Of 14 eyes receiving only sys temic therapy, vision was stable in 10, improved in one eye of a patient with brain metastases after whole-brain irradiation, and decreased in one eye of a patient who developed brain metastases. Follow-up exams at bedside were performed on three patients' eyes, in which vision could not be adequately assessed. Three patients, who will be discussed later, had late vision loss after irradiation.

Table 1.* *Effect of Treatment in 45 Patients[†]*

52 Eyes Irradiated		
Visual acuity was:		
Unchanged in	35 eyes	(67.3%)
Improved in	14 eyes	(26.9%)
Decreased in	2 eyes[‡]	(3.8%)
Unknown	1 eye	(1.9%)
14 Eyes Not Irradiated		
Visual acuity was:		
Unchanged in	10 eyes	(71.4%)
Improved in	1 eye[§]	(7.1%)
Decreased in	1 eye[‖]	(7.1%)
Unknown	2 eyes	(14.3%)

*Adapted from Mewis and Young 1982.
[†]Median follow-up time—9 months (range 1–52 months).
[‡]One patient had optic nerve metastasis, and one had inade-
quate follow-up.
[§]This patient had cortical disease causing visual loss. Brain
irradiation led to improvement.
[‖]Bilateral visual acuity decrease from brain metastases.

Asymptomatic Metastases

Of the entire series of 250 patients, 98 had no ocular complaints and were seen as part of a generalized survey of patients with metastatic disease. Nine of the 98 (9.2%) were found to have choroidal metastases in one eye. Seven of these patients were known to have other distant metastases. However, one patient was thought only to have lymph node involvement, and another had brain metastases discovered concurrently with the eye disease. Thus, choroidal metastases may give evidence of systemic spread of disease when no symptoms are present. Additionally, among the 58 patients with choroidal metastases and ocular symptoms or signs, the eye findings were the first sign of systemic dissemination in seven patients.

Eye and Systemic Dissemination

The timing of eye involvement in the course of breast cancer was investigated. The charts of all 67 patients with choroidal metastases were reviewed for evidence of pulmonary or CNS spread. Pulmonary involvement included parenchymal and pleural disease. Evidence for lesions in the brain, spinal cord, or meninges included a positive cytology, radiologic finding, or radionucleotide scan. Symptoms or seizures alone were not considered proof of CNS metastases. Among the 67 patients, 40 had pulmonary involvement (Figure 2). It preceded the ocular diagnosis in 27 patients, occurred with ocular disease in seven, and appeared after ocular disease in six. Pulmonary metastases often preceded eye disease by months to years, with a median interval of 13 months. Central nervous system disease, which was documented in 30 patients, had a distinctly different pattern. It preceded ocular disease in only two patients, coincided with ocular disease in 15, and followed in 13.

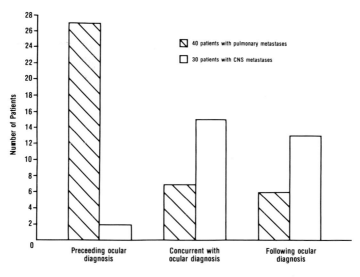

FIG. 2. Timing of systemic involvement in 67 patients with choroidal metastases (Mewis and Young 1982, with permission of Lippincott/Harper).

Late Complications

Late decreases in acuity not due to cataract occurred in three patients in this study. All three had retinal vascular abnormalities and were thought to have findings consistent with radiation retinopathy. The first patient is typical of these three women and will be described in detail.

Case 1: A 61-year-old female presented to the ophthalmology service in April 1980 because of decreased vision in the left eye. She had a history of breast carcinoma, which was diagnosed at age 57, and had developed bone metastases in October 1979. Upon examination, she was found to have 20/30 vision in the left eye and serous retinal detachment of inferior nasal quadrant. Ocular ultrasound was performed and revealed a mass in the choroid under the detachment. After the diagnosis of metastatic breast carcinoma to the choroid was made, the patient was referred for radiation. She received 2,725 rad ^{60}Co in 10 fractions over 2 weeks. By February 1981, 10 months later, her vision had improved to better than 20/25, with resolution of the detachment. However, in August 1981, 16 months after treatment, she returned complaining of another drop in vision. Her acuity in the left eye was found to be 20/40 with no new metastases. She had new fundus findings (Figure 3) consisting of two dot hemorrhages in the macula. Fluorescein angiography confirmed retinal vascular abnormalities including capillary dropout and amputated arterioles (Figure 4). Later (Figure 5) in the angiogram, more dye leakage into the macula was apparent, indicating the presence of macular edema which accounted for her vision loss. Over 9 months since this development, the patient has had no change in the fundus findings or vision. The contralateral eye has remained normal.

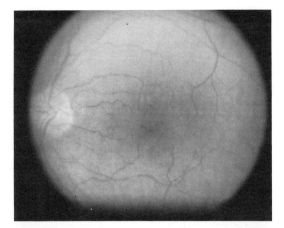

FIG. 3. Photograph of the left fundus, August 1981. Note the dot-like hemorrhages in the fovea.

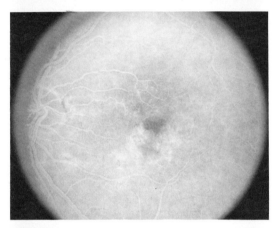

FIG. 4. In this early venous phase, the paramacular vascular abnormalities are evident. Some of the small vessels are amputated, some dilated and tortuous. Note the areas of capillary dropout.

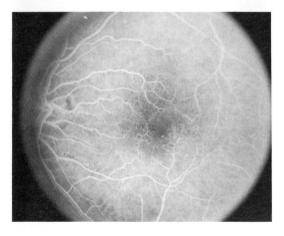

FIG. 5. In this late phase, the fluorescein dye is leaking into the retina, especially in the macular area. Such changes account for the drop in acuity.

Two additional patients have developed retinal vascular abnormalities in irradiated eyes 28 and 38 months after treatment. One patient lost all sight. There was no clinical evidence of diabetes mellitus, temporal arteritis, or carotid vascular disease in these patients. One patient had mild hypertension for which she was being treated. All patients had received 2,500 to 3,000 rad, a dose of irradiation usually considered safe for the retina (Duke-Elder and Mac Faul 1972).

DISCUSSION

The patients in this study with choroidal metastases are similar to those reported in other series (Ferry and Font 1974, Stephens and Shields 1979, Bullock and Yanes 1980) with regard to age, interval from primary to ocular involvement, and survival after ocular diagnosis. There was no marked predominance of left-versus-right eye involvement. A large number of patients (40.3%) had bilateral disease.

The metastatic lesions tend to occur in the posterior pole, an area accessible to examination with the direct ophthalmoscope. The lesions are creamy yellow plaques or mounds, single or multiple. They may have brown pigment clumping on the surface. Retinal vessels over the mass may be distorted. After radiation, definite pigment clumping over the tumor occurs.

Because of the prevalence of choroidal metastases, the oncologist should think of this as a possibility when confronted by a patient with breast cancer and vision loss. The vision loss may be gradual or sudden (sometimes a consequence of a retinal detachment involving the macula). One might advise breast carcinoma patients with disseminated disease to cover each eye once a week to check their own vision. When whole brain irradiation is planned, the eyes may be examined beforehand, so eye treatment can be given at the same time if required.

Although the choroid is the most frequent site of ocular spread, metastases to the iris, ciliary body, extraocular muscles, and orbit also occurs, but with lesser frequency. Such patients may complain of decreased vision, pain, photophobia, a distorted pupil, diplopia, or ptosis. The ptosis is due to enophathalmos from orbital involvement in scirrhous carcinoma.

Once the diagnosis of metastatic breast carcinoma to the choroid is made, even with profound vision loss, the outlook for the patient regaining sight is excellent. In this series, the majority of patients irradiated had stabilization of acuity (67.3%). This relates to the fact that many patients can see well, even 20/20, despite choroidal metastases if refracted. The choroidal mass initially causes increasing hyperopia. Improvements in the patients' other visual complaints such as distortion, blurring with their current glasses, and scotomas may be a more accurate indicator for a patient regaining sight. Fourteen eyes (26.9%) did experience a visual acuity increase after irradiation. Among 14 eyes not irradiated, no improvement in acuity could be directly attributed to medical therapy. Ten eyes did stabilize. However, four patients initially treated only with medical therapy were noted to have increasing choroidal disease and required irradiation.

Vision tends to improve over the first month after irradiation. On the other hand, large exudative retinal detachments lying over choroidal metastases can be slow to resolve. Ultrasound shows initially a flattening of the metastasis, and over the ensuing months subretinal fluid is absorbed. Surgery is not required or indicated. Dramatic improvements occur in these patients; the final visual outcome is probably limited by the length of time the detachment had been present. The retina in long-standing detachments can undergo permanent cystic changes. Thus, an ophthalmic exam and treatment for patients with symptomatic choroidal metastases, though not an emergency, should not be delayed indefinitely.

Ninety-eight patients without eye complaints were examined as part of a survey of metastatic disease. Nine (9.2%) had asymptomatic metastases, some threatening vision. Albert et al. (1967) examined 52 patients with proven metastatic breast carcinoma. They found four with choroidal metastases and three with orbital metastases. Even if only 8% or 9% of patients with disseminated breast cancer have ocular involvement, the number of individuals affected are staggering.

A significant result of this series was documentation of the time course of pulmonary and CNS spread, as compared to the eye. Pulmonary involvement, when present, usually preceded ocular disease by months. Central nervous system involvement occurred concurrently with or after choroidal diagnosis. From a circulatory standpoint, this scheme is rational. Moreover, a 3-mm choroidal metastatic deposit may be obvious long before a 1-cm frontal lobe or meningeal nodule. Even more important, the clear media of the eye permit direct observation of that 3-mm nodule for evidence of growth or stabilization. Could this not be a readily available, optimal biological test of the therapeutic efficacy of hormonal or chemotherapy?

Finally, the patients with possible late radiation retinopathy challenge our current standard therapy. No patients developed radiation-induced corneal or lens changes. One should note that radiation retinopathy in three eyes of 52 irradiated is not unfavorable odds. Also, only the long-term survivors developed these changes. With greater longevity, continuing vascular wear and tear on the retinal microcirculation, already damaged by radiation, may tip the balance toward visual loss. Considering these long-term effects, it may be time to reassess current radiotherapeutic management. There seems to be no adequate proof that a lower dose will not induce good tumor regression in the eye.

CONCLUSIONS

This study has confirmed that choroidal metastases from breast carcinoma are common and treatable and has demonstrated the following: 1) These metastases occurred in 9.2% of a series of 98 asymptomatic patients; 2) choroidal metastases tend to follow pulmonary disease and are concurrent with or appear before CNS involvement; 3) there were three patients who developed presumed radiation changes 16 to 38 months after irradiation; 4) ocular examination can help the oncologist assess successful or unsuccessful medical therapy; 5) medical therapy can restore or preserve vision in patients whose disease course spans decades.

REFERENCES

Albert, D. M., R. A. Rubenstein, and H. G. Scheie. 1967. Tumor metastasis to the eye. Part 1. Incidence in 213 adult patients with generalized malignancy. Am. J. Ophthalmol. 63:723–726.

Bloch, R. S., and S. Gartner. 1971. The incidence of ocular metastatic carcinoma. Arch. Ophthalmol. 85:673–675.

Bullock, J. D., and B. Yanes. 1980. Ophthalmic manifestations of metastatic breast cancer. Ophthalmology 87:961–973.

Duke-Elder, S., and P. A. MacFaul. 1972. Non-mechanical injuries, *in* System of Ophthalmology, vol. XIV, part 2, S. Duke-Elder, ed. C. V. Mosby Co., St. Louis, pp. 976–985.

Ferry, A. P., and R. L. Font. 1974. Carcinoma metastatic to the eye and orbit. I: A clinicopathologic study. Arch. Ophthalmol. 92:276–286.

Ferry, A. P., and R. L. Font. 1975. Carcinoma metastatic to the eye and orbit. II. A clinicopathological study of 26 patients with carcinoma metastatic to the anterior segment of the eye. Arch. Ophthalmol. 93:472–482.

Font, R. L., and A. P. Ferry. 1976. Carcinoma metastatic to the eye and orbit. III. A clinicopathologic study of 28 cases metastatic to the orbit. Cancer 38:1326–1335.

Hogan, M. J., and L. E. Zimmerman. 1962. Ophthalmic Pathology, 2nd ed. Philadelphia, W. B. Saunders Co., p. 449.

Maor, M., R. C. Chan, and S. E. Young. 1977. Radiotherapy of choroidal metastases: Breast cancer as primary site. Cancer 40:2081–2086.

Mewis, L., and S. E. Young. 1982. Breast carcinoma metastatic to the choroid. Analysis of 67 patients. Ophthalmology 89:147–151.

Nelson, C. C., B. S. Hertzberg, and G. K. Klintworth. 1982. An estimation of the number of ocular metastases in patients dying with cancer in the USA based on a histopathologic study of 650 unselected eyes. (Abstract) Invest. Ophthalmol. Vis. Sci. (Suppl) 22:75.

Stephens, R. F., and J. A. Shields. 1979. Diagnosis and management of cancer metastatic to the uvea: A study of 70 cases. Ophthalmology 86:1336–1349.

Current Controversies in Breast Cancer, edited
by F. C. Ames, G. R. Blumenschein, and E. D. Montague.
University of Texas Press, Austin © 1984.

Trends in Management of Cancer of the Breast in Community Hospital Practice

Leonard M. Toonkel, M.D., Ivor Fix, M.D., F.A.C.R.,
Lawrence H. Jacobson, M.D., and Carl B. Wallach, B.S.

*Department of Radiation Therapy, Mount Sinai Medical Center,
University of Miami School of Medicine, Miami Beach, Florida*

Even prior to the widespread availability of megavoltage radiation therapy equipment in the 1960s, the vast majority of women with cancer of the breast have been treated initially in the community hospital setting. While ongoing prospective studies and retrospective evaluations from major academic medical centers in this country and abroad are attempting to define the best management for regionally localized disease, community surgeons have been steadily limiting the extent of their initial operations. Clinical grounds for performing lesser surgery include stage of disease, age and suitability of the patient for radical surgery, and, perhaps most importantly, the patient's desire to preserve her breast. This study represents the experience of the Radiation Therapy Department of a large community hospital over the past 16 years in the initial treatment of localized breast cancer following various surgical procedures. Our previous analysis of postmastectomy radiation therapy (Toonkel et al. 1982) is reevaluated and comparisons made between this group of patients and those receiving lesser surgical procedures.

MATERIALS AND METHODS

One thousand five hundred nine patients received postoperative radiation therapy following surgical procedures ranging from incisional biopsy to classical radical mastectomy. Radiotherapy techniques included peripheral lymphatic irradiation or peripheral lymphatic irradiation plus chest wall or breast irradiation. A distribution of patients according to type of surgery and radiation therapy technique employed is given in Figure 1. Figure 2 relates the frequency of surgical procedures employed to the year of referral for the study period from January 1966 through December 1981.

Details of our postmastectomy radiation therapy techniques have been previously described (Toonkel et al. 1982). Similar techniques have been employed for postoperative radiation therapy for the patient with an intact breast. In general, opposing tangential fields were used to subtend the volume of the breast and underlying chest wall for a tumor dose of 4,500–5,000 rad delivered in 20–25 fractions over

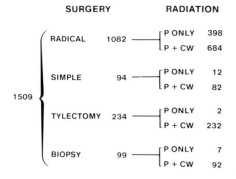

FIG. 1. Distribution of patients to the various surgical and radiotherapeutic groups. P = peripheral lymphatic irradiation; CW = chest wall irradiation; B = breast irradiation.

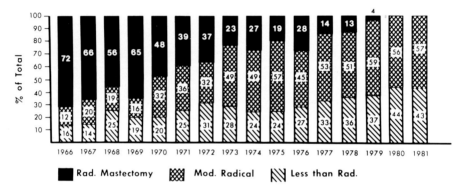

FIG. 2. Referral pattern (January 1966 to December 1981): percentage of patients treated yearly by surgical technique (Mount Sinai Medical Center Department of Radiation Therapy).

4–5 weeks employing a ^{60}Co apparatus or 4 MeV linear accelerator. Bolus was not used for the treatment of the intact breast. The internal mammary chain was usually treated with a separate en face field receiving 4,500–5,000 rad given dose during the same time period. Some patients, however, had their internal mammary node chains encompassed by the tangential fields designed to treat the breast and underlying chest wall. The supraclavicular nodes received the same dose as that given to the internal mammary nodes. A posterior axillary field was used to equalize the stated dose at the midplane of the axilla and the given dose to the supraclavicular nodes in most cases. A boost to the incision or quadrant of origin of the primary tumor was given to most patients. This consisted of 500–1,500 rad with superficial x-ray therapy, ^{60}Co at a reduced source to skin distance, or (rarely) interstitial implants.

All patients were staged retrospectively at the time of analysis according to the current AJC staging system (American Joint Commission for Cancer Staging and End Results Reporting 1978), with one exception. Patients with primary tumors between 2.0 and 5.0 cm in maximum diameter and negative axillae (T2NO) were classified as having stage I disease.

For comparing results of treatment methods, patients treated either by classical radical mastectomy or modified radical mastectomy were considered as having had radical surgery. Since all of these patients had undergone axillary dissections, their staging was based upon pathologic findings. Of the 94 patients treated by simple mastectomy, 30 had some form of axillary staging procedure. The remainder were staged clinically. Patients having less than mastectomy (i.e., partial mastectomy or lumpectomy) but at least removal of all gross tumor within the breast were placed in the tylectomy group. Of 234 patients in this group, 102 also had axillary sampling or dissections. Staging of the axillae was clinical but based upon axillary pathology when this information was available. Clinical axillary staging was employed for 99 patients who had biopsies of their primary tumors only.

Follow-up time for the entire series ranges from 6 months to 198 months, with a mean follow-up of 83 months and a median follow-up of 70 months. The mean follow-up time for the radical surgery group is 87 months. For the tylectomy group the mean follow-up is 50 months.

The mean age at diagnosis for the entire series is 61.6 years. The median age is 63.3 years. The mean age for the radical surgery group is 59.6 years, 58.4 years for the peripheral lymphatic irradiation group, and 60.3 years for the peripheral lymphatic and chest wall group. The mean age for patients treated by simple mastectomy was 65.7 years. For the tylectomy group, the mean age is 68.6 years. Patients treated by biopsy only had a mean age of 62.6 years. Figure 3 relates the type of surgical procedure employed to the decade of age at diagnosis.

For stage II patients in the radical surgery group receiving peripheral lymphatic irradiation only, the average number of involved axillary lymph nodes was 4.4. Stage II radical surgery patients in the peripheral lymphatic and chest wall radiotherapy group had an average of 6.7 involved nodes per patient. This difference was as expected based upon our selection of patients at greater risk of local recurrence

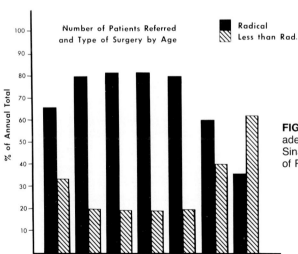

FIG. 3. Surgical technique by decade of age at diagnosis (Mount Sinai Medical Center Department of Radiation Therapy).

for additional treatment to the chest wall. Stage III patients in the radical surgery group had an 80% rate of axillary nodal involvement. Twenty-three of 27 (85%) patients in the peripheral lymphatic irradiation group had axillary involvement compared to 201 of 254 (79%) in the peripheral lymphatic plus chest wall irradiation group.

STATISTICAL ANALYSIS

Life-table analysis was computed by the actuarial method described by Berkson and Gage (1950) to provide curves comparing stage of initial disease, survival, relapse-free survival, and local control among the various surgical and radiotherapy groups. No modifications were used to correct for mean age differences. While statistical significance has limited implications in retrospective nonrandomized analyses, probability values (*P*) were calculated using the Lee-Desu statistic (Lee and Desu 1972).

RESULTS

The actuarial survival curve for the entire series is given in Figure 4. The 5-, 10-, and 15-year survival rates are 62%, 43%, and 33%, respectively. Figure 5 provides actuarial relapse-free survival by stage, regardless of treatment techniques. The 10-year relapse-free survival rates for stages I, II, and III disease are 57%, 45%, and 31%.

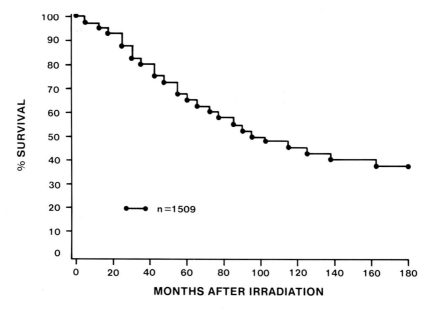

FIG. 4. Actuarial survival of entire patient population.

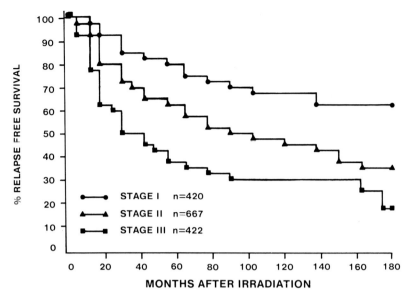

FIG. 5. Relapse-free survival for entire series by stage of disease.

The 1,082 patients who had radical surgery were evaluated as to whether the postoperative radiotherapy fields included the peripheral lymphatics only or the peripheral lymphatics and chest wall. The main indication for postoperative radiotherapy for patients with stage I disease was a medial or central location of the primary tumor within the breast. The 5- and 10-year survival rates for 147 patients receiving peripheral lymphatic irradiation only are 85% and 60%, respectively. The corresponding figures for 74 patients receiving both peripheral lymphatic and chest wall irradiation are 90% and 76%. While these differences are not statistically significant, similar advantage was seen in relapse-free survival and local control for stage I patients receiving chest wall irradiation.

While limited axillary disease has been an indication for internal mammary and supraclavicular irradiation, stage II patients with more extensive disease received elective chest wall irradiation as well. Five- and 10-year survival figures for 224 stage II patients receiving peripheral lymphatic treatment only are 55% and 38%, compared with 72% and 58% for 355 patients treated with peripheral lymphatic plus chest wall irradiation. This result was statistically significant ($P = .002$) (Figure 6). Again, differences favoring the chest wall group are seen in disease-free survival and local control.

Only 27 stage III patients received peripheral lymphatic irradiation alone. Their 5- and 10-year survival probabilities of 34% and 18% are considerably less than those seen for 255 patients receiving comprehensive irradiation of the peripheral lymphatics and chest wall (51% and 36%). Similar differences are seen for disease-

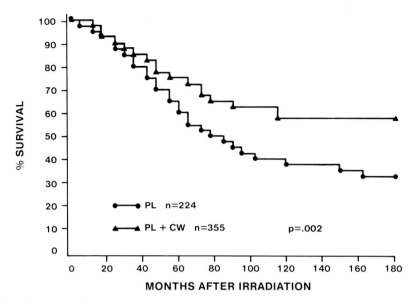

FIG. 6. Survival analysis, stage II, radical surgery: Peripheral lymphatic (PL) versus peripheral lymphatic and chest wall (PL + CW) irradiation (p = probability).

free survival. The combined 5- and 10-year local control rate is 62% for the peripheral lymphatic group and 79% for the chest wall group.

Figure 7 provides relapse-free survival rates for both radical mastectomy groups and the tylectomy group. The lack of segregation according to stage biases the radical mastectomy group, in that more stage I patients received peripheral lymphatic irradiation only and almost all of the stage III patients were in the peripheral lymphatic plus chest wall irradiation group. In the same way, earlier stage patients were less likely to be treated by conservation surgery.

Because patients in the radical mastectomy group receiving peripheral lymphatic and chest wall irradiation had improved survival, disease-free survival, and local control rates, and received radiation therapy comparable to that of patients treated by less than mastectomy, this group was used in the stage-by-stage comparisons. The disease-free survival rates for stage I patients treated by radical mastectomy, simple mastectomy, or tylectomy are essentially identical, as shown in Figure 8. All groups received postoperative radiation therapy to the peripheral lymphatics and chest wall or breast.

Figure 9 provides disease-free survival analysis for stage II patients. Again almost identical 5- and 10-year disease-free survival rates are seen for the radical surgery and tylectomy groups. The number of patients treated by simple mastectomy is small.

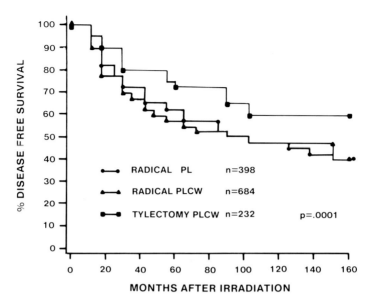

FIG. 7. Relapse-free survival for stages I, II, & III: Radical surgery with peripheral lymphatic (PL) irradiation versus radical surgery with peripheral lymphatic plus chest wall (PLCW) irradiation versus tylectomy with peripheral lymphatic and breast irradiation.

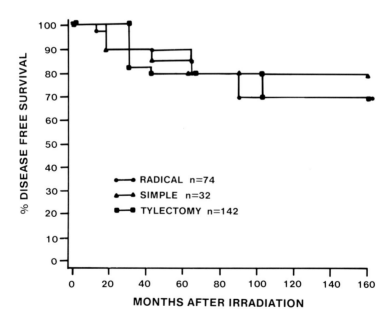

FIG. 8. Relapse-free survival, stage I. Comprehensive postoperative irradiation: Radical mastectomy versus simple mastectomy versus tylectomy.

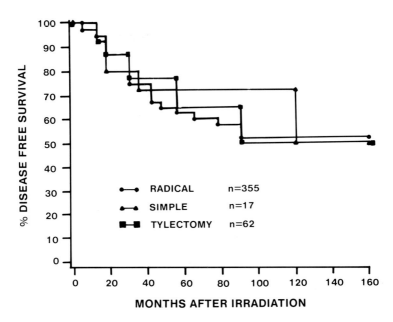

FIG. 9. Relapse-free survival, stage II. Comprehensive postoperative irradiation: Radical mastectomy versus simple mastectomy versus tylectomy.

By combining stages I and II, larger patient numbers in each group are achieved and the bias induced by the lack of surgical staging of the axilla in the majority of patients not subjected to radical surgery is removed. Figure 10 provides actuarial survival analysis for all four surgical groups receiving comprehensive postoperative irradiation. The 5- and 10-year survival rates of 72% and 53% for the tylectomy group compare with the 65% and 50% figures seen for the radical mastectomy series. Disease-free survival, which may be a more useful comparison because of the marked age difference between the surgical groups, is shown in Figure 11. The 74% five-year figure and 60% ten-year figure for the tylectomy group can be contrasted with 5- and 10-year disease-free survivals of only 54% and 48% for the radical mastectomy group. Patients treated by biopsy only had very poor survival and disease-free survival. Local and regional control were comparable for patients treated by tylectomy, radical mastectomy, or simple mastectomy, but were achieved in only 55% of patients who were treated only with biopsy of their primary tumor (Figure 12).

Only 28 stage III patients were treated by tylectomy, with a maximum follow-up of 96 months. The 5-year disease-free survival and local control rates of 62% and 91% for these patients compares with 39% and 80% for 255 patients treated by radical surgery and comprehensive postoperative radiation therapy.

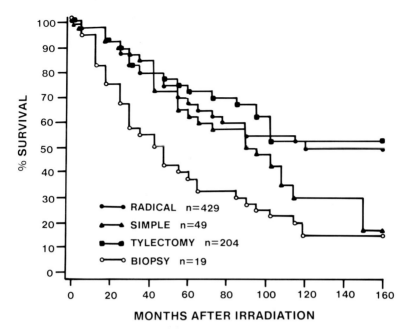

FIG. 10. Actuarial survival, stages I and II. Comprehensive postoperative irradiation: Radical mastectomy versus simple mastectomy versus tylectomy versus biopsy.

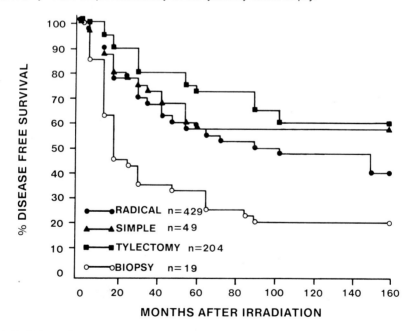

FIG. 11. Relapse-free survival, stages I and II. Comprehensive postoperative irradiation: Radical mastectomy versus simple mastectomy versus tylectomy versus biopsy.

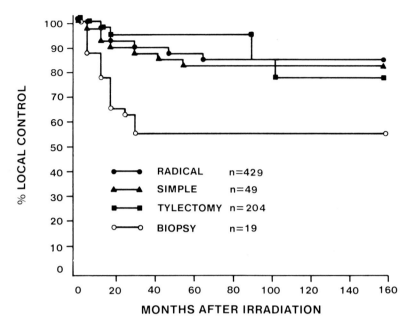

FIG. 12. Local control analysis, stages I and II. Comprehensive postoperative irradiation: Radical mastectomy versus simple mastectomy versus tylectomy versus biopsy.

DISCUSSION AND CONCLUSIONS

Recent theories regarding the natural history of breast cancer based upon biologic predeterminism may diminish the role of aggressive local therapy (Fisher et al. 1980). It is apparent, however, from many studies that increasing the scope of regional therapy with surgical or radiotherapeutic treatment of the internal mammary nodes is of benefit for certain subsets of patients (Lacour et al. 1976, Høst and Brennhovd 1977, Fletcher and Montague 1978, Montague and Fletcher 1980, Wallgren et al. 1980, Regnier et al. 1982, Roseman and James 1982). In our radical mastectomy series of over 1000 patients, the addition of chest wall irradiation to the postoperative treatment of the internal mammary chain and supraclavicular fossa results in improved survival rates for patients who have large primary tumors or involved axillary lymph nodes despite a selection process that reserves chest wall therapy for more advanced disease. These data imply the existence of a subset of patients with residual regional disease who do not have occult systemic spread or whose total tumor cell burden is reduced sufficiently by regional therapy to allow host defense mechanisms to control their systemic micrometastases.

In the early years of this review the classical radical mastectomy was the most commonly prescribed surgical procedure for localized disease. Two trends could be seen in the surgical techniques employed. The first was a phasing out of the classical radical mastectomy in favor of the modified operation, which spares the pectoral musculature. This trend was relatively rapid despite the fact that no randomized controlled series were ever reported to demonstrate equivalent cure rates with either procedure. The second trend has been a gradual increase over the years in the use of even more conservative operations. Since 1956, when Mustakallio of Finland reported equivalent results with tumorectomy and roentgen therapy compared to more radical surgical procedures, many studies in this country and abroad have been published showing equivalent results of radical surgery to conservative surgery and irradiation (Peters 1967, Rissanen 1969, Crile and Hoerr 1971, Wise et al. 1971, Mustakallio 1972, Calle et al. 1973, Papillon 1974, Lavigne and Desaive 1975, Prosnitz and Goldenberg 1975, Harris et al. 1978, Montague et al. 1979, Chu et al. 1980, Pierquin et al. 1980, Amalric et al. 1982, Clark et al. 1982). In fact, only one study (the Guy's Hospital experience) showed inferior results for tumorectomy and radiation therapy in stage II patients. These patients however had clinically involved axillary nodes that were not removed, and were irradiated with doses considered insufficient for control of even microscopic disease, let alone gross residual tumor (Atkins et al. 1972).

The improved relapse-free survival rates with adjuvant chemotherapy for premenopausal patients with limited axillary involvement gives additional importance to the axillary dissection and raises the question of interaction of radiation therapy and chemotherapy. In a randomized study from Milan comparing quadrantectomy, axillary dissection, and radiotherapy with radical mastectomy, patients in both groups who had positive axillary nodes received chemotherapy with cyclophosphamide, methotrexate, and fluorouracil and showed equivalent actuarial survival and relapse-free rates (Veronesi et al. 1981).

Our study is unique in that the surgery was not performed by a single surgeon or surgical group but instead by many surgeons with a wide variety of backgrounds and techniques. The radiation therapy, on the other hand, has been under the direction of the same physician (I.F.) for the entire study period, and the techniques employed have been relatively standard. The local control rate (breast and surrounding lymph nodes) in our series is 95% at 5 years for stages I and II patients treated by tylectomy and radiation therapy. This compares with 96% in the series at The University of Texas M. D. Anderson Hospital and Tumor Institute at Houston, where similar techniques were employed (Montague et al. 1979). These techniques are based on the philosophy that the initial treatment for localized breast cancer should be radical. As moderate doses of radiation therapy have been shown to control subclinical disease (Montague and Fletcher 1980), excision of the primary tumor and palpable axillary lymph nodes followed by comprehensive irradiation of the remaining breast tissue, underlying chest wall, and peripheral lymphatics constitutes a radical approach.

This is not a report of a randomized prospective series, and the surgical groups reported on differ in both age and follow-up time. This study was undertaken, however, to demonstrate trends in the surgical management of localized breast cancer and determine if comparable control rates were achieved in community practice. Our results are in accord with the published findings of major centers employing radical surgery, radical surgery plus adjuvant chemotherapy, or conservative surgical approaches (Bonadonna and Valagussa 1981, Amalric et al. 1982, Tapley et al. 1982). As relapse-free survival rates for our patients having less than radical mastectomy and comprehensive postoperative radiotherapy are at least as good as similarly staged patients subjected to radical surgery followed by similar postoperative irradiation, we can conclude that patients with localized breast cancer in our community who elect breast-conserving surgery do not jeopardize their expectation of cure.

ACKNOWLEDGMENTS

The authors wish to acknowledge the support of the many referring physicians of the south Florida area who provided follow-up information on their patients. The authors also acknowledge that without the support of the entire clerical, technical, and nursing personnel of the Department of Radiation Therapy, this study would not have been possible.

REFERENCES

Amalric, R., F. Santamaria, F. Robert, J. Seigle, C. Altschuler, J. M. Kurtz, J. M. Spitalier, H. Brandone, Y. Ayme, J. F. Pollet, C. Burmeister, and K. Abed. 1982. Radiation therapy with or without primary limited surgery for operable breast cancer: A 20 year experience at the Mareilles Cancer Institute. Cancer 49:30–34.

American Joint Commission for Cancer Staging and End-results Reporting. 1978. Manual for Staging of Cancer. Whiting Press, Chicago, pp. 101–108.

Atkins, H., J. L. Hayward, D. J. Klugman, and A. A. Wayte. 1972. Treatment of early breast cancer: A report after ten years of a clinical trial. Br. Med. J. 2:423–429.

Berkson, I., and R. Gage. 1950. Calculation of survival rates for cancer. Proc. Mayo Clin. 25:270.

Bonadonna, G., and P. Valagussa. 1981. Dose-response effect of adjuvant chemotherapy in breast cancer. N. Engl. J. Med. 304:10–15.

Calle, R., J. P. Pilleron, and P. Schlienger. 1973. Therapeutiques "a visee conservatrice" des epitheliomas mammaires. Bull. Cancer 60:217–234.

Chu, A. M., O. Cope, R. Russo, C. C. Wang, M. Shultz, C. A. Want, and G. Rodkey. 1980. Treatment of early stage breast cancer by limited surgery and radical irradiation. Int. J. Radiat. Oncol. Biol. Phys. 6:25–30.

Clark, R. M., R. H. Wilkinson, L. J. Mahoney, J. G. Reid, and W. D. MacDonald. 1982. Breast cancer: A 21-year experience with conservative surgery and radiation. Int. J. Radiat. Oncol. Biol. Phys. 8:967–975.

Crile, Jr., G., and S. O. Hoerr. 1971. Results of treatment of carcinoma of the breast by local excision. Surg. Gynecol. Obstet. 132:780.

Fisher, B., C. Redmond, E. R. Fisher, and participating NSABP investigators. 1980. The contribution of recent NSABP clinical trials of primary breast cancer therapy to an understanding of tumor biopsy—an overview of findings. Cancer 46:1009–1025.

Fletcher, G. H., and E. D. Montague. 1978. Does adequate irradiation of the internal mammary chain and supraclavicular nodes improve survival rates? Int. J. Radiat. Oncol. Biol. Phys. 4:481–492.

Harris, J. R., M. B. Levene, and S. Hellman. 1978. Results of treating Stage I and II carcinoma of the breast with primary radiation therapy. Cancer Treat. Rep. 62:985–991.

Høst, H., and I. O. Brennhovd. 1977. The effect of postoperative radiotherapy in breast cancer. Int. J. Radiat. Oncol. Biol. Phys. 2:1061–1067.

Lacour, J. L., P. Bucalassi, E. Cacers, G. Jacobelli, T. Koszarowski, M. Le, C. Rumeau-Rouquette, and U. Veronesi. 1976. Radical mastectomy versus radical mastectomy plus internal mammary dissection: Five-year results of an international cooperative study. Cancer 37:206–214.

Lavigne, J., and C. Desaive. 1975. Cancer of the breast. A study of prognostic factors as a guide in selecting cases for conservative treatment. Acta Chir. Belg. 74:63–81.

Lee, E., and M. Desu. 1972. A computer program for comparing K samples with right censored data. Comput. Programs Biomed. 2:315–321.

Montague, E. D., and G. H. Fletcher. 1980. The curative value of irradiation in the treatment of nondisseminated breast cancer. Cancer 46:995–998.

Montague, E. D., A. E. Gutierrez, J. L. Barker, N. duV. Tapley, and G. H. Fletcher. 1979. Conservation surgery and irradiation for the treatment of favorable breast cancer. Cancer 43:1058–1061.

Mustakallio, S. 1954. Treatment of breast cancer by tumor extirpation and roentgen therapy instead of radical operation. J. Fac. Radiologists 6:23.

Mustakallio, S. 1972. Conservative treatment of breast carcinoma: review of 25 years follow-up. Clin. Radiol. 23:110.

Papillon, J. 1974. Conservative treatment of breast cancer by tumorectomy + irradiation, *in* Current Concepts in Breast Cancer and Tumor Immunology, Joseph P. Castro, ed. Medical Examination Pub. Co., Flushing, New York, pp. 117–134.

Peters, M. V. 1967. Wedge resection and irradiation. An effective treatment in early breast cancer. JAMA 200:134–135.

Pierquin, B., R. Owen, C. Maylin, Y. Otmezguine, M. Raynal, W. Mueller, and S. Hannoun. 1980. Radical Radiation of breast cancer. Int. J. Radiat. Oncol. Biol. Phys. 6:17–24.

Prosnitz, L., and I. Goldenberg. 1975. Radiation therapy as primary treatment for early stage carcinoma of the breast. Cancer 35:1587–1596.

Regnier, R., T. H. Nguyen, D. Balikdjian, J. Lustman-Marechal, P. Smets, H. Darquennes, and J. Henry. 1982. Experience of telecobalt therapy in operable breast cancer at J. Bordet Institute (1969–1975). Int. J. Radiat. Oncol. Biol. Phys. 8:1517–1523.

Rissanen, P. M. 1969. A comparison of conservative and radical surgery combined with radiotherapy in the treatment of stage I carcinoma of the breast. Br. J. Radiol. 42:423–426.

Roseman, J. M., and A. G. James. 1982. The significance of the internal mammary lymph nodes in medially located breast cancer. Cancer 50:1426–1429.

Tapley, N. DuV., W. J. Spanos, G. H. Fletcher, E. D. Montague, S. Schell, and M. J. Oswald. 1982. Results in patients with breast cancer treated by radical mastectomy and postoperative irradiation with no adjuvant chemotherapy. Cancer 49:1316–1319.

Toonkel, L. M., I. Fix, L. H. Jacobson, J. J. Schneider, and C. B. Wallach. 1982. Postoperative radiation therapy for carcinoma of the breast: Improved results with elective irradiation of the chest wall. Int. J. Radiat. Oncol. Biol. Phys. 8:977–982.

Veronesi, U., R. Saccozzi, M. DelVecchio, A. Banfi, C. Clemente, .M. Delena, G. Gallus, M. Greco, A. Luini, E. Marubini, G. Muscolino, F. Rilke, B. Salvadore, A. Zecchini, and R. Zucali. 1981. Comparing radical mastectomy with quadrantectomy, axillary dissection, and radiotherapy in patients with small cancers of the breast. N. Engl. J. Med. 305:6–11.

Wallgren, A., O. Arner, J. Bergstrom, B. Blomstedt, P. Granberg, L. Karstrom, L. Raf, and C. Silversward. 1980. The value of preoperative radiotherapy in operable mammary cancer. Int. J. Radiat. Oncol. Biol. Phys. 6:287–290.

Wise, L., A. Y. Mason, and C. V. Ackerman. 1971. Local excision and irradiation: An alternative method for the treatment of early mammary cancer. Ann. Surg. 174:393–401.

NEW STAGING AND PROGNOSTIC FACTORS IN BREAST CANCER

Current Controversies in Breast Cancer, edited
by F. C. Ames, G. R. Blumenschein, and E. D. Montague.
University of Texas Press, Austin © 1984.

The Use of Monoclonal Antibodies Specific for the gp52 of Mouse Mammary Tumor Virus as Indicators of Human Disease

Lionel A. Manson, Ph.D.,* Anne Tax, Ph.D.,* and
Henry F. Sears, M.D.†

*The Wistar Institute of Anatomy and Biology, Philadelphia, Pennsylvania, and
†The Fox Chase Cancer Center, Philadelphia, Pennsylvania

As part of a long-range research goal assessing the role of the immune response in the progressive growth of malignant neoplasms, we are studying whether tumor-associated antigens on growing tumor cells in a syngeneic host can trigger humoral and cell-mediated responses (Manson 1981). As an example of a tumor system etiologically associated with a viral agent, we have focused on mammary tumors of the mouse. Some inbred mouse lines have a high incidence of mammary tumors (approaching 100%), whereas others have a very low incidence of mammary tumors (less than 1%). Bittner (1936) demonstrated that the factor that was associated with the high spontaneous incidence in the mouse was an agent that was transmitted through the milk, subsequently characterized and named Mouse Mammary Tumor Virus (MMTV, "milk factor"). High incidence and early occurrence of mammary tumors in mice are associated with the presence of this particle (B particle) in milk. In addition to the presence of the "milk factor," various other physiological parameters such as hormonal and genetic, affect the rate of appearance of the neoplasms.

To determine the role of immune response on the growth of murine mammary tumors, tumor-associated antigens displayed to the hosts' immune system were identified by the monoclonal antibody technology. Hybridomas from spleens from animals carrying tumors that secrete MMTV produced specific tumor-related monoclonal antibodies of two kinds. One group (IIIA1 and VE7 are representatives) was directed against gp52, a 52,000 dalton glycoprotein that constitutes the knobs seen on the surface of the viral particle and is the major envelope glycoprotein of the virus. The other group, (IIB5 and IC12) reacted specifically with tumor cells secreting the virus but did not precipitate any viral or cellular protein from labeled tumor cells or labeled virus particles (Tax and Manson 1981). No hybridomas were found secreting monoclonal antibodies against other components of the virus particle, gp68, gp34, p28, p14, or p12 (Moore et al. 1979). In more recent experiments, both IIB5 and IC12 were shown to be directed against detergent-sensitive epitopes on the MMTV gp52. We concluded that gp52 of the MMTV particle is a major immunogen in the tumor-bearing host.

Other laboratories have documented similarities between human and mouse tumor-cell antigens related to MMTV. A proportion of women with breast cancer have circulating antibodies against MMTV antigens. How these antibodies relate to the human disease process is the focus of a long-range study, the first phase of which is to determine the characteristics of the human immunogen producing these antibodies and whether this immunogen contains epitopes that are homologous to those expressed on the gp52 glycoprotein of the MMTV. This paper describes these efforts and those directed at defining what epitope(s) of the MMTV gp52 particle is recognized by the human antibody.

MONOCLONAL ANTIBODIES

Anti-gp52 MMTV monoclonal antibodies (MAB) used in this study are IIIA1 (IgG3) and VE7 (IgG3) obtained from a tumor-bearing mouse and IIB5 (IgG1), IC12 (IgM), and IVC11 (IgM) obtained from an immunized rat. All have light chains of the κ type. The two mouse MAB bind Protein A, and the three rat MAB do not.

The antibodies IIB5 and IC12 did not immunoprecipitate materials from a labeled virus or labeled cells in the early experiments (Tax and Manson 1981). In such experiments, labeled cells or viruses normally are first dissociated with a nonionic detergent, NP-40, and then aliquots of the solubilized preparation are used in immunoprecipitation protocols. It has since been found (Manson and Tax 1983) that when MAB IIB5 or IC12 were added to the labeled virus preparation and allowed to bind and detergent was added after the MAB were bound, then the gp52 peak did appear after immunoprecipitation on sodium dodecyl sulfate polyacrylamide gel electrophoresis. The amount of detergent used did not prevent the combination of gp52 epitopes with MAB, IIIA1, VE7, and IVC11; detergent is generally considered not to be a denaturing material (Crumpton and Parkhouse 1972) at the concentration used (0.1%). Since gp52 is a membrane protein, there is likely to be a hydrophobic region in the native molecule in which detergent molecules might congregate and thus prevent access of MAB to epitopes present in this region. It would appear that the epitopes for IIB5 and IC12 fall into this category and therefore are conformational peptide epitopes. Whether the epitopes for the other three MAB are protein or carbohydrate is not yet certain.

Attempts have been made to estimate whether any of these five MAB are directed against unique epitopes and whether these epitopes are close to each other on the gp52 molecule. Using a variety of experiments involving labeling one MAB and testing the others to see if they compete with each other in binding assays or in binding using labeled Protein A as a probe, it is reasonably certain that IVC11, IIB5, and IC12 represent distinct epitopes, although IIB5 and IC12 may be close to each other on the gp52 molecule. The epitopes against which the other two MAB, IIIA1 and VE7, are directed are distinct from the three rat MAB, and are different from each other; however, again they may be close to each other on the gp52 molecule. The data reported in this study have been obtained using the IIIA1 and VE7 MAB.

BLOCKING ASSAY

All of the data contained in this report were obtained using a radioimmunoassay (RIA) in a blocking mode (Manson et al. 1978). In this assay, the solid phase consists of purified tissue-culture raised C3H-MMTV particles bound covalently to filter paper discs. The discs are then placed in the wells of a 96-well microtiter plate and the assay carried out as described. In a blocking mode protocol, 50 λ of a dilution of human serum is added to the well for 2 hours. To the well are then added 50 λ of a 1:100 dilution of a tissue-culture supernatant fluid of hybridoma IIIA1 or VE7. The incubation is continued for another 4 hours at room temperature. The contents of the wells are washed out, and a 100 λ aliquot of a ^{125}I antimouse Fab protein is added (Cancro and Klinman 1981) containing approximately 100,000 cpm (1–2 ng of antimouse Fab protein). After an overnight incubation at room temperature, the wells are again washed, and the discs are dried for 10 minutes in a stream of warm air, transferred to test tubes, and counted in a γ-spectrometer. The degree to which the human serum sample decreases the amount of MAB bound to the MMTV disc is compared to control discs that were not exposed to human serum, and this is reported in the tables as a percent of inhibition. Normal pools of goat, rabbit, calf, fetal calf, and horse sera contain no blocking substances detectable in such an assay when the sera are present at the 10% level. The antimouse Fab protein used in this study reacts equally well with mouse IgG, IgM, and IgA.

RESULTS

The capacities of human sera from a variety of sources to block the binding of IIIA1 and VE7 with C3H-MMTV discs in the RIA are shown in Table 1. Because of the higher blocking activity found with blood-donor sera with IIIA1 than with VE7, we have set a higher value (25%) as the maximum blocking activity below which any activity will be considered normal (in the tables this is termed "negative"). Using these criteria, one control was positive with IIIA1, and none with VE7. Only three sera have been tested thus far from patients with advanced melanoma; two were negative and one was positive for IIIA1, and all three were negative for VE7. Of great interest were the results found with sera from patients who had been diagnosed as having benign breast disease. Four showed a high blocking activity when tested with IIIA1, and 11 when tested with VE7. Three of the four that were positive with IIIA1 were also positive with VE7.

In Table 2, are shown cumulative data obtained over a period of 6 months testing, and the number of times each serum was tested is indicated. Patients #578, #580, and #661 were negative with IIIA1, and #285, #581, and #661 were negative with VE7. As can be seen from the table, #285 and #661 have been assayed a number of times, whereas #581 has only been tested three times and only once with VE7.

At a recent meeting on "Monoclonal Antibodies and Breast Cancer," in Washington, D.C., it was reported by Schlom that many of his MAB that were derived from mice immunized with malignant breast tissue (Egan and Henson 1982) also reacted with colon cancer tissue. We therefore tested a number of sera from patients with

Table 1. *Assay for Blocking Substances In Human Sera with Anti-MMTV gp52 Monoclonal Antibodies*

Source of Sera	No. of Pts.	IIIA1*		VE7[†]	
		1:10	1:20	1:10	1:20
Blood donor	12	14	19 ± 8	7	8 ± 8.6
Pts. with melanoma	2	8 ± 7	6 ± 5	0	3
Pts. with melanoma	1	32	26	5	2
Pts. with congenital nevus	1	14	22	3	5
Pts. with benign breast disease	25	19 ± 7	15 ± 8	19 ± 7	16 ± 7

*>25% inhibition with IIIA1 at a 1:20 dilution is positive.
[†]>15% inhibition with VE7 at a 1:20 dilution is positive.

Table 2. *Mammary Tumor Sera*

Pt. No.	No. of Experiments	% Inhibition			
		IIIA1*		VE7[†]	
		1:10	1:20	1:10	1:20
CEA2	4	34 ± 4	28 ± 5	21	29
55	4	44 ± 4	30 ± 2	30	24
125	2	45	39		20
285	6	16 ± 7	29 ± 15	10	1
318	3	38	41	9	26
578	2	17	21	7	23
579	2	31	39	8	18
580	5	24 ± 12	17 ± 11	32	17
581	3	30	40	0	0
582	10	29 ± 16	27 ± 19	28 ± 12	25 ± 8
661	5	24 ± 14	23 ± 9	8	1

*>25% inhibition with IIIA1 at a 1:20 dilution is positive.
[†]>15% inhibition with VE7 at a 1:20 dilution is positive.

colon cancer with IIIA1 and VE7. As the data in Table 3 show, five of seven were positive with IIIA1, whereas only two of seven were positive with VE7. Both sera positive with VE7 were also positive with IIIA1.

DISCUSSION

In inbred lines of mice, a high incidence and early occurrence of mammary tumors is associated with the presence of the infectious MMTV B particle in milk transmitted from the mother to the young. Mouse mammary tumor virus is an RNA-containing retrovirus, different and distinct from C-type retroviruses. DNA probes made of MMTV RNA have shown that the genomes of all inbred lines of mice, regardless of whether they have a high or low incidence of mammary tumors con-

Table 3. *Colon Cancer Pts.' Sera*

Pt. No.	No. of Experiments	% Inhibition			
		IIIA1*		VE7†	
		1:10	1:20	1:10	1:20
WCDK	3	38	32	7	3
F.P.	3	21	16	0	6
NO	3	41	41	10	7
131	3	38	13	3	6
156	6	38 ± 6	41 + 2	14 + 9	21 + 18
195	6	37 ± 1	37 ± 7	11 ± 4	11 ± 2
223	7	38 ± 2	42 ± 1	12 ± 11	16 ± 17

* >25% inhibition for IIIA1 at a 1:20 dilution is positive.
† >15% inhibition for VE7 at a 1:20 dilution is positive.

tain four to seven copies of the sequences per genome. In a most recent study (Callahan et al. 1982a), two types of MMTV-related sequences found in mouse genomes were described, the α-type, detected using high-stringency nucleic acid hybridization conditions, and the β-type, detected using lower stringency hybridization conditions. Inbred laboratory mice all have α-type sequences. The β-type sequences have been found in all strains of feral mice, some of whom were claimed to be free of MMTV-like sequences. In this study, these were shown to be free of any α-type sequences. The probes used contained the *env* region that is known to code for the major envelope virus proteins of MMTV gp52 and gp36. If one translates these findings into expectations of what the gene products in each case might be, then the α-type gene product ought to resemble the parent gp52 amino acid sequences greatly, whereas the β-type sequence might translate into sequences that resemble the gp52 peptide but would show distinct differences as well.

In parallel to these studies, we are using MAB as indicators of what may be the gene products of such sequences. In a study just completed (Tax, Ewert, and Manson 1983) we have found the VE7 epitope expressed on the surface membranes of a subpopulation of both C3H (MMTV+) and C57BL/6 (MMTV-) B spleen cells. The molecule carrying the VE7 epitope behaved in the membrane independently of the membrane immunoglobulin in capping tests. Thus, in the mouse we can use MAB as a tool to study gene expression by detecting the presence of the gene product. Whether the VE7 epitope is part of a gp52-like molecule in the membranes of the B cells has not yet been determined.

Evidence suggesting that MMTV-like antigens have an association with breast cancer in humans comes mainly from three laboratories. From Spiegelman's laboratory have come a series of papers (Keydar et al. 1978, Mesa-Tejada et al. 1978, Ohno et al. 1979, Spiegelman et al. 1980) demonstrating a high frequency of positive staining of paraffin sections obtained from patients with breast cancer using an indirect immunoperoxidase technique. The reagent used in this study was an IgG preparation made from a rabbit anti-RIII MMTV serum. In their most recent review of the data, 212 out of 447 patients' sections were found to be positive (47.4%). The antibodies that gave the positive reaction were directed against antigenic determinants found on the peptide portions of the gp52 of RIII and of C3H MMTV. Only one positive reaction was seen in sections from 99 patients with other malignancies.

The second laboratory that has provided positive data linking breast cancer and MMTV antigens is that of Sarkar (Witkin et al. 1980, Sarkar 1980). Using an enzyme-linked immunoassay (ELISA) with purified RIII MMTV as the solid phase, 14 out of 54 sera (26%) from patients with breast cancer showed significant binding levels to MMTV; seven out of 58 benign sera (12%) were positive, and six out of 63 normal sera (10%) were positive. The sera were also tested for virolytic activity against MMTV by assaying for the release of reverse transcriptase. Again, the antibodies in the human sera responsible for the virolytic activity were absorbed by MMTV.

The results obtained by these two laboratories showed that anti-gp52 antibodies react with substances found in breast cancer sections and that these substances may be immunogenic in man. The third study of importance to note is that of Dion et al. 1980. They processed a pool of human milk obtained from approximately 300 separate donors for a B particle-rich fraction. They obtained a human milk protein that resembled the B particle of mouse milk biochemically and immunologically. Whereas the goat anti-MMTV serum reacted with a 55,000 dalton glycoprotein from RIII MMTV, the analogous molecule obtained from the human preparation that reacted with the same sera was a 58,000 dalton glycoprotein. The two glycoproteins shared common sequences when tryptic peptide maps were prepared, but they also differed significantly so that it was clear that the two glycoproteins were not identical. This study established that there was a human structural analogue to mouse gp52 but did not establish whether this human analogue had a physiological function.

The data reported in this study are an interim report of an analysis of the expression of "gp52 human analogue" (if there is one) as it appears in sera of normal controls and patients with various malignant diseases. The analytic tool we are using in this analysis are MAB directed against epitopes found on the gp52 of C3H-MMTV. All of the MAB used in this study have also been tested against the gp55 of RIII-MMTV (Dion personal communication) and were found to react. There are two major serotypes of MMTV; one is represented by C3H-MMTV; the other is represented by RIII-MMTV (Massey et al. 1980). Thus, the MAB we are using are likely to be capable of detecting common sequences that might exist on gene products of even β-type MMTV-like DNA sequences. While these studies were ongoing, a most significant study was published. Callahan et al. 1982b have reported that sequences related to the MMTV genome have been detected in human cellular DNA, both normal and malignant. The probe containing the *env* DNA sequences hybridized with DNA from human liver, human placenta, and human mammary adenocarcinoma but not with salmon sperm DNA or chicken embryo DNA. It is therefore not unreasonable to expect that these sequences might result in the production of the appropriate gene product. The finding that in the human genome the sequences belong to the β-type rather than the α-type would lead us to look for the expression in human cells of some epitopes in common with those found in the mouse, but we should also expect that the human gene products could contain unique regions not to be found in the mouse. It is for this reason that we will have to postpone drawing conclusions on the true significance of data such as those reported in this study until more information is obtained on the reactivities seen with other MAB already available and as yet to be produced.

CONCLUSIONS

The following conclusions can be drawn from the results of this study: (1) Human sera have been tested for substances (antigen and/or antibody) that block the interaction of two anti-gp52 MMTV MAB (IIIA1 and VE7) with purified MMTV particles. (2) Sera from normal blood donors block IIIA1 much more frequently than VE7. Whether this means that there is a normal amount of IIIA1-reacting material present at all times is not clear. (3) Eight of 11 sera of a group of patients with metastatic breast cancer block IIIA1 and VE7 to a significantly higher degree than do sera from normal blood donors. (4) Of a group of seven sera from patients with colon cancer, five blocked IIIA1, whereas only two blocked VE7. (5) Twenty-five sera from patients with benign breast disease were tested. Of these, four blocked IIIA1, 11 blocked VE7, and three of the four that were positive for IIIA1 were also positive for VE7. (6) Additional studies using monoclonal antibodies directed against epitopes found on different regions of the gp52 molecule of MMTV are being carried out with these human sera.

ACKNOWLEDGMENTS

We would like to thank Ms. Anita Guarini, Ms. Jennifer Kennedy, and Mrs. Holly Savage for their excellent technical assistance.

This investigation was supported by Grant Number CA 10815 awarded by the National Cancer Institute, U.S. Department of Health and Human Services and Grant Number IM 309 awarded by the American Cancer Society.

REFERENCES

Bittner, J. J. 1936. Some possible effects of nursing on the mammary tumor incidence in mice. Science 84:162.

Callahan, R., W. Drohan, D. Gallahan, L. D'Hoostelaere, and M. Potter. 1982a. Novel class of mouse mammary tumor virus-related DNA sequences found in all species of *Mus*, including mice lacking the virus proviral genome. Proc. Natl. Acad. Sci. USA 79:4113–4117.

Callahan, R., W. Drohan, S. Tronick, and J. Schlom. 1982b. Detection and cloning of human DNA sequences related to the mouse mammary tumor virus genome. Proc. Natl. Acad. Sci. USA 79:5503–5507.

Cancro, M. P., and N. R. Klinman. 1981. B cell repertoire ontogeny: Heritable but dissimilar development of parental and F₁ repertoires. J. Immunol. 126:1160–1164.

Crumpton, M. J., and R. M. E. Parkhouse. 1972. Comparison of the effects of various detergents on antigen-antibody interaction. FEBS Lett. 22:210–212.

Dion, A. S., D. C. Farwell, A. A. Pomenti, and A. J. Girardi. 1980. A human protein related to the major envelope protein of murine mammary tumor virus: Identification and characterization. Proc. Natl. Acad. Sci. USA 77:1301–1305.

Egan, M. L., and D. E. Henson. 1982. Monoclonal antibodies and breast cancer. JNCI 68:338–340.

Keydar, I., R. Mesa-Tejada, M. Ramanarayanan, T. Ohno, C. Fenoglio, R. Hu, and S. Spiegelman. 1978. Detection of viral proteins in mouse mammary tumors by immunoperoxidase staining of paraffin sections. Proc. Natl. Acad. Sci. USA 75:1524–1528.

Manson, L. A. 1981. The role of cell-surface antigens in progressive tumor growth (Immunological surveillance re-revisited), *in* Current Trends in Histocompatibility, R. A. Reisfeld and S. Ferrone, eds., vol. 2. Plenum Publishing Corp., New York, pp. 105–112.

Manson, L. A. and A. Tax. 1983. A viral coat glycoprotein (gp52 MUMTV) has detergent-sensitive and detergent resistant epitopes in the same molecule. Molec. Immunol., in press.

Manson, L. A., E. Verastegui-Cerdan, and R. Sporer. 1978. A quantitative disc radioimmunoassay for antibodies directed against membrane-associated antigens, *in* Current Topics in Microbiology and Immunology, F. Melchers, M. Potter, and N. Warner, eds., vol. 81. Springer-Verlag, New York, pp. 232–234.

Massey, R. J., L. O. Arthur, R. C. Nowinski, and G. Schochetman. 1980. Monoclonal antibodies identify individual determinants on mouse mammary tumor virus glycoprotein gp52 with group, class, or type specificity. J. Virol. 34:635–643.

Mesa-Tejada, R., I. Keydar, M. Ramanarayanan, T. Ohno, C. Fenoglio, and S. Spiegelman. 1978. Detection in human breast carcinomas of an antigen immunologically related to a group-specific antigen of mouse mammary tumor virus. Proc. Natl. Acad. Sci. USA 75:1529–1533.

Moore, D. H., C. A. Long, J. B. Sheffield, A. S. Dion, and E. Y. Lasfargues. 1979. Mammary tumor viruses. Adv. Cancer Res. 29:347–418.

Ohno, T., R. Mesa-Tejada, I. Keydar, M. Ramanarayanan, J. Bausch, and S. Spiegelman. 1979. Human breast carcinoma antigen is immunologically related to the polypeptide of the group-specific glycoprotein of mouse mammary tumor virus. Proc. Natl. Acad. Sci. USA 76:2460–2464.

Sarkar, N. H. 1980. Type B virus and human breast cancer, *in* The Role of Viruses in Human Cancer, G. Giraldo and E. Beth, eds., vol. 1. Elsevier North Holland, Inc., New York, pp. 207–235.

Spiegelman, S., R. Mesa-Tejada, T. Ohno, M. Ramanarayanan, R. Nayak, J. Bausch, C. Fenoglio, and I. Keydar. 1980. The presence and clinical implications of a virus-related protein in human breast cancer, *in* Viruses in Naturally Occurring Cancers, vol. 7. Cold Spring Harbor, Cold Spring Harbor, New York, pp. 1149–1167.

Tax, A., D. Ewert, and L. A. Manson. 1983. An antigen cross-reactive with gp52 of mammary tumor virus is expressed on a B-cell subpopulation of mice. J. Immunol. 130:2368–2371.

Tax, A., and L. A. Manson. 1981. Monoclonal antibodies against antigens displayed on a progressively growing mammary tumor. Proc. Natl. Acad. Sci. USA 78:529–533.

Witkin, S. S., N. H. Sarkar, D. W. Kinne, R. A. Good, and N. K. Day. 1980. Antibodies reactive with the mouse mammary tumor virus in sera of breast cancer patients. Int. J. Cancer 25:721–725.

Current Controversies in Breast Cancer, edited
by F. C. Ames, G. R. Blumenschein, and E. D. Montague.
University of Texas Press, Austin © 1984.

A Sensitive Solid-Phase Enzyme Immunoassay for Human Estrogen Receptor

Chris Nolan, Ph.D., Louise W. Przywara, Ph.D., Larry S. Miller,
Ph.D., Victor Suduikis, B.S., and Joseph T. Tomita, Ph.D.

Abbott Laboratories, North Chicago, Illinois

The utility of estrogen receptor (ER) determinations in breast cancers as an aid to patient management and as an indicator of prognosis is well established (McGuire et al. 1975, DeSombre et al. 1979). Until now, measurement of ER in the clinical laboratory has been performed by steroid binding assays, which use radiolabeled estradiol to detect the receptor. These assays, which have been reviewed by Chamness and McGuire (1979), include the dextran-coated charcoal (DCC) and sucrose density gradient assays. Although the steroid binding assays have been very useful, they have some important drawbacks: (1) the methods are rather difficult and cumbersome, and this precludes their use in many clinical laboratories; (2) as routinely run, they measure only available receptor, i.e., that not occupied by endogeneous estrogens—thus, the level of receptor measured is dependent upon the hormonal status of the patient; (3) there is generally poor correlation between assay values obtained in different laboratories (Oxley et al. 1982).

The preparation of monoclonal antibodies to human ER by Greene et al. (1980) made possible the development of an immunoassay for human ER, and preliminary results obtained with an immunoradiometric assay (IRMA) using two rat monoclonal antibodies to human ER, D547SPγ and D75P3γ, have been reported (Jensen et al. 1982, Greene and Jensen 1982). Previous studies of these antibodies (Greene et al. 1980, Jensen et al. 1982, Greene and Jensen, 1982) have shown that they will bind both the cytoplasmic and nuclear forms of human ER from breast cancer tissue and both the receptor-estrogen complex and the unoccupied cytoplasmic receptor. Moreover, both antibodies will bind to the ER molecule at the same time, showing that they are directed toward different determinants on the receptor molecule. Further specificity studies demonstrated that, although both antibodies cross-react with ER from other mammalian species, neither cross-reacts with human receptors for progestins, androgens, or glucocorticoids. These properties indicate these antibodies are well suited for use in an immunoassay.

We have developed a solid-phase, "sandwich" type enzyme immunoassay (EIA) for human ER using these two monoclonal antibodies. The following is a report on our preliminary studies with this assay.

METHODS

Estrogen Receptor EIA

A description of the ER-EIA procedure is given in Figure 1, and the assay protocol is outlined in Table 1. The two antibodies used in the assay are rat monoclonal antibodies to MCF-7 cell ER prepared as previously described (Greene et al. 1980). As shown in Table 1, 0.2 ml of ER standard solution or 0.1 ml of specimen (e.g., cytosol) plus 0.1 ml of specimen diluent were used in the assay, and the results are expressed in fmol ER/0.2 ml of standard or fmol ER/0.1 ml of specimen. In cases where cytosol protein concentrations were determined, results are given in fmol ER/mg cytosol protein.

The first two incubation steps (Table 1) were performed in 20- or 60-well plastic reaction trays (Abbott). The beads were transferred to 12 x 75 mm plastic tubes for the enzyme-substrate reaction, and the measurement of A_{492nm} and data reduction were performed on a Quantum I spectrophotometer (Abbott).

Sample Preparation

Breast cancer tissues, received frozen on dry ice and stored at −70°C, were pulverized with a Thermovac tissue pulverizer that had been chilled with liquid nitrogen; the tissues were then homogenized in cold (2°−4°C) buffer (2 ml/gm of

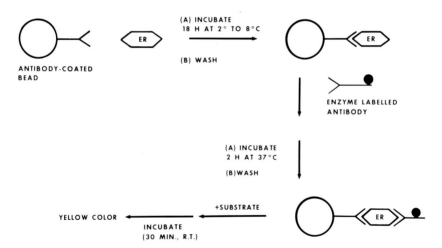

FIG. 1. Schematic diagram of the solid-phase, "sandwich" type enzyme immunoassay for estrogen receptor (ER). The sample containing ER is incubated with a .25-inch diameter plastic bead coated with the first antibody (D547Spγ). After washing, the resulting bead-bound ER-antibody complex is incubated with the second antibody (D75P3γ) conjugated with horseradish peroxidase. The bead is washed to remove excess conjugate, and the enzyme-tagged ER-antibody complex is incubated with enzyme substrate solution (H_2O_2 and orthophenylenediamine). The reaction is stopped with 1 N H_2SO_4, and the A_{492nm} is measured.

Table 1. *Estrogen Receptor EIA* Protocol*

First Incubation
1. To reaction tray wells add
   a. 0.2 ml of standard or 0.1 ml cytosol plus 0.1 ml specimen diluent.
   b. Anti-ER-coated beads.
2. Incubate at 2°–8°C overnight (18 ± 2 hours).
3. Aspirate and wash beads.

Second Incubation
1. Add 0.2 ml of anti-ER:peroxidase conjugate to wells.
2. Incubate for 2 hours at 37°C
3. Aspirate and wash beads with water.

Enzyme Reaction
1. Transfer beads to assay tubes and add 0.3 ml of enzyme substrate solution to each.
2. Incubate for 30 minutes at room temperature.
3. Add 1.0 ml of 1 N H_2SO_4 to each tube and mix.
4. Measure A_{492nm}.

*ER = estrogen receptor; EIA = enzyme immunoassay.

pulverized tissue) with a Tekmar Tissumizer (three 3-second bursts with the SDT-100EN probe, with 30-second cooling intervals in an ice bath between bursts). The homogenizing buffer was either TED (10 mM Tris·HCl, 1.5 mM EDTA, and 0.5 mM dithiothreitol, pH 7.4), or PMTGCG (10 mM sodium phosphate, pH 7.5, containing monothioglycerol [0.108 gm/L], cortisol [1.7×10^{-7} M], and glycerol [10%, V/V]). The homogenates were centrifuged at 105,000 x g for 1 hour at 4°C. The cytosol fractions were collected and assayed the same day.

Comparison of the EIA and DCC Assays for ER

Comparison of the EIA and DCC assays was made with breast cancer cytosols in the laboratory of Interlab Associates, Miami, Florida, using their routine DCC assay for ER. The assay was a seven-point assay using ³H-estradiol at final concentrations ranging from 0.1 to 1.6 nM, with duplicate determinations at each concentration. Labeling was performed overnight (19 hours) at 4°C, the binding data were corrected for nonspecific binding (that not inhibited by a 200-fold excess of diethylstilbestrol), and ER values and dissociation constants were determined from Scatchard plots of the data (Scatchard 1949).

The EIA was run on duplicate 0.1-ml aliquots of undiluted cytosol and, when enough cytosol was available, on cytosol aliquots diluted threefold with homogenizing buffer.

Breast cancer tissue samples were assayed by the two methods in the order they were received in the laboratory; the only exceptions were those samples too small to permit assay by both methods. Cytosols were prepared as described above. Cytosolic protein concentrations were determined independently (separate dilutions) for the two ER assays by the method of Lowry et al. (1951) with bovine serum albumin as the standard.

RESULTS AND DISCUSSION

Performance Characteristics of Estrogen Receptor EIA

A standard curve for the ER-EIA is shown in Figure 2. The curve is essentially linear over the assay range of 0-250 fmol of ER. Since 0.1-ml aliquots of specimen (cytosol) are used in the assay, this gives a range of 0-250 fmol/0.1 ml or 0-2500 fmol/ml of cytosol. For higher ER concentrations, dilution of the sample is required. The volume of undiluted cytosol required for a single determination (0.1 ml) is equivalent to approximately 33 mg of breast cancer tissue when 2 ml of homogenizing buffer/gm of tissue is used, or about 20 mg of tissue when 4 ml of buffer/gm of tissue is used.

Figure 3 shows the results of a study of the effects of sample dilution, using MCF-7 cell cytosol as sample, on the ER values obtained by EIA. As can be seen, the ER values correlate well with the reciprocal of the dilution ($r=0.999$) over a range of dilutions of 4- to 640-fold. Similar results were obtained with a breast cancer tissue cytosol sample diluted over a range of 2- to 1728-fold (Figure 4) ($r=0.9970$).

To estimate the sensitivity of the EIA, ER standards were run in replicates of four on each of 4 days, and the ER value corresponding to the A_{492nm} value two standard deviations away from the zero standard absorbance value was taken as the limit of sensitivity. The average value was 1.1 fmol/0.1 ml, with an upper limit of 1.7 fmol/0.1 ml. This is consistent with the results in Figure 3, which indicate a sensitivity of

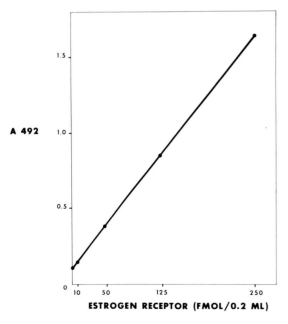

FIG. 2. Estrogen receptor enzyme immunoassay standard curve. The standards contained 0-250 fmol of ER in a total volume of 0.2 ml.

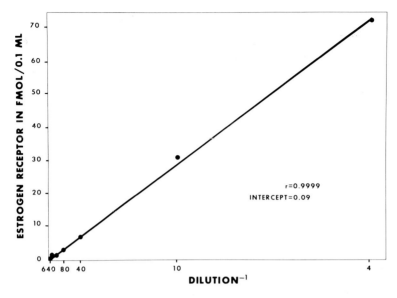

FIG. 3. Estrogen receptor concentrations of dilutions of MCF-7 cell cytosol, as measured by the enzyme immunoassay as a function of cytosol dilution. Freshly prepared cytosol was diluted as indicated with the zero standard, and 0.2 ml of each dilution was assayed in duplicate. The curve was drawn by least squares linear regression analysis of the data.

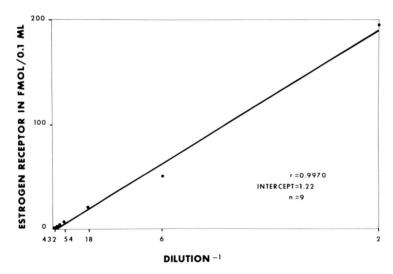

FIG. 4. Estrogen receptor concentrations of dilutions of a breast cancer cytosol, as measured by the enzyme immunoassay as a function of cytosol dilution. Freshly prepared cytosol was diluted and assayed, and the data plotted as described in the legend to Figure 3.

Table 2. *ER-EIA* Inter-Assay Reproducibility[†]*

Specimen Number	Number of Assays	fmol ER/0.1 ml (mean)	SD[‡]	CV (%)[‡]
1	5	145	8.7	6.0
2	4	50.6	2.1	4.1
3	5	5.6	0.2	3.5
Control	5	32.7	1.7	5.1

*ER = estrogen receptor; EIA = enzyme immunoassay.
[†]The assays were run by one technician in duplicate on each of 5 days. Specimens were MCF-7 cell cytosol preparations. Specimen 2 was inadvertently omitted on day 5.
[‡]SD = standard deviation; CV = coefficients of variation.

≤1.7 fmol/0.1 ml of specimen, since the ER values obtained for the 40-, 80-, and 160-fold dilutions, all of which fell on the curve, were 6.9, 3.4, and 1.7 fmol/0.1 ml. For a cytosol sample with a protein concentration of 10 mg/ml, 1.1 to 1.7 fmol ER/0.1 ml would be equivalent to 1.1 to 1.7 fmol/mg protein. This is below 3 fmol/mg, the lowest cut-off point between ER-positive and ER-negative breast cancer tissues.

A 5-day interassay reproducibility study was performed with the EIA, using samples prepared from MCF-7 cell cytosol (Table 2). Over a range of 5.6 to 145 fmol ER/0.1 ml, the coefficients of variation (CV) ranged from 3.5% to 6.0%.

The results of recovery studies with the EIA are shown in Table 3. In this experiment the recovery of various concentrations of ER added to a breast cancer cytosol was determined. As can be seen, recovery of added receptor at concentrations ranging from 4.7 to 133.4 fmol/0.1 ml ranged from 105% to 112% of control values.

Table 3. *Recovery of Added Estrogen Receptor from Breast Cancer Tissue Cytosol with the ER-EIA* Procedure[†]*

From Zero Standard	ER Recovered (fmol/0.1 ml) From Tissue Cytosol Uncorrected	Corrected[‡]	% Recovery from Tissue Cytosol[§]
133.4	151.2	150.0	112
44.4	49.4	48.2	109
14.8	17.4	16.2	109
4.7	6.2	5.0	105
0.0	1.2	0.0	—

*ER = estrogen receptor; EIA = enzyme immunoassay.
[†]The ER-EIA zero standard and an ER-poor (1.2 fmol ER/0.1 ml) breast cancer cytosol were spiked with different amounts of MCF-7 cytosol, and the samples were assayed in duplicate by the EIA. The volume of MCF-7 cytosol added to the samples was ≤6% of the total volume in every case.
[‡]Corrected for endogenous ER (1.2 fmol/0.1 ml).
[§]Recoveries are relative to the corresponding spiked zero standard.

Correlation of EIA and DCC Assay Values

To further evaluate the EIA, freshly prepared breast cancer cytosols were assayed by both the EIA and a multipoint DCC assay for ER, and the results were compared. A plot of the values, expressed in fmol ER/mg cytosol protein, obtained with 54 cytosols (Figure 5) shows a good correlation between the two methods ($r=0.96$). Protein determinations were run on separate dilutions of the cytosols for the two ER assays, and the variations seen (Figure 5) reflect variations in the protein assays as well as the receptor assays. The slope of the curve in Figure 5 is 2.0, which means that, on the average, the EIA values were twice as high as the DCC values. When the factor of 2 is taken into account, all values were in agreement with respect to ER-positive ($\geq$ 3 fmol/mg of protein) or ER-negative ($<$ 3 fmol/mg) status except one, which was weakly positive (13 fmol/mg) by the DCC assay and negative (not detectable) by the EIA. Lack of sufficient cytosol prevented us from repeating the assay of this sample by either method to confirm the results.

In addition to these 54 samples, there were 10 cytosols in which the ER concentrations were so high that they were beyond the range of one or both assays at the dilutions used. The values were in agreement, in that high values were obtained by

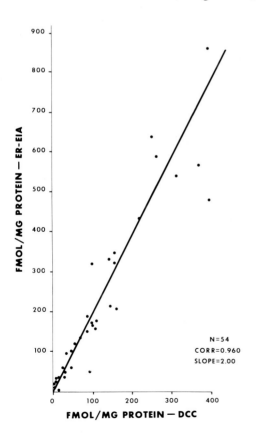

FIG. 5. Correlation of estrogen receptor enzyme immunoassay values with results obtained with a multipoint dextran-coated charcoal (DCC) assay on 54 freshly prepared breast cancer cytosols. The curve was drawn by least-squares linear regression analysis of the data.

both assays. Thus, the two assays were in agreement with respect to ER status in 63/64 samples.

Of the 54 breast cancer cytosols compared in Figure 5, 21 were in TED buffer and 33 in PMTGCG buffer. When only the cytosols in the Tris buffer are compared, as in Figure 5, $r=0.99$ and the slope is 2.3; comparing only the cytosols in the phosphate buffer, the corresponding values are 0.96 and 2.0. Although the number of samples is relatively small, these results indicate that the correlation between the two methods is good with either buffer and that there is no significant difference in the results obtained with the two buffers.

When enough cytosol was available, the EIA was performed on both the undiluted cytosol and a threefold dilution in the homogenizing buffer. Of these, the values of both dilutions fell within the range of the assay in 32 of the 54 cytosols compared in Figure 5. A plot of the values obtained with the undiluted samples (on the abscissa) against those obtained with the diluted samples (on the ordinate) gave $r=0.99$ and a slope of 0.91 (not shown).

An earlier comparison by Jensen and co-workers (Jensen et al. 1982, Greene and Jensen 1982) of their IRMA assay for ER with their sucrose density gradient (SDG) assay on 18 breast cancer cytosol samples showed a 98% correlation between the two assays and agreement with respect to the ER status of the breast cancer in 18/18 cases. Thus, together the EIA and IRMA assays, which used the same two monoclonal antibodies, agree with the steroid binding assays with respect to the ER status of the sample in 81/82 cases. A plot of the ER values obtained with the IRMA assay (on the ordinate) against those obtained with the SDG assay (on the abscissa) gave a slope near unity (0.94). This indicates that the slope of 2.0 obtained in the plot of the EIA values against the DCC values in Figure 5 was not a result of any differences inherent in the two assays due to the differences in the means of detecting the receptor. The higher values obtained with the EIA relative to the DCC assay may be largely attributable to differences in the DCC assay used in the comparative study and the one used in our own laboratory to assign the ER concentration to the EIA-ER standard.

CONCLUSIONS

The results of these preliminary studies with the ER-EIA and the earlier studies with the IRMA assay for ER (Jensen et al. 1982, Greene and Jensen 1982) show very good correlations between the immunoassays and steroid binding assays. These results, together with the sensitivity and precision of the EIA, its ease of use, and the shorter time required relative to the steroid binding assays, indicate that the EIA is an attractive alternative to the steroid binding assays. Further evaluation of the EIA is in progress.

ACKNOWLEDGMENTS

We thank Sosamma George, Bonnie Moore, and Sally Weitendorf for excellent technical assistance. We gratefully acknowledge Dr. Julio Cortes and Ms. Suzy Pixley of Interlab Associates, Miami, for their generous help in part of these studies.

REFERENCES

Chamness, G. C., and W. L. McGuire. 1979. Steroid receptor assay methods in human breast cancer, *in* Steroid Receptors in the Management of Breast Cancer, vol. 1, E. B. Thompson and M. E. Lippman, eds. CRC Press, Boca Raton, Florida, pp. 3–30.

DeSombre, E. R., P. P. Carbone, E. V. Jensen, W. L. McGuire, S. A. Wells, Jr., J. L. Wittliff, and M. B. Lipsett. 1979. Steroid receptors in breast cancer. N. Engl. J. Med. 301:1011–1012.

Greene, G. L., C. Nolan, J. P. Engler, and E. V. Jensen. 1980. Monoclonal antibodies to human estrogen receptor. Proc. Natl. Acad. Sci. USA 77:5115–5119.

Greene, G. L., and E. V. Jensen. 1982. Monoclonal antibodies as probes for estrogen receptor detection and characterization. J. Steroid Biochem. 16:353–359.

Jensen, E. V., G. L. Greene, L. E. Closs, E. R. DeSombre, and M. Nadji. 1982. Receptors reconsidered: A 20-year perspective. Rec. Prog. Horm. Res. 38:1–40.

Lowry, O. H., N. J. Rosebrough, A. L. Farr, and R. J. Randall. 1951. Protein measurement with the Folin phenol reagent. J. Biol. Chem. 193:265–275.

McGuire, W. L., P. P. Carbone, M. E. Sears, and G. C. Escher. 1975. Estrogen receptors in human breast cancer: An overview, *in* Estrogen Receptors in Human Breast Cancer, W. L. McGuire, P. P. Carbone, and E. P. Vollmer, eds. Raven Press, New York, pp. 1–7.

Oxley, D. K., G. T. Haven, J. L. Wittliff, and D. Gilbo. 1982. Precision in estrogen and progesterone receptor assays. Results of the first CAP survey. Am. J. Clin. Pathol. 78 (Suppl.):587–596.

Scatchard, G. 1949. The attraction of proteins for small molecules and ions. Ann. N.Y. Acad. Sci. 51:660–672.

Current Controversies in Breast Cancer, edited
by F. C. Ames, G. R. Blumenschein, and E. D. Montague.
University of Texas Press, Austin © 1984.

Serial Bone Scans For Assessing Therapeutic Response in Bony Metastasis of Breast Cancer

E. Edmund Kim, M.D.,*† Carlos R. Gutierrez, M.D.,* Thomas P. Haynie, M.D.,† and Anthony G. Bledin, M.D.†

Department of Radiology, The University of Texas Medical School at Houston, Houston, Texas, and †Department of Internal Medicine, The University of Texas M. D. Anderson Hospital and Tumor Institute at Houston, Houston, Texas

Many clinical studies have compared the relative efficiency of the radiographic bone survey and the radionuclide bone scan in the detection of bone metastases (Osmond et al. 1975, O'Mara 1976, Citrin et al. 1977). These studies agree that the bone scan is a more sensitive indicator of the presence of bone metastases than the radiograph. A destructive lesion in trabecular bone must be greater than 1.5 cm in diameter with at least 50% of bone mineral removed before any abnormality will be detected radiographically (Edelstyn et al. 1967). In patients with early bone involvement, radiographs are rarely abnormal, while a significant number of cases of occult bone metastases can be identified by bone scanning. In patients with advanced disease, comparative studies have shown a significantly increased number of lesions seen on the bone scan when compared with those seen on the radiograph (Citrin et al. 1981).

However, there has been controversy over the relative value of serial bone scans and radiographs in evaluating the response of bone metastasis of breast cancer to systemic therapy (Bitran et al. 1980, Citrin et al. 1981, Libshitz and Hortobagyi 1981). In order to evaluate our experience, serial bone scans and radiographs of patients with breast cancer and bone metastases were retrospectively analyzed.

MATERIALS AND METHODS

Sixty patients with metastatic breast cancer (stage IV) were selected from the patients referred to the Nuclear Medicine Clinics of The University of Texas M. D. Anderson Hospital and Tumor Institute at Houston (55 patients) and Hermann Hospital (5 patients), also in Houston, during the last quarter of 1981 and first quarter of 1982 for retrospective analysis. These patients had had multiple previous bone scintigrams and were returning for follow-up. All patients had histologically proven carcinoma of the breast and were receiving hormonal therapy or chemotherapeutic agents (usually a combination of cyclophosphamide, Adriamycin or methotrexate,

Table 1. *Criteria for Response of Bone Metastases to Systemic Therapy*

A. Improvement
Bone scan
Significant reduction of abnormally increased radioactivity without new lesion when compared with initial scan.
X-ray
Sclerotic rim around osteolytic lesion without new lesion → filling-in with blastic response → fading blastic area.
Fading of osteoblastic lesion without new lesion.
B. Worsening
Bone scan
Significant increase of abnormal uptake of radioactivity when compared with initial scan.
Appearance of new lesion.
X-ray
Increased size of osteolytic or mixed lesion.
Increased area of osteoblastic lesion.
Destruction of sclerotic response in previous lesion.
Appearance of new lesion.
C. Mixed
Bone scan and X-ray
Combination of improvement and worsening.
D. No change

and 5-fluorouracil) or both during the evaluation periods ranging from 12–96 months (average 38 months).

Serial bone scans (every 3–12 months with an average of 6.7 months) were performed using 15 mCi of [99mTc] phosphate compounds and a Total Body Hybrid Scanner (Cleon, Union Carbide Corp.) to obtain whole body anterior and posterior images for all patients. The five patients at Hermann Hospital had follow-up studies with a large field-of-view gamma camera (Technicare). More frequent conventional x-ray bone surveys (every 3–12 months, average 5.7 months for complete survey, and every 1–12 months, average 3.1 months for limited survey) were obtained in these patients.

Comparable bone scans and radiographs were reevaluated by one observer to correlate reported positive lesions on one modality with the other. The criteria in assessing response of bony metastasis on bone scans or radiographs is outlined in Table 1.

RESULTS

In the 60 patients (age range 36–79 years, median 61 years) with advanced breast carcinoma, a total of 252 metastatic bony lesions were found by serial bone scans or radiographs or both. Sixty-nine lesions (mostly in the rib cage, spine, and pelvis) detected initially only on scans, but later showing as abnormalities on x-ray also

Table 2. *Comparison of Bone Scans and X-rays in Assessment of Overall Response in Bony Metastases in 60 Breast Cancer Patients*

A. Overall Response:

I*−18; W†−7; M‡−28; N§−7

B. Preferred Modality for Response:

scan	x-ray	same
44	3	13

*Improvement.
†Worsening.
‡Mixed.
§No change.

compared with 16 lesions (mostly in skull and pubis) detected initially only on x-ray but later appearing on scans. Six pelvic lesions were found only on radiographs and 6 rib lesions on scans, but none of these 12 lesions were ever seen on both modalities. These sites never developed clinical metastases on follow-up and were therefore classified "false-positive."

Overall response in 60 patients revealed improvement in 18, worsening in 7, mixed response in 28, and no change in 7. The scan was judged a better modality for assessing overall response in 44 patients (Table 2) because of its ability to detect new lesions earlier and minimal changes and to show fading or intensification that correlated with clinical response or progression. Radiographs showed minimal changes of many osteoblastic or mixed lesions. In 3 patients, x-ray was preferred in osteolytic lesions showing sclerotic response, and in 13 patients the two modalities were equal.

In 125 comparable lesions detected by scan and x-ray (Table 3), on x-ray examination 48% were radiolucent (osteolytic) lesions, 34% were radiodense (osteoblas-

Table 3. *Comparison of Bone Scans and X-Rays in Assessment of Response in 125 Comparable Metastatic Lesions*

Type of Lesion By X-Ray	Overall Lesion Response					Preferred Modality		
	I*	W†	M‡	N§	Total (%)	Scan	X-ray	Same
Osteolytic	37	10	7	6	60 (48%)	24	20	16
Osteoblastic	25	8	4	6	43 (34%)	37	6	0
Mixed	8	5	1	8	22 (18%)	14	6	2

*Improvement.
†Worsening.
‡Mixed.
§No change.

tic), and 18% were mixed. Comparison of response by type of lesion revealed that in instances in which the modalities differed the scan was only slightly preferred over x-ray bone survey for evaluating response of osteolytic lesions (24 to 20), while osteoblastic or mixed lesions were much better evaluated on bone scans (37 to 6 and 14 to 6). Representative cases are illustrated in Figures 1, 2, 3, and 4.

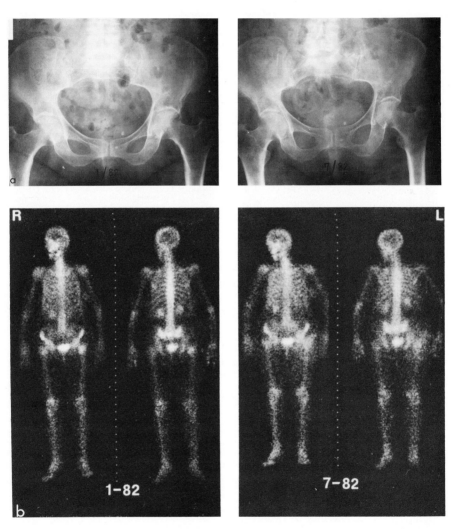

FIG. 1. A 66-year-old woman 7 months after right mastectomy for adenocarcinoma of the breast. **A.** Frontal radiograph of the anatomic pelvis shows an osteolytic lesion in the medial portion of left intertrochanteric ridge that demonstrates slightly sclerotic response after chemotherapy on the follow-up study. **B.** Whole-body image of the bone scan shows a focal increased activity in the left trochanteric region that is markedly diminished on follow-up scan. No new lesion is noted.

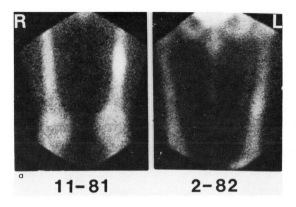

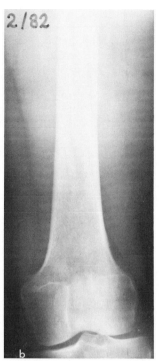

FIG. 2. A 74-year-old woman with an infiltrating carcinoma of the left breast had negative preoperative studies for metastatic lesion. **A.** Six-month follow-up bone scan demonstrates a metastatic lesion in the left femoral shaft, in addition to multiple rib lesions. Corresponding radiograph was essentially negative. Three months later with chemotherapy, follow-up bone scan shows a significant reduction of increased radioactivity in the left femur. **B.** Radiograph reveals an osteolytic or mixed lesion.

DISCUSSION

Metastatic disease of bone from breast cancer is usually due to hematogenous spread, although a carcinoma of the breast may involve the rib cage by direct extension. The skull, spine, ribs, shoulder, and pelvic girdles, and proximal ends of the long bone are most frequently involved. Bone metastases frequently occur rapidly: in one series, 50% of patients developed metastases by 12 months, and in another, 75% developed them by 18 months (McNeil et al. 1978).

Tumor cells are first deposited within the sinusoids of the red marrow and grow to surround and destroy trabecular bone. Eventually they invade and may destroy the cortex of the bone, often resulting in pathologic fracture. It has been suggested that the initial mechanism is osteoclast activation followed at a later stage by direct tumor-associated, prostaglandin-mediated osteolysis (Bennett et al. 1975, Galasko 1976).

Bone destruction due to metastatic breast cancer is associated almost invariably with attempts at repair (Galasko 1976). The most frequent radiographic abnormality in breast cancer patients with bone metastases is a desctructive area seen in trabecular bone. Mixed lytic and blastic lesions are frequently seen in patients with metastatic breast cancer and are prevalent in patients having previously received hor-

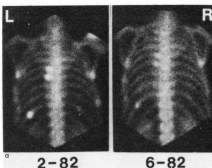

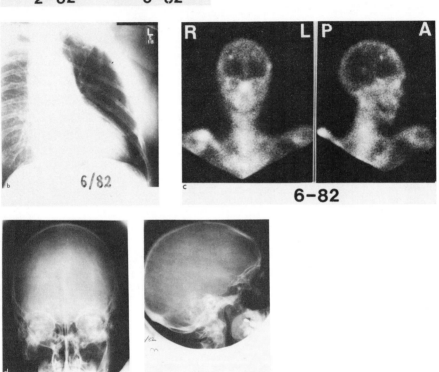

FIG. 3. A 61-year-old woman with an infiltrating ductal adenocarcinoma of the right breast was found to have disseminated metastatic lesions on 6-month follow-up studies. **A.** (left) Posterior image of the chest shows multiple lesions in the posterior ribs and scapula inferior tips. (right) Four months later. **B.** Healing fractures are seen on rib radiographs. Comparable bone scan shows an improvement of metastatic rib lesions. **C.** Lesions in the frontal skull are seen on camera image. **D.** Lesions in frontal skull are seen on radiographs.

monal or chemotherapy. The variable appearance of lesions on x-ray may cause major difficulty in interpretation of therapeutic response (Citrin et al. 1981).

In contrast to the radiograph that demonstrates the net result of bone destruction and repair, the bone scan is based on the dynamic response of bone to the disease process. Tumor destruction of bone results in local increase in bone blood flow and osteoblastic activity due to reactive new bone formation, as demonstrated on the scan. The greater the reactive process, the more intense is the abnormality seen on the bone scan (Charkes et al. 1968).

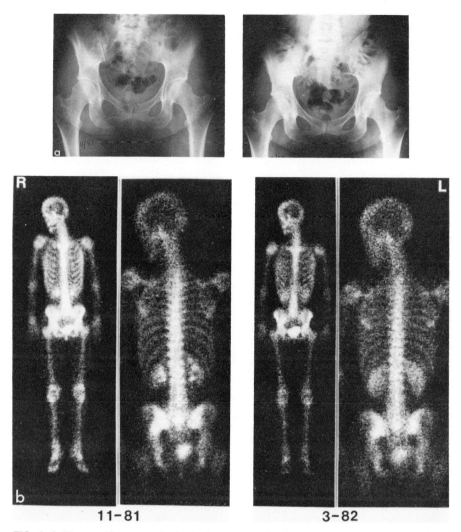

11-81   3-82

FIG. 4. A 65-year-old woman who had a lumpectomy for right breast carcinoma was found to have multiple bony metastases on 6-month follow-up. **A.** Pelvic frontal radiographs at the same time as the bone scans show an osteoblastic lesion in the right ilium, which is increased on follow-up study **B.** Whole-body bone scan 6 months later, after chemotherapy, reveals only lesions in the right ilium and sacrum. A follow-up 4 months later shows slight reduction of abnormally increased activity suggesting an improvement.

Bone scans should have a predominant role in the assessment of response to systemic therapy in patients with disseminated breast cancer. When bone metastases heal under the influence of treatment, avidity for radiopharmaceuticals ceases with normalization of the bone scan, and when metastases progress the response in new bone formation results in increased uptake of radioactivity. In the present study, bonc scans dctcctcd morc ncw lcsions and demonstrated earlier changes of healing or progression of disease than did x-rays. With radiographs, it was difficult to detect early lesions in trabecular bone, and there were no significant or only very delayed changes in healing osteoblastic or mixed lesions.

In conclusion, serial bone scans should be the primary modality to assess the response of bone metastasis to systemic therapy in breast cancer patients. Radiographs are complementary in evaluation of sclerotic response of osteolytic lesions.

ACKNOWLEDGMENT

We thank Mrs. Betty Hornung for reviewing and Mrs. Linda Watts and Mrs. Catherine Kenig for typing this manuscript.

REFERENCES

Bennett, A., J. S. Simpson, A. MacDonald, and I. F. Stamford. 1975. Breast cancer, prostaglandins, and bone metastases. Lancet 1:1218–1220.

Bitran, J. D., C. Berkerman, and R. K. Desser. 1980. The predictive value of serial bone scans assessing response to chemotherapy in advanced breast cancer. Cancer 45:1562–1568.

Charkes, N. D., I. Young, and D. M. Sklaroff. 1968. The pathologic basis of the strontium bone scan. JAMA 206:2482–2485.

Citrin, D. L., R. G. Bessent, and W. R. Greig. 1977. A comparison of sensitivity and accuracy of the ^{99m}Tc phosphate bone scan and skeletal radiograph in the diagnosis of bone metastases. Clin. Radiol. 28:107–111.

Citrin, D. L., C. Hougen, W. Zweibel, S. Schlise, B. Pruitt, W. Ershler, T. E. Davis, J. Harberg, and A. I. Cohen. 1981. The use of serial bone scans in assessing response to bone metastases to systemic treatment. Cancer 47:680–685.

Edelystyn, G. A., P. J. Gillespie, and E. S. Grebbell. 1967. The radiological demonstration of osseous metastases: experimental observations. Clin. Radiol. 18:158–164.

Galasko, C. S. B. 1976. Mechanisms of bone destruction in the development of skeletal metastases. Nature 263:507–510.

Libshitz, H. I., and G. N. Hortobagyi. 1981. Radiographic evaluation of therapeutic response in bony metastases of breast cancer. Skeletal Radiol. 7:159–165.

McNeil, B. J., P. D. Pace, and E. B. Gray. 1978. Preoperative and follow-up bone scans in patients with primary carcinoma of the breast. Surg. Gynecol. Obstet. 147:745–750.

O'Mara, R. E. 1976. Skeletal scanning in neoplastic disease. Cancer 37:480–484.

Osmond, J. D., H. P. Pendergrass, and M. S. Potsaid. 1975. Accuracy of ^{99m}Tc-diphosphonate bone scans and roentgenograms in the detection of prostate, breast, and lung carcinoma metastases. AJR 125:972–977.

Current Controversies in Breast Cancer, edited
by F. C. Ames, G. R. Blumenschein, and E. D. Montague.
University of Texas Press, Austin © 1984.

Membrane External Proteins and the Metastatic Ability of Breast Cancer

G. V. Sherbet, D.Sc., M. R. C. Path.,
and M. S. Lakshmi, M.Sc., Ph.D.

*Cancer Research Unit, University of Newcastle upon Tyne,
Royal Victoria Infirmary, Newcastle upon Tyne, England*

The development of tumors, their dissemination, and the formation of distant metastatic deposits can be described as a series of events beginning with the inception of the primary tumor. This is followed by an avascular phase of growth. For successful establishment, the primary tumor requires vascularization, which tumors are known to induce. When blood vessels of adequate diameter are formed in association with the tumor, it may invade and release individual cells or clumps of cells into the vascular and lymphatic systems. A majority of these circulating tumor cells are destroyed. The surviving cells may be distributed to distant organs. The tumor cells extravasate into the parenchyma of the organ in which they may eventually form metastatic deposits.

The cell membrane plays important and varied roles in the processes of tumor dissemination, as in tumor cell detachment, entry into and exit from the vascular and lymphatic systems, and evasion of immune surveillance, and in the interaction of the tumor cell with tissues of the target organ. Furthermore, glycoprotein/protein components of the cell membrane may be intricately involved in the various processes. It is possible, therefore, that membrane external components may provide useful markers for the metastatic potential of tumors (Sherbet 1982, Nicolson 1982).

The metastatic ability of carcinomas of the breast has been the subject of our investigations over the past several years. This intractable topic has led to the development of several techniques for studying the malignant properties of the carcinomas. We describe here the expression of two groups of membrane external proteins in a series of nonmalignant and malignant tumors of the breast. The expression of these appears to be related to the degree of malignancy of the tumors, as determined by the epigenetic grading test which is a new bioassay developed in the course of this investigation, tumor histology, and the metastatic outcome of the disease.

MATERIALS AND METHODS

Breast Tumors Investigated

Fibrocystic hyperplasias, fibroadenomas, and carcinomas of the breast were investigated in this study. The specimens were supplied by the Royal Victoria Infirmary, Newcastle General Hospital, and University College School of Medicine.

Tumor Cell Cultures

Tumor specimens were collected within 30 minutes after excision from patients and used to initiate cell cultures as described previously (Sherbet and Lakshmi 1974a; Wildridge and Sherbet 1981). The tumor tissue was dissected free of fat and capsular and necrotic material. The remaining tumor tissue was washed in saline, finely chopped with scissors and No. 22 (Swann-Morton) flat scalpel blades, and placed in 25-cm^2 culture flasks (Nunc-Flow Labs.) with 10 ml of growth medium. The growth medium consisted of Eagle's minimum essential medium containing 20 mM of Hepes buffer and supplemented with 10% (v/v) foetal bovine serum, 10% (v/v) heat-inactivated horse serum, 0.03% (w/v) NaHCO$_3$, 0.36 mM glutamine, and antibiotics (0.025% (w/v) streptomycin sulphate, 500 units/ml penicillin G, and 60 units/ml Mycostatin). The flasks were equilibrated with 5% CO$_2$ in air. The explants of tumor tissue were allowed to settle and adhere to the substratum at 37°C. Epithelial cells grew out radially from the explants. At this stage, the adherent pieces were detached by gentle shaking, and the epithelial cell cultures allowed to grow at 37°C. The cells were subcultured at confluence as follows: They were harvested with the aid of 0.25% (w/v) trypsin and 0.02% EDTA in phosphate buffered saline (PBS) without calcium and magnesium and were washed twice in growth medium. Then 10^6 viable cells suspended in 25-ml growth medium were inoculated into 75-cm^2 culture flasks and incubated at 37°C.

Cell cultures at early passages were used in the investigation. In all cultures, epithelial cells predominated, the cells being identifiable by their morphology and tendency to form coherent sheets (Figure 1). The use of early passages ensured that only small numbers of fibroblasts or their precursors were present among the epithelial cells.

Radioiodination of Monolayer Cultures

Subconfluent monolayer cell cultures were used for the radioiodination of surface proteins. The cell monolayer was incubated in PBS pH 7.2 for 30 minutes at 37°C. This was followed by a final rinse in PBS to wash off adherent serum proteins. This procedure would be expected to remove the majority of adherent serum proteins, but it is possible that some strongly adherent proteins may have remained absorbed to the cell surface. On the other hand, certain weakly bound peripheral proteins may have been removed, although this would seem unlikely.

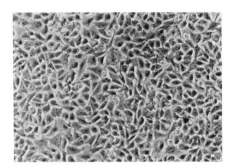

FIG. 1. Morphology of a carcinoma in tissue culture (x 40). (Reproduced from Wildridge and Sherbet 1981, with permission of The Macmillan Press Ltd.)

The cell surface proteins were then labeled by lactoperoxidase catalysed radio-iodination (Hynes 1973). To each culture flask, 2 ml of PBS containing 5 mM of glucose were added. Carrier-free [^{125}I] NaI (Radiochemical Centre, Amersham), glucose oxidase (Boehringer), and lactoperoxidase (Calbiochem) were used at 1 mCi, 2.5 μg, and 1 IU respectively per flask. The constituents were mixed gently, and the flasks were left at room temperature for 10 minutes, with occasional gentle shaking. The reaction was terminated by the addition of 5 ml of phosphate buffered iodine (PBI) containing 0.137 M NaI and 2 mM phenylmethyl sulphonyl fluoride (PMSF) (proteinase inhibitor). The iodinated monolayer was washed three times in PBI-PMSF solution. The cells were scraped off using a polypropylene 'policeman' and solubilised in 0.3 ml of 0.01 M sodium phosphate buffer, pH 7.0, containing 1% (w/v) sodium dodecyl sulphate (SDS), 1% (w/v) mercaptoethanol, and 2 mM PMSF, by incubation for 10 minutes in a boiling water bath. To each extract was added 0.1 gm of sucrose. The extracts were stored at -20°C.

Thirty-microliter aliquots of extracts of the labeled material were separated by electrophoresis in 6.0% (w/v) cylindrical polyacrylamide gels (4 mm x 8 cm), containing 200 mM sodium phosphate buffer, pH 7.2, 0.2% (w/v) SDS, and 0.5% bromophenol blue (Guy et al. 1977). Six replicate gels were run of each labeled extract. After electrophoresis, 1-mm thick slices of the gels were prepared. The radioactive content of each slice was counted in a Nuclear Enterprises 1600 gamma counter and expressed as a percentage of total activity recovered. Standard molecular weight markers (B.D.H.) in the range of 56,000–280,000 daltons were used in electrophoretic analysis and for the estimation of the molecular weights of the labeled proteins.

Epigenetic Grading

The epigenetic grading tests were performed by cultivating in vitro 16- to 18-hour-old chick embryo blastoderms, as described by New (1955). Pieces of the tumor tissue to be investigated were implanted between the ectodermal and endodermal layers of the blastoderm (approximately 25 per tumor sample) according to the technique of Waddington (1932). The embryos containing the implanted test tissues were incubated for 24 hours. At the end of this incubation period, the embryos were examined morphologically and fixed, embedded in wax, serially sectioned, and stained for assessing the induction of embryonic cell responses by the test cells.

The responses were scored as described previously (Sherbet and Lakshmi 1974b). The histogenetic responses from the ectoderm and the endoderm were scored for the frequency of occurrence as well as the intensity of the responses.

In order to eliminate any subconscious bias, epigenetic grading was done before the histologic data on the tumors were collated.

Histology

The histology reports for the tumors were obtained from the Departments of Pathology of the above-mentioned hospitals.

Follow-Up of Patients

The follow-up reports of the patients were also made available by the hospitals. The patients had been followed up at 6-month intervals.

RESULTS AND DISCUSSION

Several differences were noticed in the pattern of membrane external proteins of cells derived from fibrocystic hyperplasias and fibroadenomas. Typical electrophoretic patterns are given in Figure 2. The most remarkable difference related to the occurrence of two groups of proteins of average molecular weights of 265×10^3 and 233×10^3. The protein with a molecular weight of 265×10^3 occurred in both cystic hyperplasias examined and in four-fifths of the fibroadenomas. The 233×10^3 component occurred as a well-defined peak in three-fifths of the carcinomas (Table 1), but there was no statistically significant quantitative difference between these proteins found in fibroadenomas and carcinomas. However, the ratio of $265 \times 10^3/233 \times 10^3$ was higher in the fibroadenoma group than in the carcinoma group (Table 2). In other words, the 265×10^3 peak was less in the carcinomas than in the fibroadenomas.

In histologically proven carcinomas, the $265 \times 10^3/233 \times 10^3$ ratio showed much variation (Wildridge and Sherbet 1981). Therefore we considered the possibility that this variation may be related to the degree of malignancy, i.e. the ability of tumors to disseminate and form metastatic deposits. The primary tumors were tested by the epigenetic grading test. This bioassay, which is dependent upon the proliferative and differentiative responses induced by tumor tissues from early chick embryos, has shown that the more malignant a tumor the greater is the intensity of induction of differentiative responses (Sherbet and Lakshmi, 1974c, 1978, 1980). Previous investigations had shown that the epigenetic scale of malignancy is divisible into three sections, comprising, in Group I (low-grade tumors), nonmetastatic

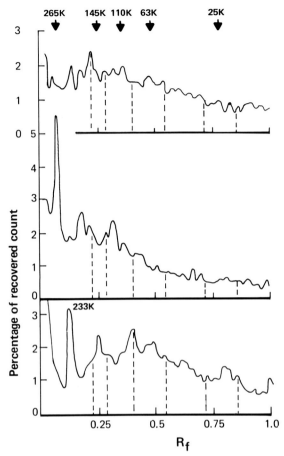

FIG. 2. Electrophoretic patterns of radioiodinated membrane external proteins of a cystic hyperplasia (top), fibroadenoma (middle), and a carcinoma (bottom) (R_f = electrophoretic mobility of protein relative to marker dye). (Reproduced from Wildridge and Sherbet 1981, with permission of The Macmillan Press Ltd.)

tumors such as some well-differentiated Morris hepatomas, fibrocystic hyperplasias, and reactive gliosis tissue. Group II formed a narrow zone composed of benign tumors and tumors of low malignancy. In Group III could be found metastatic hamster lymphosarcomas, human astrocytomas of Kernohan Grade III-IV, and a majority of carcinomas of the breast (Figure 3). A recent investigation has revealed that the incidence of metastases was significantly higher in Group III than in Groups I and II (Sherbet 1982; Lakshmi and Sherbet 1982). There was no dramatic time difference in the appearance of secondary tumors. Therefore, this apparent correlation between the incidence of metastases and their epigenetic grade cannot be attributed to the growth characteristics of the primary tumor but probably is due to the dissemination achieved by the primary tumor. It would appear, therefore, that the location of a given tumor on the epigenetic scale reflects its malignancy reasonably accurately.

In the present series of tumors investigated, the epigenetic grading was restricted

Table 1. *Cell Surface Proteins of Breast Tumors*[*]

Tumor Identification	Tumor Type	Major Components (approximate molecular weight)			
		265×10^3	233×10^3	145×10^3	63×10^3
EBA	fibrocystic	+[†]		+	+
VHG	hyperplasia	+		+	
MAT	fibroadenoma	?		+	
AFH		+		+	+
JFE		+		+	
MEA		+		+	
WRA		+		?	
MCP	carcinoma		?	+	+
HOR			+	+	+
AME			+	+	+
BAS			?	+	+
MCF			+	?	?

[*] Adapted from Wildridge and Sherbet 1981.
[†] The + sign indicates the presence of a well-defined peak of incorporation of radioiodine.

Table 2. *Distribution of Radioactivity Associated with Cell Surface Components of Fibroadenomas and Carcinomas of the Breast*[*]

Tumor Identification	Type	Mean Total Counts Recovered Per Gel $\times 10^{-3}$	$265^{†} \times 10^3$	233×10^3	$\dfrac{265 \times 10^3}{233 \times 10^3}$
			% Radioactivity		
MAT		26.3	5.6 ± 0.9	2.80 ± 0.8	2.0
MEA		27.5	10.07 ± 0.5	1.74 ± 0.8	5.79
JFE	fibroadenoma	47.5	11.92 ± 1.8	2.38 ± 0.9	5.01
WRA		34.9	6.77 ± 1.4	2.22 ± 0.9	3.05
AFH		17.0	11.97 ± 1.5	2.27 ± 0.9	5.27
MCP		52.6	3.83 ± 0.7	1.50 ± 0.5	2.55
AME		121.3	4.47 ± 0.3	3.27 ± 0.7	1.37
BAS	carcinoma	23.5	3.72 ± 0.2	1.29 ± 0.2	2.88
HOR		84.1	9.27 ± 2.8	5.79 ± 2.0	1.60
MCF		28.3	4.07 ± 0.5	2.44 ± 0.2	1.67
Probability values in the Mann-Whitney test			0.016	N.S.	0.016

[*] Adapted from Wildridge and Sherbet 1981.
[†] Approximate molecular weight.

to a determination of the histogenetic differentiative responses alone. It may be seen from Table 3 that there is an inverse relationship between the ratio of occurrence of $265 \times 10^3/233 \times 10^3$ proteins and the histogenetic score that the tumor tissue produced in epigenetic grading tests (Lakshmi et al. 1982). This correlation was statistically significant ($r = -0.775$, $P < 0.025$). The results of these tests may therefore be interpreted as indicating that lower $265 \times 10^3/233 \times 10^3$ ratios may be associated with a higher intrinsic malignancy of the carcinomas.

THE DISTRIBUTION OF SOME NEOPLASMS ON THE EPIGENETIC SCALE

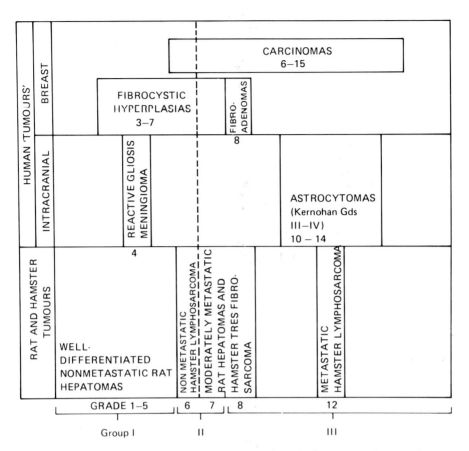

FIG. 3. The distribution of neoplasms on the epigenetic scale. Based on various publications from the authors' laboratory. (Reproduced from Sherbet 1982, with permission of Academic Press.)

The natural extension of this work was to follow up the patients and record the course of the disease and the incidence of metastases, if any. Preliminary indications are that high $265 \times 10^3/233 \times 10^3$ ratios may be associated with longer disease-free intervals than low $265 \times 10^3/233 \times 10^3$ ratios. Admittedly, the present investigation concerns only a small number of breast tumors. Nonetheless, it may be noted that for fibroadenomas the $265 \times 10^3/233 \times 10^3$ ratio is between 3 and 6. The ratio for the carcinomas varied from 1.3 to 3.0. There is an overlap in the middle in which there are two cases: a recurrent fibroadenoma and a carcinoma that metastasized to the liver after 3 years. With these exceptions in mind, we would suggest that the lower the $265 \times 10^3/233 \times 10^3$ ratio, the greater seems to be the metastatic ability of the

Table 3. *Relationship Between the Relative Expression of Surface Proteins 265 × 10³/233 × 10³ and Histogenetic Scores of Some Human Breast Tumors**

Patient	% ^{125}I Incorporation[†] 265 × 10³/233[‡] × 10³	Histogenetic Score
BAI	4.29	0
MCP	2.55	3
VG	2.30	5
MAT	2.0	5
MCF	1.67	6
BAS	2.88	8
AME	1.37	9
HOR	1.6	10

*Adapted from Sherbet 1982.

[†]Cell surface proteins were labeled with ^{125}I using lactoperoxidase-mediated radioiodination method. The proteins were then separated by polyacrylamide gel electrophoresis. The values given in column 2 represent ratios of percentage of recovered count in proteins of molecular weights of 265 × 10³ and 233 × 10³. The correlation between histogenetic grading and the ratio of incorporation of ^{125}I into 265 × 10³ and 233 × 10³ components was significant ($r = -0.775$, $P < 0.025$).

[‡]Approximate molecular weights.

carcinoma. It is needless to emphasize that this remains to be established in a large number of cases, but indications to date are that the degree of expression of the two groups of proteins is related to tumor histology, the degree of malignancy as determined in bioassay, and the metastatic outcome of the disease.

ACKNOWLEDGMENTS

We thank Professor I. D. A. Johnston, Mr. R. G. Wilson, and Dr. P. A. Riley for supplying tumor specimens for investigation, and the staff of the Pathology Departments of Newcastle General Hospital, Royal Victoria Infirmary, Newcastle upon Tyne, and University College School of Medicine, London, for providing histology reports. This work was supported by the North of England Council of the Cancer Research Campaign.

REFERENCES

Guy, D., A. L. Latner, and G. A. Turner. 1977. Radioiodination studies of tumour cell surface proteins after different disaggregation procedures. Br. J. Cancer 36:166–172.

Hynes, R. O. 1973. Alteration of cell surface proteins by viral transformation and by proteolysis. Proc. Natl. Acad. Sci. USA 70:3170–3174.

Lakshmi, M. S., A. L. Latner, and G. V. Sherbet. 1982. The role of cell surface proteins in the induction of histogenetic differentiative responses by some human breast tumours and hamster tumours implanted into chick embryos. Exp. Cell Biol. 50: 169–179.

Lakshmi, M. S., and G. V. Sherbet. 1982. The value of epigenetic grading in the determination of the metastatic potential of carcinomas of the breast. Anticancer Res. 3: 181–184.

New, D. A. T. 1955. A new technique for the cultivation of chick embryos *in vitro*. J. Embryol. Exp. Morphol. 3: 326–331.

Nicolson, G. L. 1982. Cell surface properties of metastatic tumour cells, *in* Tumour Invasion and Metastasis, L. A. Liotta and I. R. Hart, eds. Martinus Nijhoff, The Hague, pp. 57–79.

Sherbet, G. V. 1982. The Biology of Tumour Malignancy. Academic Press, London, pp. 100– 124.

Sherbet, G. V., and M. S. Lakshmi. 1974a. The surface properties of some human intracranial tumours in relation to their malignancy. Oncology 29: 335–347.

Sherbet, G. V., and M. S. Lakshmi. 1974b. Tumor grading by implantation in chick embryo. I. Grading of minimum-deviation hepatomas. JNCI 52: 681–685.

Sherbet, G. V., and M. S. Lakshmi. 1974c. Tumor grading by implantation in chick embryo. II. Grading of some human astrocytomas. JNCI 52: 687–692.

Sherbet, G. V., and M. S. Lakshmi. 1978. Malignancy and prognosis evaluated by an embryonic system. Grading of breast tumours. Eur. J. Cancer 14: 415–420.

Sherbet, G. V., and M. S. Lakshmi. 1980. A possibility of predicting metastatic ability of tumours by implantation in chick embryos, *in* Metastasis: Clinical and Experimental Aspects, K. Hellman, P. Hilgard, and S. Eccles, eds. Martinus Nijhoff, The Hague, pp. 38–44.

Waddington, C. H. 1932. Experiments on the development of chick and duck embryos in vitro. Proc. R. Soc. Lond. [Biol] 221: 179–230.

Wildridge, M., and G. V. Sherbet. 1981. Possible surface protein markers for breast cancer. Br. J. Cancer 43: 118–121.

Current Controversies in Breast Cancer, edited
by F. C. Ames, G. R. Blumenschein, and E. D. Montague.
University of Texas Press, Austin © 1984.

Role of Carcinoembryonic Antigen for Follow-Up of Breast Cancer Patients

Gabriel N. Hortobagyi, M.D.,* Herbert A. Fritsche, Jr., Ph.D.,†
Abdul W. Mughal, M.B., B.S.,* Aman U. Buzdar, M.B., B.S.,*
Hwee-Yong Yap, M.D.,* and George R. Blumenschein, M.D.*

*From the Departments of *Internal Medicine and †Laboratory Medicine, The University of
Texas M. D. Anderson Hospital and Tumor Institute at Houston, Houston, Texas*

It is a well-known fact that elevated carcinoembryonic antigen (CEA) levels in plasma and other biological fluids occur in patients with various solid tumors (Martin et al. 1976). Depending on the distribution of organ sites involved by metastasis, elevated CEA concentrations are present in 30% to 80% of patients with metastatic breast cancer (Tormey et al. 1977). We have analyzed our data from serial measurements of plasma CEA concentrations in patients with metastatic breast cancer who are undergoing treatment with combination chemotherapy programs. Our main goal was to assess the value of fluctuations in CEA levels as they are related to changes in clinical status; i.e., we attempted to determine whether changes in CEA levels can be used as an additional modality to evaluate the effectiveness of systemic therapy.

MATERIALS AND METHODS

The charts of 298 patients with metastatic breast cancer treated with combination chemotherapy were reviewed. None of these patients had received prior systemic treatment. The combination used for this trial was 5-fluorouracil, doxorubicin, and cyclophosphamide (FAC) followed by 5-fluorouracil, methotrexate, and cyclophosphamide (CMF) maintenance therapy after doxorubicin was discontinued (Legha et al. 1982, Hortobagyi et al. 1982). Patients with estrogen receptor (ER) positive or ER unknown tumors were also treated with tamoxifen starting 6 to 8 weeks before the initiation of combination chemotherapy. Patients who failed to respond to this combination or in whom progressive disease developed after an initial response were removed from the study. All patients had clearly measurable disease.

The initial workup included a patient history, physical examination, hematologic survey, SMA-12, chest x-ray, liver scan, bone scan, and radiographic bone survey as well as other imaging techniques appropriate for special areas of metastasis. Clinical response to therapy was evaluated according to the criteria published by the

International Union Against Cancer (Hayward et al. 1977). One hundred sixty-seven of the 298 patients had a baseline and at least one follow-up CEA-level determination, and only these patients were entered in the trial. In most patients, plasma CEA levels were measured at 4- to 8-week intervals by means of a direct competitive protein-binding assay (Fritsche et al. 1980). The normal values for this assay were less than 6 ng/ml for nonsmokers and less than 10 ng/ml for smokers. The coefficient of variation was 12% at the lower ranges where sample dilution is not necessary. The chi-square test was used to compare the variables in different patient subgroups. The Kaplan and Meier (Kaplan and Meier 1958) method was used to calculate and plot curves for duration of response and survival, and differences between curves were assessed by a two-tailed Wilcoxon test (Gehan 1965).

RESULTS

The pretreatment CEA titer was normal in 83 patients and abnormal in 84 (50%). We did not find serial measurement of CEA values useful in patients in whom the pretreatment CEA was within normal limits. Only five of 35 (14%) patients in this group who showed evidence of progressive metastatic disease had a subsequent elevation of CEA level that correlated with progression; therefore, the sensitivity of CEA monitoring in this group of patients is very low.

In the 84 patients with elevated pretreatment CEA levels, the median concentration was 26 ng/ml (range 6.7 to 1,447 ng/ml). Seventy (83%) patients achieved an objective remission during chemotherapy. In 66 of the 70 (94%) patients who responded to therapy, a concomitant decrease in CEA level was noted. Of 11 patients in whom metastatic disease remained stable during therapy, the plasma CEA level decreased in eight and increased in three. In three patients in whom disease continued to progress after the initiation of chemotherapy, the CEA levels increased. Analysis of various pretreatment clinical factors and CEA levels revealed a correlation between higher CEA levels and increasing tumor burden according to the number of organ sites involved. The CEA concentration was highest in patients with bone, bone marrow, or liver metastases and lowest in patients with soft tissue lesions.

Plasma CEA levels returned to normal in 48 of 70 (68%) patients who responded but in 18 patients decreased and never returned to normal. The duration of remission was significantly longer in the first group (20 months) than in the second group (8 months) ($P = 0.002$) (Figure 1). A similar advantage in length of tumor control was observed in the few patients with clinically stable disease whose CEA levels returned to normal.

Progressive disease occurred in 37 of the 70 patients in whom an objective remission was achieved. Thirty-one patients had elevated plasma CEA levels at the time of progression, and 27 (87%) of these showed elevation in relation to the remission levels. In three of the four patients with no evidence of elevated CEA level at the time of progression, recurrent disease was confined to the brain. In all seven patients in whom initially only stability of disease was achieved with chemotherapy

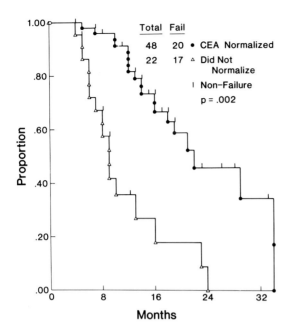

FIG. 1. Duration of remission in patients with complete and partial normalization of carcinoembryonic antigen (CEA) levels.

and in whom progressive disease subsequently developed, CEA levels increased. Plasma CEA levels increased before progression became clinically evident in 67% of the patients. The increased levels of the marker occurred from 1 to 13 months prior to clinical detection (median time, 3 months).

The plasma CEA levels increased in 13 patients during the initial 4 to 8 weeks of chemotherapy and then progressively decreased in nine of these patients. All nine patients achieved an objective clinical remission, while, in the other four, increasing CEA levels soon correlated with clinical progression.

We attempted to quantify the minimum change in CEA concentration necessary to obtain correlation with changes in clinical course and found the highest correlation when two consecutive decreases or increases in CEA concentration were greater than 12% of the initial value (coefficient of variation). When these criteria were strictly adhered to, changes in CEA level correlated with clinical changes in all but one patient.

DISCUSSION

The experience described in this paper shows that CEA levels become elevated in a substantial number of patients with metastatic breast cancer. The likelihood of increasing CEA levels is higher in patients with liver, bone, or bone marrow metastatic disease than in patients with soft tissue metastatic disease only. Since response to thcrapy is often more difficult to assess in patients with liver or bone metastases, the discovery of abnormal CEA levels in this subgroup of patients is especially useful.

Our results also have shown that serial changes in CEA levels during chemotherapy in patients with metastatic breast cancer correlate with clinical response or progression of disease in the majority, especially when two or more sequential CEA-level determinations are made. In many patients, gradual, sustained increases in CEA levels precede by weeks or months clinically detectable evidence of progression. This lead time may allow early confirmation of progressive disease, discontinuation of therapy that is no longer useful, and institution of more effective modalities of treatment. Our data confirm those reported by Lokich (1978) and Tormey et al. (1977).

Additional information was derived from our investigation. We found the prognostic value of the degree of CEA normalization to be clearly demonstrated. In patients whose CEA levels returned to normal during systemic therapy, the period of disease control was extended, reflecting a more complete biologic response to treatment than in patients in whom only partial normalization of CEA levels was observed. The early, transient rise in CEA concentration in nine patients who subsequently responded to therapy suggests that during the initial part of systemic treatment frequent CEA determinations may uncover early evidence of progressive disease. Such a finding should be confirmed by the appropriate clinical tests or examination.

Based on our observations and those of other investigators, we recommend that a baseline CEA level be obtained in all patients with metastatic breast cancer. When the initial CEA level is found to be elevated, changes in clinical status can be effectively monitored by sequential measurements every 4 to 8 weeks. Furthermore, it might be useful to measure CEA concentrations at frequent intervals during the first 4 to 8 weeks. At this time, we are of the opinion that CEA level is the single most useful biologic marker for monitoring changes in disease pattern in patients with metastatic breast cancer.

ACKNOWLEDGMENTS

This investigation was supported in part by Grant Number 5T32 CA 9163-05 awarded by the National Cancer Institute, U.S. Department of Health and Human Services.

REFERENCES

Fritsche, H. A., C. K. Tashima, W. L. Collingsworth, A. Geitner, and J. Van Oort. 1980. A direct competitive binding radioimmunoassay for CEA. J. Immunol. Methods 35:115–128.

Gehan, E. A. 1965. A generalized Wilcoxon test for comparing arbitrarily single-censored samples. Biometrika 52:204–223.

Hayward, J. L., P. Carbone, A. C. Heuson, S. Kumoka, A. Segaloff, and R. D. Reubens. 1977. Assessment of response to therapy in advanced breast cancer. Cancer 39:1289–1294.

Hortobagyi, G., G. Blumenschein, D. Frye, A. Buzdar, H-Y. Yap, F. Schell, and B. Barnes. 1982. A prospective randomized study of hormone-chemotherapy with or without Pseudomonas vaccine in metastatic breast cancer. (Abstract) Proc. Am. Soc. Clin. Oncol. 1:81.

Kaplan, E. L., and P. Meier. 1958. Nonparametric estimation from incomplete observation. J. Am. Statist. Soc. 53:457–481.

Legha, S., G. Blumenschein, G. Hortobagyi, A. Buzdar, H. Yap, and G. Bodey. 1982. Treatment of metastatic breast carcinoma using a combination of 5-fluorouracil, Adriamycin, cyclophosphamide, and tamoxifen. (Abstract) Proc. Soc. Clin. Oncol. 1:78.

Lokich, J. J., N. Zamcheck, and M. Lowenstein. 1978. Sequential carcinoembryonic antigen levels in the therapy of metastatic breast cancer. A predictor and monitor of response and relapse. Ann. Intern. Med. 89:902–906.

Martin, E. W., Jr., W. E. Kibby, L. DiVecchia, G. Anderson, P. Catalano, and J. P. Minton. 1976. Carcinoembryonic antigen, clinical and historical aspects. Cancer 37:62–81.

Tormey, D. C., T. P. Waalkes, J. J. Snyder, and R. M. Simon. 1977. Biological markers in breast carcinoma. III. Clinical correlations with carcinoembryonic antigen. Cancer 39:2397–2404.

SYSTEMIC THERAPEUTIC TRIALS FOR STAGES II AND IV BREAST CANCER

Current Controversies in Breast Cancer, edited
by F. C. Ames, G. R. Blumenschein, and E. D. Montague.
University of Texas Press, Austin © 1984.

Statistical Considerations for Historical Controlled Adjuvant Studies With Application to FAC-BCG Study in Breast Cancer

Edmund A. Gehan, Ph.D.,* Terry L. Smith, B.S.,*
and Aman U. Buzdar, M.D.†

*Departments of *Biomathematics and †Internal Medicine, The University of Texas
M. D. Anderson Hospital and Tumor Institute at Houston, Houston, Texas*

At this conference, reports have been given on both randomized and nonrandomized studies of adjuvant chemotherapy or hormonal treatment for patients with stage II or stage III breast cancer. Bonadonna et al. (1983, see pages 631 to 647, this volume) and Fisher et al. (1983, see pages 159 to 169, this volume) have given reports of randomized studies, and Buzdar et al. (1983, see pages 171 to 184, this volume) have reported on a nonrandomized study of 5-fluorouracil, Adriamycin, cyclophosphamide, and bacillus Calmette Guerin (FAC-BCG) as adjuvant treatment.

Our objective is to discuss general principles relating to the design of adjuvant studies in breast cancer, using as an example the nonrandomized FAC-BCG adjuvant study by Buzdar et al. (1978). We do not advocate a particular viewpoint in the controversy regarding randomized versus nonrandomized studies, but we have provided some discussion of considerations that affect whether a particular adjuvant study should be randomized or not.

ISSUES IN PLANNING ADJUVANT STUDIES

Table 1 lists the major medical and statistical issues one should consider in planning a study of adjuvant treatment for breast cancer. Moon (1979) has previously discussed comparability of treatments and size of study for adjuvant breast cancer studies.

From a medical viewpoint, clearly one must choose the treatments to be compared, the types of patients to be studied, and the major endpoints for evaluation (usually relapse-free survival or overall survival, or both). From a statistical viewpoint, one should specify the difference in endpoints to be detected, the desired statistical significance level, and the desired power of the test of the difference between treatments. Having specified these characteristics, one can then determine the number of patients to be studied on each treatment if the study is randomized

Table 1. *General Considerations for Adjuvant Studies in Breast Cancer*

Issues in Planning
> Medical: choice of treatments, types of patients, end points for evaluation
> Statistical: difference in end points to be detected, significance level, power of test
> Medical Statistical: knowledge of prognostic factors, one- versus two-sided test, randomized or historical control groups

Special Features
> Treatment comparison: $T_1 + T_2$ versus T_1*
> Patient is well at start. End point: disease-free survival, overall survival
> Subgroups of patients: identify subgroups that may benefit from adjuvant treatment

---

*T_1 = standard, T_2 = adjuvant treatment.

(Gehan and Schneiderman 1982), or if it is not (Makuch and Simon 1979). To utilize the tables of sample size in either of these articles, one can test for differences in the proportions of patients either relapse-free or surviving for a given time after the start of study, say 2 years. Alternatively, sample size can be determined for comparing characteristics of the survival curves (George and Desu 1974).

A combined medical-statistical issue (Table 1) is knowledge of prognostic factors. If patient characteristics that influence disease-free survival are known, e.g., number of positive nodes, stage of cancer, and size of tumor, then one might use a statistical model that includes these features to adjust the comparison of treatments for possible differences in the distribution of patients who have these prognostic features.

The decision to use one- or two-sided statistical tests is of substantial importance, since differences between treatments that are statistically significant at $P = .10$ in the two-sided test would be statistically significant at $P = .05$ in the one-sided test. Significance levels for one-sided tests are precisely half those for two-sided tests that demonstrate the same amount of difference between treatments. Ordinarily, the one-sided test is relevant for adjuvant studies, since, as indicated in the lower portion of Table 1, the explicit objective is to determine whether the adjuvant treatment (T_2) when added to the standard treatment (T_1) is as or more effective than T_1 alone. Failure to demonstrate an advantage of $T_1 + T_2$ over T_1 would mean that T_1 was the preferred treatment; it is not necessary to demonstrate $T_1 + T_2$ is significantly inferior to T_1. Thus, the hypothesis to be tested in an adjuvant study is inherently one-sided.

A special feature of an adjuvant study is that the patient is presumed to be well at the start of the study and the objective is to maintain the patient in that state, while in the usual cancer clinical trial the patient is presumed to be ill and the objective is to cause a reduction in size or disappearance of a tumor.

A further feature of adjuvant trials might be termed the "subgroups of patients' problems," which has been discussed by Higgins (1978). It may be that the adjuvant treatment is beneficial, but only for a certain subgroup of patients (e.g., those patients who have some residual tumor) that may constitute only a small portion of the patients entered in the trial. The therapeutic benefit of the adjuvant treatment may

Table 2. *Reasons to Consider Randomized Control Group for Breast Cancer Adjuvant Studies*

1. Unbiased allocation of patients to treatments.
2. Comparable patients on each treatment (on the average).
3. Unbiased estimation of treatment effects.
4. Endpoints may take a long time to observe.
5. Inferences can be based on randomized models.
6. Randomized studies are "more convincing."

not be evident unless sufficient patients from the subgroup who can potentially benefit from the adjuvant treatment have been included.

Reasons for a Randomized Control Group

Table 2 lists the reasons for considering using a randomized control group in breast cancer adjuvant studies. If the assignment of treatment is properly randomized, there is no possibility of such investigator bias as allocating patients with more favorable prognoses to a particular treatment. On the average, patients in each treatment group are thus comparable with respect to major prognostic features, especially if they have also been stratified according to known prognostic features prior to randomization. For example, patients might be stratified by stage of disease and menopausal status, then randomized to treatments within each stratification category.

If the endpoints in an adjuvant study will take a very long time to observe, say 5 years or more, then in a nonrandomized study it would be less likely that one could use a control group consisting of patients treated in the past, since an assumption must be made that there have been no changes in the criteria for diagnosis, use of supportive therapy, determination of relapse, and other aspects (except treatment) that may affect outcome.

Finally, some have argued that randomized studies are more convincing than non-randomized studies. This argument may be based largely upon the research philosophy of clinical investigators, since it is our belief that confirmatory studies, whether randomized or nonrandomized, convince skeptics. Indeed, one could give examples of individual randomized and nonrandomized studies that were extremely controversial. The most important point is to conduct the study properly, regardless of whether it is randomized.

Reasons to Consider Historical Control Group

Table 3 gives the reasons for considering a historical control group in adjuvant studies of breast cancer (Gehan and Freireich 1981). Ultimately, all real knowledge must be based on historical evidence, even that resulting from randomized studies. All studies, when completed, become part of a historical data base. If a large series of historical control patients are available at a particular institution, then its use in a

Table 3. *Reasons to Consider Historical Control Group for Breast Cancer Adjuvant Studies*

1. All knowledge is based on historical evidence; series of historical control patients are available.
2. Number of patients needed is approximately four times larger for randomized study than for nonrandomized study with equivalent statistical significance level and power.
3. Prognostic factors are known for stage II, III patients: number of positive nodes, stage, menopausal status, size of tumor.
4. Adjuvant studies generally test whether treatment is beneficial or not, creating ethical problem for randomized study.
5. Adjuvant treatment would be expected to have moderate to large effect on disease-free survival and survival.

clinical trial should seriously be considered. If this group is not to be used for a formal clinical trial, it still provides a basis for evaluating current clinical experience.

An important point favoring nonrandomized studies is that they require only one-fourth the number of patients required by randomized studies with equivalent statistical features, i.e., difference in response rates to be detected, statistical significance level, and power (Gehan and Freireich 1974). Consequently, it is possible to do a relatively small nonrandomized study and obtain results quickly. The crucial assumption required is that outcomes using the standard treatment are well known. Confirmatory studies can be conducted if interesting results are obtained.

To utilize properly a historical control series of patients, one must know the patient characteristics related to prognosis. For example, prognosis for patients with stage II or stage III breast cancer is related to number of positive nodes, menopausal status, and size of tumor. Knowledge of these prognostic features permits their use in statistical models and makes it possible to test for treatment differences after adjusting for differences in prognostic features.

Depending on the adjuvant treatment being studied, an ethical problem may confront those conducting a randomized study. In clinical cancer research there are continuing efforts to find better treatments. If preliminary studies suggest moderate to large expected benefit from the adjuvant treatment, then it would not be ethical to enter a new patient into a randomized study. The ethical basis for the randomized study depends on having equivalent evidence favoring each of the treatments. If the hypothesis being tested in the clinical trial is whether the adjuvant treatment is better than the standard treatment, then the one-sided nature of the hypothesis vitiates the ethical basis for the randomized study. The larger the expected positive benefit from the adjuvant treatment, the more difficult it becomes to ask for informed consent from a potential patient in a randomized study.

EXAMPLE OF HISTORICAL CONTROLLED
ADJUVANT STUDY IN BREAST CANCER PATIENTS

A study of adjuvant treatment with FAC-BCG was conducted in breast cancer patients at The University of Texas M.D. Anderson Hospital and Tumor Institute at Houston between 1972 and 1976, and reported by Buzdar et al. (1978). All patients had stage II or stage III breast cancer and had one or more histologically positive axillary lymph nodes. Patients in the historical control group were treated in 1972 and 1973, and all received definitive surgery; some also received x-ray therapy. Patients in the adjuvant treatment group received surgery plus FAC-BCG beginning in January 1974 and continuing to October 1976. Subsequently, a randomized study has been conducted comparing adjuvant treatment with FAC to FAC-BCG. The historical control group had 151 patients and the adjuvant treatment group had 131 patients. The major endpoints for evaluation were disease-free survival and overall survival, both measured from time of surgery.

Patients were not comparable between groups with respect to distribution of prognostic features. The control group was favored with respect to age and menopausal status, since there was a higher percentage of patients over age 50 (68% versus 52%) and perimenopausal or postmenopausal (75% versus 58%) in the control versus the adjuvant treatment groups. Patients in the FAC-BCG group were favored with respect to size of tumor, stage of disease, and type of surgery. There was a lower percentage of patients in the FAC-BCG group with primary tumors larger than 5 cm (15% versus 26%) and a lower percentage with stage III disease (25% versus 40%). A higher percentage received radical or modified radical mastectomies than did those in the control group (85% versus 55%). The distribution of the number of positive nodes was about the same in each group.

Since the groups of patients were not strictly comparable, Cox's regression model (Cox 1972) was utilized to test for differences between treatment groups, adjusting for prognostic features. Fitting the regression model to the disease-free survival data from the 151 control patients in a forward stepwise fashion resulted in the following regression model:

$$\ln \left\{ \frac{\lambda_i(t)}{\lambda_o(t)} \right\} = .110 \text{ (no. nodes} - 6.16) + .8122 \text{ (stage} - 2.39) \\ + .8720 \text{ (menopausal status} - .26)$$

where $\lambda_j(t)$ is the hazard function at time t (roughly the risk of relapse per unit time). When $j = i$ the hazard is for the ith patient with a given set of prognostic features, and when $j = 0$ the hazard is for a patient with average values of the prognostic features. The codes for the prognostic variables were: number of involved nodes $(2 = < 4, 7 = 4\text{-}10, 12 = > 10)$, stage of disease $(2 = II, 3 = III)$, and menopausal status $(1 = \text{premenopausal}, 0 = \text{other})$. Favorable values are small number of positive nodes, stage II disease, and postmenopausal status.

The model was then fitted to the combined data from FAC-BCG and control patients to test whether adjuvant FAC-BCG treatment influenced disease-free survival. Type of treatment $(O = \text{historical control}, 1 = \text{FAC-BCG})$ was included as a variable in the model in addition to number of involved nodes, stage of disease, and menopausal status. The equation obtained by fitting the model in forward stepwise fashion was:

$$\ln \left\{ \frac{\lambda_i(t)}{\lambda_o(t)} \right\} = 1.6982 \text{ (treatment} - .47) + .0965 \text{ (no nodes} - 8.34) \\ + .8616 \text{ (menopausal status} - .33) + .6563 \text{ (stage} - 2.33).$$

All four variables entered the regression model at a statistically significant level: type of treatment ($P < .01$), number of involved nodes ($P = .01$), menopausal status ($P = .01$), and stage of disease ($P = .01$). Patients receiving surgery alone have approximately 5.5 times the risk of relapse per unit time as patients receiving FAC-BCG. Fitting the regression model resulted in the conclusion that FAC-BCG is significantly better than no adjuvant treatment for disease-free survival, after adjustment for differences between groups in the number of involved nodes, menopausal status, and stage of disease. At the most recent analysis (June 1982), an estimated 72% of patients in the FAC-BCG group and 53% in the control group were free of disease 3 years after surgery.

Since this study involved historical patients, several additional questions, whose answers would justify the conclusion reached, were investigated: Do the results depend on the choice of variables in the forward stepwise regression procedure? Do results appear better in the FAC-BCG group because the disease-free survival experience was inferior in the control group and not representative of other control groups of patients? Was there evidence that prognosis was improving with time within the control group, so that one might conclude that the improved disease-free survival was simply the next step in a natural progression? The answer to all of these questions is "No," and more detailed consideration of them is given in Gehan et al. (1980). Consequently, the conclusion that FAC-BCG adjuvant treatment prolongs disease-free survival is justified, despite differences in prognostic features between the two groups of patients. A similar analysis leads to the conclusion that adjuvant FAC-BCG also favorably influences overall survival subsequent to surgery.

EVIDENCE FOR CURABILITY OF BREAST CANCER PATIENTS

Table 4 gives the estimated percentages for controls and FAC-BCG-treated patients who are disease free. These percentages are classified by stage of disease and year after surgery. There is a statistically significant advantage in disease-free survival for patients receiving adjuvant treatment with FAC-BCG both for patients with stage II disease ($P = .01$) and with stage III disease ($P = .03$). There is some evidence of a "plateau effect" (i.e., no further relapses after about 6 years in the FAC-BCG-treated patients and 8 years in stage II control patients).

Table 4. *Estimated Percentages of Stage II and III Patients Disease-Free at Given Times After Treatment with Surgery Alone or Surgery + FAC-BCG**

Stage	Adjuvant Treatment	No. of Patients	No. of Relapses	Percentages of Patients Disease-free at Year					Evidence of Plateau Effect
				1	2	4	6	8	
II	FAC-BCG	153	49	98	91	75	62	62	Yes
II	None	117	72	95	70	52	41	28	Yes
III	FAC-BCG	69	41	88	70	44	37	37	Yes
III	None	69	48	75	52	35	29	27	No

*FAC = 5-fluorouracil, Adriamycin, cyclophosphamide; BCG = bacillus Calmette Guerin.

Table 5. *Evidence for Curability of Patients on Plateau of Curve*

Type of Patient	No. of Patients on Plateau	Last Relapse (Month)	Estimated Relapse Rate Per Month	Patient Months of Observation After Last Relapse	Probability of No Relapses if No Cures
Stage II-control	29	95	.012	389	.01
Stage III-control	0	118	.020	0	–
Stage II-FAC*	24	71	.008	166	.26
Stage III-FAC	10	73	.012	82	.37

*FAC = 5-fluorouracil, Adriamycin, cyclophosphamide.

A number of different statistical distributions have been considered that might characterize the disease-free survival of the stage II and III treated patients. Using the methodology given in Gehan and Siddiqui (1973), it was found that a very simple survival distribution, the exponential, provided a good fit to the data for both stage II and stage III control and FAC-BCG-treated patients. Up until the last relapse, the data are consistent with a constant risk of relapse per month after surgery.

Table 5 contains the evidence for curability of the patients on the "plateau" of the curves. In the stage II patients receiving adjuvant FAC treatment, the relapse rate is 0.8% per month up to the last relapse at the 71st month, and there are 24 patients who are disease-free after 71 months. In the column labeled "Patient Months of Observation After Last Relapse," note that these 24 patients have been observed for a total of 166 patient months after 71 months. If one assumes that the relapse rate after 71 months is the same as it was before, 0.8% per month, then the probability calculated in the last column of the table, $P = .26$, gives the probability of no relapses in the observed set of data. This calculated probability can be interpreted as a statistical significance level for testing the null hypothesis of no change in relapse rate after 71 months versus the alternative of a lower relapse rate. Hence, the evidence for curability or a lower relapse rate in stage II FAC-treated patients is not very strong.

In fact, from the table, the strongest evidence for a significantly lowered relapse rate after the time of last relapse occurs among patients in the stage II control group. The relapse rate prior to 95 months was 1.2% per month, but there have been no relapses since the 95th month in 29 patients who have been observed for a total of 389 months. The calculated value $P = .01$ suggests strongly that the relapse rate after 95 months is significantly less than 1.2%, and, since there have been no relapses, the results are consistent with a 0% relapse rate. Strictly speaking, one cannot conclude that these patients are "cured," but the evidence strongly suggests a significantly lowered relapse rate after 95 months.

Note that for both stage II and stage III patients treated with adjuvant FAC, the probabilities in the last column of Table 4 are not extremely unlikely. Consequently, further observation of the FAC-treated patients is necessary to determine whether any cures have been obtained. Since relapses have been observed at least up to 6 years, it suggests that patients cannot be considered cured at least until they have been disease free for that time.

REFERENCES

Bonadonna, G. 1983. Operable breast cancer: The challenge of adjuvant chemotherapy, *in* Current Controversies in Breast Center (The University of Texas M. D. Anderson Hospital and Tumor Institute at Houston 26th Annual Clinical Conference, 1982). University of Texas Press, Austin, pp. 631–647.

Buzdar, A. U., J. Gutterman, G. R. Blumenschein, G. N. Hortobagyi, C. Tashima, T. L. Smith, E. M. Hersh, E. J Freireich, and E. A. Gehan. 1978. Intensive postoperative chemoimmuno-therapy for patients with stage II and III breast cancer. Cancer 41:1064–1075.

Buzdar, A. U., T. L. Smith, G. R. Blumenschein, G. N. Hortobagyi, H.-Y. Yap, E. M. Hersh, and E. A. Gehan. 1983. Adjuvant therapy for stage II or III breast cancer: UT M. D. Anderson Hospital Experience, *in* Current Controversies in Breast Cancer (The University of Texas M. D. Anderson Hospital and Tumor Institute at Houston 26th Annual Clinical Conference, 1982). University of Texas Press, Austin, pp. 171–184.

Cox, D. R. 1972. Regression models and lifetables. J. Royal Statist. Soc. 34:187–220.

Fisher, B. 1983. Adjunctive hormonal therapy for stage II breast cancer, *in* Current Controversies in Breast Cancer (The University of Texas M. D. Anderson Hospital and Tumor Institute at Houston 26th Annual Clinical Conference, 1982). University of Texas Press, Austin, pp. 159–169.

Gehan, E. A., and E. J Freireich. 1974. Nonrandomized controls in cancer clinical trials: A rational basis for use of historical controls. Semin. Oncol. 8:430–436.

Gehan, E. A., and E. J Freireich. 1981. Cancer clinical trials: A rational basis for use of historical controls. Semin. Oncol. 8:430–436.

Gehan, E. A., T. L. Smith, and A. U. Buzdar. 1980. Use of prognostic factors in analysis of historical control studies. Cancer Treat. Rep. 28:373–379.

Gehan, E. A., and M. A. Schneiderman. 1982. Experimental design of clinical trials, *in* Cancer Medicine, 2nd edition, J. F. Holland and E. Frei III, eds. Lea and Febiger, Philadelphia, pp. 531–554.

Gehan, E. A., and M. M. Siddiqui. 1973. Simple regression methods for survival time studies. J. Am. Stat. Assoc. 68:848–856.

George, S. L., and M. M. Desu. 1974. Planning the size and duration of a clinical trial: Studying the time to some critical event. J. Chron. Dis. 27:15–24.

Higgins, G. A. 1978. Special problems in the evaluation of results in adjuvant trials of cancer treatment. J. Surg. Oncol. 10:321–326.

Makuch, R., and R. Simon. 1979. Sample size consideration for nonrandomized comparative studies. J. Chron. Dis. 33:175–181.

Moon, T. E. 1979. Statistical design of adjuvant trials, *in* Adjuvant Therapy of Cancer II (2nd International Conference on the Adjuvant Therapy of Cancer, March 1979). Grune and Stratton, New York, pp. 87–96.

Current Controversies in Breast Cancer, edited
by F. C. Ames, G. R. Blumenschein, and E. D. Montague.
University of Texas Press, Austin © 1984.

Chemotherapy Compared to Chemotherapy Plus Hormonal Therapy in the Treatment of Postmenopausal Women with Advanced Breast Cancer: An Interim Report

Michael C. Perry, M.D.,* Carl G. Kardinal, M.D.,† Vivian Weinberg, M.S.,‡ Sandra Ginsberg, M.D.,§ and William Wood, M.D.∥

Department of Medicine, University of Missouri Health Sciences Center, Columbia, Missouri, †Department of Medicine, Ochsner Clinic and Alton Ochsner Medical Foundation, New Orleans, Louisiana, ‡Cancer and Leukemia Group B Statistical Office, Brookline, Massachusetts, §Department of Medicine, State University of New York, Syracuse, New York, ∥Department of Surgery, Massachusetts General Hospital, Boston, Massachusetts

Although they present a homogenous picture under the microscope, breast carcinomas actually comprise several distinct populations. Some cells may be sensitive to endocrine therapy, some to chemotherapy, and some to both. The likelihood of response to a given therapy is determined by the relative proportion of cells sensitive to that treatment. If the fraction of tumor cells sensitive to both endocrine and chemotherapy is large, then an additive effect may be seen. This assumes that the two forms of therapy do not interact with one another, either biochemically, biologically, or pharmacologically. An interaction may reduce the efficacy of combined therapy rather than enhance it.

Although both hormonal therapy and chemotherapy can produce acceptable response rates, including complete remissions, these responses are temporary, and few, if any, patients are cured. Since neither form of therapy is sufficient by itself, and the two seem to work by different modes of action, Cancer and Leukemia Group B (CALGB) elected to combine the two to see if an increased response rate and improved response duration would be seen.

Our previous CALGB study demonstrated that the combination of cyclophosphamide, Adriamycin, 5-fluorouracil (5-FU), vincristine, and prednisone (CAFVP) was superior to the widely used combination of cyclophosphamide, methotrexate, 5-FU, vincristine, and prednisone (CMFVP) therapy that substitutes methotrexate for Adriamycin (Aisner et al. 1981). In that study, the cyclophosphamide, Adriamycin, and 5-fluorouracil (CAF) combination gave results similar to CAFVP and was less toxic. Tamoxifen was chosen as the hormonal agent because of its demonstrated efficacy in postmenopausal women with breast cancer and its relative lack of toxicity (Ingle et al. 1981).

ELIGIBILITY

Eligibility requirements for this study included: histologically documented carcinoma of the breast that was surgically incurable (stage IV), locally recurrent, or metastatic; measurable disease; a CALGB performance score of three or less; and age less than 75 years. Patients were considered naturally postmenopausal if at least 6 months had elapsed since the last menstrual period. At least 3 weeks had to have elapsed since previous radiation therapy. Patients had to have a white blood cell count of $\geq 4,000/\mu l$, platelets $\geq 100,000/\mu l$, a blood urea nitrogen count of < 20 mg/dl, creatinine of < 1.5 mg/dl, and normal values for serum glutamic oxaloacetic transaminase (SGOT) and bilirubin, unless abnormal values resulted from metastatic involvement. Informed consent was required. Patients were eligible after receiving adjuvant chemotherapy if it had been discontinued for at least 6 months at the time of protocol entry.

Patients were ineligible if they did not satisfy the criteria above or had a second primary neoplasm other than cured basal cell carcinoma of the skin or carcinoma in situ of the cervix. They were also excluded if they had malignant mammary tumors other than carcinoma or a coexisting medical or psychiatric disease that would not permit the patient to give informed consent or undergo therapy. A history of myocardial infarction within the 6 months prior to entry on protocol, congestive heart failure requiring digitalis, or angina were all causes for exclusion. Radiation therapy to 50% or more of the bony pelvis and lumbar spine or palliative radiotherapy to more than two sites of metastatic disease also rendered a patient ineligible. Patients who had suffered relapse while receiving adjuvant therapy or who had been previously treated with chemotherapy or hormonal therapy were ineligible.

STRATIFICATION

Patients were stratified according to estrogen-receptor (ER) status, dominant disease site, and prior (adjuvant) therapy status (Table 1). The protocol recommended the use of the dextran-coated charcoal ER assay. Values of ≥ 7 fmol/mg/protein were considered positive, and < 7 negative. When no ER assay was performed, the patient was considered ER unknown. When possible, the ER assay was performed on tissue obtained from a metastatic site at the time of protocol entry. If this was not possible, patients were stratified according to the ER determination made on the primary tumor.

Patients were classified as having either visceral or other (osseous or soft tissue) dominant disease when they entered the study. Visceral metastases included disease in the liver, pulmonary parenchyma, pleura, brain, or bone marrow. Osseous disease indicated metastases in bone. Soft-tissue disease was defined as local recurrence in the skin or lymph nodes or inoperable (stage IV) breast cancer. When multiple sites were involved, visceral disease was dominant over others for stratification purposes. Patients who had received prior adjuvant therapy were placed in a separate stratum.

Table 1. *Stratifications*

1. Estrogen receptor (ER) status
    a. ER-negative   <7 fmol/mg protein
    b. ER-positive   ≥7 fmol/mg protein
    c. ER-unknown   test not performed
2. Dominant site of metastatic disease
    a. Visceral
    b. Osseous
    c. Soft tissue
3. Prior therapy
    a. No prior therapy
    b. Prior adjuvant chemotherapy

TREATMENT

Patients were randomized to receive either CAF chemotherapy or CAF plus tamoxifen. Chemotherapy was given in 28-day cycles: a 14-day period of drug administration followed by a 14-day rest period (Figure 1). Patients received cyclophosphamide, 100 mg/m² orally for days 1 through 14 of each cycle, plus Adriamycin, 25 mg/m², and 5-FU, 500 mg/m² intravenously on days 1 and 8 of each cycle. Pa-

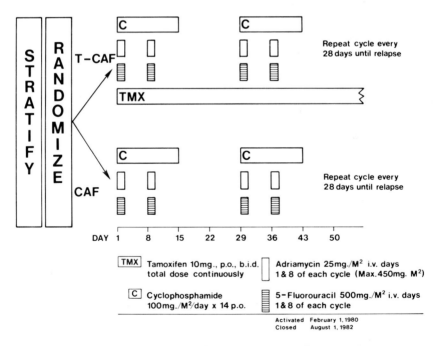

FIG. 1. Schema of Cancer and Leukemia Group B Study 8081. Treatment of postmenopausal women with metastatic breast cancer. (T-CAF = Tamoxifen plus cyclophosphamide, Adriamycin, and 5-fluorouracil; CAF = cyclophosphamide, Adriamycin, and 5-fluorouracil)

tients in regimen one also received tamoxifen, 10 mg twice daily continuously. Dose calculations were based on the patient's ideal body weight or actual weight, whichever was lower. After a total cumulative dose of 450 mg/m^2 of Adriamycin had been reached, methotrexate was substituted at a dose of 40 mg/m^2 (30 mg/m^2 for patients older than 60 years).

Dose modifications for cyclophosphamide, Adriamycin, and 5-FU were based on the total white blood cell count and platelet count on the day of treatment. Reductions were also made for elevations of serum bilirubin and SGOT and for the occurrence of stomatitis, diarrhea, or cystitis.

RESPONSE CRITERIA

A complete response (CR) required 100% disappearance of all signs and symptoms attributable to the tumor, including the disappearance of all measurable lesions for at least 1 month and the appearance of no new lesions. For bony disease, CR meant recalcification of all osteolytic lesions.

A partial response (PR) indicated a 50–99% reduction in the sum of the products of the two largest perpendicular diameters of all measured lesions without deterioration in performance. This had to last at least 1 month without the appearance of new lesions or the enlargement of existing ones. For bony metastases, a PR was considered present when partial recalcification of osteolytic lesions occurred without new osteolytic lesions.

Stable disease was considered present when tumor size was reduced less than 50% or increased less than 25% over the original measurements. For bone lesions this meant no change. In addition, no new lesions could appear.

Progressive disease (PD) indicated the appearance of new lesions subsequently proven to be metastases. When the sum of the products of the two largest perpendicular diameters increased by 25% over that obtained at the time of maximum regression, the patient was considered to have progressive disease. Progression of osteolytic lesions or the appearance of new osteolytic lesions on x-ray also constituted progression of disease.

For patients achieving an objective response, the date that the tumor met the criteria was the onset of response. Response duration was calculated from the onset of CR or PR until the documentation of progression. Patients were evaluated after two courses (8 weeks) of therapy. If there was evidence of progressive disease, the patient was considered a treatment failure and taken off protocol. Responding patients or those with stable disease continued on therapy until there was evidence of tumor progression or prohibitive drug toxicity.

ANCILLARY THERAPY

Once the patient was started on protocol, palliative radiation was not administered, except for cranial radiation for documented intracranial metastases. Chemotherapy was not withheld when patients required such radiation.

STATISTICAL METHODS

Treatment assignment was done by Latin square design, balancing within and across institutions for each stratum. In performing the analyses, differences in pretreatment characteristics and response frequencies were evaluated using the chi square technique for contingency tables. Differences in remission duration were evaluated by the generalized Wilcoxon test. Multivariate regression analyses were performed using Cox's multiple linear logistic model.

RESULTS

From February 1, 1980, to August 1, 1982, 246 patients were enrolled in this study. Fourteen cases were not evaluable because of pending data, leaving 232 evaluable patients. These were evenly divided between the two treatment groups; the comparability of the two treatment groups is seen in Table 2.

The two groups were similar with regard to type of menopause, age at diagnosis, type of initial breast surgery, prior adjuvant therapy, performance score at entry, ER status, and site of first recurrence. The one major difference in the two groups was the dominant site of disease; the CAF-treated group consisted of more patients with osseous dominant disease (32% vs 17% for the group receiving tamoxifen plus CAF (T-CAF), $P = .02$). There was a higher frequency of patients with visceral dominant disease randomized to receive T-CAF.

Of the 116 patients on the T-CAF regimen, 18 (15.5%) achieved CR, and 47

Table 2. *Comparability of Treatment Groups*

	T-CAF	CAF
Total eligible	120	126
Number evaluable	116	116
Dominant site of metastases		
Visceral	71%	59%
Osseous	17%	32%
Soft tissue	12%	9%
Estrogen receptor (ER) status		
ER-negative	33%	32.5%
ER-positive	29%	35%
ER-unknown	38%	32.5%
Prior therapy		
Adjuvant chemotherapy	11%	14%
No prior therapy	89%	86%
Performance status		
0–1	71%	79%
2–3	29%	21%
Type of menopause		
Natural	59%	64%
Surgical	21%	21%
Median age	55.3 years	56.9 years

Table 3. *Overall Frequency of Response**

Therapy	N	CR	PR	S	PD	% CR + PR
T-CAF	116	18 (15.5%)	47 (40.5%)	26	25	56
CAF	116	16 (14%)	43 (37%)	31	26	51

$P = .43$

*Abbreviations are as follows: N = number of evaluable cases; CR = complete response; PR = partial response; S = stable; PD = progressive disease; T-CAF = tamoxifen plus cyclophosphamide, Adriamycin, and 5-fluorouracil; CAF = cyclophosphamide, Adriamycin and 5-fluorouracil.

(40.5%) had PR (Table 3). In the CAF-treated group there were 16 (14%) with CR and 43 (37%) with PR. There was no difference in CR rates ($P = .71$) or in CR plus PR rates ($P = .43$) between the two groups.

The patients were also analyzed by ER status (Table 4). The response rate (CR + PR) for ER-negative patients treated with T-CAF was 54%, and for those treated with CAF, 70%. There was no difference between the two programs ($P = .14$). For ER-positive patients, the response rate for T-CAF patients was 47% and for those receiving CAF, 50% ($P = .80$). Estrogen receptor-unknown patients exhibited a significantly higher frequency of response when tamoxifen was added to CAF (T-CAF 65%, CAF 33%, $P = .004$). This reflects a higher frequency of PR in the T-CAF group (21 vs 8 in the CAF group), but the reason for the unexpected low-response frequency with CAF in this group is not clear.

Response rates were virtually identical in the T-CAF program for ER-positive and ER-negative patients and of borderline statistical significance in the CAF group. Estrogen receptor-positive patients treated with CAF had a response rate of 50% while ER-negative patients had a response of 70% ($P = .07$).

When analyzed by dominant disease site (Table 5), patients with visceral dominant disease had a response rate of 51% in both T-CAF and CAF-treated groups ($P = .95$). Patients with osseous disease had a response rate of 55% in the T-CAF

Table 4. *Response by Estrogen-Receptor Status**

	T-CAF (CR + PR/Total)	CAF (CR + PR/Total)	P
ER-negative	9 + 12/39 = 54%	4 + 22/37 = 70%[†]	.14
ER-positive	2 + 14/34 = 47%	7 + 13/40 = 50%[†]	.80
ER-unknown	7 + 21/43 = 65%	5 + 8/39 = 33%	.004

*Abbreviations are as follows: ER = estrogen receptor; T-CAF = tamoxifen plus cyclophosphamide, Adriamycin, and 5-fluorouracil; CAF = cyclophosphamide, Adriamycin, and 5-fluorouracil; CR = complete response; PR = partial response; P = probability.
[†]$P = .07$.

Table 5. *Response by Dominant Site of Metastatic Disease**

	T-CAF (CR + PR/Total)	CAF (CR + PR/Total)	P
Visceral	15 + 27/82 = 51%	9 + 26/69 = 51%	.95
Osseous	1 + 10/20 = 55%	4 + 15/38 + 50%	.72
Soft tissue	2 + 10/14 = 86%	3 + 2/9 = 56%	.11

*Abbreviations are as follows: T-CAF = tamoxifen plus cyclophosphamide, Adriamycin, and 5-fluorouracil; CAF = cyclophosphamide, Adriamycin, and 5-fluorouracil; CR = complete response; PR = partial response; P = probability.

Table 6. *Response by Prior Adjuvant Chemotherapy**

	T-CAF (CR + PR/Total)	CAF (CR + PR/Total)	P
No prior chemotherapy	17 + 43/103 = 58%	13 + 38/99 = 51%	.34
Prior adjuvant chemotherapy[†]	1 + 4/13 = 38%	3 + 5/17 = 47%	.26

*Abbreviations are as follows: T-CAF = tamoxifen plus cyclophosphamide, Adriamycin, and 5-fluorouracil; CR = complete response; PR = partial response.
[†]Adjuvant chemotherapy completed more than 6 months prior to protocol entry.

group and 50% in the CAF group ($P = .72$). For soft-tissue disease, the response rate was 86% for T-CAF and 56% for CAF ($P = .11$). Thus, despite the difference in distribution of site of dominant disease, there was no difference in response to either therapy within each of the categories.

Table 6 compares the response to T-CAF and to CAF of those patients with previous chemotherapy and those without prior therapy. For patients with prior adjuvant chemotherapy, response rates were 38% in the T-CAF group and 47% in the CAF group ($P = .26$). The previously untreated group receiving T-CAF had a 58% response rate, and those receiving CAF a 51% rate ($P = .34$).

A multivariate analysis was performed to determine which factor, or combination of factors, might predict response. The factors considered in various combinations were: Randomized therapy with or without tamoxifen; the presence or absence of bone metastases or visceral metastases; having or having not received mastectomy or prior radiation therapy; a performance score of 0–1 or 2–3; age at diagnosis < 50 vs > 50; and ER status. The existence of bone metastases ($P = .009$) and previous treatment with radiation therapy ($P = .037$) significantly adversely influenced the frequency of response.

TOXICITY

The side effects of therapy consisted of mild to moderate myelosuppression, nausea and vomiting, alopecia, and stomatitis. Toxicity was similar in the two groups, and no additional side effects appeared to be caused by tamoxifen.

Table 7. *Duration of Response*: Preliminary Data[†]*

	Median	% Responders in Remission at 12 Months
T-CAF	17.3 months	59%
CAF	14.6 months	56%

*Follow-up to 20 months.
[†] Abbreviations are as follows: T-CAF = tamoxifen plus cyclophosphamide, Adriamycin, and 5-fluorouracil; CAF = cyclophosphamide, Adriamycin, and 5-fluorouracil.

REMISSION DURATION

So far, follow-up is insufficient to permit a reliable comparison of remission duration in the two treatment groups. This analysis reflects all available data from activation on February 1, 1980, through November 12, 1981, with a maximum study time of 22 months. At 6 months after achieving response, 77% of the patients receiving T-CAF were in remission (33 patients still at risk), as were 81% receiving CAF (22 patients still at risk). At 12 months of follow-up, 59% of the patients responding to T-CAF remain in remission, as do 56% of the responders to CAF. Median duration of response is 17.3 months for T-CAF and 14.6 months for CAF (Table 7). These estimates are preliminary because of the high frequency of censoring. An update of the study should evaluate completely remission duration. Currently, no differences in remission duration appear to be associated with type of therapy or with ER status (negative vs positive) within each treatment group.

DISCUSSION

Osborne (1981) has suggested three reasons for the failure of combined hormonal therapy and chemotherapy to exert a major impact on tumor cell kill: 1) a large fraction of tumor cells may be resistant to both treatments; 2) a small fraction of the cells present may be sensitive to only one of the modalities (a large fraction of tumor cells may be sensitive to either therapy, thus minimizing the effect of a combined approach); or 3) an interaction between the treatments themselves may result in an adverse, or at least less than maximally additive, effect on cell kill.

It is conceivable that endocrine therapy is cell-cycle specific. After treatment with tamoxifen, a progressively larger fraction of tumor cells accumulates in the G_1 phase of the cell cycle, an unfavorable position for most chemotherapeutic agents. Thus, combined chemoendocrine therapy may not be additive but may be less efficacious than the two modalities used separately.

Although it has been argued that patients with ER-negative tumors have a higher response rate to chemotherapy (Lippman et al. 1978), others have disputed this claim (Kiang et al. 1978). In this study, response was similar for ER-positive and ER-negative patients to either T-CAF or CAF.

Other published studies of the use of combined chemohormonal therapy in post-menopausal women are not easily compared to the present study because of the use of differing types of chemotherapy or hormonal therapy, failure to stratify by ER status, small numbers of patients enrolled, or the use of an historical, rather than concomitant, control group. Cocconi et al. (1982) performed a similar study on 133 postmenopausal patients using CMF with or without tamoxifen. It is of note that 42% of the patients in this study had received prior endocrine therapy. Response rates were greater in the group receiving tamoxifen, but neither the duration of response nor overall survival were prolonged. Mouridsen et al. (1980) reported a similar trial of CMF with or without tamoxifen in 150 patients and also reported a significant advantage to the combined therapy group. The use of the less effective CMF chemotherapy combination may have permitted any effect of tamoxifen to become apparent. Conversely, our use of the more potent CAF therapy may have obliterated any effect of the tamoxifen.

An interesting sidelight is that patients who had completed adjuvant chemotherapy more than 6 months prior to entry on protocol responded to chemotherapy on relapse with acceptable response rates, despite the fact that almost all of this group had received prior CMF therapy, a program similar to the CAF used in this protocol. This suggests that patients may suffer relapse after adjuvant therapy due to kinetic reasons, rather than intrinsic drug resistance.

CONCLUSION

This study shows that no benefit accrued from adding the antiestrogen, tamoxifen, to CMF. Specifically, there was no difference in CR or PR or in length of remission duration. This lack of additional benefit was seen in all sites of dominant disease, even in patients with positive ER assays. The failure of this combination to be synergestic may reflect an effect of tamoxifen on tumor cell kinetics that interferes with the activity of the chemotherapeutic agents.

ACKNOWLEDGEMENTS

This investigation was supported by grant number 5 R10 CA12046, awarded by the National Cancer Institute, U.S. Department of Health and Human Services.

The authors wish to acknowledge the investigators of Cancer and Leukemia Group B who entered patients in the study. Dr. James Witliff of the University of Louisville provided quality control of the estrogen receptor assay. Editorial comments were provided by Susan Bentzinger, Ph.D., Richard L. Schilsky, M.D., and John Yarbro, M.D. Mrs. Mary Lou Wolfe prepared the manuscript.

REFERENCES

Aisner, J., V. Weinberg, M. Perloff, R. Weiss, P. Raich, M. Perry, and P. H. Wiernik. 1981. Chemoimmunotherapy for advanced breast cancer: A randomized comparison of six combinations (CMF, CAF, vs CAFVP) each with or without MER immunotherapy. A CALGB Study. (Abstract) Amer. Soc. Clin. Onc. 22:443.

Cocconi, G., V. DeLisi, C. Boni, P. Magnani, M. Bertusi, A. Ravaioli, and E. Giovannetti. 1982. Tamoxifen in combination with or following chemotherapy in advanced breast cancer: Results of a randomized prospective study, *in* The Role of Tamoxifen in Breast Cancer, S. Iacobelli, M. E. Lippman, G. R. Della Cuna, eds. Raven Press, New York, pp 35–43.

Ingle, J. N., D. L. Ahmann, S. J. Green, J. H. Edmonson, H. F. Bisel, L. K. Kvols, W. C. Nichols, E. T. Creagan, R. G. Hahn, J. Rubin, and S. Frytak. 1981. Randomized clinical trial of diethylstilbestrol versus tamoxifen in post-menopausal women with advanced breast cancer. N. Engl. J. Med. 304:16–21.

Kiang, D. T., D. M. Frenning, A. I. Goldman, V. F. Ascensao, and B. J. Kennedy. 1978. Estrogen receptors and responses to chemotherapy and hormonal therapy in advanced breast cancer. N. Engl. J. Med. 299:1330–1334.

Lippman, M. E., J. C. Allegra, E. B. Thompson, R. Simon, S. Barlock, L. Green, K. K. Huff, H. M. T. Do, S. C. Aitken, and R. Warren. 1978. The relation between estrogen receptors and response rate to cytotoxic chemotherapy in advanced breast cancer. N. Engl. J. Med. 298:1223–1228.

Mouridsen, H. T., T. Palshof, E. Engelsman, and R. Sylvester. 1980. CMF versus CMF plus tamoxifen in advanced breast cancer in post-menopausal women. An EORTC trial, *in* Breast Cancer: Experimental and Clinical Aspects, H. T. Mouridsen and T. Palshof, eds. Pergamon Press, Oxford, pp 119–123.

Osborne, C. K. 1981. Combined chemo-hormonal therapy in breast cancer: A hypothesis. Breast Cancer Res. Treat. 1:121–123.

Current Controversies in Breast Cancer, edited
by F. C. Ames, G. R. Blumenschein, and E. D. Montague.
University of Texas Press, Austin © 1984.

Chemotherapy of Brain Metastases in Breast Cancer

Dutzu Rosner, M.D.

Department of Breast Surgery, Roswell Park Memorial Institute, Buffalo, New York

Metastasis to the brain from breast carcinoma is considered usually an ominous development. The median survival in untreated patients is less than 2 months (Lang and Slater 1964, Posner 1977). Most of the patients who show brain metastasis are treated with radiation therapy and corticosteroids as palliative therapy. Whole brain irradiation, the standard initial therapy for brain metastasis, gives a neurological control of the disease with a transient limited palliation. However, the overall survival is limited in these patients by the presence of widespread disseminated metastatic disease. Most of these patients die as a result of progressive extracranial systemic disease rather than from neurologic causes. The survival in these patients is limited and ranges from 2.5 to 7.5 months. (Order et al. 1968, Horton et al. 1971, Nisce et al. 1971, Montana et al. 1972). In the experience of the Radiation Therapy Oncology group, over 1,000 patients with brain metastasis have been reviewed, and of these only 15% survived 1 year (Hendrickson 1977). The addition of corticosteroids to irradiation of the brain as treatment for these patients did not influence the overall response and survival (Horton et al. 1971, Nisce et al. 1971). Surgical excision of brain metastases has limited indication because a solitary lesion is exceedingly rare (Wilson 1977).

The use of chemotherapeutic agents in the management of brain tumors has been limited for years because it was assumed that the standard antineoplastic drugs administered systemically are unable to permeate the "intact" blood-brain barrier (BBB).

The present prospective pilot clinical trial was undertaken to test the efficacy of systemic chemotherapy alone in improving survival by controlling the brain metastases and associated extracranial disease. The protocol design was based upon: a) The presence of extracranial metastases in almost all patients (99%) with brain metastases; b) the fact that the major cause of death in the majority of these patients is due to extracranial disease; c) the fact that many patients whose brain metastases are improved by radiation therapy succumb to systemic disease; d) objective responses observed in patients with brain metastases following systemic chemotherapy, as well as in patients with other extracranial disease; e) experimental and clinical investigations of primary and metastatic brain tumors suggesting that some agents who fail to cross the intact BBB, may penetrate it under certain circumstances. (Vick and Bigner 1972, Bourke et al. 1973, Vick et al. 1977).

Our clinical experience in 71 patients with brain metastases from breast cancer treated initially by systemic chemotherapy suggests new areas for fruitful investigations in the management of brain metastases.

METHODS OF DIAGNOSIS AND EVALUATION

From 1970 to 1982 we have treated with systemic chemotherapy, as first therapeutic modality, 71 consecutive patients who have had symptomatic central nervous system (CNS) metastases with clinical neurologic findings.

The diagnosis of brain metastasis was made after initial clinical suspicion and was documented by radionuclide brain scan or computerized axial tomography (CT) scan or both in 61 of 65 patients who received the scan. The other four patients with negative scans were treated according to clinical criteria alone, as were the six patients, not receiving scans, but with poor clinical conditions (critical status, paranoia, confusion, etc.). Before 1977, 43 of 49 patients were studied by brain scan, and after 1977 twenty-two patients were studied by CT scan, either alone or in conjunction with contrast enhancement. Ten patients wre studied by both methods. Cerebral angiography was limited to five patients in whom surgical intervention was considered. This procedure identified the brain metastases in four of the five patients. Electroencephalograms were taken in nine patients and were abnormal in six. Lumbar punctures were not performed in the presence of mass lesions detected on brain or CT scan.

Twenty-three of 71 patients included in this study who died in our hospital had an autopsy examination.

While the general performance status has been recorded, the patients were also classified according to neurologic functional status into four classes (Order et al. 1968, Hendrickson 1977): Class 1—minor neurologic findings are present. The patient is able to work; Class 2—neurologic findings are present but are not a major factor. No hospitalization is required; however, nursing care may be required; Class 3—major neurologic findings are present. Hospitalization is required; Class 4—the patient has a profound neurologic deficit and may suffer coma. Hospitalization is essential.

Clinical improvement was defined as a decrease in posttreatment neurologic functional status of at least one class over the pretreatment classification. Partial objective response (PR) of brain metastases was defined as a 50% reduction in the two dimensional measurements of the brain lesion(s). Complete response (CR) required a complete disappearance of metastatic brain deposit detected by the radionuclide brain or CT scans. The response of extracranial metastases was assessed by the criteria outlined by the International Union Against Cancer (Hayward et al. 1977). Survival times were calculated from the time of initiation of chemotherapy for brain metastases.

CHARACTERISTICS OF PATIENTS

At the time of diagnosis of brain metastasis, most patients had active systemic disease outside the nervous system (Table 1). Extracranial metastases were present in 69 of our 71 patients. The most frequent sites involved were bone and soft tissue (61% for both sites), followed by pleuropulmonary (51%), liver (25%), and mediastinal and spinal cord (4%, for both sites).

Metastases were present in two sites in 16 patients, three sites in 27 patients, and four or more sites in 26 patients. Brain metastases alone were present in only two patients.

The brain was the first site of metastasis in 17 patients (24%). Only two of these 17 patients presented with brain metastases alone. The other 15 patients had associated extracranial metastases at the time of diagnosis. Of the other 54 patients, the brain was the second, third, or fourth site in 30, 16, and 8 patients, respectively.

Sixty-five percent of the patients (46 of 71) were actively receiving systemic therapy for metastatic disease when they developed brain metastases. About half of these patients showed response to prior hormonal therapy or chemotherapy for extracranial disease. Two patients were first treated outside of our department by irradiation to the whole brain; in one patient irradiation followed surgical excision of a solitary lesion. Both patients did not respond. Twenty-three patients received no prior systemic therapy for metastatic disease.

Table 1. *Characteristics of 71 Patients with Brain Metastases (BM) From Breast Cancer*

	Median	Range	
Age at diagnosis of BM (years)	51	32–75	
Time of onset of BM from other metastasis	14	1–49	
	Number of Patients*		
Therapy prior to diagnosis of BM			
None	23		
Systemic therapy for extracranial metastases			
(total)	46		
hormonaltherapy	20		
chemotherapy	26		
	Number of Patients/ Total Number		Percent
Brain metastasis only	2/71		2.8
Brain metastasis with extracranial metastases	69/71		97.2
Associated extracranial metastases			
Osseous	43/71		60.6
Soft-tissue	43/71		60.6
Pleuropulmonary	36/71		50.7
Liver	18/71		25.3
Mediastinal	3/71		4.2
Spinal Cord	3/71		4.2

*Two patients were first treated by whole-brain irradiation.

Table 2. *Brain Metastases From Breast Cancer in 71 Patients:*
Neurologic Symptoms and Signs

Cerebral (total)	68	*Cranial Nerve (total)*	30
Headache	33	Diplopia	9
Change in mental status (total)	29	Blurry vision	9
confusion	19	Papilledema	4
lethargy	12	Facial palsy	5
disorientation	10	Tongue deviation	3
personality changes	8	*Mixed (cerebral, cranial nerve, spinal root)*	
semicoma-terminal	7	Dysarthria	5
loss memory or reason	5	Bladder and bowel dysfunction	3
difficulty concentrating	3	Generalized weakness	6
Seizures	25	Hemiparesis	2
Gait disturbances	24	No symptoms	3
Dizziness	15		
Nausea and vomiting	9		

The median age, at the time of diagnosis of brain metastasis, was 51, with a range from 32 to 75 years. The median time between the onset of extracranial metastasis and the diagnosis of brain involvement was 14 months.

The symptoms and signs exhibited by the 71 patients, which were attributed to central nervous system (CNS) metastasis, are shown in Table 2. Headaches (49%) and changes in mental status (43%) were the most frequent symptoms encountered, followed by focal seizures (35%) and gait disturbances (34%).

TREATMENT PROGRAMS

Combination chemotherapy regimens used in this study were similar to those regimens currently applied in our department for all metastatic breast cancer patients.

Thirty-seven patients were given a three-drug regimen consisting of: cyclophosphamide (CTX), 150 mg/m^2, and 5-fluorouracil (5FU), 300 mg/m^2, both given intravenously (IV) daily for 5 days with courses given every 5 weeks, and prednisone (PRD), given orally daily and tapered weekly from 40 mg to 10 mg daily as maintenance. Twenty-five patients received a five-drug combination: 5FU, 500 mg, methotrexate (MTX), 25 mg, vincristine (VCR), 1 mg, all given IV once weekly; CTX, 100 mg, given orally daily; and PRD, given orally as in the three-drug regimen. Nine patients received MTX-VCR-PRD, with similar dosages and schedule as described in the five-drug regimen.

Twenty patients who failed or suffered relapse after first-line CTX-5FU-PRD were treated subsequently with the five-day combination (CTX-5FU-PRD-MTX-VCR), and three other patients received the MTX-VCR-PRD combination as a second-line chemotherapy for CNS involvement. Nine patients who failed or suffered relapse following the five-drug regimen received CTX + Adriamycin (ADR) + PRD:

CTX, 400 mg/m², and ADR, 40 mg/m², both given IV day 1, courses given every 4 weeks; and PRD administered in above regimens.

Following exhaustion of active systemic chemotherapy, radiation therapy to the whole brain (3,000–4,000 rad) was given in 11 patients who failed or suffered relapse after chemotherapy.

RESULTS OF CHEMOTHERAPY

Combination chemotherapy used in 71 patients with brain metastasis from breast carcinoma proved to be effective in half of the patients treated. Thirty-six of 71 patients (51%) showed an objective response. There were eight patients with CR, 28 patients with PR, three patients with stable disease, and 32 patients who failed to respond. Since in the first period of study, positive brain scans may have been caused by involvement of the skull and dural or leptomeningeal metastases, the results are analyzed in two separate groups. Twenty-four of 49 patients (49%) responded in the first group studied by brain scan, and 12 of 22 (54%) in the second group studied by CT scan ($P > 0.1$). The rate of response was similar regardless of whether the brain was the first, second, third, or fourth site to be involved (Table 3).

The response to chemotherapy was similar to the whole group in the subset of 23 patients who had the diagnosis of brain metastasis confirmed also by autopsy: 13 of 23 patients (56%) responded.

The response was also related to the specific chemotherapeutic regimen. Primary chemotherapy of brain metastases yielded responses in 20 of 37 patients (54%) treated with CTX-5FU-PRD, 13 of 25 patients (52%) receiving CTX-5FU-PRD-MTX-VCR, and three of nine patients (33%) in the group of patients treated with MTX-VCR-PRD.

Our experience shows also that patients who developed recurrent neurologic symptoms and relapse of brain metastases can be treated again successfully with further chemotherapy. Secondary chemotherapy yielded responses in 15 of 23 patients (65%) treated with CTX-5FU-PRD-MTX-VCR or MTX-VCR-PRD, and in five of nine patients (55%) treated with CTX-ADR-PRD.

Table 3. *Response of Brain Metastases (BM) to Systemic Chemotherapy in 71 Patients*

Presenting BM*	1st Group 1970–1976	2nd Group 1977–1981	Total	
Primary	4/8† (50.0)‡	5/ 9 (55.5)	9/17 (52.9)	
Secondary	10/22 (45.4)	5/ 8 (62.5)	15/30 (50.0)	
Tertiary	4/11 (36.4)	2/ 5 (40.0)	6/16 (37.5)	
Quaternary	6/8 (75.0)	–	6/8 (75.0)	
Total	24/49 (48.9)	12/22 (54.5)	36/71 (50.7)	$P > 0.1$

*Primary = brain first organ involved; secondary, tertiary, quaternary = brain 2nd, 3rd, or 4th organ involved.
†Number of responders/total number of patients.
‡Number in parentheses are percentages.

The rate of response in patients with associated extracranial metastases was 63% in soft tissue, 51% in pleuropulmonary, 50% in osseous, and 47% in liver metastases. These objective responses were similar to those obtained by us in treating extracranial metastases with these regimens. (Rosner et al. 1979, Rosner and Nemoto 1979).

The median duration of remission in 36 patients responding to chemotherapy was 10 months, ranging from 5 to 74 months.

All 36 responding patients presented a clinical improvement of CNS symptoms and neurologic functional status. Seventeen patients became totally asymptomatic resuming a normal life during the period of remission. The other 19 patients showed an improvement in neurologic status of at least one neurologic class.

The addition of irradiation to the whole brain in 11 patients who failed or suffered relapse following exhaustion of chemotherapy modality did not influence the overall response rate or survival. There were two of 11 patients who responded to irradiation for 5 and 10 months, respectively. Following the initiation of irradiation, nine of 11 patients did not respond to radiation therapy and died: four patients died within one month, three patients within 2 months, and two patients within 3 months.

The median survival from the time of initiation of chemotherapy for brain metastases was 13.1 months (range 5 to 74 months) for responders and 3.0 months for nonresponding patients ($P < 0.0001$). In the group of 34 responding patients, there were 18 long-term survivors, with a median survival time of 18 months (range 13 to 74 months).

AUTOPSY FINDINGS

The diagnosis of CNS metastasis was confirmed in 22 of 23 patients (Rosner et al. 1983). At autopsy, involvement of cerebrum, cerebellum, pons, and basal ganglia was present in 14 patients. These involvements were associated with the dura in four patients, leptomeninges in three patients, and both dura and leptomeninges in two patients. Dural or leptomeningeal metastatases alone were present in three patients. Tumor necrosis was found in four responding patients. Pituitary gland involvement in association with dura involvement was found in one patient. Central nervous system metastases were not identified at the time of autopsy in only one of these 23 patients. It is worth noticing that in two patients with negative brain scans, treated on clinical evidence, viable brain metastases were found in one nonresponding patient, and a necrotic tumor was found in the other patient who responded to chemotherapy. Nuclear changes and proliferation of gemistocytes identified in two patients, were considered as repair processes following chemotherapy. A central necrotic cavity surrounded by viable tumor was found in three of 14 patients.

Extracranial metastases were present at the time of autopsy in all 23 patients: pleuropulmonary 78% (18/23), bones 74% (17/23), soft tissue 57% (13/23), liver 52% (12/23), and others 30% (7/23). The cause of death in these 23 autopsied patients with CNS metastases was due to respiratory failure 43% (10/23), followed by CNS death 39% (9/23), liver failure 13% (3/23), and kidney failure 4% (1/23).

DISCUSSION

Our experience shows that brain metastases of breast cancer origin are at least as responsive to chemotherapeutic drugs as are extracranial metastases. Fifty-one percent of our patients with brain metastasis treated systemically with combination chemotherapy showed an objective response with partial or complete disappearance of CNS metastases.

Our data suggest that the chemotherapeutic agents used, do enter the metastatic lesions and induce tumor response in those lesions in the brain, dura, and lep tomeninges. Since the presence of associated extracranial metastases in patients with CNS involvement limits the length of life (Hendrickson 1977, Caincross et al. 1980) and therefore requires systemic chemotherapy, it seems that the survival might be improved by using systemic chemotherapy either alone, as our experience shows, or in association with radiation therapy as demonstrated by other investigators (Casimir et al. 1981, Logothetis et al. 1982).

The use of chemotherapy alone in the management of brain metastases has been limited for years because it was assumed that nonlipid-soluble cytotoxic drugs have a restricted accessibility to the brain metastases due to the "intact" BBB in these patients. This thinking is almost inaccurate since brain tumors are diagnosed by using radioisotopes or radioopaque compounds that usually do not cross the BBB.

Numerous investigators have shown that in pathologic circumstances the BBB function is partially or totally lost (Vick and Bigner 1972, Bourke et al. 1973, Vick et al. 1977), suggesting that tumor growth circumvents the blood-brain barrier, probably by neovascularization (Ushio et al. 1977).

Pharmacokinetic studies with different antineoplastic agents, i.e. bleomycin and cisplatin (Hasegawa et al. 1979), 5FU (Mukherjee et al. 1963, Bourke et al. 1973, Levin et al. 1972), and CTX (Ushio et al. 1977), showed that "lipid solubility" of the drug is not mandatory for penetration of the BBB. These drugs, thought not to cross the BBB, have shown higher concentrations in brain tumors than in adjacent normal brain.

Our experience suggests that chemotherapy is an effective therapy in the management of brain metastases from breast cancer.

Our results, as well as those of other investigators, signal the need for reconsidering the use of chemotherapy for CNS metastases to improve patient response and ultimately prolong survival.

Further prospective randomized trials on a large number of patients need to be conducted to determine the role of chemotherapy alone in comparison to chemotherapy in association with radiation and hormone therapy.

REFERENCES

Bourke, R. S., C. R. West, G. Chheda, and D. B. Tower. 1973. Kinetics of entry and distribution of 5-Fluorouracil in cerebrospinal fluid and brain following intravenous injection in a primate. Cancer Res. 33:1735–1746.

Caincross, J. G., J. H. Kim, and J. B. Posner. 1980. Radiation therapy for brain metastases. Ann. Neurol. 7:529–541.

Casimir, M., H. Y. Yap, A. Distefano, G. N. Hortobayi, and G. R. Blumenschein. 1981. The influence of combined modality treatment on the survival of breast cancer patients with brain metastases. (Abstract) Proc. Am. Soc. Clin. Oncol. 22:442.

Hasegawa, H., W. S. Shapiro, and J. B. Posner. 1979. Chemotherapy of experimental metastatic brain tumors in female wistar rats. Cancer Res. 39:2691–2697.

Hayward, J. L., R. D. Rubens, P. P. Carbone, J. C. Heuson, S. Kumaoka, and A. Segaloff. 1977. Assessment of response to therapy in advanced breast cancer. Br. J. Cancer 35:292–298.

Hendrickson, F. R. 1977. The optimum schedule for palliative radiotherapy for metastatic brain cancer. Int. J. Radiat. Oncol. Biol. Phys. 2:165–168.

Horton, J., D. H. Baxter, and K. B. Olson. 1971. The management of metastases to the brain by irradiation and corticosteroids. Am. J. Roentgenol. 2:334–336.

Lang, E. F., and J. Slater. 1964. Metastatic brain tumor: Results of surgical and nonsurgical treatment. Surg. Clin. North Am. 44:865–872.

Levin, V. A., M. Chadwick, and A. D. Little. 1972. Distribution of 5-fluorouracil-2-^{14}C and its metabolites in a murine glioma. JNCI 49:1577–1584.

Logothetis, C. J., M. L. Samuels, and A. Trindale. 1982. The management of brain metastases in germ cell tumors. Cancer 49:12–18.

Montana, G. S., W. F. Meacham, and W. L. Caldwell. 1972. Brain irradiation for metastatic disease of lung origin. Cancer 29:1477–1480.

Mukherjee, K. L., A. R. Curreri, M. Javid, and C. Heidelberger. 1963. Studies on fluorinated pyrimidines XVII. Tissue distribution of 5-fluorouracil-2-C^{14} and 5-Fluoro-2′-deoxyuridine in cancer patients. Cancer Res. 23:67–77.

Nisce, L. Z., B. S. Hilaris, and F. C. Chu. 1971. A review of experience with irradiation of brain metastases. Am. J. Roentgenol. 3:329–333.

Order, S. E., S. Hellman, C. F. Von Essen, and M. H. Kligerman. 1968. Improvement in quality of survival following whole-brain irradiation for brain metastases. Radiology 91:149–153.

Posner, J. B. 1977. Management of central nervous system metastases. Semin. Oncol. 4:81–91.

Rosner, D., M. Sneyderman, and T. Nemoto. 1979. Potentiating role of previously administered agents in the combination chemotherapy of breast cancer. Oncology 36:160–163.

Rosner, D., and T. Nemoto. 1979. Sequence for developing optimal combination chemotherapy of metastatic breast cancer. Eur. J. Cancer 15:1197–1201.

Rosner, D., T. Nemoto, J. Pickren, and W. Lane. 1983. Management of brain metastases from breast cancer by combination chemotherapy. Journal of Neuro-Oncology 1:131–137.

Ushio, Y., J. B. Posner, and W. R. Shapiro. 1977. Chemotherapy of experimental meningeal carcinomatosis. Cancer Res. 37:1232–1237.

Vick, N. A., and D. D. Bigner. 1972. Microvascular abnormalities in virally-induced canine brain tumors: Structural bases for altered blood-brain barrier function. J. Neurol. Sci. 17:29–39.

Vick, N. A., J. D. Khandekar, and D. D. Bigner. 1977. Chemotherapy of brain tumors: The "blood-brain barrier" is not a factor. Arch. Neurol. 34:523–526.

Wilson, C. B. 1977. Brain metastases: The basis for surgical selection. Int. J. Radiat. Oncol. Biol. Phys. 2:169–197.

Current Controversies in Breast Cancer, edited
by F. C. Ames, G. R. Blumenschein, and E. D. Montague.
University of Texas Press, Austin © 1984.

FAC vs L-PAM Chemotherapy for Adjuvant Treatment of Breast Cancer in Postmenopausal Women

M. A. Simmonds, M.D., A. Lipton, M.D., H. A. Harvey, M.D.,
D. White, R.N., J. Stryker, M.D., R. Dixon, M.D.,
J. Meloy, M.D., and S. Hoffman, M.D.

*Central Pennsylvania Oncology Group, M. S. Hershey Medical Center of the
Pennsylvania State University, University Park, Pennsylvania*

One of the conceptual advances in the treatment of breast cancer in the past decade has been the use of chemotherapy as an adjuvant. Observations of the natural history of the disease after radical surgery led to the appreciation that micrometastases are present in most patients at the time of presentation. The question then arose as to whether chemotherapy given immediately following mastectomy could prolong the disease-free interval and perhaps prolong survival. Many thousands of women have now been enrolled in various trials to try to answer this question.

This is a report of a study performed by the Central Pennsylvania Oncology Group from 1978 through 1980. At the time this trial was designed, the first large multiinstitutional adjuvant study in breast cancer had just been reported (Fisher 1977). This report by the National Surgical Adjuvant Breast Project (NSABP) claimed that there was an advantage for the use of 1-phenylalanine mustard (L-PAM) compared to placebo. Another ongoing trial that had considerable promise, conducted at The University of Texas M. D. Anderson Hospital and Tumor Institute at Houston, was the adjuvant use of 5-fluorouracil, Adriamycin, and cyclophosphamide (Cytoxan) (FAC), the most active combination for advanced disease (Buzdar et al. 1978). These reports led the Central Pennsylvania Oncology Group to design a study to compare L-PAM to the FAC combination in a multiinstitutional prospective randomized trial. Preliminary results have been reported elsewhere (Simmonds et al. 1981a, 1981b). This report is based on a median duration of follow-up of 42 months.

MATERIALS AND METHODS

Selection of Patients and Stratification

Postmenopausal women under the age of 80 with stage II breast cancer were eligible for this study. Menopause was defined as no menses for at least 6 months or postmenopausal levels of follicular stimulating hormonc (FSH) and leutinizing hormone (LH). Postoperative radiation therapy was permitted prior to randomization. Patients with a history of heart disease were omitted from this study.

To account for the major factors known to affect recurrence of breast cancer, patients were stratified according to estrogen receptor status, number of involved nodes, and whether they received postoperative radiation therapy. Estrogen receptor levels were not determined routinely in all hospitals at the time this study was begun. Results of these levels, if performed, were noted, and patients were stratified as either positive (per control of each laboratory), negative, or unknown. Patients were further grouped as having one to three or four or more positive nodes. For inclusion in this study, patients could have no evidence of distant metastasis by abnormalities of liver enzyme levels, chest x-ray, bone scan, or liver scan. Patients were started on chemotherapy within 10 weeks of surgery. All patients gave written informed consent.

Treatment Design

Patients randomized to receive the single agent received L-PAM 0.15 mg/kg/day for 5 days by mouth every 6 weeks for 2 years. Patients randomized to receive the combination chemotherapy received 5-fluorouracil 400 mg/m^2 intravenously on days 1 and 8, Adriamycin 40 mg/m^2 intravenously on day 1 only, and Cytoxan 400 mg/m^2 on day 1 only. The cycle was repeated every 28 days for 2 years. When the total Adriamycin dose reached 320 mg/m^2, methotrexate was substituted at a dose of 30 mg/m^2.

A complete blood count was performed on day 1. If the white blood cell count was $<$ 3500/mm^3 or the platelet count was $<$ 100,000/mm^3 the doses were reduced by 50%. If the white blood cell count was $<$ 3000/mm^3 or the platelet count $<$ 75,000/mm^3 the drugs were withheld until the counts recovered. Therapy was then restarted at full doses.

Patients were taken off the study if they developed recurrent disease. At the end of 2 years of treatment, chest x-rays, bone scans, liver scans, and mammograms were performed.

Patients were entered on study from January 1978 through June 1979. Fifteen investigators from nine institutions in Central Pennsylvania entered patients. A total of 54 patients were randomized, but because one patient never received chemotherapy, the study included a total of 53 evaluable patients.

RESULTS

Patient Characteristics

Of 53 evaluable patients, 24 received L-PAM and 29 received FAC. In the L-PAM group, six patients had one to three positive nodes, and 18 had four or more positive nodes. In the FAC group, nine patients had one to three positive nodes, and

Table 1. *Characteristics of 53 Study Patients**

Patient Characteristics	L-PAM	FAC
No. evaluable patients	24	29
Nodal status		
1–3 nodes positive	6	9
>4 nodes positive	18	20
Estrogen receptor		
Positive	6	10
Negative	6	7
Unknown	12	12
P.O.[†] radiotherapy	7	7

*Mean duration of follow-up is 42 months.
[†]Postoperative.

20 had four or more positive nodes. Thus, the groups were equally balanced, but there was a preponderance of four or more nodes in both groups. Estrogen receptor levels were considered positive in six patients in the L-PAM group and in 10 patients in the FAC group. Receptor levels were negative in six of the L-PAM patients and in seven of the FAC patients. Hormone receptor levels were not measured in 12 patients in each group. Seven patients from each group received postoperative radiation therapy (Table 1).

The patients have been followed from 24 to 60 months, with a median duration of follow-up of 42 months. All patients have completed chemotherapy.

Recurrences

At the time of this analysis, there had been 12 recurrences in the L-PAM group and 11 recurrences in the FAC group. From the time of the analysis 1 year ago, there have been no further recurrences. At present, there have been seven deaths in the L-PAM group and 10 deaths in the FAC group. There was one death in the L-PAM group from acute myelogenous leukemia 14 months after the drug was stopped. One patient in the FAC group died from a cerebrovascular accident, but she had no evidence of breast cancer at the time. The other deaths were all due to metastatic breast cancer.

Most of the recurrences were among patients who had four or more positive nodes in each treatment group (Table 2). Ten of 12 recurrences in the L-PAM group and nine of 11 recurrences in the FAC group appeared in patients who had more than four nodes involved by breast cancer at the outset. In patients with recurrent disease, the mean number of positive nodes was 9.3 and 9.1 in the L-PAM and FAC groups, respectively. The mean number of positive nodes in the patients still free of recurrence at this time is 5.5 and 4.5, respectively.

The sites of recurrence were comparable in the two groups. No patients who received chest radiotherapy suffered relapse in the chest wall. There was a case of a

Table 2. *Characteristics of Patients with Recurrence*

Patient Characteristics	L-PAM	FAC
Nodal status of patients with recurrence		
1–3 nodes positive	2	2
>4 nodes positive	10	9
Sites of recurrence		
Bone	4	1
Chest wall	2	2
Multiple	5	7
2nd breast	1	1

second breast primary cancer in each group. At the time of recurrence, many patients had evidence of disease in multiple sites.

Survival

The median disease-free survival was 36 months in the L-PAM group and 43 months in the FAC group. The projected disease-free survival at 5 years is 47% in the L-PAM group and 54% in the FAC group. As determined by the Wilcoxon method, this difference is not statistically significant ($P = 0.326$).

The median overall survival was 38 months in the L-PAM group and 35 months in the FAC group. The projected overall survival at 5 years is 63% in the L-PAM group and 62% in the FAC group. There is no statistical difference between the two ($P = 0.974$).

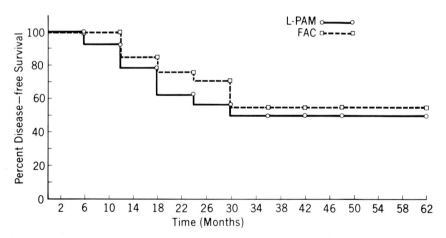

FIG. 1. Disease-free survival from time of surgery. (L-PAM = 1-phenylalanine mustard; FAC = 5-fluorouracil, Adriamycin, and cyclophosphamide)

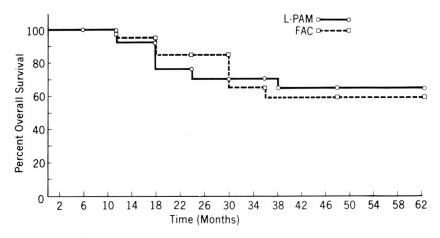

FIG. 2. Overall survival from time of surgery. (L-PAM = 1-phenylalanine mustard; FAC = 5-fluorouracil, Adriamycin, and cyclophosphamide)

Toxicity

In the adjuvant setting, the toxicity of drugs is important for a patient's compliance to the treatment. In the group receiving the Adriamycin-containing combination chemotherapy there was considerably more nausea and vomiting than in the L-PAM group (Table 3). Alopecia was almost universal in the FAC group. Hemotologic toxicity was exactly comparable in the two groups, and 12 patients in the L-PAM group and nine patients in the FAC group had to have some modification of dose for this reason. However, 54% of the L-PAM group and 76% of the FAC group received greater than 80% of the maximum dose. An additional patient had a maculopapular rash and hypotension associated with two consecutive courses of L-PAM. One patient receiving Adriamycin had reactivation of radiation erythema over the chest wall. No clinical cardiac toxicity was noted, although no specific cardiac monitoring was performed.

Table 3. *Toxicity*

Patient Characteristics	L-PAM	FAC
N/V	2	11
Stomatitis	0	3
Hematologic toxicity	12	11
No. change dose	12	9
Other	1 allergic reaction	1 Adriamycin recall
No toxicity	6	5

*Nausea and vomiting.

CONCLUSION AND DISCUSSION

In this group of 53 postmenopausal patients, the Adriamycin-containing chemotherapy FAC, did not delay recurrences of breast carcinoma or improve survival over that of L-PAM. No significant difference could be demonstrated in three subsequent analyses at 30 months, 36 months, and 42 months. Even though the number of patients in this trial is smaller than the two trials after which it was patterned, the statistical power of the results precludes any true differences.

The doses of chemotherapy in both treatment groups are exactly comparable to the trials from the NSABP and The University of Texas M. D. Anderson Hospital and Tumor Institute at Houston. Adequate doses were actually delivered, as evidenced by hematologic toxicity. Over 80% of the maximum dose was delivered to 75% of the FAC group and to 54% of the L-PAM group.

It is important to note that there was a great preponderance of patients with four or more positive nodes. In this study there was a greater proportion of patients in the group with advanced nodal disease than in both the NSABP and the U.T. M. D. Anderson Hospital trials. Furthermore, review of the pathology reports of the patients in this study who subsequently developed recurrences revealed that many of their primary tumors had more anaplasia and less differentiation than the tumors of patients who are now free of recurrence. One possible explanation of the results of this study is that unfavorable prognostic factors, such as a high degree of nodal involvement and a low degree of differentiation, could outweigh the ability of chemotherapy to eradicate micrometastases.

REFERENCES

Buzdar, A. U., J. U. Gutterman, G. R. Blumenschein, G. N. Hortobagyi, C. K. Tashima, T. L. Smith, E. M. Hersh, E. J. Freireich, and E. A. Gehan. 1978. Intensive postoperative chemoimmunotherapy for patients with stage II and stage III breast cancer. Cancer 41:1064–1075.

Fisher, B., A. Glass, C. Redmond, E. Fisher, D. B. Barton, E. Such, P. Carbone, S. Economou, D. R. Foster, R. Frelick, H. Lerner, M. Levitt, R. Margolese, J. MacFarlane, D. Plotkin, H. Shibata, H. Volk, and other cooperating investigators. 1977. L-Phenylalanine mustard (L-PAM) in the management of primary breast cancer. Cancer 39:2883–2903.

Simmonds, M. A., A. Lipton, H. A. Harvey, D. White, J. Stryker, R. Dixon, J. Meloy, and S. Hoffman. 1981a. FAC vs L-PAM chemotherapy for adjuvant treatment of breast cancer in postmenopausal women. (Abstract) Third International Conference on the Adjuvant Therapy of Cancer, Tucson, Arizona.

Simmonds, M. A., A. Lipton, H. A. Harvey, D. White, J. Stryker, R. Dixon, J. Meloy, and S. Hoffman. 1981b. FAC vs L-PAM chemotherapy for adjuvant treatment of breast cancer in postmenopausal women. Eastern Pennsylvania Region American College of Physicians, White Haven, Pennsylvania.

Current Controversies in Breast Cancer, edited
by F. C. Ames, G. R. Blumenschein, and E. D. Montague.
University of Texas Press, Austin © 1984.

Adjuvant Therapy of Breast Cancer: Southwest Oncology Group Experience

Saul E. Rivkin, M.D.,* Harold Glucksberg, M.D.,*
and Mary Foulkes, Ph.D.†

*The Tumor Institute of The Swedish Hospital Medical Center, Seattle, Washington, and
†Southwest Oncology Group, Houston, Texas*

The disease-free and overall survival of women with operable breast cancer with positive axillary nodes has not improved over the past several decades despite a variety of locoregional approaches. The prognosis has not been significantly affected by the extent of surgery (Kaae and Johansen 1967, Lacour et al. 1976) or the administration of postoperative radiation therapy (Stjernsward 1977). Although several factors, including the size of the primary tumor (Fisher et al. 1969, Say and Donegan 1974) and the estrogen receptor status (McGuire 1975) are of prognostic importance, the status of the axillary lymph nodes (Fisher 1972) remains the most important prognostic factor. Approximately 50% of women with one to three and 75% with four or more involved axillary nodes have tumor recurrence within 5 years of initial treatment (Fisher 1972, Valagussa et al. 1978). Clearly, locoregional therapy is not adequate or curative in most women with axillary nodal metastases.

Most women with involved axillary nodes are not cured with local measures because of microscopic deposits of tumor present at sites distant from the primary tumor at the time of initial treatment. Therefore, only treatment, such as hormonal manipulation or chemotherapy, reaching these distant sites can affect disease-free survival in these women. The results of early trials with adjuvant chemotherapy (THIO-tepa, etc.) have been conflicting but generally disappointing (Fisher et al. 1975b, Tormey 1975). However, these early trials involved short courses of chemotherapy, since they were aimed at eradicating malignant cells dislodged at the time of surgery. The currently accepted hypothesis, i.e., that micrometastases have already formed at the time of initial treatment, calls for a prolonged course of systemic treatment to eradicate these deposits (Schabel 1977).

In 1975 and 1976, the preliminary results of two controlled trials involving long-term adjuvant chemotherapy were reported. The National Surgical Adjuvant Breast Project (NSABP) reported on the efficacy of melphalan (L-Pam) (Fisher et al. 1975a), and Bonadonna (Bonadonna et al. 1976) reported on the efficacy of cyclic cyclophosphamide, methotrexate, and 5-fluorouracil (CMF) versus surgery alone in women with operable breast cancer and histologically involved axillary nodes. The promising preliminary results of these two controlled studies prompted the Southwest Oncology Group (SWOG) to compare combination versus single-agent adjuvant chemotherapy in women at high risk for relapse after locoregional therapy. Continuous rather than intermittent combination chemotherapy was used because the former was more effective in a SWOG study in women with metastatic breast cancer (Hoogstraten et al. 1976).

This study evaluates the relative efficacy of continuous CMFVP (cyclophosphamide, methotrexate, 5-fluorouracil, vincristine, and prednisone) and L-Pam in terms of disease-free and total survival and short- and long-term toxicity in women with operable breast cancer with histologically involved axillary nodes. This report is an update of data previously reported, with a mean follow-up of 5 years (Glucksberg et al. 1982).

PATIENTS AND METHODS

Selection of Patients

All women who had modified or radical mastectomies, one or more nodes positive on histologic examination, and no evidence of metastatic disease were eligible for this study provided they fulfilled specific criteria described in the protocol. These included primary and axillary neoplasm completely removed as confirmed by the pathologic report, tumors confined to the breast and axilla, tumors moveable in relation to the underlying muscle and chest wall, axillary nodes moveable in relation to the chest wall and neurovascular bundle, no preoperative arm edema, a leukocyte count $\geq$ 4000, a platelet count $\geq$ 100,000, a blood urea nitrogen (BUN) $\leq$ 25 mg/100 ml. Patients with inflammatory carcinoma or skin ulcerations larger than 2 cm were excluded from the study. T_3 lesions were included if there was no fixation. Chemotherapy was initiated within 42 days after mastectomy.

This study was carried out on patients from 32 institutions affiliated with SWOG. Patients signed informed consents stating they would receive either single-agent or combination chemotherapy after mastectomy.

Pretherapy Studies

All patients underwent the following studies: bone scan, complete blood count, chest x-rays, and measures of transaminase, alkaline phosphatase, bilirubin, BUN, serum creatinine, serum calcium, and phosphorus levels. Liver and brain scans were obtained if symptoms, signs, or laboratory tests suggested possible metastases at these sites. Most patients also had mammography or xerography of the opposite breast.

Experimental Design

Stratification was done according to menopausal status, number of involved axillary nodes (1–3 and $\geq$ 4), and whether postoperative radiation was going to be administered. Patients were randomized to receive either 2 years of melphalan or 1 year of CMFVP. Treatment was begun 1 to 6 weeks after mastectomy.

Treatment

Adjuvant melphalan treatment consisted of 5 mg/m^2 daily by mouth for 5 days every 6 weeks for 2 years. CMFVP treatment consisted of cyclophosphamide 60 mg/m^2 daily by mouth, methotrexate 15 mg/m^2 intravenously weekly, and 5-fluorouracil (5-FU) 300 mg/m^2 intravenously weekly, all for 1 year. Vincristine 0.625 mg/m^2 was administered intravenously weekly for 10 weeks; prednisone, 30 mg/m^2 by mouth, was given daily for days 1–14, 20 mg/m^2 daily for days 15–28, and 10 mg/m^2 for days 29–42, and discontinued thereafter. Drug doses were modified according to the presence and degree of toxicity.

Postoperative Radiation

Radiation was an option available to the primary physician and his patient to facilitate accrual on this study. The dose schedule and radiation fields were not standardized. Most patients received radiation to the supraclavicular and internal mammary nodal areas. Some also received radiation to the anterior chest wall. When postoperative radiotherapy was used, it was started 10 weeks after combination chemotherapy or after three courses of melphalan had been administered. Twenty-six fully evaluable (18%) patients on the CMFVP arm and 39 (23%) patients on the melphalan arm received radiation.

Follow-up Studies

While receiving chemotherapy, patients received a monthly physical examination and a complete blood count at each clinic visit. During the treatment period, transaminase, alkaline phosphatase, serum calcium and phosphorus, serum creatinine and BUN data were obtained every 3 months, a chest x-ray every 3 months, and a bone scan every 12 months. After treatment was completed, the above blood tests were obtained every 3 months, a chest x-ray every 3–6 months, and a bone scan and mammogram every year.

Statistical Analysis

Statistical analysis of this study was based on time to first evidence of treatment failure, represented by local, regional, or distant recurrence and survival time. All patients with treatment failures were followed until death, and the survival curves include both fully and partially evaluable patients. Disease-free interval and survival curves were plotted using the life-table method of Kaplan and Meier (Kaplan and Meier 1958). A two-tailed generalized Wilcoxon test (Gehan 1965) was used to test for the differences between disease-free interval and survival curves. Three hundred sixty-two fully and partially evaluable patients were analyzed, 188 on the

L-Pam arm and 174 on the CMFVP arm. Comparing the two treatment groups with respect to age, race, tumor location, tumor size, and menopausal status revealed that the randomization generated treatment groups comparable with respect to these patient characteristics.

RESULTS

Table 1 shows recurrence patterns for fully and partially evaluable patients in the two treatment arms, both overall and within patient subgroups. The median follow-up time for these patients is approximately 60 months, and the minimum is 46 months. The difference in the overall rate of recurrence between CMFVP and melphalan (22% versus 41%) is highly significant ($P = .002$). The difference in the observed proportion of treatment failures is also highly significant in favor of CMFVP compared to melphalan for the following subgroups: premenopausal women 19% versus 44% ($P = .002$); postmenopausal women 25% versus 39% ($P = .003$); women with 1–3 involved axillary nodes 10% versus 25% ($P = .017$); and women with four or more involved axillary nodes 32% versus 52% ($P = .002$). In the analysis of recurrence by menopausal status and number of involved nodes (1–3 and $\geqslant 4$), there are differences favoring CMFVP in all subgroups.

Figure 1 shows Kaplan-Meier estimates of the time to treatment failure (disease-free interval) of both fully (FE) and partially (PE) evaluable patients on the two treatment arms. The 5-year disease-free interval is 70% for CMFVP compared to 53% for melphalan ($P = .002$).

Length of survival from onset of chemotherapy for all patients is shown in Figure 2. The life-table estimate of survival at 5 years is 73% for CMFVP and 56% for melphalan. There is a significant difference in survival in favor of CMFVP over melphalan ($P = .002$).

Figure 3 compares the disease-free interval by menopausal status. The 5-year disease-free interval is equal in both premenopausal and postmenopausal CMFVP patients (70% versus 68%). The 5-year disease-free interval of premenopausal pa-

Table 1. *Characteristics of Women Treated with CMFVP and Melphalan, with Observed Treatment Failures*

| | Recurrences | | | | |
| Patient Characteristics | Melphalan | | CMFVP* | | Two-Tailed P-Value |
	No.	(%)	No.	(%)	
Total	78/188	41	39/173	22	.002
Nodal status					
1–3	18/72	25	8/77	10	.017
$\geqslant 4$	60/116	52	31/96	32	.002
Menopausal status					
Premenopausal	35/79	44	13/68	19	.002
Postmenopausal	43/109	39	26/105	25	.003

*CMFVP = cyclophosphamide, methotrexate, 5-fluorouracil, vincristine, and prednisone.

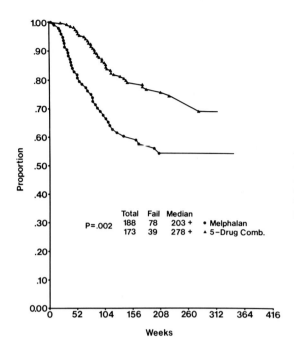

FIG. 1. Treatment failure time distribution for all fully and partially evaluable patients. Abbreviations are as follows: 5-Drug Comb. = cyclophosphamide, methotrexate, 5-fluorouracil, vincristine, and prednisone; *P* = probability.

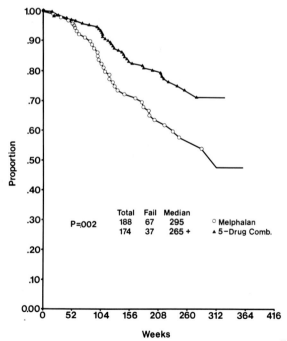

FIG. 2. Overall survival in fully and partially evaluable patients treated with melphalan and cyclophosphamide, methotrexate, 5-fluorouracil, vincristine, and prednisone (CMFVP). Abbreviations are as follows: *P* = probability; 5-Drug Comb. = CMFVP.

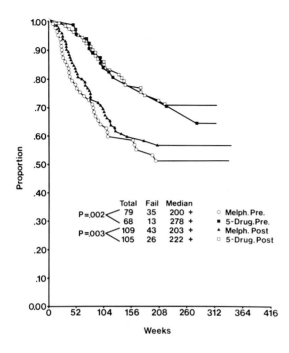

FIG. 3. Treatment failure time distribution in fully and partially evaluable pre- and postmenopausal patients. Abbreviations are as follows: P = probability; melph. = melphalan; 5-Drug = cyclophosphamide, methotrexate, 5-fluorouracil, vincristine, and prednisone; Pre. = premenopausal; Post. = postmenopausal.

tients treated with melphalan is 50%, and 55% for postmenopausal patients. Both premenopausal and postmenopausal patients treated with CMFVP have significantly longer disease-free intervals compared to those treated with melphalan (P = .002 for premenopausal and P = .003 for postmenopausal patients).

Figure 4 compares the length of total survival by menopausal status. The 5-year survival for both premenopausal and postmenopausal patients treated with CMFVP is identical at 73%. The 5-year survival for premenopausal patients treated with melphalan is 51%, and 58% for postmenopausal patients. Both premenopausal and postmenopausal patients treated with CMFVP have a significantly longer survival than those treated with melphalan (P = .021 for premenopausal; P = .037 for postmenopausal).

Figure 5 is the disease-free interval by nodal status. The CMFVP-treated group has a 5-year disease-free interval of 88%, compared to 73% for patients treated with melphalan (P = .017). The lower two curves represent patients with a larger tumor burden with four or more involved axillary nodes, and again the difference with CMFVP treatment is highly significant. The 5-year disease free interval is 60% for CMFVP and 40% for melphalan (P = .002).

The length of survival by number of involved axillary nodes is shown in Figure 6. The 5-year survival of patients treated with CMFVP is 81%, compared to 67% for melphalan. This is not a significant difference in survival. The reason for this is twofold: 1) In the CMFVP group four patients died of unrelated causes; 2) in the

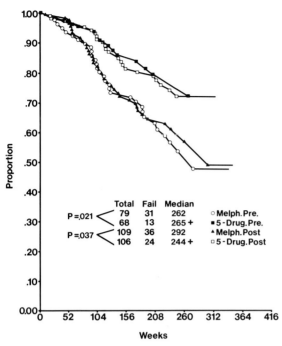

FIG. 4. Survival in fully and partially evaluable pre- and post-menopausal patients. Abbreviations are as follows: P = probability; Melph. = melphalan; 5-Drug = cyclophosphamide, methotrexate, 5-fluorouracil, vincristine, and prednisone; Pre. = premenopausal; Post. = postmenopausal.

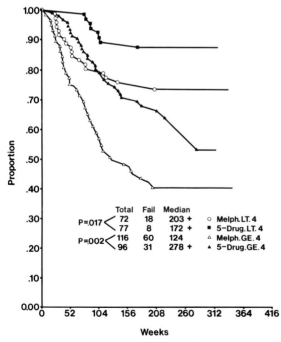

FIG. 5. Treatment failure time distribution in fully and partially evaluable patients with 1–3 and ⩾ 4 involved axillary nodes. Lower two curves represent latter group of patients. Abbreviations are as follows: P = probability; Melph. = melphalan; 5-Drug = cyclophosphamide, methotrexate, 5-fluorouracil, vincristine, prednisone; Lt. 4 = < 4 positive nodes; GE. 4 = ⩾ 4 positive nodes.

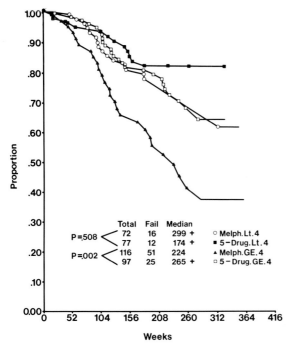

FIG. 6. Survival in fully and partially evaluable patients with 1–3 and ⩾ 4 involved axillary nodes. Abbreviations are as follows: P = probability; Melph. = melphalan; 5- Drug = cyclophosphamide, methotrexate, 5-fluorouracil, vincristine, and prednisone; LT. 4 = < 4 positive nodes; GE. 4 = ⩾ 4 positive nodes.

	Total	Fail	Median	
P =.508	72	16	299 +	○ Melph.Lt.4
	77	12	174 +	■ 5−Drug.Lt.4
P =.002	116	51	224	▲ Melph.GE.4
	97	25	265 +	□ 5−Drug.GE.4

melphalan group those patients relapsing with local recurrence were effectively salvaged with CMFVP and local radiation.

Patients with four or more involved axillary nodes have a 67% survival at 5 years when treated with CMFVP, compared to 41% when treated with melphalan ($P = .002$).

Toxicity

The side effects of both treatment arms are shown in Table 2. Nausea, vomiting, and malaise were more prominent with CMFVP than with melphalan. Cystitis, mucositis, and alopecia only occurred in patients treated with CMFVP. The eight patients who developed hemorrhagic cystitis secondary to cyclophosphamide were switched to chlorambucil. Approximately 40% of women treated with CMFVP developed significant alopecia. Leukopenia was a frequent complication in both treatment arms but was usually mild to moderate in degree. Less than 10% of patients on either treatment arm developed leukocyte counts < 2,500 or platelet counts < 50,000.

Subjective and objective toxicity, while more prominent in the CMFVP group, was acceptable with both treatment arms. The low patient dropout rate (5.3%) and the rarity of severe leukopenia reflect the acceptable toxicity of both treatment arms.

Table 2. *Side Effects*

Manifestation	CMFVP* (%)	Melphalan (%)
Leukopenia[†]		
3,999 − 2,500	39	22
< 2,500	10	5
Thrombocytopenia[‡]		
99,000 − 50,000	6	7
< 50,000	1	2
Alopecia	40	0
Cystitis	5	0
Mucositis	16	0

*CMFVP = cyclophosphamide, methotrexate, 5-fluorouracil, vincristine, and prednisone.
[†]Leukocyte/mm^3.
[‡]Platelets/mm^3.

DISCUSSION

With a median follow-up of 5 years, our data show that women with operable breast cancer and histologically involved axillary nodes treated with continuous CMFVP show a significantly longer disease-free and total survival than those treated with intermittent melphalan. This decrease in recurrence is demonstrated in both premenopausal and postmenopausal women, resulting in prolonged total survival. Women with four or more involved axillary nodes have decreased recurrences and prolonged total survival when treated with CMFVP than when treated with melphalan. Patients with one to three involved axillary nodes had a longer disease-free survival, but total survival was not significantly different because of deaths due to other causes and salvage therapy of local recurrences with surgery, radiotherapy, and chemotherapy.

In summary, we believe the data at this time do not support the use of melphalan as adjuvant therapy in operable breast cancer with histologically involved axillary nodes. Based on our preliminary data, our present treatment for these patients is continuous CMFVP.

ACKNOWLEDGMENTS

This investigation was supported by the following grant numbers awarded by the National Cancer Institute, U.S. Department of Health and Human Services: CA-20319, CA-03096, CA-12644, CA-13238, CA-22416, CA-22411, CA-04915, CA-04920, CA-13392, CA-16957, CA-16385, CA-03389, CA-21116, CA-12213, CA-27057, CA-14028, CA-04919, CA-22433, CA-12014, and CA-16943, and by Foreign Research Agreement 03-054-N.

REFERENCES

Bonadonna, G., E. Brusamolino, P. Valagussa, A. Rossi, L. Brugnatelli, C. Brambilla, M. De Lena, G. Tancini, E. Bajetta, R. Musumeci, and U. Veronesi. 1976. Combination chemotherapy as an adjuvant treatment in operable breast cancer. N. Engl. J. Med. 294:405–410.

Fisher, B. 1972. Surgical adjuvant therapy for breast cancer. Cancer 30:1556–1564.

Fisher, B., P. Carbone, S. G. Economou, R. Frelick, A. Glass, H. Lerner, C. Redmond, M. Zelen, P. Band, D. Katrych, N. Wolmark, and E. R. Fisher. 1975a. 1-Phenylalanine mustard (L-PAM) in the management of primary breast cancer: A report of early findings. N. Engl. J. Med. 292:117–122.

Fisher, B., N. H. Slack, and I. D. J. Bross. 1969. Cancer of the breast: Size of neoplasm and prognosis. Cancer 24:1071–1080.

Fisher, B., N. Slack, D. Katrych, and N. Wolmark. 1975b. Ten-year follow-up results of patients with carcinoma of the breast in a cooperative clinical trial evaluating surgical adjuvant chemotherapy. Surg. Gynecol. Obstet. 140:528–534.

Gehan, E. A. 1965. A generalized Wilcoxon test for comparing arbitrarily single-censored samples. Biometrika 52:203–223.

Glucksberg, H., S. E. Rivkin, S. Rasmussen, B. Tranum, N. Gad-el-Mawla, J. Costanzi, B. Hoogstraten, J. Athens, T. Maloney, J. McCracken, and C. Vaughn, 1982. Combination chemotherapy (CMFVP) versus 1-phenylalanine mustard (L-PAM) for operable breast cancer with positive axillary nodes: A Southwest Oncology Group study. Cancer 50:423–434.

Hoogstraten, B., S. L. George, B. Samal, S. E. Rivkin, J. J. Costanzi, J. D. Bonnet, T. Thigpen, and H. Braine. 1976. Combination chemotherapy and Adriamycin in patients with advanced breast cancer: A Southwest Oncology Group study. Cancer 38:13–20.

Kaae, S., and H. Johansen. 1967. Prognostic factors in breast cancer, *in* Proceedings of First Ten-ovus Symposium, Welsh National School of Medicine, Cardiff, Wales, A. P. M. Forrest and P. B. Kunkler, eds. E. S. Livingstone, Edinburgh, pp. 93–102.

Kaplan, E. L., and P. Meier. 1958. Nonparametric estimation from incomplete observations. J. Am. Stat. Assoc. 53:457–481.

Lacour, J., P. Bucalossi, and E. Caceres. 1976. Radical mastectomy vs. radical mastectomy plus internal mammary dissection: Five-year results of an international cooperative study. Cancer 37:206–214.

McGuire, W. L. 1975. Current status of estrogen receptors in human breast cancer. Cancer 36:638–644.

Say, C. C., and W. L. Donegan. 1974. Invasive carcinoma of the breast: Prognostic significance of tumor size and involved axillary lymph nodes. Cancer 34:468–471.

Schabel, F. M., Jr. 1977. Rationale for adjuvant chemotherapy. Cancer 39:2875–2882.

Stjernsward, J. 1977. Adjuvant radiotherapy trials of breast cancer. Cancer 39:2846–2867.

Tormey, D. C. 1975. Combined chemotherapy and surgery in breast cancer: A review. Cancer 36:881–892.

Valagussa, P., G. Bonadonna, and U. Veronesi. 1978. Patterns of relapse and survival following radical mastectomy: Analysis of 716 consecutive patients. Cancer 41:1170–1178.

Current Controversies in Breast Cancer, edited
by F. C. Ames, G. R. Blumenschein, and E. D. Montague.
University of Texas Press, Austin © 1984.

Sequential Systemic Therapy for Increased Survival in Metastatic Breast Cancer

Dutzu Rosner, M.D.

Department of Breast Surgery, Roswell Park Memorial Institute, Buffalo, New York

The standard chemotherapeutic regimens for the treatment of metastatic breast cancer such as the three-drug combination of cyclophosphamide (C), methotrexate (M), and 5-fluorouracil (F) (CMF) or five-drug regimen, CMF, vincristine (V), and prednisone (P) (CMFVP), or Adriamycin (A) combinations, AC or FAC, have produced a high initial response (50–70%) with a similar duration of remission. However, the overall survival of patients receiving these combinations was not significantly prolonged when compared to those receiving less aggressive therapy (Chlebowski et al. 1979, Powles et al. 1980).

During the past years, most oncologists have favored more aggressive chemotherapy regimens with the aim of obtaining a potential "cure" for metastatic breast cancer. In many instances, the trend has been toward exhaustion of the most available active drugs in the first-line chemotherapy, almost to the exclusion of endocrine manipulations regardless of the estrogen-receptor (ER) status. It has been well recognized that prior chemotherapy diminishes the rates of remissions in second-line chemo- or hormonotherapy due to cross-resistance to subsequent regimens, to more advanced disease present, to cumulative toxic effects, and to many other factors (Rosencweig et al. 1979).

The sequence of therapy aimed at producing remission and prolongation of life has evolved empirically, and most of the second-line systemic therapies are less effective.

During the past decade, we have attempted to develop an optimal sequential therapy in the management of metastatic breast cancer in order to increase the number of responses and ultimately prolong survival. Our efforts have been directed toward avoiding premature exhaustion of therapeutic modalities.

In the present study, the sequential approach of endocrine therapy followed by chemotherapy was investigated in ER positive or ER unknown patients, and chemotherapy alone was studied in ER-negative patients. At the same time, the concept of recycling previously used drugs and adding new drugs in sequential regimens as a form of salvage therapy was investigated in patients receiving chemotherapy.

PATIENT SELECTION

One hundred seventy-six patients with progressive metastatic breast cancer and measurable disease were included in this study. An expected survival of at least 2 months was required for eligibility in order to evaluate this long-range projected sequential study. Patients who received prior chemotherapy more than 2 months, either adjuvant or palliative, were excluded from this study. Patients with central nervous system (CNS) metastases and patients with active heart disease, history of congestive heart failure, or myocardial infarction less than 6 months prior to entry into the study were also excluded.

All patients were evaluated and followed by clinical, radiologic, biochemical, and hemotologic examinations and scans of bones and liver when indicated, performed every 8 to 10 weeks during therapy. Regression of metastatic disease was assessed by the criteria outlined by the International Union Against Cancer for metastatic breast cancer (Hayward et al. 1977).

The selection of patients for this study was done according to ER status (Figure 1). Patients with ER positive were assigned first to hormonal manipulations.

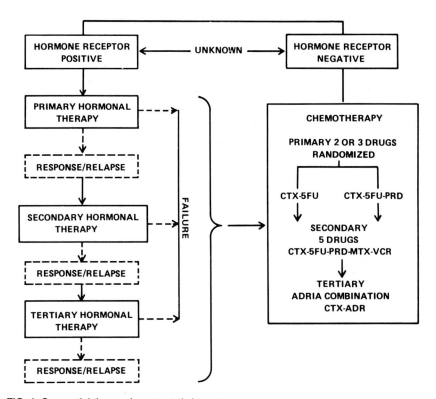

FIG. 1. Sequential therapy in metastatic breast cancer.

Estrogen-receptor negative patients received systemic chemotherapy. Patients with ER unknown were allocated either to hormono-chemotherapy or chemotherapy alone according to their clinical and performance status. All patients receiving chemotherapy were randomized to receive the two- or three-drug regimen, CF or CFP, as first-line chemotherapy. At the time of relapse or failure, patients were moved as assigned to the second- or third-line chemotherapy, consisting of the five-drug regimen, CFPMV, and the Adriamycin combination, (AC). This study was started in May 1977, and patient accession was terminated in September 1981, with a follow-up of 14 to 64 months or to death of patients.

DETAILS OF DRUG TREATMENT

A. Cyclophosphamide and 5-fluorouracil in the two- and three-drug regimens were given at 150 mg/m^2 and 300 mg/m^2, respectively, both by direct intravenous (IV) injection on each of 5 successive days; the courses were repeated every 5 weeks. Prednisone in the three-drug regimen was tapered weekly from 40 to 10 mg taken orally and daily.

B. The five-drug regimen, CFPMV, was given as follows: F, 500 mg; M, 25 mg; and V, 1 mg, taken IV weekly; C, 50 mg twice daily orally; and P, orally as in the three-drug regimen.

C. The AC combination was given as follows: A, 40 mg/m^2 by direct infusion; and C, 400 mg/m^2. Adriamycin-cyclophosphamide courses were repeated every 4 weeks. When the maximum dose of A, 500 mg/m^2, was reached, the patient was maintained on C at the same dosage and schedule until relapse.

RESPONSE TO THERAPY

Results of the hormonotherapy are shown in Table 1. A total of 98 patients with ER positive or ER unknown were entered into the primary hormonal study. Forty-three of 98 patients responded to the first-line hormonal manipulations: 19 of 34 (56%) premenopausal patients to bilateral salpingo-oophorectomy; 12 of 26 (46%)

Table 1. *Response to Sequential Hormonotherapy in ER-Positive and ER-Unknown Patients**

Therapy[†]	First Line	Second Line	Third Line	Total
BSO	19/34 (56)[‡]	0/1 (0)	–	19/35 (54)
ADX	12/26 (46)	13/24 (54)	3/7 (43)	28/57 (49)
TMX	7/23 (30)	7/18 (39)	3/10 (30)	17/51 (33)
Additive hormones, others	5/15 (33)	2/4 (50)	0/8 (0)	7/27 (26)
TOTAL	43/98 (44)	22/47 (47)	6/25 (24)	71/170 (42)

*Responding patients underwent sequentially one or more hormonal manipulations.
[†]BSO = bilateral salpingo-oophorectomy; ADX = adrenalectomy; TMX = tamoxifen, additive hormones, others (androgens, progesterones, etc.).
[‡]Number of responders/total number of patients; number in parentheses are percentages.

Table 2. *Response to Sequential Combination Chemotherapy Regimens* *
in 176 Metastatic Breast Cancer Patients

	CF			CFP			
First line	48/89	(54)[†]		52/87	(60)	100/176	(57)
			CFPMV				
Second line	27/55	(49)		16/37	(43)	43/92	(47)
			CA				
Third line	7/19	(37)		4/14	(29)	11/33	(33)

*CF = cyclophosphamide and 5-fluorouracil; CFP = CF plus prednisone; CFPMV = CFP plus methotrexate and vincristine; CA = cyclophosphamide and Adriamycin.
[†]Number of responders/total number of patients; numbers in parentheses are percentages.

postmenopausal patients to adrenalectomy; and seven of 23 (30%) to tamoxifen. Five of 15 patients (33%) responded to other additive hormones (progesterone; androgen compounds). Forty-three responding patients and four nonresponding patients to first-line hormonal manipulations were receiving second-line hormonal therapy. Twenty-two of 47 (47%) showed further responses. Twenty-five patients who suffered relapse received third-line hormonal therapy, and six patients had objective remission (24%).

Results of Sequential Chemotherapy

The best objective responses to each regimen given sequentially are tabulated in Table 2. All regimens used sequentially were effective and noncross-resistant: 48 of 89 (54%) and 52 of 87 (60%) responded to primary CF and CFP ($P > 0.01$); 43 of

Table 3. *Dominant Metastasis in Patients Responding to First-Line Combination Chemotherapy with Two or Three Drugs* *: Randomized Study

	No. of Responders/ Total Patients[‡]	
Specific Site	CTX–5FU	CTX–5FU–PRD
Visceral	26/60 (43%)	33/59 (56%)
Central nervous system[†]	–	–
Liver	11/32	21/31
Pleuropulmonary	10/20	5/14
Mediastinal esophageal obstruction	3/5	3/5
Peritoneal-retroperitoneal	2/3	4/9
Osseous	13/16 (81%)	11/18 (61%)
Soft Tissue	9/13 (69%)	8/10 (80%)
Totals	48/89 (54%)	52/87 (60%)

*CTX = cyclophosphamide; 5FU = fluorouracil; PRD = prednisone.
[†]Excluded from this study.
[‡]$P > 0.1$

Table 4. *Dominant Metastasis in Patients Responding to Second-Line Combination Chemotherapy*

Specific Site	No. of Responders/Total Patients		
	Post-CTX-5FU	Post-CTX-5FU PRD	Totals[†]
Visceral	20/44	12/32	32/76
Central nervous system	0/2	1/2	1/4
Liver	9/21	4/22	13/43
Pleuropulmonary	10/17	4/5	14/22
Mediastinal esophageal obstruction	1/2	1/1	2/3
Peritoneal-retroperitoneal	0/2	2/2	2/4
Osseous	4/6	2/3	6/9
Soft Tissue	3/5	2/2	5/7
Totals	27/55 (49%)	16/37 (43%)	43/92 (47%)

*CTX = cyclophosphamide; 5FU = 5-flourouracil; PRD = prednisone.
[†]$P < .075$.

92 (47%) to second-line CFPMV; and 11 of 33 (33%) to the third-line chemotherapy. The median duration of remission was 11, 12, 8, and 10 months in each group respectively. The responses related to predominant site in first-line and second-line chemotherapy are shown in Tables 3 and 4.

The presence or absence of ER did not predict, or correlate with, the responses to chemotherapy. In the first-line chemotherapy, there were no significant differences ($P > 0.10$): 36 of 54 (67%) ER negative, 29 of 55 (53%) ER unknown, and 35 of 67 (52%) ER positive patients had objective responses to the two- (CF) or three-drug (CFP) combination (Table 5).

LENGTH OF SURVIVAL

The survival rates in this study were updated per October 1982. One hundred forty-two patients of 176 entered in this study died. Seven patients were lost to follow-up. Eight patients withdrew from the study. Nineteen patients are still re-

Table 5. *Response to Primary Combination Chemotherapy Regimen* as Related to Estrogen Receptor (ER) Status Randomized Study*

ER Status	CF	CFP		Total[‡]	
Negative	19/29 (65)[†]	17/25 (68)		36/54	(67)
Unknown	17/28 (61)	12/27 (44)		29/55	(53)
Positive	12/32 (38)	23/35 (66)	$P < 0.05$	35/67	(52)
Total	48/89 (54)	52/87 (60)		100/176	(57)

*CF = cyclophosphamide and 5-flourouracil; CFP = CF + prednisone.
[†]Number of responders/total number of patients; numbers in parenthesis are percentages.
[‡]$P > 0.1$.

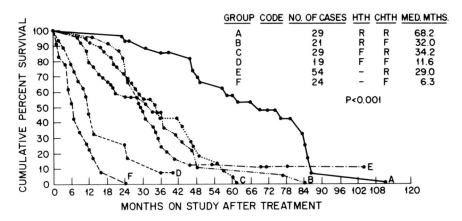

FIG. 2. Survival according to the type of treatment in metastatic breast cancer. (HTH = hormonotherapy; CHTH = chemotherapy; MED. MTHS. = median months; R = response; F = failure; P = probability)

ceiving chemotherapy: five patients receiving first-line chemotherapy, seven patients receiving CFPMV as second-line, and seven patients receiving CA as third-line.

The sequential use of these three noncross-resistant regimens secured further objective responses and prolonged survival (Figure 2). In 29 patients responding to sequential endocrine manipulation and chemotherapy, the median survival from the onset of metastasis was 68.2 months, in contrast to 32.0 months in 21 patients responding only to hormonal manipulations and 34.2 months in 29 patients responding only to chemotherapy ($P < 0.001$). Nineteen patients failing both modalities presented a median survival of 11.6 months. In 78 patients who received only chemotherapy, without prior endocrine treatment, the survival in 54 who responded was significantly longer (29.0 months) than in 24 patients who failed (6.3 months) ($P < 0.001$). There were no significant differences in survival in both groups CF → CFPMV → CA or CFP → CFPMV → CA. The median survival from the onset of metastasis was 28.3 and 30.1 months in each group respectively ($P > 0.1$).

DISCUSSION

The present data confirm our previous studies, in which we were able to demonstrate that a two- or three-drug regimen is as effective as five-drug combination chemotherapy (Rosner et al. 1976, Rosner et al. 1978). Furthermore, we have found that the five-drug regimen used as second-line chemotherapy retains its effectiveness, even if used after CF or CFP. In a prior study, we have shown that the five-drug combination of CFPMV was significantly more effective than the MV or MVP regimens used after the patient has had CF or CFP (Rosner et al. 1979). Our findings suggest that the previously used drugs, C and F, may enhance the drug effects of M and V given as secondary chemotherapy in the five-drug regimen. The same potentiating effect was noticed in the third-line chemotherapy in which the use of C enhanced the effectiveness of A. In a prior randomized trial in which A alone was used in the second- and third-line chemotherapy following the CFP regimen, the response to A was 16% (Rosner et al. 1974). The previously used drugs, C and F, seemed to enhance the effect of the newly added drugs, MVP and A, in subsequent combinations.

Recycling previously used drugs in effective noncross-resistant regimens provides the opportunity for further responses and significantly prolongs the survival. Other investigators have shown that retreatment with the same chemotherapeutic agents at high doses results in objective remission in 40% of the patients (Buzdar et al. 1981).

The exploitation of this potentiating effect of previously used drugs in subsequent regimens may provide significant improvements over treatment options now available.

Our study has demonstrated antitumor activity for each of the chemotherapy combinations used sequentially, as first- (CF or CFP), second- (CFPMV), or third- (CA) line chemotherapy. Furthermore, it was shown that these regimens are effective and noncross-resistant. The use of initial regimens of less aggressive nature offered responses similar to those obtained with more aggressive combinations. Using a less aggressive regimen avoids premature exhaustion of most active drugs available (Rosner and Nemoto, 1979).

In an ongoing randomized study we have attempted to determine whether the duration of response and survival of patients with metastatic breast cancer can be altered by changing the order of sequential combination chemotherapy regimens, either starting with a five-drug regimen or an Adriamycin combination or a three-drug regimen. Each of the three combinations in this study (CFP-CFPMV-CA) has been used in three groups as a primary, secondary, or tertiary form of chemotherapy.

Our present study confirms our previous observations (Rosner et al. 1980) that the presence or absence of ER in metastatic breast cancer does not predict the response to chemotherapy. This lack of correlation between the ER status and response to cytotoxic chemotherapy has many implications for the therapy of patients with metastatic breast cancer. Patients with ER-positive or ER-unknown tumors can benefit initially from the use of endocrine therapy without precluding further response to chemotherapy at the time of relapse or failure of the disease. The best survival in our series was observed in the subset of patients responding to both modalities, endocrine and chemotherapy. Manni et al. (1981) showed that sequential endocrine therapy and chemotherapy is highly effective in the treatment of advanced breast cancer and offers prolonged survival to patients with hormone responsive tumors. Legha et al. (1979), in analyzing a group of patients with metastatic breast cancer who achieved CR with combination chemotherapy, founded the longest remission in a subset of patients treated with oophorectomy and chemotherapy.

In an incurable disease, in which improvement of life quality of patients is of prime importance and all therapies are palliative, the rational approach would be to offer more therapeutic modalities given sequentially in the presence of progressive metastatic disease.

Our data suggest that more than one treatment strategy will be required to optimize survival of patients with metastatic breast cancer (Rosner 1982, Rosner and Nemoto 1982).

The use of subsequent modalities (hormonal and chemotherapy), as well as recycling previously used drugs in effective noncross-resistant regimens, provides the opportunity for further responses and significantly prolongs the survival by avoiding premature exhaustion of therapeutic modalities.

REFERENCES

Buzdar, A., S. S. Legha, G. N. Hortobagyi, H-Y. Yap, C. L. Wiseman, A. Distefano, F. C. Schell, B. C. Barnes, L. T. Campos, and G. R. Blumenschein. 1981. Management of breast cancer patients failing adjuvant chemotherapy with Adriamycin-containing regimens. Cancer 47:2798–2802.

Chlebowski, R. T., I. E. Lowell, R. P. Pugh, L. Sadoff, R. Hestorff, J. M. Wiener, and J. R. Bateman. 1979. Survival of patients with metastatic breast cancer treated with either combination or sequential chemotherapy. Cancer Res. 39:4503–4506.

Hayward, J. L., R. D. Rubens, P. Carbone, J. C. Heuson, S. Kumaoka, and A. Segaloff. 1977. Assessment of response to therapy in advanced breast cancer. Br. J. Cancer 35:292–298.

Legha, S. S., A. Buzdar, T. L. Smith, G. Hortobagyi, K. Swenerton, G. Blumenschein, E. A. Gehan, G. Bodey, and E. J Freireich. 1979. Complete remission in metastatic breast cancer treated with combination drug therapy. Ann. Intern. Med. 91:847–852.

Manni, A., O. H. Pearson, J. S. Marshall, and B. M. Arafah. 1981. Sequential endocrine therapy and chemotherapy in metastatic breast cancer: Effects on survival. Breast Cancer Research and Treatment 1:97–103.

Powles, T. J., I. E. Smith, H. T. Ford, R. C. Coombes, J. M. Jones, and J. C. Gazet. 1980. Failure of chemotherapy to prolong survival in a group of patients with metastatic breast cancer. Lancet 1:580–582.

Rosencweig, M., M. J. Staquet, D. D. Von Hoff, J. C. Heuson, and F. M. Muggia. 1979. Prognostic factors for the response to chemotherapy in advanced breast cancer. Cancer Clin. Trials 2:165–169.

Rosner, D. 1982. Recycling prior used drugs in sequential combination chemotherapy enhances response and survival in metastatic breast cancer. (Abstract) Proc. Am. Soc. Clin. Oncol. 1:72.

Rosner, D., T. Dao, J. Horton, T. Cunningham, R. Diaz, S. Taylor, G. Rosenbaum, and V. Vatanasapt. 1974. Randomized study of Adriamycin (ADM) vs. combined therapy (FCP) vs. adrenalectomy (ADX) in breast cancer. (Abstract) Proc. Am. Soc. Clin. Oncol. 15:63.

Rosner, D., and T. Nemoto. 1979. Sequence for developing optimal combination chemotherapy of metastatic breast cancer. Eur. J. Cancer 15:1197–1201.

Rosner, D., and T. Nemoto. 1982. Optimal sequential chemotherapy for metastatic breast cancer: Effects on survival. Current Chemotherapy and Immunotherapy 2:1488–1490.

Rosner, D., T. Nemoto, and T. Dao. 1976. Combination chemotherapy in the treatment of advanced breast cancer. J. Surg. Oncol. 8:465–469.

Rosner, D., T. Nemoto, and T. Dao. 1978. Combination chemotherapy with five, three, or two agents in metastatic breast cancer. Current Chemotherapy and Immunotherapy 2:1067–1069.

Rosner, D., T. Nemoto, and J. Uribe. 1980. Estrogen receptors and responses to combination chemotherapy in metastatic breast cancer: Results of a prospective randomized study. Current Chemotherapy and Infectious Disease 2:1672–1673.

Rosner, D., M. Sneiderman, and T. Nemoto. 1979. Potentiating role of previously administered agents in the combination chemotherapy of breast cancer. Oncology 36:160–163.

CYTOKINETIC AND CYTOMETRIC MEASUREMENTS IN BREAST CANCER

Current Controversies in Breast Cancer, edited
by F. C. Ames, G. R. Blumenschein, and E. D. Montague.
University of Texas Press, Austin © 1984.

Tumor Cell Kinetic Studies in Animal Models Can Aid the Design of Human Tumor Treatments

Lewis M. Schiffer, M.D., and Paul G. Braunschweiger, Ph.D.

Department of Experimental Therapeutics, AMC Cancer Research Center and Hospital, Lakewood, Colorado

It is rare for a novel idea or technique to proceed directly from its original biologic application, usually tissue culture, to human usage without first undergoing extensive studies in intact animals, yet clinicians have been known to downgrade small-animal studies as being "nonapplicable" to humans. This appears to be a common occurrence in grant application peer reviews and reflects a generally poor understanding of the nature of in vivo animal studies. When performed properly, small-animal studies can be every bit as enlightening as human clinical trials, although one must be cognizant of species differences and differences in tumor biology. The advantage of animal studies lies in the fact that the investigator is working with intact physiologic, biochemical, and hormonal systems, with all the variables they imply. In tumor work one also has the immunologic background of the host, tumor heterogeneity, and tumor vascular aberrations to contend with. Rather than representing a myriad of uncontrolled variables, these animal systems, when appropriately applied, can be used expeditiously in experiments that are logistically difficult or impossible to do in a clinical setting. Background information on some clinical concepts derived from chemotherapy studies with animals has recently been reviewed (Goldin and Schabel 1981).

The studies presented here represent one aspect of tumor biology studies in intact animals and were planned so that the conceptual aspects of the results could be extrapolated and tested in a clinical setting.

METHODS

The methods we have developed over the years have been fully published. Briefly, they consist of treating intact animals that have solid tumors with a variety of drugs or physical insults, or both, and then sampling the tumors by excisional biopsy to determine changes in cell kinetic parameters. Analysis of these changes then allows us to identify intervals that, from a kinetic standpoint, could be efficacious for sequencing subsequent treatments. In studies designed to assess the significance of these kinetic changes for the design of therapeutic strategies, our goals have been tumor size reduction, regrowth delay, or animal survival, depending upon the experiment. The cell kinetic techniques used in these studies were designed to have potential clinical application if tumor biopsy specimens were available. Thus, all kinetic studies are done after the biopsy and do not entail giving animals isotopically lableled compounds. The tumors used usually represent late-stage disease, where the tumor growth rate is decelerating (i.e., the plateau of the Gompertzian curve). Drug availability, intratumor drug distribution, and tumor heterogeneity cannot, obviously, be controlled. However, this scenario mimics the clinical situation in which patients are treated with antitumor agents.

The in vitro cell kinetic techniques we utilize are: ^{3}H-TdR labeling index (TLI) (Braunschweiger et al. 1976), the passage of cells from S to G2 phase (which in unperturbed systems can be used to estimate DNA synthesis time) (Braunschweiger et al. 1976), and the PDP index (PDPI), an estimate of tumor growth fraction (GF) (Nelson and Schiffer 1973, Schiffer et al. 1976b). The latter stands for primer-dependent DNA polymerase index, and in unperturbed systems reliably estimates tumor GF. When available, measurements of mitotic index and calculations of average cell cycle time and potential doubling of the tumor can be performed. Since kinetic endpoints are determined by autoradiography, a lag time of 1 to 14 days is usual. At about the same time we were developing these techniques, other investigators were developing flow microfluorometry systems and applications. These systems are faster than autoradiographic analysis and can often produce similar kinetic data. For solid tumors, however, this method must be used with tissue dispersion, cell separation, and labeling techniques.

UNPERTURBED SYSTEMS

As part of the initial evaluation of in vitro techniques, we studied extensively the kinetics of the C3H/He spontaneous mouse mammary tumor (Braunschweiger et al. 1977). We have characterized this system, using hundreds of animals, with tumors of different sizes and ages. There is clear evidence of gross tumor heterogeneity in tumor cell kinetics as measured by our techniques, despite the similarity of the highly inbred host. This has profound significance for the clinic, since one can expect much greater variation in human tumor kinetics. In fact, in our studies of human tumors (Schiffer et al. 1979) this was confirmed (Table 1). Imagine the expected variation of response when one treats with S-phase active agents 100 patients who have mammary tumors when the fraction of cells in S phase varies from < 1% to 35%. If nothing else, our studies make one pause to consider the usual rationale in treatment designs and how to improve them.

Other findings produced by our techniques in this unperturbed system include correlation of cell kinetic patterns with tumor growth characteristics and correlations among the cell kinetic characteristics themselves (Braunschweiger et al. 1977). These had been speculated upon, but were never really shown to exist in a large group of similar tumors. Several examples of these correlations are shown

Table 1. *Measure of Mammary Tumor Cell Kinetic Heterogeneity** *in Rodent Models and Human Tumors*

Tumor	TLI[†]	DNA Synthesis Time	Growth Fraction (PDP Index)	Cell Cycle Time
Transplantable				
C3H/S102F	1.4	1.1	1.3	1.3
C3H/67-A	2.3	1.2	1.6	2.3
13762/F344[‡]	1.4	1.1	1.2	1.3
First-generation				
C3H/HeJ[§]	3.9		2.8	
Spontaneous				
C3H/HeJ	2.3	1.3	2.1	1.8
CD8F₁	4.4		6.3	
DMBA/SD[‡]	6.3	1.5	4.1	3.6
Human, primary	68.6	1.7	35.1	31.4
Human, metastatic	3.8	1.5	8.2	3.6

*Maximum value/minimum value in a series of individual tumors.
[†]3H-TdR labeling index.
[‡]Rat tumors.
[§]Values depend upon the kinetics of spontaneous C3H/HeJ tumors that were transplanted.

below. In Figure 1, it can be seen that the TLI of the tumor cell population increases as the volume doubling time decreases. Figure 2 shows that there is a direct relationship between TLI and the growth fraction, as estimated by the PDPI. While these results do not directly aid in designing human treatments, they have been verified in human tumors and should give the clinician reason to pause to consider their implications (Schiffer et al. 1979).

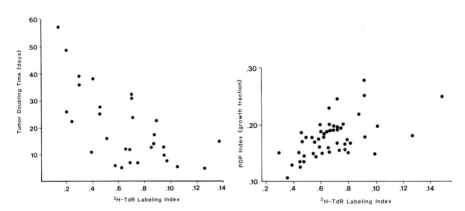

FIG. 1. Relationship between tumor doubling time (days) and ³H-TdR labeling index in spontaneous C3H/HeJ mammary tumors.

FIG. 2. Relationship between PDP index (growth fraction) and ³H-TdR labeling index in spontaneous C3H/HeJ mammary tumors.

Treatment Value of Unperturbed Cell Kinetics

If one could take a biopsy specimen of a human tumor and, on the basis of one or more tests, accurately determine whether the tumor would respond to a specific treatment, one could design individual treatment programs. We addressed this problem with two animal tumor models, the spontaneous C3H/HeJ and the dimethylbenzanthracene (DMBA) induced mammary tumor of the Sprague-Dawley rat.

The experimental approach was to perform needle biopsies of primary tumors, perform in vitro cell kinetic assays on the biopsy specimens, and then 3 days later treat the tumor-bearing animals with either 5-fluorouracil, cyclophosphamide, methotrexate, doxorubicin, or vincristine. Prior to biopsy the volumetric tumor doubling time was determined for each tumor. After drug treatment, tumor response was assessed by percent tumor regression, rate of tumor regression, rate of tumor regrowth, and regrowth delay.

The response parameters were then compared with the pretreatment kinetic parameters, tumor doubling time, TLI, PDPI, potential doubling time, cell cycle time, and cell loss to detect significant prognostic correlations. The responses of at least 45 tumors of each type were assessed for each drug studied.

The results indicated that the response of mammary tumors to chemotherapeutic agents is extremely heterogeneous. Pretreatment cell kinetic parameters may be useful as prognostic indicators of initial treatment efficacy for some agents. For example, in C3H/HeJ spontaneous mammary tumors, the TLI was predictive for response to doxorubicin, vincristine, methotrexate, and 5-fluorouracil, but not for cyclophosphamide. In DMBA-induced tumors, a good response to doxorubicin and vincristine was correlated with a high TLI. Doxorubicin, vincristine, and 5-fluorouracil were most often correlated with one or more kinetic parameters, while the responses to cyclophosphamide and methotrexate usually did not correlate well with the pretreatment cell kinetics. Our data for doxorubicin, vincristine, and 5-fluorouracil do indicate that the rapidly proliferating tumors (i.e., high TLI, high GF, and short Tc) are most responsive to therapy. The data would also seem to indicate that pretreatment cell kinetics is not the only, and probably not the main, determinant of chemosensitivity. These data indicate to us that pretreatment analysis of human tumor cell kinetics may have some treatment value (depending upon the tumor and the drugs involved), but that verification would be required from patient biopsy specimens. This would entail a major clinical study involving hundreds of patients, and it is doubtful that it could be accomplished today. A repeat of the animal study, using different models, might be an appropriate follow-up experiment.

TREATMENT-INDUCED PERTURBATIONS IN ANIMAL MODELS

The administration of an insult to a tumor-bearing animal, whether it be an antineoplastic drug, radiation, or other agent, generally causes suppression of tumor cell proliferation followed by a period of relative quiescence, followed by an interval of proliferative recovery. The magnitude and timing of these stages are insult, dose, tumor, and host dependent.

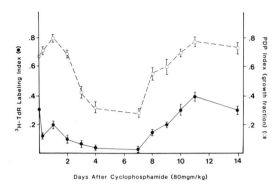

FIG. 3. Sequence of cell kinetic changes in 13762 mammary tumor in Fischer 344 rat following a single dose of 80 mg/kg cyclophosphamide. ³H-TdR labeling index (●), and PDP index growth fraction (○).

For example, the 13762 mammary tumor in the Fischer 344 rat was, at one time, considered a model for human mammary tumors because it responded to similar drugs. However, unlike human tumors, it is rapidly growing with a high GF, a high TLI, and a short cell cycle time (Braunschweiger and Schiffer 1978b). Administration of cyclophosphamide, at a dose of 80 mg/kg, causes marked reduction in tumor volume and a profound change in the tumor cell kinetics (Figure 3). Recovery is measurable by our techniques by day 8 after initial treatment, and recovery peaks at day 11.

The growth of the C3H/He spontaneous mammary tumor can be suppressed by administration of high-dose corticosteroids (Braunschweiger et al. 1978). The mechanism of action appears to be blockade of tumor cells in the G1 phase. There is a reduction of TLI of about 50% caused by methylprednisilone given every 12 hours. When the methylprednisilone is withdrawn, there is a large increase in the number of tumor cells found in S phase (Figure 4, lower portion). This increase of

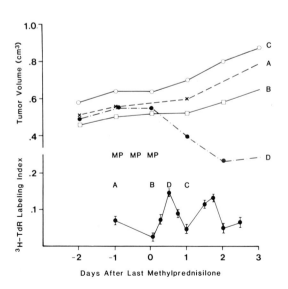

FIG. 4. Lower portion: Sequence of changes of ³H-TdR labeling index in spontaneous C3H/HeJ mammary tumors after administration of methylprednisilone (MP), 10 mg/kg q 12 hours. Upper portion: Tumor volume changes, measured by caliper in (A) control animals (X); (B) animals treated with MP, then methotrexate (MTX), 6 mg/kg, and 5-fluorouracil (5-FU), 42 mg/kg, 2 hours after the last MP (□); (C) animals treated with MP and then MTX + 5-FU 24 hours after the last MP (○); (D) animals treated with MP and then MTX + 5-FU 12 hours after the last MP (●).

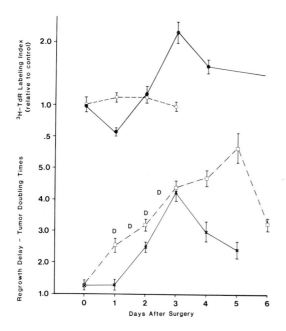

FIG. 5. Upper portion: Sequence of changes of ³H-TdR labeling index (TLI) (relative to control) in residual tumor after surgical removal of ¾ of first-generation mammary tumor (●). (○) represents TLI changes in tumor after sham surgery. Lower portion: Regrowth delay (X), expressed in tumor doubling time, in the same system when vincristine, 1 mg/kg, and 5-fluorouracil, 84 mg/kg, were given at various days after surgery. Peak regrowth delay corresponds with peak TLI after surgery. Regrowth delays from surgery alone have been subtracted. Regrowth delay in the same system but with dexamethasone (D), 10 mg/kg q 12 hours × 4 doses (□), results in suppression of peak proliferation recovery for 2 days.

cells in S phase is probably not caused by new cellular growth but by a cohort of G1-blocked cells moving into S phase.

Surgical removal of part of a first-generation transplanted C3H/He mammary tumor causes a short diminution of TLI followed by a marked increase in TLI over surgical control values (Braunschweiger et al. 1982). The peak TLI varies with the amount of tumor removed and the tumor-host model utilized for study. For example, ¾ removal results in peak proliferative recovery at 3 days after surgery (Figure 5, upper portion).

Treatment Planning Using Perturbed Cell Kinetics

An extremely important observation made in conjunction with the above studies is that sequential treatment with the same or different agents at the time of proliferative recovery, or at the time of progression of G1-blocked cells, results in considerably better tumor control than if treatments were administered at other times. Using the three examples mentioned previously, we observed the following.

In the case of 13762 tumor, administration of another dose of cyclophosphamide at 9 days (when reproliferation is proceeding) results in a complete response (CR) rate of 80% and 30% long-term survivors (LTS) (greater than 100 days), rather than the 25% CR and 5% LTS produced by a single dose (Braunschweiger and Schiffer 1978b). Administration of another dose of cyclophosphamide in another 9 days results in 100% CR and 100% LTS. Design of a curative schedule with this drug is made possible by using cell kinetic techniques and could not easily have been achieved by trial and error alone.

In the C3H/He spontaneous tumor model treated with methylprednisilone, there was a peak of cells in S phase 12 hours after stopping the corticosteroid. When the animals were treated with cytotoxic drugs (in this case methotrexate, 6 mg/kg, and 5-fluorouracil, 42 mg/kg) at various times after stopping the corticosteroid, the best response (60% tumor regression) was seen at 12 hours, corresponding to the peak of cells in S phase (Figure 4, upper portion). There was exquisite time sensitivity, with no significant responses seen at the times of administration of the last steroid or at 24 hours after cessation of the steroid (Braunschweiger et al. 1978).

A similar finding is noted with the last example. Administration of vincristine (1 mg/kg) and 5-fluorouracil (84 mg/kg) in combination at various times after ¾ surgical removal of first-generation mammary tumor results in the best regrowth delay, by a factor of almost 4, at 3 days after surgery (Figure 5, lower portion)—the time of peak proliferative recovery (Braunschweiger et al. 1982). This timing can be extended by administering corticosteroids (dexamethasone) after surgery to suppress proliferation.

Similar observations using other drugs and insults, and in other tumor systems, have been made (Schiffer et al. 1976a, Braunschweiger and Schiffer 1978a, Schiffer et al. 1978, Stragand et al. 1979, Braunschweiger et al. 1979, Braunschweiger and Schiffer 1979, Braunschweiger and Schiffer 1980a, Braunschweiger and Schiffer 1980b, Braunschweiger et al. 1981, Braunschweiger and Schiffer 1981, Braunschweiger et al. 1982, Stragand et al. 1982). These results provide the conceptual rationale for testing kinetically based time sequencing strategies at the clinical level. The major problem, of course, is logistical in that state-of-the-art direct tumor measurements require multiple biopsies. While these could be performed in some patients with easily accessible lesions, the vast majority of situations demand either a noninvasive means to detect tumor cell proliferation or mathematical models and reliable chemosensitivity assays to predict proliferative recovery time lines. Both avenues of investigation are being explored by us and other investigators. Studies by Lippman et al. (1982) and Allegra et al. (1982) using tamoxifen to suppress proliferation and an estrogen (Premarin) to subsequently rescue the cells blocked in G1, followed by cytotoxic drugs to kill cells moving in a cohort through S phase, have been completed or are in progress. Livingston and Groppe, together with us (personal communication), designed a clinical study using high-dose prednisone followed by cyclophosphamide, doxorubicin, and tamoxifen, which was based on the results from our animal studies mentioned above. It is being evaluated by the Southwest Oncology Group.

CONCLUSIONS

It is clear that there are potential alternatives to the presently accepted rationale for the design of therapeutic strategies. These alternatives, which utilize the same drugs but are administered sequentially in a logical fashion, can best be explored and tested in animal models prior to human evaluation. A prematurely conducted clinical trial purporting to test kinetically based sequential therapy may meet with failure not because the conceptual aspects of the animal work are flawed, but because logistical considerations and biologic uncertainties were applied incorrectly or arbitrarily. Although we have used changes in cell kinetic parameters to model timed-sequential strategies, other biologic phenomena associated with cytotoxic perturbation and recovery may prove equally cogent, logistically easier, and of increased clinical utility.

ACKNOWLEDGMENTS

These investigations were supported by Grants CA 27233, CA 26020, and BCTF contracts CB-43899 and CB-74083, awarded by the National Cancer Institute, U.S. Department of Health and Human Services.

REFERENCES

Allegra, J. C., T. M. Woodcock, S. P. Richman, K. I. Bland, and J. L. Wittliff. 1982. A phase II evaluation of tamoxifen, Premarin, methotrexate and 5-fluorouracil in stage IV breast cancer. (Abstract 1037) J. Cell. Biochem., Supp 6:367.

Braunschweiger, P. G., L. Poulakos, and L. M. Schiffer. 1976. In vitro labeling and gold activation autoradiography for determination of labeling index and DNA synthesis times of solid tumors. Cancer Res. 36:1748–1753.

Braunschweiger, P. G., L. Poulakos, and L. M. Schiffer. 1977. Cell kinetics in vivo and in vitro for C3H/He spontaneous mammary tumors. JNCI 59:1197–1204.

Braunschweiger, P. G., L. L. Schenken, and L. M. Schiffer. 1979. The cytokinetic basis for the design of efficacious radiotherapy protocols. Int. J. Radiat. Oncol. Biol. Phys. 5:37–47.

Braunschweiger, P. G., L. L. Schenken, and L. M. Schiffer. 1981. Kinetically directed combination therapy with Adriamycin and x-irradiation in a mammary tumor model. Int. J. Radiat. Oncol. Biol. Phys. 7:747–754.

Braunschweiger, P.G., and L. M. Schiffer. 1978a. Cell kinetics after vincristine treatment of C3H/He spontaneous mammary tumors: Implications for therapy. JNCI 60:1043–1048.

Braunschweiger, P. G., and L. M. Schiffer. 1978b. Therapeutic implications of cell kinetic changes after cyclophosphamide treatment in "spontaneous" and "transplantable" mammary tumors. Cancer Treat. Rep. 62:727–736.

Braunschweiger, P. G., and L. M. Schiffer. 1979. The effect of methylprednisolone on the cell kinetic response of C3H/HeJ mammary tumors to cyclophosphamide and Adriamycin. Cancer Res. 39:3812–3815.

Braunschweiger, P. G., and L. M. Schiffer. 1980a. The effect of Adriamycin on the cell kinetics of 13762 rat mammary tumors and implications for therapy. Cancer Treat. Rep. 64:293–300.

Braunschweiger, P. G., and L. M. Schiffer. 1980b. Cell kinetically based combination chemotherapy of T1699 mammary tumors with Adriamycin and cyclophosphamide. Cancer Res. 40:737–743.

Braunschweiger, P. G., and L. M. Schiffer. 1981. Antiproliferative effects of corticosteroids in C3H/HeJ mammary tumors and implications for sequential combination chemotherapy. Cancer Res. 41:3324–3330.

Braunschweiger, P. G., L. M. Schiffer, and S. Betancourt. 1982. Tumor cell proliferation and sequential chemotherapy after partial tumor resection in C3H/HeJ mammary tumors. Breast Cancer Research and Treatment 2:323–329.

Braunschweiger, P. G., J. J. Stragand, and L. M. Schiffer. 1978. Effect of methylprednisolone on cell proliferation in C3H/HeJ spontaneous mammary tumors. Cancer Res. 38:4510–4514.

Goldin, A., and F. M. Schabel. 1981. Clinical concepts derived from animal chemotherapy studies. Cancer Treat. Rep. 65:11–19.

Lippman, M. E., J. Cassidy, M. Wesley, and R. C. Young. 1982. A randomized attempt to increase the efficacy of cytotoxic chemotherapy in metastatic breast cancer by hormonal synchronization. (Abstract) Am. Soc. Clin. Oncol. 1:79.

Nelson, J. S. R., and L. M. Schiffer. 1973. Autoradiographic detection of DNA polymerase containing nuclei in sarcoma 180 ascites cells. Cell Tissue Kinet. 6:45–54.

Schiffer, L. M., P. G. Braunschweiger, and L. Poulakos. 1976a. Rapid methods for utilizing cell kinetics for treatment in the C3H/He spontaneous mammary tumor: Effects of vincristine. Cancer Treat. Rep. 60:1913–1924.

Schiffer, L. M., P. G. Braunschweiger, and J. J. Stragand. 1978. Tumor cell population kinetics following noncurative treatment, *in* Antibiotics and Chemotherapy, Fundamentals in Cancer Chemotherapy, (Tenth International Congress of Chemotherapy, 1977) S. Karger, Basel, Switzerland, pp. 148–156.

Schiffer, L. M., P. G. Braunschweiger, J. J. Stragand, and L. Poulakos. 1979. The cell kinetics of human mammary cancers. Cancer 43:1707–1719.

Schiffer, L. M., A. M. Markoe, and J. S. R. Nelson. 1976b. Estimation of tumor growth fraction in murine tumors by the primer-available DNA-dependent DNA polymerase assay. Cancer Res. 36:2415–2418.

Stragand, J. J., P. G. Braunschweiger, A. A. Pollice, and L. M. Schiffer. 1979. Cell kinetic alterations in murine mammary tumors following fasting and refeeding. Eur. J. Cancer 15:281–286.

Stragand, J. J., B. Drewinko, B. Barlogie, N. Papadopoulous, and R. A. White. 1982. Serial analysis of melanoma growth kinetics in a patient receiving bleomycin and procarbazine therapy: Comparison of tumor volume, flow cytometry and thymidine labeling techniques. Cancer Treat. Rep. 66:529–534.

Current Controversies in Breast Cancer, edited
by F. C. Ames, G. R. Blumenschein, and E. D. Montague.
University of Texas Press, Austin © 1984.

Cytokinetic Analysis of Breast Carcinoma: Implications for Adjuvant Cytotoxic Therapy for Patients with Negative Nodes

John S. Meyer, M.D.

*Department of Pathology, The Jewish Hospital of St. Louis, St. Louis, Missouri, and
Washington University School of Medicine, St. Louis, Missouri*

Breast carcinomas can be classified into several types morphologically, but a large group is difficult to subdivide and has been referred to as "infiltrating ductal carcinoma." This term has often been loosely applied in that not all carcinomas so designated form ductal structures. Presumably the carcinomas are all derived from ducts, but even from this point of view the term "ductal" can be confusing because it can mean the larger, postlobular ducts as distinguished from the smaller, terminal ductal coil of the lobule, which often is referred to simply as the "lobule." Therefore, we prefer to designate the large residual group of infiltrating carcinomas, as suggested by Fisher and associates (Fisher et al. 1975), as "carcinoma, not otherwise specified" (NOS).

Most of the special types of infiltrating carcinoma of the breast have distinctive clinical characteristics that affect patient survival patterns. Adenocystic and tubular carcinomas rarely metastasize, even to regional lymph nodes (Friedman and Oberman 1970, Deos and Norris 1982, McDivitt et al. 1982), nor do mucinous and papillary carcinomas (Haagensen 1971a, Fisher et al. 1980a). Controversy exists about the relative malignancy of infiltrating lobular (small cell) and medullary carcinomas, but relapses of medullary carcinomas appear to be restricted to a period of approximately 5 years after mastectomy (Ridolfi et al. 1977), whereas the rate of relapse for infiltrating lobular carcinoma does not differ strikingly from that of infiltrating breast carcinomas in general (Adair et al. 1974, Ashikari et al. 1973, Haagensen 1971b).

Beyond the histologic type of the carcinoma, microscopic characteristics including invasiveness, nuclear characteristics, and cell to cell relations (histologic differentiation) have been examined to determine patient prognosis (Black et al. 1975, Nealon et al. 1979). A problem that arises is lack of an objective grading system for these characteristics, which leads to variability among observers (Delides et al. 1982). The most powerful prognostic finding obtained by pathologic examination has been the axillary lymph node status (Fisher et al. 1980b). While the number of

Table 1. *Relapse Rates for Patients with No Lymph Node Metastases in Radical or Modified Radical Mastectomy Specimens*

Author	No. of Pts.	Interval at Risk	Percent Survival*	
			Relapse-free	Unconditional
Albano et al. 1979	62	5 yr.	77%	70%
Crowe et al. 1982	510	5 yr.	76%	
Fisher et al. 1980b	266	5 yr.	87%	
Lacour et al. 1976	631	5 yr.	87%	
Nealon et al. 1979	203	5 yr.	71%	
Nemoto et al. 1980	1,608	5 yr.	65%	
Sears et al. 1982	275	5 yr.	82%	
Schottenfeld et al. 1976	147	5 yr.		86%
Valagussa et al. 1978	335	5 yr.	79%	
Albano et al. 1979	62	10 yr.	55%	46%
Haagensen 1971c	484	10 yr.		75%
Schottenfeld et al. 1976	147	10 yr.		71%
Valagussa et al. 1978	335	10 yr.	72%	

*Mean of 5-year relapse-free survival rates = 78%.

axillary lymph nodes containing metastases correlates inversely with relapse-free survival rates, nearly one-half of mastectomy specimens reveal no nodal metastases. If one or more nodes contain metastases, the probability of short-term relapse is sufficient to merit trials of systemic therapy.

A good deal of experimental evidence exists to show that cytotoxic agents kill neoplastic cells according to first-order kinetics, meaning that a given dose will kill a given fraction of any number of cells present. Large numbers of cells are eliminated with more difficulty than small numbers (Skipper 1971, Schabel 1977). Therefore, adjuvant cytotoxic treatment of breast carcinoma should succeed most often in populations of patients with few residual neoplastic cells. Measurements of numbers of residual cells after local primary treatment of breast carcinoma have not been made, but intuition suggests that the number would increase as evidence of local spread increased. Smaller residual burdens should be present after primary local treatment in patients with no pathologically detectable axillary metastases than in patients with axillary metastases. This concept is reinforced by higher success rates with adjuvant cytotoxic therapy in patients with one to three positive axillary nodes in comparison to those with more than three (Bonadonna and Valagussa 1981). With these considerations in mind, the group most likely to be cured by adjuvant cytotoxic therapy would appear to be patients with negative nodes who nevertheless are destined to experience relapse. However, the relapse-free survival rates for these patients within 5 years after radical surgical treatment in recent studies have been 65% to 87% (Table 1). A method for identification of a high-risk subset is needed. We will review evidence indicating that most of the patients destined to relapse early have carcinomas with high proliferative indices.

PROLIFERATIVE RATE MEASURED BY THYMIDINE LABELING OR FLOW CYTOMETRY

The S-phase duration of breast carcinomas and of most human neoplasms appears to be approximately 18 hours, whereas the duration of morphologically recognizable mitosis is only about 1 hour. Therefore, a tumor contains more than 10 times as many S-phase cells as mitotic figures. In the case of most breast carcinomas, the mitotic count is too low for accurate quantitation. This difficulty is compounded by the risk of confusing nuclear artifacts with mitoses. A thymidine labeling index (TLI) derived from a sample of 2,000 cells gives more reliable information than is obtainable from a mitotic count of 10,000 cells (Table 2).

The TLI is performed on fresh tissue by incubation with tritiated thymidine, [³H]dThd. We have found 2 hours to be the optimum duration of incubation at 37°C in balanced salt solution with agitation. Adequate uptake of the labeled DNA precursor is insured by presence of an agent to block thymidylate synthetase, such as 5-fluoro-2'-deoxyuridine (Dörmer et al. 1975, Meyer and Facher 1977). Hyperbaric oxygen at 3 to 4 atm is necessary to ensure uptake beneath the surface of the tissue slices (Fabrikant et al. 1969). The slices, which must be less than 1-mm thick, are cut freehand from the viable periphery of the tumor, and the details of the procedure are carried out as described previously (Meyer and Connor, 1977).

The TLI of breast carcinoma reflects the method used in its measurement. When hyperbaric oxygen and a thymidylate synthetase blocker were not used, the means have been relatively low, but a wide spread of values has still been obtained (Table 3). All studies of the TLI of primary breast carcinomas agree that the TLI is lognormally distributed (Figure 1). High TLI have consistently been associated with youth and premenopausal status (Meyer et al. 1978, Schiffer et al. 1979, Meyer and Hixon 1979, Bertuzzi et al. 1981), but these variables are not major determinants of the TLI, and broad distributions occur in various age and menopausal groups. We have recently analyzed our data from 278 patients and have found no significant relationship between the TLI of the breast carcinoma and the date of the menstrual cycle in 48 premenopausal patients of known menstrual phase. A consistent significant in-

Table 2. *Comparison of Mitotic Index (MI) with Thymidine Labeling Index (TLI) in Breast Carcinoma**

Type of Carcinoma	% MI	% TLI
Adenocystic	0.10	0.62
Infiltrating lobular	0.00	0.75
NOS†	0.08	5.17
NOS	0.29	13.9
Medullary	0.34	14.9

*MI based on count of 10,000 cells; TLI on count of 2,000 cells.
†Carcinoma not otherwise specified ("infiltrating ductal carcinoma").

Table 3. *Reported TLI* of Primary Breast Carcinomas*

Author	No. of Pts.	Method[†]	% TLI Mean	% TLI Geometric Mean	% TLI Median	% TLI Range
Bertuzzi et al. 1981	357	1			2.7	0.01–41
Straus et al. 1980	23	4	6.8			
Sklarew et al. 1977	56	1[‡]	2.4			
Schiffer et al. 1979	67	1[‡]	5.6		4.7	0.50–35
Tubiana et al. 1981	128	1		1.0		
Meyer et al. 1979	128	2	3.7	2.2	2.2	0.04–19
Meyer et al. 1983	278	3	6.7	4.2	4.5	0.05–36

*Thymidine labeling index.
[†] In vitro slices, neither hyperbaric oxygen (HBO) nor thymidylate synthetase blocker (TSB). 2: In vitro slices, HBO. 3: In vitro slices, HBO + TSB. 4: In vivo, neither HBO nor TSB; heavily weighted toward advanced clinical stages.
[‡] Dissociated cells rather than slices.

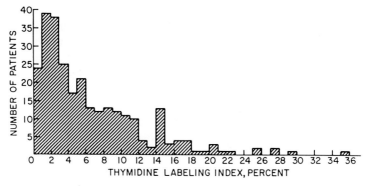

FIG. 1. Distribution of thymidine labeling index of primary breast carcinomas in 278 female patients analyzed in the author's laboratory. Exposure to [³H]dThd was for 2 hours at 37°C in presence of 3 atm oxygen and 1 umol/liter 5-fluoro-2′-deoxyuridine.

verse relationship between content of estrogen receptors (ER) and the TLI of breast carcinoma (Meyer et al. 1978, Silvestrini et al. 1979, Nordenskjöld et al. 1980) can account for the shorter relapse-free intervals that have been noted for ER-negative tumors by several observers (Knight et al. 1977, Maynard et al. 1978, Rich et al. 1978, Meyer et al., in press).

The TLI of breast carcinoma relates consistently to certain histologic characteristics. It has been low in carcinomas with minimal nuclear anaplasia, particularly in those of the mucinous, adenocystic, and tubular types, and in most infiltrating lobular (small cell) carcinomas, but it has been consistently high in medullary carcinomas (Table 4). In the NOS carcinomas, increasing nuclear anaplasia is associated with increasing TLI (Meyer and Hixon 1979, Meyer et al., 1983). The TLI has not shown a significant correlation with size of the primary tumor or the number

Table 4. *Breast Carcinoma Histologic Type and TLI**

Histologic Type	No. Pts.	% TLI Geometric Mean	Range
Adenocystic	3	1.1	0.57–3.9
Mucinous	11	1.0	0.05–2.8
Lobular (small cell)	28	1.5	0.05–9.2
Papillary	2	1.5	0.70–3.1
Tubular	5	1.3	0.40–2.5
Medullary and atypical medullary	23	14.7	7.8–36
NOS[†]	106	4.7	0.09–27
All types	178	4.2	0.05–36

*Thymidine labeling index.
[†]Carcinoma not otherwise specified ("infiltrating ductal carcinoma").

of positive axillary lymph nodes (Meyer et al. 1978, Schiffer et al. 1979, Meyer and Hixon 1979, Tubiana et al. 1981).

Our recent measurements of breast carcinoma thymidine labeling indices contradict earlier impressions that breast carcinomas generally have low proliferative rates. Inclusion of hyperbaric oxygen and blockage of thymidylate synthetase in the labeling regimen result in higher geometric mean and median TLI (Table 3). The effect appears to be principally on the more rapidly proliferating tumors. With and without thymidylate synthetase inhibition, we noted comparable TLI in lobular (small cell), adenocystic, and tubular carcinomas, but, with inhibition, TLI of medullary and NOS carcinomas were distinctly higher (Meyer and Hixon 1979, Meyer et al. 1978).

Flow cytometric DNA measurements have yielded S-phase fraction (SPF) estimates of consistently greater magnitude than reported TLI for breast carcinomas (Table 5). The higher flow cytometric values could reflect detection of cells arrested during the S phase, but scant evidence for S-phase arrest exists. In the inner zones of human spheroid cultures adjacent to the necrotic centers, S-phase arrest could not

Table 5. *DNA Flow Cytometry of Infiltrating Breast Carcinomas*

Source	No. of Pts.	% S-Phase Fraction (SPF) Mean ± Standard Error	Median	Range
Olszewski et al. 1981*	90	9.1 ± 0.7		
Kute et al. 1981*	70	13.7 ± 0.8		
Raber et al. 1982[†]	46	13.2	12.7	2.0–30.5
Author's unpublished data[†]	46	13.4 ± 1.4		2.2–42.3

*Primary operable carcinomas only.
[†]Both primary and metastatic carcinomas.

be demonstrated, and the TLI remained similar to the SPF measured by flow cytometry (Wibe et al. 1981). Under these circumstances of deprivation of nutrients and oxygen, all segments of the cell cycle are prolonged, and in some cases slowing of DNA synthesis could cause [^{3}H]dThd uptakes to fall below the threshold of detection. Nonetheless, the higher SPF values by flow cytometry, in comparison to TLI, more likely result from a combination of other factors. Flow cytometric SPF means based on mixtures of primary and metastatic carcinomas should reflect the higher proliferative rates of metastatic carcinomas (Meyer and Lee 1980). We note that the flow cytometric mean of Olszewski et al. (1981), from primary operable tumors only, is closer to the thymidine labeling results than are the other means obtained by flow cytometry. However, we have compared TLI with SPF measured by flow cytometry in a series of breast carcinomas and have observed a consistent excess of the flow cytometric results over those of thymidine labeling (unpublished data). Furthermore, we have observed the same differences for benign breast tissues. Since S-phase arrest would appear to be unlikely in normal tissues, we believe that our flow cytometric SPF measurements may be erroneously high. Presence of fluorescent debris and binding of dye to cytoplasmic components could be sources of error.

Despite possible technical problems inherent in flow cytometric DNA measurements of breast carcinomas, flow cytometric SPF measurements have shown correlations with histologic features (Olszewski et al. 1981) or ER content (Olszewski et al. 1981, Kute et al. 1981, Raber et al. 1982) of breast carcinoma similar to those established by thymidine labeling. Furthermore, the various flow cytometric studies provide a consensus that breast carcinomas with increased DNA content per cell (DNA index > 1) have decreased rates of ER positivity and higher SPF than those with DNA index = 1 (Bichel et al. 1982) and that an increased DNA index appears to be associated with an increased rate of relapse after primary therapy (Auer et al. 1980).

IMPLICATIONS OF BREAST CARCINOMA CELL KINETICS FOR ADJUVANT CYTOTOXIC CHEMOTHERAPY

The broad spectrum of proliferative indices of primary, infiltrating breast carcinomas implies widely varying growth rates. The actual growth rate of a tumor depends on the rate of cell production and the rate of cell loss by death or transport from the tumor. The rate of production of cells is related to both the SPF or TLI and the S-phase duration (T_s). Steel (1977) has presented a thorough study of these interrelationships. In general, the growth rate of carcinomas and malignant neoplasms slows as the population of cells increases. The cells accumulate at approximately an exponential rate when the tumor is very small, but then the rate of increase plateaus and eventually may become close to zero. This pattern resembles the plot of a Gompertz function (Laird 1964, Simpson-Herren and Lloyd 1970). The principal reason for the slowing of growth of most tumors is increased rates of cell loss (Steel 1977, de Lacroix and Lennartz 1981). The growth fraction (fraction of viable cells in the

Table 6. *Proliferative Index* and Potential* *Doubling Time* $(T_{D_{pot}})^\dagger$

Index (%)	$T_{D_{pot}}$ (days)
0.12	500
0.60	100
1.2	50
4.55	13
6.0	10
12	5
20	3
30	2

*Thymidine labeling index or S-phase fraction.
†Based on $T_s = 18$ hours.

replicative cycle) may decrease, and the T_s may increase during growth (de Lacroix and Lennartz 1981). The latter changes would have counterbalancing effects on the TLI. Since no significant relationship between TLI and size of breast carcinomas has been observed, we believe that the TLI of clinically apparent carcinomas probably are similar to those of microscopic, preclinical tumors. This belief is supported by our unpublished observation that the TLI of the intraductal and infiltrative components of breast carcinomas are similar.

Measurements available at this time suggest that the T_s of breast carcinoma cells approximate 18 hours (Meyer 1981). The formula $T_c = 0.8 \, (T_s/\text{TLI})$ (Steel 1977) can be used to calculate the cell cycle time (T_c), which would approximate the time for doubling of the neoplastic cells if all daughter cells survived in situ and remained in the cell cycle. The resulting theoretical doubling times (T_{Dpot}) that correspond to various TLI are given in Table 6. Because of decreasing growth fraction and increasing rates of cell loss, this relationship would seldom hold true for the rate of cellular accumulation in clinically detectable tumors (Meyer 1981), but it might approximate the conditions in a very small metastasis.

With these ideas in mind, we might construct a model relating the behavior of breast carcinoma under cytotoxic chemotherapy to the TLI. In order to keep the model simple, we would assume no dispersion of cycle-phase durations, no cell loss, a growth fraction of 100%, no kinetic selectivity of chemotherapy, no carry-over or kinetic effects of chemotherapy, and no development of resistant clones. The number of cells is calculated according to $N = N_0 e^{\ln 2(t)}$ in which N is the number at a given time, N_0 is the number at a prior time, e is the base of natural logarithms, and t = the elapsed time divided by T_D. If the cytotoxic therapy were given once monthly and killed 90% of the neoplastic cells each time, the result for selected TLI would be as depicted in Figure 2. One might conceive of the cure of microscopic deposits of breast carcinomas with median TLI (4.55%) and one million cells present if the long duration of therapy required did not permit emergence of resistant cell lines. With a TLI of 1.2% and one million cells at the start of therapy, a micrometastasis might be cured in 7 months. A carcinoma with TLI = 6.64%

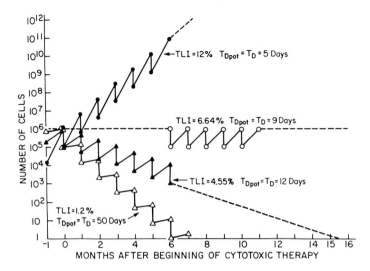

FIG. 2. Simple model relating thymidine labeling index (TLI) to number of neoplastic cells in deposits of breast carcinomas during cytotoxic chemotherapy. The therapy is given once monthly beginning at month zero with resultant one log kill each time. Other assumptions are given in the text. (T_D = doubling time; T_{Dpot} = potential doubling time)

would only be stabilized. Therapy of carcinomas with higher TLI would fail because of kinetic relapse. To prevent kinetic relapse, either a change in schedule or more effective drugs would be needed. The frequency of therapy necessary to achieve stabilization in this model for different TLI is given in Table 7.

The assumptions on which the model is based obviously are not tenable at all

Table 7. *Results from Simple Model of Kinetic Relapse with One Log Kill per Course of Cytotoxic Drugs**

% TLI[†]	$T_{D_{pot}}$[‡] $= T_D$[§] (days)	Treatment Interval for Stabilization (days)
0.12	500	1,660
0.60	100	332
1.2	50	166
4.55	13	43
6.0	10	33
12	5	16
20	3	10
30	2	6

* Assumptions on which this simplified model are based are
   given in the text.
† Thymidine labeling index.
‡ Potential doubling time.
§ Actual doubling time.

times. We would expect changes in cell kinetic variables over time, and size and kinetic characteristics of the tumors should affect cytotoxic cell kill. Nonetheless, the model may help to illustrate ways in which breast carcinoma cell kinetics could affect the success of cytotoxic adjuvant chemotherapy.

SELECTION OF HIGH-RISK GROUP

Histologic assessment, particularly of degree of nuclear anaplasia, ER assay, and the proliferative index have been advanced as means of selection of a population at high risk of early relapse from the group of breast carcinoma patients with negative nodes. Histologic grading systems have elements of subjectivity that impair reproducibility. In most, but not all, studies the ER-negative group of breast carcinomas has shown significantly higher rates of early relapse than the ER-positive group (Table 8). The ER assay therefore may be useful in making the selection.

The inverse association between breast carcinoma ER content and proliferative activity reflected by TLI or SPF is an evident explanation for the prognostic value of ER content. Tubiana et al. (1981), Meyer and Hixon (1979), and Straus and Moran (1980) demonstrated that the TLI is a significant, independent prognostic variable for operable breast carcinoma patients. Two publications (Gentili et al. 1981, Silvestrini et al. 1982) have extended this observation specifically to the group with negative nodes (Table 8). Multivariate analysis of our group of 117 patients with negative nodes showed that the probability of early relapse following mastectomy with axillary lymph node dissection was strongly related to the TLI. Addition of the ER-assay result did not significantly improve prognostic accuracy. Furthermore, in the entire group of operable patients, with negative and positive nodes, the TLI was able to discriminate significantly between groups at high and low risk of early relapse within each ER group. When the patients were first divided by median TLI and then by ER status, the added prognostic effect of ER was only of borderline significance in the low-TLI group and was not significant in the high-TLI group. The probability of relapse within 4 years of primary surgical treatment in the operable group with negative nodes approximated 15% for the subgroup with below-median TLI and 50% for the subgroup with above-median TLI.

We believe that the proliferative index, either TLI or SPF by flow cytometry, is likely to provide the best method of selection of a high-risk group of breast carcinoma patients with negative nodes for adjuvant cytotoxic therapy and that current evidence warrants a trial of such therapy for the group with above-median proliferative indices. These patients will consist of a rather homogeneous kinetic group with rapid rates of neoplastic cellular replication. Therefore, we would advocate a relatively short period of intensive cytotoxic therapy with short intervals between exposure to the cytotoxic agents. A regimen of this type achieved relatively good success in patients with positive nodes (Glucksberg et al. 1982). Comparable or even superior success, because of the possibility of lower tumor cell burdens, could be expected in the patients with negative nodes.

Table 8. *Cytosol ER*, TLI[†], and Relapse-Free Survival of Operable Breast Carcinoma Patients*

Author and Tumor Status	No. of Pts.	Interval of Observation	% Disease-Free[‡]	Significance Value
Knight et al. 1977				
ER-negative	54	18 mo.	63%	<0.05
ER-positive	91	18 mo.	87%	
Maynard et al. 1978				
ER-negative	22	36 mo.	62%	<0.05
ER-positive	130	36 mo.	68%	
Allegra et al. 1979				
ER-negative	79	23 mo.	70%	0.001
ER-positive	103	23 mo.	92%	
Hähnel et al. 1979				
ER-negative	158	30 mo.	~60%	<0.05
ER-positive	177	30 mo.	~66%	
Blamey et al. 1980				
ER-negative	94	3 yr.	58%	N.S.
ER-positive	112	3 yr.	62%	
Furmanski et al. 1980				
ER-negative	219	30 mo.	58%	0.003
ER-positive	203	30 mo.	82%	
Hilf et al. 1980				
ER-negative	56	24 mo.	44%	N.S.
ER-positive	36	24 mo.	54%	
Samaan et al. 1981				
ER-negative	117	3 yr.	76%	<0.05
ER-positive	100	3 yr.	46%	
Westerberg et al. 1980				
ER-negative	70	24 mo.	73%	
ER-positive, low	67	24 mo.	82%	0.03
ER-positive, intermediate	65	24 mo.	85%	
ER-positive, high	68	24 mo.	90%	
Shapiro and Schifeling 1982				
ER-negative	152		82%	N.S.
ER-positive	150		88%	
Sears et al. 1982				
Node-negative only				
ER-negative	68	4 yr.	76%	N.S.
ER-positive	87	4 yr.	87%	
Meyer et al. 1983				
ER-negative	78	3 yr.	50%	0.0001
ER-positive	114	3 yr.	78%	
Tubiana et al. 1982[§]				
TLI high	21	6 yr.	48%	
TLI intermediate	84	6 yr.	55%	<0.05
TLI low	19	6 yr.	79%	
Meyer and Hixon 1979				
TLI above median	57	3 yr.	67%	0.002
TLI below median	62	3 yr.	90%	
Silvestrini et al. 1982[§]				
Node-negative only				
TLI above median	~80	5 yr.	72%	<0.05
TLI below median	~80	5 yr.	90%	

Table 8. *continued*

Author and Tumor Status	No. of Pts.	Interval of Observation	% Disease-Free[‡]	Significance Value
Premenopausal only				
TLI above median	~39	5 yr.	39%	<0.05
TLI below median	~39	5 yr.	88%	
Meyer et al. 1983[#]				
All patients				
TLI above median	115	3 yr.	52%	0.0001
TLI below median	112	3 yr.	85%	
Node-negative				
TLI above median	59	3 yr.	55%	0.0001
TLI below median	58	3 yr.	90%	

[*] Estrogen receptor.
[†] Thymidine labeling index.
[‡] Some figures are approximations from interpretation of relapse-free survival graphs.
[§] In vitro thymidine labeling, neither hyperbaric oxygen nor block of thymidylate synthetase.
[‖] In vitro thymidine labeling, hyperbaric oxygen, no block of thymidylate synthetase.
[#] In vitro thymidine labeling, hyperbaric oxygen, and 5-fluoro-2'-deoxyuridine.

ACKNOWLEDGMENTS

Robert E. Connor, M.D., B. Ramanath Rao, Ph.D., Sue C. Stevens, Ph.D., Walter C. Bauer, M.D., Barbara Hixon, B.S., Jeannette Y. Lee, Ph.D., M. Martha McCrate, B.S., and Ellen Friedman, M.S., participated in the investigations of proliferative indices and receptor assays of breast carcinomas. Rhoda Facher, B.S., Jean Dale, B.S., Laura Googin, B.S., Nancy MacPherson, B.S., Nancy Vandillen, B.S., and Harold Briggs provided technical assistance. Meredith Hammer typed the manuscript. The Jewish Hospital of St. Louis, American Cancer Society Grant 4268IM, and a general research supporting grant from the National Institutes of Health provided financial support.

REFERENCES

Adair, R., J. Berg, L. Joubert, and G. F. Robbins. 1974. Long-term follow-up of breast cancer patients: The 30-year report. Cancer 33:1145–1150.

Albano, W. A., C. D. Hanf, and C. H. Organ, Jr. 1979. Natural history of lymph-node-negative breast cancer. Surgery 86:574–576.

Allegra, J. C., M. E. Lippman, R. Simon, E. B. Thompson, A. Barlock, L. Green, K. K. Huff, H. M. Do, S. C. Aitken, and R. Warren. 1979. The association between steroid hormone receptor status and disease free interval in breast cancer. Cancer Treat. Rep. 8:1271–1277.

Ashikari, R., A. G. Huvos, J. A. Urban, and G. F. Robbins. 1973. Infiltrating lobular carcinoma of the breast. Cancer 31:110–116.

Auer, G. U., T. O. Caspersson, and A. S. Wallgren. 1980. DNA content and survival in mammary carcinoma. Anal. Quant. Cytol. 2:161–165.

Bertuzzi, A., M. G. Diadone, G. Di Fronzo, and R. Silvestrini. 1981. Relationship among estrogen receptors, proliferative activity and menopausal status in breast cancer. Breast Cancer Res. Treat. 1:253–262.

Bichel, P., H. S. Poulsen, and J. Anderson. 1982. Estrogen receptor content and ploidy of human mammary carcinoma. Cancer 50:1771–1774.

Black, M. M., T. H. C. Barclay, and B. F. Hankey. 1975. Prognosis in breast cancer utilizing histologic characteristics of the primary tumor. Cancer 36:2048–2055.

Blamey, R. W., H. M. Bishop, J. R. S. Blake, P. J. Doyle, C. W. Elston, J. L. Haybittle, R. I. Nicholson, and K. Griffiths. 1980. Relationship between primary breast tumor receptor status and patient survival. Cancer 46:2765–2769.

Bonadonna, G., and P. Valagussa. 1981. Dose-response effect of adjuvant chemotherapy in breast cancer. N. Engl. J. Med. 304:10–15.

Crowe, J. P., C. A. Hubay, O. H. Pearson, J. S. Marshall, J. Rosenblatt, E. G. Mansour, R. E. Hermann, J. C. Jones, W. J. Flynn, W. L. McGuire, and participating investigators. 1982. Estrogen receptor as a prognostic indicator for stage I breast cancer patients. Breast Cancer Res. Treat. 2:171–176.

de Lacroix, F. W., and K. J. Lennartz. 1981. Changes in the proliferation characteristics of a solid transplantable tumour of the mouse with time after transplantation. Cell Tissue Kinet. 14:135–142.

Delides, G. S., G. Garas, and G. Georgouli. 1982. Intralaboratory variations in the grading of breast carcinoma. Arch. Pathol. Lab. Med. 106:126–128.

Deos, P. H., and H. J. Norris. 1982. Well-differentiated (tubular) carcinoma of the breast. A clinicopathologic study of 145 pure and mixed cases. Am. J. Clin. Pathol. 78:1–7.

Dörmer, P., W. Brinkmann, R. Born, and G. G. Steel. 1975. Rate and time of DNA synthesis of individual Chinese hamster cells. Cell Tissue Kinet. 8:399–412.

Fabrikant, J. I., C. L. Wisseman III, and M. J. Vitak. 1969. The kinetics of cellular proliferation in normal and malignant tissues. II. An in vitro method for incorporation of tritiated thymidine in human tissues. Radiology 92:1309–1320.

Fisher, E. R., R. M. Gregorio, and B. Fisher. 1975. The pathology of invasive breast cancer. A syllabus derived from findings of the National Surgical Adjuvant Breast Project (Protocol No. 4). Cancer 36:1–85.

Fisher, E. R., A. S. Palekar, C. Redmond, B. Barton, and B. Fisher. 1980a. Pathologic findings from the National Surgical Adjuvant Breast Project (Protocol No. 4). VI. Invasive papillary cancer. Am. J. Clin. Pathol. 73:314–322.

Fisher, E. R., C. Redmond, and B. Fisher. 1980b. Pathologic findings from the National Surgical Adjuvant Breast Project (Protocol No. 4). VI. Discriminants for five-year treatment failure. Cancer 46:908–918.

Friedman, B. A., and H. A. Oberman. 1970. Adenoid cystic carcinoma of the breast. Am. J. Clin. Pathol. 54:1–14.

Furmanski, P., D. E. Saunders, S. C. Brooks, M. A. Rich, and The Breast Cancer Prognostic Study Clinical and Pathology Associates. 1980. The prognostic value of estrogen receptor determinations in patients with primary breast cancer: an update. Cancer 46:2794–2796.

Gentili, C., O. Sanfilippo, and R. Silvestrini. 1981. Cell proliferation and its relationship to clinical features and relapse in breast cancers. Cancer 48:974–979.

Glucksberg, H., S. E. Rivkin, S. Rasmussen, B. Tranum, N. Gad-el-Mawla, J. Costanzi, B. Hoogstraten, J. Athens, T. Maloney, J. McCracken, and C. Vaughn. 1982. Combination chemotherapy (CMFVP) versus L-phenylalanine mustard (L-PAM) for operable breast cancer with positive axillary nodes. A Southwest Oncology Group Study. Cancer 50:423–434.

Haagensen, C. D. 1971a. Diseases of the Breast, 2nd ed., Revised Reprint. W. B. Saunders Co., Philadelphia, pp. 590–594.

Haagensen, C. D. 1971b. Diseases of the Breast, 2nd ed., Revised Reprint. W. B. Saunders Co., Philadelphia, pp. 520–527.

Haagensen, C. D. 1971c. Diseases of the Breast, 2nd ed., Revised Reprint. W. B. Saunders Co., Philadelphia, p. 706.

Hähnel, R., T. Woodings, and A. B. Vivian. 1979. Prognostic value of estrogen receptors in primary breast cancer. Cancer 44:671–675.

Hilf, R., M. L. Feldstein, S. L. Gibson, and E. D. Savlov. 1980. The relative importance of estrogen receptor analysis as a prognostic factor for recurrence or response to chemotherapy in women with breast cancer. Cancer 45:1993–2000.

Knight, W., III, R. B. Livingston, E. J. Gregory, and W. L. McGuire. 1977. Estrogen receptor as an independent prognostic factor for recurrence in breast cancer. Cancer Res. 37:4669–4671.

Kute, T. E., H. B. Muss, D. Anderson, K. Crumb, B. Miller, D. Burns, and L. A. Dube. 1981. Relationship of steroid receptor, cell kinetics, and clinical status in patients with breast cancer. Cancer Res. 41:3524–3529.

Lacour, J., P. Bucalossi, E. Cacers, G. Jacobelli, T. Koszarowski, M. Le, C. Rumeau-Rouquette, and U. Veronesi. 1976. Radical mastectomy versus radical mastectomy plus internal mammary dissection. Five-year results of an international cooperative study. Cancer 37:206–214.

Laird, A. K. 1964. Dynamics of tumor growth. Br. J. Cancer 18:490–502.

Maynard, P. V., R. W. Blamey, C. W. Elston, J. L. Haybittle, and K. Griffiths. 1978. Estrogen receptor assay in primary breast cancer and early recurrence of the disease. Cancer Res. 38:4292–4295.

McDivitt, R. W., W. Boyce, and D. Gersell. 1982. Tubular carcinoma of the breast. Clinical and pathological observations concerning 135 cases. Am. J. Surg. Pathol. 6:401–411.

Meyer, J. S. 1981. Growth and cell kinetic measurements in human tumors. Pathol. Annu. 16, No. 2:53–81.

Meyer, J. S., W. C. Bauer, and B. R. Rao. 1978. Subpopulations of breast carcinoma defined by S-phase fraction, morphology, and estrogen receptor content. Lab. Invest. 39:225–235.

Meyer, J. S., and R. E. Connor. 1977. In vitro labeling of solid tissues with tritiated thymidine for autoradiographic detection of S-phase nuclei. Stain Technol. 52:185–195.

Meyer, J. S., and R. Facher. 1977. Thymidine labeling index of human breast carcinoma. Enhancement of in vitro labeling by 5-fluorouracil and 5-fluoro-2'-deoxyuridine. Cancer 39:2524–2532.

Meyer, J. S., E. Friedman, M. M. McCrate, and W. C. Bauer. 1983. Prediction of early course of breast carcinoma by thymidine labeling. Cancer 51:1879–1886.

Meyer, J. S., and B. Hixon. 1979. Advanced stage and early relapse of breast carcinomas associated with high thymidine labeling indices. Cancer Res. 39:4042–4047.

Meyer, J. S., and J. Y. Lee. 1980. Relationships of S-phase fraction of breast carcinoma in relapse to duration of remission, estrogen receptor content, therapeutic responsiveness, and duration of survival. Cancer Res. 40:1890–1896.

Nealon, T. F., Jr., A. Nkongho, C. Grossi, and J. Gillooley. 1979. Pathologic identification of poor prognosis stage I ($T_1N_0M_0$) cancer of the breast. Ann. Surg. 190:129–132.

Nemoto, T., J. Vana, R. N. Bedwani, H. W. Baker, F. H. McGregor, and G. P. Murphy. 1980. Management and survival of female breast cancer: results of a national survey by the American College of Surgeons. Cancer 45:2917–2924.

Nordenskjöld, B., L. Skoog, A. Wallgren, C. Silverswärd, S. Gustafsson, B.-M. Ljung, H. Westerberg, J.-A. Gustafsson, and O. Wrange. 1980. Measurements of DNA synthesis and estrogen receptor in needle aspirates as powerful methods in the management of breast carcinoma. Adv. Enzyme. Regul. 19:489–496.

Olszewski, W., Z. Darzynkiewicz, P. P. Rosen, M. D. Schwartz, and M. R. Melamed. 1981. Flow cytometry of breast carcinoma: II. Relation of tumor cell cycle distribution to histology and estrogen receptor. Cancer 48:985–988.

Raber, M. N., B. Barlogie, J. Latreille, C. Bedrossian, H. Fritsche, and G. Blumenschein. 1982. Ploidy, proliferative activity, and estrogen receptor content in human breast cancer. Cytometry 3:36–41.

Rich, M. A., P. Furmanski, and S. C. Brooks. 1978. Prognostic value of estrogen receptor determinations in patients with breast cancer. Cancer Res. 38:4296–4298.

Ridolfi, R. L., P. P. Rosen, A. Port, D. Kinne, and V. Mike. 1977. Medullary carcinoma of the breast. A clinicopathologic study with 10-year follow-up. Cancer 40:1365–1386.

Samaan, N. A., A. U. Buzdar, K. A. Aldinger, P. N. Schultz, K.-P. Yang, M. M. Romsdahl, and R. Martin. 1981. Estrogen receptor: a prognostic factor in breast cancer. Cancer 47:554–560.

Sears, H. F., C. Janus, W. Levy, R. Hopson, R. Creech, and P. Grotzinger. 1982. Breast cancer without axillary metastases. Are there high-risk biologic subpopulations? Cancer 50:1820–1827.

Schabel, F. M. 1977. Surgical adjuvant chemotherapy of metastatic murine tumors. Cancer 40:558–568.

Schiffer, L. M., P. G. Braunschweiger, J. J. Stragand, and L. Poulakos. 1979. The cell kinetics of human mammary cancers. Cancer 43:1707–1719.

Schottenfield, D., A. G. Nash, G. F. Robbins, and E. J. Beattie, Jr. 1976. Ten-year results of the treatment of primary operable breast carcinoma. A summary of 304 patients evaluated by the TNM system. Cancer 38:1101–1107.

Shapiro, C. M., and D. Schifeling. 1982. Prognostic value of the estrogen receptor level in pathologic stage I and II adenocarcinoma of the breast. J. Surg. Oncol. 19:119–121.

Silvestrini, R., M. G. Diadone, and A. Bertuzzi. 1982. Prognostic importance of proliferative activity alone or in combination with estrogen receptors (ER) in node-negative (N-) breast cancers. (Abstract) Proc. Am. Soc. Clin. Oncol. 1:83.

Silvestrini, R., M. G. Diadone, and G. Di Fronzo. 1979. Relationship between proliferative activity and estrogen receptors in breast cancer. Cancer 44:665–670.

Simpson-Herren, L., and H. H. Lloyd. 1970. Kinetic parameters and growth curves for experimental tumor systems. Cancer Chemother. Rep. 54:143–174.

Skipper, H. E. 1971. Kinetics of mammary tumor cell growth and implications for therapy. Cancer 28:1479–1499.

Sklarew, R. J., J. Hoffman, and J. Post. 1977. A rapid in vitro method for measuring cell proliferation in human breast cancer. Cancer 40:2299–2302.

Steel, G. G. 1977. Growth Kinetics of Tumors. Clarendon Press, Oxford.

Straus, M. M., and R. E. Moran. 1980. The cell cycle kinetics of human breast cancer. Cancer 46:2634–2639.

Tubiana, M., M. J. Pajovic, A. Renaud, G. Contesso, N. Chavaudra, J. Gioanni, and E. P. Malaise. 1981. Kinetic parameters and the course of the disease in breast cancer. Cancer 47:937–943.

Valagussa, P., G. Bonadonna, and U. Veronesi. 1978. Patterns of relapse and survival following radical mastectomy. Analysis of 716 consecutive patients. Cancer 41:1170–1178.

Westerberg, H., S. A. Gustafsson, B. Nordenskjöld, C. Silverswärd, and A. Wallgren. 1980. Estrogen receptor level and other factors in early recurrence of breast cancer. Int. J. Cancer 26:429–433.

Wibe, E., T. Lindmo, and O.Kaalhus. 1981. Cell kinetic characteristics in different parts of multicellular spheroids of human origin. Cell Tissue Kinet. 14:639–651.

Current Controversies in Breast Cancer, edited
by F. C. Ames, G. R. Blumenschein, and E. D. Montague.
University of Texas Press, Austin © 1984.

Applications of Flow Cytometry in Human Breast Cancer

Martin N. Raber, M.D.,* Barthel Barlogie, M.D.,† Tod S. Johnson, Ph.D.,† and Nguyen T. Van, Ph.D.‡

Department of Medicine, The University of Texas Medical School at Houston, Houston, Texas, and the Departments of †Developmental Therapeutics and ‡Laboratory Medicine, The University of Texas M. D. Anderson Hospital and Tumor Institute at Houston, Houston, Texas

The prognosis of patients with primary breast cancer classically rests on the pathologic stage (size of primary tumor and number of positive lymph nodes) at the time of diagnosis (Henny and DeVita 1978). Although one can classify tumors on the basis of their degree of cytologic differentiation or histologic degree of invasiveness, aside from the subgroup of carcinoma in situ this information adds little to management decisions.

Over the last few years, however, attention has turned to the study of biochemical markers that might help explain the variable behavior of seemingly similar breast tumors. Part of the impetus for this work has come from the demonstration of the importance of estrogen receptor (ER) in determining both the response to hormonal therapy (McGuire et al. 1975) and the overall prognosis of patients with breast cancer (Knight et al. 1977, Allegra et al. 1979). In this sense, ER is not a tumor marker specific for breast cancer; however, the knowledge of its presence helps in the selection of therapeutic strategies. In this report we will attempt to define other cellular probes available for the characterization of breast cancer and comment on their possible roles in determining the prognosis of both primary and metastatic breast cancer. These probes are both phenotypic and genotypic, and can serve as well to describe the cell cycle kinetics of tumors. We will also review current attempts to better define and quantitate ER in human breast tumors.

DNA CONTENT ANALYSIS

It has long been known that genotype abnormalities play a major role in the malignant process. Clonal proliferation of cells having abnormal karyotypes is considered synonymous with malignancy (Norwell 1974), and karyotypic abnormalities in some cancers have been shown to have important prognostic implications (Trujillo et al. 1974).

The idea that genotypic information could be obtained by measuring the DNA content of cells is not new, yet many investigators are today actively studying the importance of DNA content measurements using new technology. Studies based on histologic sections stained using the Feulgin technique have shown that survival is better in patients whose tumors have near normal DNA contents when compared to those whose tumors have high DNA contents (Atkin 1972, Auer et al. 1980).

Automated flow cytometry (FCM) is a technique of measuring fluorescence or other biophysical properties in single cells rapidly. In conjunction with a DNA-specific fluorescent dye it can be used to rapidly determine the DNA content of a large number of cells (Barlogie et al. 1980, Laerum and Farsund 1981). This analysis provides two pieces of useful information. First, one can determine the "modal DNA content," that is, the DNA content of the majority of cells. This can be compared to the modal DNA content of a population of normal cells and, if different, defines a genotypic abnormality. We have chosen to express this abnormality as the DNA index, which is defined as the ratio of tumor to normal DNA content (Barlogie et al. 1980). Thus, a diploid sample would have a DNA index (DI) of 1, while a tetraploid sample would have a DI of 2.

A number of authors have performed such analyses of human breast cancer, and the results of these studies are given in Table 1. Over 400 cases have been reported, with an incidence of abnormal DNA content ranging from 44% to 90% (mean 75%). It is probable that in breast cancer, as in other solid tumors, with further refinement in cell preparation, staining technology, and instrumentation, the incidence of aneuploidy will approach 100%.

The advantage of FCM determination of DNA content is not that it is of greater inherent value than classic cytogenic evaluation, but that it provides a rapid, quantitative, and objective measurement of DNA content amenable to interphase non-dividing cells. The importance of DNA content abnormality is not yet clear. Most of the studies listed in Table 1 have appeared within the last few years, and follow-up on these patients is, for the most part, too early or unknown. These studies and our own suggest that ploidy abnormality is greater and more common in poorly differentiated and ER-negative tumors (Raber et al. 1982b). Conflicting results regarding its relationship to stage of disease have been reported, and in our own study there was no difference in ploidy between patients with primary tumors and those with metastatic disease. Thornthwaite (1982) has reported that 2-year survival in 79 patients was 100% for diploid tumors and 67% for aneuploid hyper diploid tumors (DI > 1). In our own population of patients who had primary tumors, patients with diploid tumors separated by stage at presentation, also fared better, with a mean follow-up of 36 months. However, the number of relapses is small, and since only 15% of tumors in our series are diploid, it is difficult to draw statistically significant conclusions. Clearly, only a large study with long follow-up will tell us if these suggestions of improved prognosis with diploid disease are valid, and, if so, whether they are of independent significance. There is little reason to expect, however, that FCM DNA content analysis results will be different from those of the Feulgen technique studies mentioned earlier, which have demonstrated prolonged survival for patients with diploid and near diploid disease.

Table 1. *Flow Cytometric Studies of Cellular DNA Content in Human Breast Cancer*

Author	No. Pts.	% Aneuploid	Mean %S*	Relationship ER† & %S	Relationship ER & DI‡	Comment
Kute (1981)	70	44	13	ER+ -low %S	↑ aneuploidy ER−	no relation stage of disease
Olszewski (1981)	92	85	9	ER+ -low %S	↑ aneuploidy ER−	↑ aneuploidy anaplasia
Raber (1982b)	80	85	13.2	ER+ -low %S	↑ aneuploidy ER−	↑ aneuploidy anaplasia
Moran (1982)	64	90	–	ER+ -low %S	↑ aneuploidy	↑ aneuploidy anaplasia ↑ aneuploidy ↑ stage
Thornthwaite (1982)	79	79	–	–	–	diploid survival >aneuploid
Frankfort (1982)	25	72	–	–	–	–
Total	410	76				

*%S = Percent cells in S phase.
†ER = Estrogen receptor.
‡DI = DNA index.

DESCRIPTION OF THE CELL CYCLE

As is the case with cytogenetic karyotyping, classic techniques for evaluating events in the cell cycle are laborious and not easily adapted for routine analyses. Nevertheless, studies by a number of authors have shown that the thymidine labeling index (TLI) of human breast cancer tumors can be measured and has prognostic significance in predicting the disease-free interval and survival of patients with primary breast cancer (Meyer and Lee 1980, Meyer 1982). Other studies have also suggested that breast tumors with high TLI are more responsive to chemotherapy than those with low TLI (Sulkes et al. 1979). TLI appears to be lower in ER-positive than in ER-negative tumors (Meyer et al. 1976, Silvistrini et al. 1979).

Since cells increase their DNA contents during S phase (the DNA content of G2 and mitotic cells is twice that of G1 and G0 cells), cellular DNA content measurement not only gives us an appreciation of ploidy but also reveals the position of each cell in the cell cycle. Thus, one can calculate the percentage of cells in the S phase compartment of the cell cycle (%S), which should be similar to the TLI. In fact, it is usually higher than the TLI, probably because slowly cycling cells in S phase will incorporate little thymidine during a relatively brief exposure (Ford and Shakney 1977). As is the case with ploidy determination, there is good agreement between laboratories for values of %S (Table 1), but the prognostic value of this measurement remains unclear.

Most workers also have reported low values for %S in ER-positive tumors, a finding that confirms the studies based on labeling indices. However, in all subgroups studied there is a wide range of values for %S, and ER positivity does not guarantee low proliferative activity. This disparity may explain why some patients with ER-positive tumors have short disease-free intervals.

In our own laboratory, of 32 patients with primary tumors studied in 1979, 13 have suffered relapse. Overall, tumors in patients who have relapsed had higher %S than tumors in those who remain disease free (14.9% vs. 12.3%). This difference was most striking, however, in the negative node subset (16.3% vs. 9.8%). Although in most studies ER-positive tumors have significantly lower values for %S than ER-negative tumors, this difference in disease-free interval was present in both ER-positive and ER-negative subsets.

While this patient population is small and the results preliminary, we believe that as other laboratories gain sufficient follow-up of the patients already studied, flow-measured %S will have a prognostic value similar to that attributed to TLI, and it will also have the advantage of being more easily and reproducibly measured.

OTHER FLOW CYTOMETRIC PROBES

Size, Protein, RNA Content

Using FCM, one can assess cell size by forward-angle light scatter, and protein content or RNA content can be measured with specific fluorescent dyes. It is likely

Table 2. *Cellular RNA Content in Human Breast Cancer*

Mean RNA index	1.40 ± 0.92
(83 cases)	
DNA index	RNA index
≤1	1.11
1.01–1.5	1.52
>1.5	1.86
Proliferative activity (%S)	
<7	1.22
8–16	1.40
>16	1.48
ER* content	
O	1.47
borderline	1.25
positive	1.08

*Estrogen receptor.

that these three parameters are interrelated. In our own laboratory, we have chosen to measure cellular RNA content using the metachromatic dye acridine orange (Traganos et al. 1977). This dye simultaneously stains DNA and RNA. We have studied 83 patients who have primary breast cancer. RNA content is expressed as the RNA index (the ratio of tumor modal RNA content to normal lymphocyte RNA content). Using this measure, we have correlated RNA index values with ploidy and proliferative activity (Table 2). For the group as a whole, the mean RNA index was 1.4 ± .92 (1.0 would be the RNA index of normal lymphocytes). The RNA index values are increased in tumors with higher DNA content abnormalities, higher %S and in ER-negative tumors, all of which support the concept of increased RNA in cells more actively synthesizing DNA. While in multiple myeloma increased RNA content is a marker of differentiation (Latreille et al. 1982), in breast cancer ER-positive tumors have lower RNA content; and RNA content appears to be related to proliferative activity (Table 2). The prognostic value of this measurement as an independent variable cannot yet be assessed.

Hormone Receptor Content

It has been evident for some time that FCM analysis of ER content in single cells would be a powerful tool for investigating the heterogeneity of receptor expression in breast cancer, as well as a means of dissecting out the response of subsets of breast cancer cells to hormonal and chemotherapeutic manipulations. Our own work in this area has been directed to the application of a fluorescent probe for the estrogen receptor, 17 β FITC-estradiol synthesized and kindly provided by Dr. George Barrows at the University of Louisville (Barrows et al. 1978). Using FCM, we have demonstrated that this compound is a good ligand for the receptor and have begun preliminary studies in human tumors and cell culture systems (Raber et al. 1982a). Figure 1 shows an ER-positive tumor that has been stained with the fluorescent

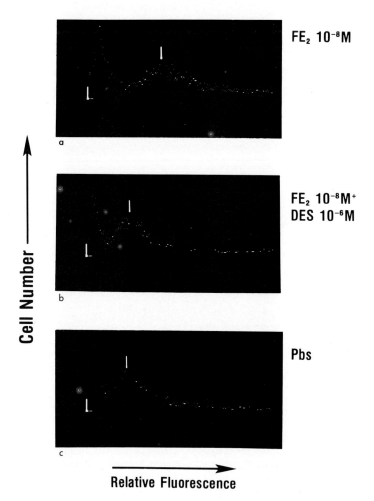

FE₂ 10⁻⁸M

FE₂ 10⁻⁸M⁺
DES 10⁻⁶M

Pbs

Relative Fluorescence

FIG. 1A. Relative fluorescence of cells taken from an estrogen receptor-positive human breast tumor stained with FE₂ (ethyl-succinamide 17 β estradiol-fluorescein). **B.** Similarly treated cells coinculated with a 100-fold excess of diethylstilbestrol (DES). Note that the relative fluorescence has decreased. **C.** The same cells unstained in phosphate buffered saline (Pbs). The fluorescence recorded in this panel represents background autofluorescence. The difference between the fluorescence displayed in panel A and that of panel B represents specific binding of FE₂ to the estrogen receptor.

compound; the tumor exhibits specific fluorescence that can be suppressed by co-incubation with diethylstilbestrol. We hope these studies will give us new insight into understanding the biology of hormone receptor expression.

CONCLUSIONS

In our search for better means to predict the course of each patient's disease, we must continually evaluate new probes. Having reached the limits of traditional morphology, we are entering an era where cell markers not apparent on light microscopic examination are assuming increasing importance. Estrogen receptor is a good example of such a marker. The use of FCM analysis of ploidy and proliferative activity appears to provide additional information of prognostic importance. As well, on a more basic level, the ability to quantitate ER content on a per cell basis will provide a new means of studying the biology of estrogen receptor expression.

ACKNOWLEDGMENTS

The original work described in this section was supported in part by grants CA 11520 and CA 28771 awarded by the National Cancer Institute, U.S. Department of Health and Human Services. The authors would also like to acknowledge the continued support of Dr. George Barrows of the University of Louisville, Louisville, Kentucky, for the development of fluorescent probes, and the secretarial help of Ms. Solange Blickley.

REFERENCES

Allegra, J. D., M. E. Lippman, and R. Simon. 1979. Association between studied steroid hormone receptor status and disease free interval in breast cancer. Cancer Treat. Rep. 63:1271–1279.

Atkin, N. B. 1972. Modal deoxyribonucleic acid value and survival in carcinoma of the breast. Br. Med. J. 1:271–272.

Auer, G., J. Caspersson, and A. Wallgren. 1980. DNA content and survival in mammary carcinoma. Anal. Quant. Cytol. 2:161–165.

Barlogie, B., B. Drewinko, J. Schumann, W. Göhde, G. Dosik, D. Johnston, and E. Freireich. 1980. Cellular DNA content as a marker of neoplasia in man. Am. J. Med. 69:195–203.

Barrows, G., S. Stroupe, and L. Gray. 1978. In vitro uptake and nuclear transfer of fluorescei-nated estradiol in human mammary cancer and normal endometrium. Am. J. Clin. Path. 70:330–331.

Ford, S. S., and S. E. Shakney. 1977. Lethal and sublethal effects of hydroxyurea in relation to drug concentration and duration of drug exposure in sarcoma 180 *in vitro*. Cancer Res. 37:2628–2637.

Frankfort, O. S., H. C. Slocum, R. Grecow, and Y. M. Rustum. 1982. Cytometric analysis of human solid tumors. (Abstract) Cytometry in the Clinical Laboratory, 1982 Meeting of the Engineering Foundation, Santa Barbara, California, p. 6.4.

Henney, J. E., and V. T. DeVita. 1978. Future prospective in the treatment of breast cancer. Semin. Oncol. 4:465–468.

Knight, W. A., R. B. Livingston, E. J. Gregory, and W. L. McGuire. 1977. Estrogen receptor as an independent prognostic factor for early recurrence in breast cancer. Cancer Res. 37:4669–4671.

Kute, T. E., H. B. Moss, D. Anderson, K. Crumb, B. Miller, D. Burns, and L. Dube. 1981. Relationship of steroid receptor cell kinetics and clinical status in patients with breast cancer. Cancer Res. 41:3524–3529.

Laerum, O. D., and T. Farsund. 1981. Clinical applications of flow cytometry: A review. Cytometry 2:1–13.

Latreille, J. L., B. Barlogie, D. Johnston, B. Drewinko, and R. Alexanian. 1982. Ploidy and proliferative characteristics in monoclonal gammopathies. Blood 59:43–51.

McGuire, W. L., P. Carbone, M. Sears, and G. Escher. 1975. Estrogen receptor in human breast cancer, an overview, *in* Estrogen Receptors in Breast Cancer, W. L. McGuire, P. Carbone, and E. Vallmer, eds. Raven Press, New York, p. 17.

Meyer, J. S. 1982. Cell kinetic measurements of human tumors. Hum. Pathol. 13:874–877.

Meyer, J. S., and J. Y. Lee. 1980. Relationship of S-phase fraction of breast carcinoma in relapse to duration of remission, estrogen receptor content, therapeutic responsiveness, and duration of survival. Cancer Res. 40:1890–1896.

Meyer, J. S., B. R. Rao, S. C. Stephens, and W. L. White. 1976. Low incidence of estrogen receptor in breast cancer with rapid rates of cellular replication. Cancer 40:2290–2298.

Moran, R. E., M. J. Straus, M. M. Black, E. Alvarez, M. D. Evans, and R. Evans. 1982. Flow cytometric DNA analysis of human breast tumors and comparison with clinical and pathologic parameters. (Abstract) Proc. Am. Assoc. Cancer Res. 23:33.

Norwell, P. C. 1974. Chromosome changes and the clonal evolution of cancer, *in* Chromosomes and Cancer, J. German, ed. Wiley and Sons, New York, pp. 267–285.

Olszewski, M., Z. Darzynkiewicz, P. P. Rosen, M. Schwartz, and M. Melamed. 1981. Flow cytometry of breast carcinoma: relation of DNA ploidy level to histology and estrogen receptor. Cancer 48:980–989.

Raber, M. N., B. Barlogie, G. Barrows, D. Swartzendruber, and N. T. Van. 1982a. Flow cytometric (FCM) analysis of estrogen receptor content. (Abstract) Proc. Am. Assoc. Cancer Res. 23:32.

Raber, M. N., B. Barlogie, J. Latreille, C. Bedrossian, H. Fritsche, and G. Blumenschein. 1982b. Ploidy, proliferative activity and estrogen receptor content in human breast cancer. Cytometry 3:36–41.

Silvistrini, R., M. Daidone, and G. DiFronzo. 1979. Relationship between proliferative activity and estrogen receptor in breast cancer. Cancer 44:665–670.

Sulkes, A., R. B. Livingston, and W. K. Murphy. 1979. Tritiated thymidine labeling index and response in human breast cancer. JNCI 62:513–515.

Thornthwaite, J. T., and P. B. Coolson. 1982. Comparison of steroid receptor content, DNA levels, surgical staging, and survival in human breast cancer. (Abstract) Cytometry in the Clinical Laboratory, 1982 Meeting of the Engineering Foundation, Santa Barbara, California, p. 6.9.

Traganos, F., Z. Darzynkiewicz, T. Sharpless, and M. R. Melamed. 1977. Simultaneous staining of ribonucleic and deoxyribonucleic acid on unfixed cells using acridine orange in a flow cytofluorometric system. J. Histochem. Cytochem. 25:46–56.

Trujillo, J., A. Cork, J. Hart, S. George, and E. Freireich. 1974. Clinical implications of aneuploid cytogenetic profiles in adult acute leukemia. Cancer 33:824–834.

Current Controversies in Breast Cancer, edited
by F. C. Ames, G. R. Blumenschein, and E. D. Montague.
University of Texas Press, Austin © 1984.

The Role of the Human Tumor Stem Cell Assay in the Treatment of Patients with Breast Carcinoma

V. Hug, M.D.,* G. Blumenschein, M.D.,* H. Thames, Ph.D.,† G.
Spitzer, M.D.,‡ and B. Drewinko, Ph.D.§

*Departments of *Internal Medicine, †Biomathematics,‡Developmental Therapeutics, and
§Laboratory Medicine, The University of Texas M. D. Anderson Hospital and Tumor
Institute at Houston, Houston, Texas*

The human tumor stem cell assay (Hamburger and Salmon 1977a, Hamburger and Salmon 1977b) may play a significant role in the management of patients with breast carcinoma, since approximately 75,000 women in the United States commence chemotherapy for this disease yearly and since inherent tumor sensitivity to anticancer agents is an essential requirement of effective treatment. However, the assay is incomplete in its development (Von Hoff et al. 1981, Salmon et al. 1981), and many assumptions and conclusions surrounding it may be erroneous. We have improved the culture conditions for breast tumor cells to enable tumor sensitivity determinations to anticancer agents to be made from a larger proportion of assays. We subsequently reassessed the assay for its potential to identify active antitumor drugs, and found that it may provide a major contribution to the chemotherapy of patients who have breast carcinoma.

MATERIALS AND METHODS

Cells

Breast tumor samples were obtained from primary or metastatic solid tumors or from pleural or ascitic fluids of patients with stage III or IV disease. Solid tumors were collected and placed in 10 ml of culture medium with 15% fetal calf serum (FCS). Ten units of preservative-free heparin (Fisher Scientific Co., Houston, Texas) were added to each milliliter of fluid to prevent coagulation. An informed consent form was obtained before specimens were acquired for experimentation.

Chemical Agents

Antitumor agents were obtained from the following manufacturers: Adriamycin and 4'-epi-doxorubicin, Farmitalia Carlo Erba S.D.A., Italy; mitoxantrone

(CL232,315) and bisantrene (CL216,942), American Cyanamid Company, Pearl River, New York 10965.

Breast Tumor Colony-Forming Assay

Solid tumor tissue samples were debrided and diced into 1-mm cubes with scalpels, and single cells were teased into suspension with a 25-gauge needle. The samples were then suspended in an enzyme mixture of type III collagenase (Worthington Biochemical Corporation, Freeholt, New Jersey) and deoxyribonuclease (Sigma Chemical Co., St. Louis, Missouri) at a final strength of 1.0% and 0.005%, respectively, for 16 hours at 37°C under continuous agitation. Cells obtained from malignant effusions were treated in an identical manner. After enzyme incubation, cells were washed in calcium- and magnesium-free Hank's balanced salt solution (CMF-HBSS) (K.C. Biological Incorp., Kansas City, Kansas) and set into semi-solid suspension culture, as described by Hamburger and Salmon (Hamburger and Salmon 1977a, 1977b), with the exception that a 50:50 mixture of Nutrient Mixture F12 (Ham) and Dulbecco's Modified Eagle's Medium (Gibco, Grand Island, New York) supplemented with hepes buffer and 10 μg/ml of bovine crystalline insulin (Sigma Chemical Company) was used as a plating medium for the underlayers, and alpha minimum essential medium (α-MEM) for the upper layers. Conditioned medium was obtained by combining supernatants of three established human breast cell lines (MDA-231, MDA-435, and MDA-468), and 0.2-ml aliquots were added to the underlayers. Fifteen percent of FCS was mixed with both layers in the first 50 tumor samples. In subsequent cultures the FCS in the underlayers was replaced by 10% horse serum simultaneously with the other modifications of the culture conditions, which included the addition into the underlayers of 5×10^{-7} M of 17-β-estradiol, 50 μg/ml of epidermal growth factor, and 25 μg/ml of hydrocortisone (Sigma Chemical Company). Cultures were incubated in a fully humidified atmosphere of 7% CO_2 in air at 37°C for 14 days. One control plate was fixed with 0.05 ml of 3% glutaraldehyde and stored at 4°C to serve as reference for clump contamination.

Drug Exposure

All drugs were reconstituted to a 100X stock solution with CMF-HBSS. Further dilutions were made in α-MEM with 30% FCS. Two-millileter aliquots of the 2X final concentration were stored at −70°C. At the time of experimentation, the aliquots were thawed, agar and cells were added, and one to three replicate cultures were obtained for each concentration.

Scoring of Colonies

Tumor colonies were scored with an Olympus IMT inverted microscope at 40X magnification. Aggregates with a uniform morphology of ≥ 40 cells or a diameter of $\geq$ 75 μm at 40X magnification, or both, were counted as colonies. The glu-taraldehyde-fixed plates were scored using the same criteria, and the number of clumps enumerated were deducted from the scores of the culture plates.

RESULTS

Our first attempt was to improve the in vitro growth conditions for breast tumor cells to increase the percentage of evaluable drug tests. 17-β-estradiol at 5×10^{-7} M, hydrocortisone acetate at 2.5 μg/ml, epidermal growth factor at 50 mg/ml, and horse serum at 10% were factors that stimulated the clonogenic growth of the estrogen-receptor-negative breast cell lines MDA-231, MDA-435, and MDA-468, and of the estrogen-receptor-positive line MCF-7. The combined addition of these factors into the underlayers of subsequent cultures improved by a factor of four the median plating efficiency of breast tumors (Table 1). Thus, following these modi-fications of the culture conditions, meaningful drug sensitivities of breast tumors could be determined from over twice as many assays, a figure that represents the highest reported percentage of workable assays for breast tumors (Sandbach et al. 1982). As illustrated in Tables 2 and 3, tumors that yielded adequate in vitro growth for drug sensitivity determinations were not preferentially obtained from patients favored by having either tumors responding to alternative treatment modalities, such as estrogen-receptor-positive tumors to hormones, or by having tumors highly sensitive to most anticancer agents. On the contrary, tumors from patients who had short subsequent survivals yielded better in vitro growth (Figure 1). Since the assay could identify with an accuracy of 60% to 70% effective anticancer drugs in tumors obtained from a group of patients with a 30% expected clinical response rate (Von Hoff et al. 1981, Salmon et al. 1981), and since an evaluable assay does not select for a favorable patient group, it truly provides new information to supplement em-pirical clinical knowledge.

For meaningful conduction of in vitro drug testing, we thought it necessary to normalize the in vitro activities of the agents to be tested. As reported earlier (Hug et al. 1982), we chose to measure the in vitro activity of chemotherapeutic drugs by their effects on normal bone marrow progenitor cells. Not only do these progenitor cells represent the dose-limiting host target of most anticancer agents, but their in vitro growth requirements are also similar to those of tumor progenitor cells. A 30-fold higher plating efficiency with a 100-fold lesser variation of the bone marrow progenitors further raises their suitability for internal standard. Relative sensitivities of tumor and bone marrow progenitors to anticancer drugs so normalized can be graphically described (Figure 2). Such a comparative determination of antitumor activity of several agents permits appropriate drug selection and may contribute to the rational composition of combination treatments.

By applying this approach of drug sensitivity determination to 41 primary breast tumors, we found that while with advancing disease stage the in vitro growth in-creased (Figure 1), the frequency of positive drug sensitivity declined (Table 4), an observation that correlates with the clinical experience. This is an important find-

Table 1. *Effect of Improved Culture Conditions On the In Vitro Growth of Breast Tumors**

	No. of Tumors Plated	% Tumors that Formed $\geqslant 1$ Colony	% Tumors that Formed >30 Colonies
Prior to modification	50	78	34
Subsequent to modification	78	91	73
Literature[†]	93	–	43

*All tumors were obtained from patients with advanced breast carcinoma; 51% of the specimens were solid tumors and 49% were body fluids. The percentage of tumor cells in the suspensions ranged from 5% to 95%, and the median was 60%. The median plating efficiency prior to the modifications listed in the text was 0.004 (range 0.0002–0.1100); it was 0.016 (range 0.0004–0.2300) subsequently.
[†]Sandbach, et al. 1982.

Table 2. *In Vitro Growth of Breast Tumors and Estrogen-Receptor (ER) Content (60 Patients)*

Assay Successful*	% ER-Positive	% ER-Negative
Yes	37	28
No	17	18

*Most investigators evaluate drug assays if 30 or more colonies have formed in the untreated control plates. Tumors that contained more than 10 fmol/mg cytosol protein of ER were considered ER-positive. Successful assays are equally distributed among ER-positive and ER-negative tumors (Fischer's exact test for entire table, $P = 0.47$).
[†]$\geqslant 30$ colonies per control plate.

Table 3. *In Vitro Growth of Breast Tumors and Response of Patients to Subsequent Treatment (70 Patients)**

Assay Successful[†]	% Responders	% Failures
Yes	20	31
No	17	32

*Chemotherapy was the most commonly used treatment modality, but treatment with hormones, radiation, and biological modifiers were also included. There is an equal distribution of usable and nonusable drug tests among treatment responders and treatment failures (Fischer's exact test for entire table, $P = 0.35$).
[†]$\geqslant 30$ colonies per control plate.

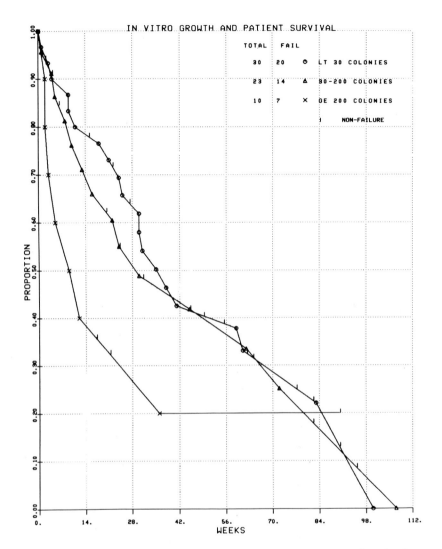

FIG. 1. The inverse relationship of plating efficiency of the in vitro tumor growth and patient survival is apparent. The upstrokes indicate patients still alive.

ing. The clinical treatment response is determined by both tumor bulk and inherent drug sensitivity. But these two factors cannot be separated, since the tumor bulk increases with advancing disease stage. In vitro, however, the tumor size is kept constant; our findings, therefore, indicate the development of true drug resistance.

Approximately 30% of breast tumors were more sensitive than normal bone marrows to the effects of each of four anthracene derivatives: 11/41 to Adriamycin,

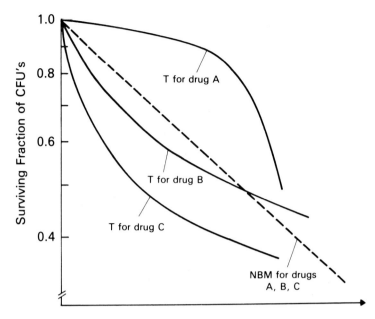

FIG. 2. Therapeutic index for tumor and bone marrow sensitivity to three anticancer agents. Graphs of this form permit rapid recognition of active agents for the treatment of individual tumors. The drug concentrations on the abscissa are normalized by their equitoxicity to normal bone marrow. (CFU = colony-forming unit, NMB = normal bone marrow, T = tumor.)

Table 4. *Change in Inherent Drug Sensitivities of Breast Tumors*
With Disease Progression and Treatment Exposure

Patient Characteristics*	Percentage of In Vitro Drug Sensitivity†
(A) Patients with no prior exposure to chemotherapy	59 (23/39)
(B) Patients failing on or suffering recurrence after adjuvant chemotherapy	54 (14/26)
(C) Patients with advanced disease stage	32 (7/22)

*Chi-square test for entire table, $P = 0.12$; A vs. B, $P = 0.75$; A vs. C, $P = 0.038$; B vs. C, $P = 0.107$.
†Absolute numbers of observations in parentheses.

5/19 to 4′-epi-doxorubicin, 10/34 mitoxantrone, and 10/33 to bisantrene. These proportions are within the range of the expected response rates to single-agent treatment with these agents. Whereas 61% of the tumors tested showed equal sensitivity to the four structurally related compounds, i.e., either sensitive to all drugs tested (32%) or resistant to all drugs tested (29%), 26 of the 41 tumors showed mixed patterns of response. These variations of in vitro sensitivity of breast tumors to different drugs are illustrated in Figure 3, where the doses of each drug necessary to kill 50% of normal bone marrow progenitors were used to compare the antitumor effects of these agents.

It remains to be determined whether, in addition to providing a means of measuring relative effects of anticancer agents on individual tumors, the use of standardized drug concentrations will also improve the accuracy of assays predicting clinical response. Elimination of false-positive predictions can be expected, since in vitro

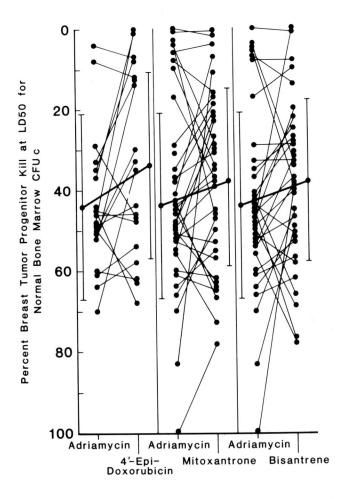

FIG. 3. Comparative effects of four anthracene derivatives on breast tumor colony-forming units. The concentration of each drug that killed 50% of normal bone marrow progenitors was determined and subsequently used to compare the cytotoxic effects of these agents on primary breast tumors. Lines connect the percentages of tumor progenitor kill on individual tumors induced by Adriamycin and by analogue.

Table 5. *Association of In Vitro Sensitivity to Adriamycin or Mitoxantrone with Clinical Response to Adriamycin or Mitoxantrone-Containing Combination Treatments**

In Vitro	Clinical[†]	
	Sensitive	Resistant
Sensitive	7	1
Resistant	3	3

*In this group of patients with an expected clinical response rate of 80%, the assay's merit is the identification of treatment failures. In this small sample, it correctly identified these in 75% of instances. This is a high proportion, since the prediction is based on the in vitro sensitivity to only one of the drugs used in the combination treatment regimens.
[†]Statistical sensitivity of resistance = 75.0%; statistical specificity of resistance = 87.5%. Previously untreated patients were given Adriamycin, 5-fluorouracil, and cyclophosphamide (7); patients failing adjuvant treatments were given Adriamycin, 5-fluorouracil, and cyclophosphamide (2); Adriamycin and vinblastine (2); or mitoxantrone, and vinblastine (3).

Table 6. *Correlation of Single-Agent Treatments, In Vitro and In Vivo**

In Vitro	Clinical[†]	
	Sensitive	Resistant
Sensitive	5	0
Resistant	0	5

*The expected clinical response rate of this group of patients is 30%. The value of the assay lies in the correct identification of active antitumor agents for individual patients. Correct in vitro identification of in vivo activity occurred twice for Adriamycin, and once each for 4'-epi-doxorubicin, bisantrene, and vinblastine.
[†]Statistical sensitivity > 80%.

cell kill is a dose-response effect for most anticancer agents, whereas false-negative predictions can be avoided if in vitro drug activity at the concentration used is assured. Our experience using the assay for predicting clinical responses is limited, but the preliminary results are encouraging (Tables 5, 6).

DISCUSSION

Individualized curative treatment for patients with early stages of breast carcinoma is the ultimate goal for in vitro identification of tumor sensitivities to anticancer agents. With respect to the human tumor stem cell assay, this implies the basic assumption that the clonogenic cells recovered and assayed for drug sensitivities in vitro are identical to those tumor progenitor cells left behind that, if left untreated, will lead to tumor recurrence. Justification of treatment guided by such an assay will require treatment results superior to the currently used empirical treatments, from which 35% to 40% of patients at risk of developing disease recurrence benefit (Buzdar et al. 1981).

Since other factors determine the clinical response to chemotherapy, even for microscopic disease, the role of in vitro determination of tumor sensitivity to anticancer agents will need to be established through appropriately designed studies. The actions of most anticancer agents are cell-cycle specific, and their physiochemical properties determine their organ distribution, which may differ between host and tumor tissue. The effect of inherent tumor sensitivity on the treatment outcome will, therefore, be difficult to assess and may vary for each tumor type. Indirect evidence is needed to define the future role of the human tumor stem cell assay in the management of patients with breast carcinoma. In this regard, our observations of changing in vitro growth properties and inherent drug sensitivities with advancing disease stage are encouraging, since they reflect the clinical experience of increasing tumor aggressiveness and decreasing drug sensitivity with tumor progression. Of particular interest is the assay's apparent capability of identifying the development of true drug resistance independent of the changing effects of tumor mass and tumor kinetics as they occur in vivo. The associations of in vitro sensitivity and clinical response are likewise promising, considering all the assay's shortcomings and the numerous other variables that determine the clinical response to chemotherapy. These observations certainly lead us to believe the assay is capable of selecting tumor cell populations identical to those that sustain in vivo tumor growth, and that, like treatment with antibiotics of bacterial infections, inherent sensitivity to anticancer agents is a major factor in successful chemotherapy. These findings should encourage further research directed at improving the quality of the assay in an attempt to make such drug tests more meaningful. For clinical usefulness, the assay has to be readily available, economical, and, most importantly, workable in all instances. Early-stage breast carcinoma will be a prime area of its application, in view of the large number of patients who currently are given chemotherapy in an attempt to cure this disease.

REFERENCES

Buzdar, A. U., T. L. Smith, G. R. Blumenschein, G. N. Hortobagyi, E. M. Hersh, and E. A. Gehan. 1981. Adjuvant chemotherapy with fluorouracil, doxorubicin, and cyclophosphamide (FAC) for stage II or III breast cancer: 5 year results, *in* Adjuvant Therapy of Cancer III, S. E. Salmon and S. E. Jones, eds. Grune and Stratton, New York, pp. 419–426.

Hamburger, A. W., and S. E. Salmon. 1977a. Primary bioassay of human tumor stem cells. Science 197:461–463.

Hamburger, A. W., and S. E. Salmon. 1977b. Primary bioassay of human myeloma stem cells. Clin. Invest. Med. 60:846–854.

Hug, V., B. Drewinko, G. Spitzer, and G. R. Blumenschein. 1982. The use of normal bone marrow GM-CFUc to enhance the predictive accuracy of the human tumor stem cell assay. J. Cell. Biochem. Suppl. 6:378.

Salmon, S. E., F. L. Meyskens, D. S. Alberts, B. Soehnlen, and L. Young. 1981. New drugs in ovarian cancer and malignant melanoma. In vitro phase II screening with the human tumor stem cell assay. Cancer Treat. Rep. 65:1–12.

Sandbach, J., D. D. VonHoff, G. Clark, A. B. Cruz, M. O'Brien, and The South Central Texas Human Tumor Cloning Group. 1982. Direct cloning of human breast cancer in soft agar culture. Cancer 50:1215–1221.

VonHoff, D. D., J. Casper, E. Bradley, J. Sandbach, and R. Rakuch. 1981. Association between human tumor colony-forming assay results and response of an individual patient's tumor to chemotherapy. Am. J. Med. 70:1027–1032.

BREAST CANCER SCREENING AND EPIDEMIOLOGY

Current Controversies in Breast Cancer, edited
by F. C. Ames, G. R. Blumenschein, and E. D. Montague.
University of Texas Press, Austin © 1984.

Risk Factors as Criteria for Inclusion in Breast Cancer Screening Programs

Lawrence J. Solin, M.D.,* Gordon F. Schwartz, M.D.,† Stephen A.
Feig, M.D.,‡ Gary S. Shaber, M.D.,‡ and Arthur S. Patchefsky,
M.D.§

*Department of Radiation Therapy, Hospital of the University of Pennsylvania,
Philadelphia, Pennsylvania, and Departments of †Surgery, ‡Radiology, and §Pathology,
Thomas Jefferson University Hospital, Philadelphia, Pennsylvania*

The value of mass screening programs for breast cancer has been the subject of considerable controversy. It has been suggested that such programs are a waste of resources if they are directed at all women. Instead, many authors have argued that mass screening programs should, therefore, be directed only at women with an identifiable risk factor in their personal or family history and exclude all women lacking such risk factors (Bailar 1977, Lemon and Thiessen 1974, Haagensen 1971, Morgan and Vakil 1976, Stark and Way 1974).

Alternatively, many studies continue to demonstrate the effectiveness of mass screening programs in detecting early breast cancers and in concomitantly increasing life expectancy. The well-known study of the Health Insurance Plan (HIP) of Greater New York showed a reduction in breast cancer mortality limited to women over age 50 and not found in women ages 40–49 (Shapiro 1977). The American Cancer Society recommends routine yearly mammography only after age 50, but yearly breast physical examination after age 40 as part of its "cancer-related checkup" (Guidelines for the Cancer Related Checkup 1980). Still others suggest benefit from mass screening in all women both over and under age 50 (Berlin 1981, Bland et al. 1981).

In 1973, the National Cancer Institute funded a cooperative study between the Thomas Jefferson University Hospital Breast Diagnostic Center (BDC) and HIP in order to evaluate effects of mammography, thermography, and clinical examination on the early detection of breast cancer in a mass screening program of asymptomatic women. The current study is a retrospective analysis of BDC data and was undertaken in order to test the efficacy of screening only women with higher risk factors for breast cancer as compared with screening all women regardless of presence or absence of risk factors. The effect of age on screening women at higher risk for breast cancer will also be discussed, as this has been a topic of considerable controversy.

MATERIAL AND METHODS

During the period 1973 to 1976, 35,367 screening examinations were performed at the BDC on 17,543 asymptomatic, self-referred women between the ages of 45 and 65. Any woman with a previous history of breast cancer was excluded from the screening program. Prior to each screening, each woman completed a detailed history form. Each screening examination consisted of a thermogram, a mammogram, and a clinical examination by a physician trained in breast examination techniques. Each thermogram and mammogram was interpreted independently by two experienced radiologists. Each case was individually reviewed after the screening, and recommendations were made by the BDC to the patient and her referring physician for either 1) 2 years' follow-up if the screen was completely negative, 2) 6 months' follow-up for rescreening if the physical examination or mammogram was equivocal or if the thermogram was abnormal, or 3) appropriate surgical procedure of biopsy or aspiration if the physical examination or mammogram was positive, regardless of thermographic findings.

A total of 249 cancers in 246 patients was found during the study period of 3 years. The records of these patients were reviewed retrospectively and are the basis of this study. A detailed analysis was undertaken with respect to family history, prior breast biopsy or surgery for benign disease, parity, menstrual history, age at first pregnancy, use of hormones or birth control pills, and final pathology from definitive cancer surgery. Increased risk was defined to include any family history of breast cancer in mother, sister, grandmother (paternal or maternal), or aunt (paternal or maternal) or cousin (paternal or maternal), or any history of prior surgical biopsy or breast procedure regardless of diagnosis. These definitions approximate, or in some cases even expand, those that have been suggested as being necessary to gain admission to a selective screening program (Bailar 1977, Guidelines for the Cancer Related Checkup 1980, Haagensen 1971, Lemon and Thiessen 1974, Morgan and Vakil 1976, Stark and Way 1974). The 246 women with breast cancer were then further analyzed with respect to the above criteria of increased risk.

RESULTS

The characteristics of the 246 women found to have breast cancer are listed in Table 1. All patients were between the ages of 44 and 67 at the time of diagnosis of breast cancer. Three patients aged 66, 66, and 67 at the time of diagnosis were aged 63, 64, and 65, respectively, at the time of their first screening. The patients were self-described as mainly white (91.5% white versus 8.5% other). Religious preference showed an increased proportion of Jews (23.6%).

A family history of breast cancer involving the patient's mother or sister was documented in only 15.0%, and any family history of breast cancer was found in only 31.7% of the women. No family history of breast cancer was found in 68.3% of the patients. A prior breast biopsy for benign breast disease was noted in only 20.3% of the women. Other previously suggested minor risk factors for breast can-

Table 1. *Patient Characteristics**

Age of diagnosis of breast cancer	range = 44–67
	(mean = 54.8)
	(median = 55)
Race	
White	91.5% (225)
Other	8.5% (21)
Religion	
Jewish	23.6% (58)
Not Jewish	76.4% (188)
Family history for breast cancer	
Negative	68.3% (168)
Mother (+)	6.9% (17)
Sister (+)	8.5% (21)
Mother or sister (+)	15.0% (37)
Any (+)	31.7% (78)
Previous breast biopsy or aspiration	
Yes	20.3% (50)
No	79.7% (196)
Menstrual history	
<30 years	9.8% (24)
30–35 years	27.6% (68)
36–40 years	43.1% (106)
>40 years	13.8% (34)
Unknown	5.7% (14)
Hormone use	
Any birth control pill or other hormone use	8.5% (21)
BCP ≥ 5 years	4.5% (11)
Pregnancy history	
Nulliparous	19.1% (47)
First pregnancy at < 20 years	8.1% (20)
First pregnancy at > 35 years	0.8% (2)
Nursing history	
Yes	40.2% (99)
No	59.8% (147)

*Total number of patients is 246.

cer are also detailed in Table 1. The relatively infrequent use of birth control pills was most likely related to the date of the screening program and the age of the women screened. These figures would probably have been markedly increased in more current studies, especially if younger women were screened.

The major risk factors of family history and previous breast biopsy are further analyzed in Tables 2a and 2b. Very few women were at risk using both criteria; only 5.7% and 2.0%, respectively, were at risk for any family history and any immediate family history plus a previous breast biopsy. The number of women without any major risk factor was surprisingly high at 53.7%. In younger women aged 44-50 years, the comparable figure was still relatively high at 44.6%.

Analysis of pathology and lymph node status (Table 3) reveals data generally comparable with other published series (Bland et al. 1981, Fisher et al. 1975). There were 249 cancers found in 246 women; three patients had bilateral syn-

Table 2a. *Profile of 246 Patients Aged 44–67 with Presence or Absence of Risk Factors*

| | | | Family History of Breast Cancer | | |
		Any (+)	M or S (+)*	M and S (−)	None (−)
Previous breast biopsy	yes	14 (5.7%)	5 (2.0%)	45 (18.3%)	36 (14.6%)
	no	64 (26.0%)	32 (13.0%)	144 (58.5%)	132 (53.7%)

*M = mother, S = sister.

Table 2b. *Profile of 65 Patients Aged 44–50 with Presence or Absence of Risk Factors*

| | | | Family History of Breast Cancer | | |
		Any (+)	M or S (+)*	M and S (−)	None (−)
Previous breast biopsy	yes	5 (7.7%)	0	13 (20.0%)	8 (12.3%)
	no	22 (33.8%)	10 (15.4%)	42 (64.6%)	29 (44.6%)

*M = mother, S = sister.

Table 3. *Surgical Pathology Results*

Histology	No.	%
Invasive ductal carcinoma:		
Medullary	6	2.4
Papillary	6	2.4
Tubular	6	2.4
Comedo	5	2.0
Mucinous	1	.4
Not otherwise specified	185	74.4
Invasive lobular carcinoma	9	3.6
Noninvasive carcinoma		
Lobular	11	4.4
Ductal	8	3.2
Unknown	12	4.8
	249*	100.0
Lymph Node (LN) Status		
Negative	103	41.9
1–3 (+)	26	10.5
≥4 (+)	11	4.5
Unspecified (+)	1	.4
Bilateral (+)	1	.4
Inoperable	5	2.0
No LN sampling	12	4.9
No LN found	1	.4
Unknown	86	35.0
	246	100.0

*Includes bilateral synchronous carcinoma in three patients.

Table 4. *Characteristics of the BDC* Screening Program*

Time of Detection[†]	No.	%
First screen (+)	178	72.4
Second screen (+)[‡]	61	24.8
(Initial (−) screen)		
Cancer found outside BDC[§]	25	10.2

*Breast Diagnostic Center of Thomas Jefferson University Hospital.
[†](+) = positive; (−) = negative.
[‡]Positive second screen 2 years after initial negative screen.
[§]Range 3–28 months (mean = 12.7 months) after initial negative BDC screen.

chronous cancers. Lymph node status was reported for each patient. Of the three patients with bilateral breast cancers, two were considered inoperable. The third had bilateral mastectomies and had bilateral positive lymph nodes at pathology. Most tumors were of ductal origin (84.0% invasive and 3.2% noninvasive); there were fewer lobular lesions (3.6% invasive and 4.4% noninvasive). Pathology from the definitive operative procedure is unknown in only 12 patients (4.8%). Lymph nodes were negative in 41.9% of the overall group, and 15.8% had at least one documented lymph node metastasis. However, the lymph node status of 86 patients (35.0%) was unknown.

Characteristics related to the screening procedure are listed in Table 4. In a majority of women (72.4%), at least one of the three screening procedures (thermogram, mammogram, or clinical examination) was positive on first screening, which led to the subsequent diagnosis of malignancy. However, a significant number of interval cancers (24.8%) were found at routine 2-year screening after an initial negative screen. In addition, 25 were patients found to have cancer outside of the BDC program following an initial negative screen, and all but one of these patients were diagnosed within 2 years of the negative BDC screen.

DISCUSSION

The definitions of increased risk characteristics were intentionally liberally interpreted in relation to the usual definitions. In designing a screening program only for women at higher risk, this interpretation minimized the number of women excluded from screening by including patients even "marginally" at higher risk. For example, a woman with an unspecified positive family history or any prior breast biopsy or aspiration, even if not for cystic disease, would be included in such a screening program.

Given the above considerations, it is striking that slightly over half (53.7%) of all cases of breast cancer would not have been detected if only selected women with higher risk characteristics were screened (Tables 2a and 2b). If only the 65 women

44   50 years of age were reviewed, again an impressively large number of cancers (44.6%) would have been missed by screening only women with higher risk factors. The increased percentage of cancers in younger women with higher risk factors could have been predicted a priori and was predominantly secondary to the higher percentage of positive family history in younger women (41.5% with any positive family history) versus the entire group (31.7%). If the stricter criteria of a positive family history in an immediate relative (i.e. mother or sister) were used, then an even greater percentage of cancers would have been missed (58.5% in the overall group and 64.6% in the group less than 50 years of age). Therefore, any mass screening program exclusively targeting women with higher risk factors would miss over half of all asymptomatic but detectable breast cancers.

We also evaluated whether the inclusion of women with any other single minor risk factor (Table 1) would substantially lower the number of cancers missed. When the 132 women (Table 2a) with negative family histories and no previous breast biopsy were examined, the most significant minor risk factors were found to be Jewish religious preference, nulliparity, and long menstrual history (more than 40 years), which reduced the number of cancers missed to 40.2%, 44.3%, and 45.1%, respectively. Therefore, the addition of any single minor risk factor to family history of breast cancer and previous breast surgery as criteria for inclusion in a selective screening program would not substantially increase the number of cancers found.

Of the patients in whom the lymph node status was known, 64.4% (103/160) of the overall group had no lymph node metastases. This figure is comparable with other published data for mass screening programs (Bland et al. 1981, Shapiro 1977) and confirms that early cancers are being detected. Of the evaluable patients 50 years of age and under, 55.6% (25/45) were without evidence of lymph node spread. Additionally, in this younger age group, there were 10.8% (7/65) noninvasive carcinomas versus 8.0% (19/237) of the evaluable lesions in the overall group. Inasmuch as early cancers are being picked up in the 45–50 age group, it appears justified to include this group for mass screening. We are unable to comment on even-younger women as they were not included in the BDC screening program. However, we feel that this is an area that should be explored in future studies.

There were 25 cancers detected outside of the BDC following a completely negative screen. All but one were found within 2 years, and 16 were found within 12 months of previous BDC screening (mean = 12.7 months). This latter group probably represents the true false-negative group (6.5%) missed during the screening examination.

The cost effectiveness of the BDC screening program was not analyzed as this was not the intent of the study. However, it should be noted that any cost-effectiveness study must weigh the consequence of missing more than half of all cancers in a limited screening program with the greater cost of an inclusive screening program aimed at all women regardless of presence or absence of higher risk factors.

In conclusion, mass screening programs that target only women with known risk factors for breast cancer miss slightly more than half of the patients with asymptomatic cancers. Therefore, the design of any such program must include all women and not just those with an identifiable risk factor in their personal or family history so that a significant number of patients with asymptomatic but detectable disease will not be excluded. These findings are equally valid in younger women aged 45–50, and, therefore, the design of mass screening programs should be extended to include women at least as young as 45 years of age.

ACKNOWLEDGMENTS

This investigation was supported in part by Grant Number N01-CN-35027, awarded by the National Cancer Institute, U.S. Department of Health and Human Services.

The authors are indebted to Mrs. Cindy Rosser for secretarial assistance and to Mrs. Carrie Solin for data collection.

REFERENCES

Bailar, J. C., III. 1977. Screening for early breast cancer: Pros and cons. Cancer 39:2783–2795.

Berlin, N. I. 1981. Breast cancer screening: The case for screening women younger than 50 years. JAMA 245:1060.

Bland, K. I., J. B. Buchanan, D. L. Mills, T. J. Kuhns, C. Moore, T. S. Spratt, and H. C. Polk, Jr. 1981. Analysis of breast cancer screening in women younger than 50 years. JAMA 245:1037–1042.

Fisher, E. R., R. M. Gregoria, B. Fisher, and participating NSABP investigators. 1975. The pathology of invasive breast cancer: A syllabus derived from findings of the NSABP (protocol 4). Cancer 36:1–85.

Guidelines for the Cancer-Related Checkup: Recommendations and Rationale. 1980. CA 30:224–232.

Haagensen, C. D. 1971. Disease of the Breast (2nd edition). W. B. Saunders, Co., Philadelphia, pp. 146–147.

Lemon, H. M., and E. U. Thiessen. 1974. Summary and recommendations of the workshop on breast cancer. Cancer 33:1740–1743, 1759–1761.

Morgan, R. W., and D. V. Vakil. 1976. Opportunities for prevention, *in* Risk Factors in Breast Cancer, B. A. Stoll, ed. Wm. Heinemann Medical Books Ltd., Great Britain, pp. 226–234.

Shapiro, S. 1977. Evidence on screening for breast cancer from a randomized trial. Cancer 39:2772–2782.

Stark, A. M., and S. Way. 1974. The screening of well women for the early detection of breast cancer using clinical examination with thermography and mammography. Cancer 33:1671–1679.

Current Controversies in Breast Cancer, edited
by F. C. Ames, G. R. Blumenschein, and E. D. Montague.
University of Texas Press, Austin © 1984.

The Current Status of Stress Telethermometry in the Detection and Monitoring of Breast Disease

Philip G. Brooks, M.D.

The University of Southern California School of Medicine, Los Angeles, California

In recent years, the progressive increase in the incidence of breast carcinoma and the persistently rising number of deaths from that disease, despite improvements in surgical, radiation, and chemotherapeutic treatments, have mandated increased efforts toward early diagnosis.

Results of studies by Shapiro et al. (1972) and Hicks et al. (1979) clearly showed improved survival resulting from breast screening and early detection methods. To reach the greatest numbers of women, the screening method should be safe, inexpensive, reasonably accurate, and simple enough for the primary care physician to interpret. Unfortunately, because of fears of radiation hazards, expense of equipment, and a limited number of trained interpreters, x-ray and ultrasound breast imaging have not succeeded as widespread screening techniques. Telethermography has had limited acceptance because of its expense. To date, contact thermography is the most widely used breast screening technique, although difficult interpretation and imprecision have retarded widespread acceptance and have prompted suggestions that it be used only with other screening methods (Shaber 1980).

Therefore, a study was begun September 1, 1978, to determine whether a new method, computer-assisted stress telethermometry, could become a more effective screening tool for primary care physicians (Brooks et al. 1983). This heat-sensing method uses a hand-held infrared sensing probe placed 1 or 2 cm away from the skin overlying the breast and passed sequentially over the nipple and eight segments of each breast while the patient is in the supine position. The patient then immerses her hands in ice water for 15 seconds, and the entire procedure is repeated. Heat emission is directly proportional to infrared radiation, and infrared measurements are recorded in 0.1°C steps by a microcomputer programmed to analyze thermal patterns. After this analysis, the computer assesses a score from 1 through 99 that approximates the relative risk of breast disease based on experience accumulated from a data base of over 21,000 tests performed on normal and diseased breasts. Within several minutes, the computer generates a three-page printed report listing the patient's historical data, the actual temperatures of the breast, as well as those of the forehead and the testing room for comparison, and a histogram depicting the heat emission patterns of the breast with areas of concern clearly marked.

Initial validation of the efficacy of stress telethermometry was reported by Snyder (1979). In a study of 315 patients with biopsy-proved disease, only 5% of the cancers fell into the lowest score grouping (so-called class I). Almost two-thirds of the cancers fell into the highest risk grouping (class III). In addition, Snyder found that the size of the lesion had no significant effect on the scores nor on the frequency of false-negative results.

MATERIALS AND METHODS

From September 1, 1978, through August 31, 1981, 1,030 patients underwent screening stress telethermometry (total of 2,012 tests; an average of almost two tests per patient). No patient in this study had palpable masses, nipple discharge, or acute breast symptoms, because those patients were not considered asymptomatic and were excluded. The indications for recommending stress telethermometry were age 35 or older, a family history of breast cancer, or a prior history of breast pathology (excluding the young patient with so-called fibrocystic breast disease symptoms and granularity).

Patients with high-risk scores or suspicious thermal patterns (irrespective of the score), or both, were referred for x-ray mammography and, when indicated, surgical consultation.

RESULTS

Table 1 shows the age distribution of the 1,030 patients screened. The surprisingly high percentage of patients under age 40 reflects the characteristics of our patient population as well as the anxiety about breast disease in younger women, who fear repeated exposure to radiation more than older women do.

Table 2 shows the distribution of the scores. The preponderance of patients in the intermediate risk category (class II) reflects the large number of patients in our practice with fibrocystic or symptomatic changes in the breast. These patients more readily accept closer monitoring and newer techniques for the detection of pathologic conditions of the breast. In a previous report of our early experience with stress telethermometry (Brooks et al. 1980), we reported that our patients had an almost threefold greater incidence of breast symptoms than did those in a normal randomized sampling of the population.

Table 1. *Age Distribution of 1,030 Patients*

Age	No.	%
Under 30	130	13
31–40	439	43
41–50	290	28
51–60	130	13
60–70	32	3
Over 70	9	1

Table 2. *Distribution of 2,012 GST* Scores*

Score	Number of Tests (%)
1−40 (class I)	438 (22)
41−80 (class II)	1190 (59)
81−99 (class III)	384 (19)

*GST = Graphic stress telethermometry.

Table 3. *Results of Mammography*

Number recommended, but refused	31
Number performed	258
Results:	
no evidence of pathology	18
fibrocystic disease	46
mammary dysplasia	191
suspicious for carcinoma	3

Table 3 shows the results of referrals for mammography. Note that 31 of 289 patients (11%) refused x-rays. The current resistance of patients to radiation is a significant factor in the assessment of mammography as a screening tool. Evaluation of the results of mammography distinctly show the value of stress telethermometry in detecting breast disease. Only 18 (6%) of these mammograms reported no evidence of disease, that is, 94% of abnormal stress telethermometries show radiographic evidence of breast pathology. This group of patients should be followed carefully, since recent data (Gautherie and Gros 1980) indicate that within 5 years of original testing 38% of patients with suspicious thermograms but negative x-ray and physical examinations ultimately develop histologically proved cancer.

Table 4 lists the results of the surgical referrals. Of the 61 patients referred for surgical consultations because of abnormal stress telethermometry, mammography, or physical examination results, half underwent observation or aspiration biopsy only. Thirty-one patients underwent surgical biopsy, and over half of those had fibroadenomata. Table 5 presents data on the six patients in whom carcinoma was diagnosed. Three of these patients were under age 50. Five of the patients under-

Table 4. *Results of Surgical Referral*

Number referred	61
Examination only	16
Aspiration biopsy only	14
Surgical biopsies done	31
fibroadenoma	17
mammary dysplasia	7
lipoma	2
carcinoma	5

Table 5. *Carcinomas Diagnosed*

Pts.	Age	GST* Scores	Mammography Results	Pathologic Diagnosis	Date of Surgery	Tumor Size	Positive Nodes	Miscellaneous
1.	60	81,85	negative	infiltrating ductal CA	7/79	0.3 cm	?	biopsy after nipple bleeding lumpectomy, radiation
2.	48	99	negative	infiltrating ductal CA	2/80	1.0 cm	none	very dense breasts
3.	30	77	not done	medullary CA	1/80	2.0 cm	none	biopsy of mass found 4 months after GST
4.	51	80	not done	infiltrating ductal CA	12/80	1.3 cm	none	biopsy of ill-defined thickening
5.	58	35†	positive	infiltrating ductal CA	9/79	1.2 cm	none	developed mass 3 months after normal GST
6.	48	46,75	negative then suspicious	infiltrating ductal CA	8/81	1.0 cm	none	serial GSTs show progression of abnormality

*GST = Graphic stress telethermometry.
†Score on newest algorithm: 82.

went modified radical mastectomies; the sixth (No. 1) refused this procedure and opted for lumpectomy and radiation therapy instead. None of the five who underwent mastectomy had positive lymph nodes. Patient No. 5 originally had an overall score in the low-risk category. Three months later, a mammogram was obtained because of increased breast thickening; on the basis of the mammogram, carcinoma was suspected and confirmed on biopsy. No other false-negative stress telethermometries have occurred in this study, nor have any occurred among the 481 patients whose stress telethermometry results were reported in our earlier study (Brooks et al. 1980), which has 36 or more months of follow-up. Finally, the average size of the five lesions detected by stress telethermometry was 1.1 cm.

DISCUSSION

Stress telethermometry, because of its noninvasive nature, its relatively low cost to the patient, and its lack of direct contact with the breast, is an acceptable office procedure. The fact that it is computer read and includes a superficial vasoconstrictive stress test obviates many of the problems with high percentages of false-positive results and subjective interpretations that accompany other heat-sensing methods.

Because stress telethermometry measures function instead of structure, and because of the computer-assisted display of the thermal emission pattern and risk score, we have been able to use this technique to monitor changes in breast function. Confirming the original report by Minton et al. (1979) that patients with fibrocystic breast disease showed dramatic improvement when caffeine was eliminated from the diet, we were able to monitor this improvement objectively in 66 patients (Brooks et al. 1981). In that study, stress telethermometry scores improved by almost 34%, while stress telethermometry patterns became less atypical in 85% of the subjects after only 6 months of caffeine restriction.

Another attempt at diminishing symptoms and signs of fibrocystic disease was reported by London et al. (1978), wherein vitamin E was used with good success in a small number of patients. Again, we tried to document objectively the effects of this therapy upon the course of fibrocystic disease. To date, 28 patients have been studied for a minimum of 6 months of treatment with 600 IU of vitamin E daily. Our preliminary results have been far less striking than those in the caffeine study. After 6 months of treatment with vitamin E, there was an average improvement in over-all GST scores of 7 points (8.3%) (Table 6). This figure is not statistically significant. Furthermore, there were as many patients with no change as those who improved

Table 6. *Vitamin E and Fibrocystic Breast Disease*
Stress Teletherometry Scores

Before therapy	(avg.)	77.2
6 mos. after therapy	(avg.)	70.4
Percent change		8.3%

Table 7. *Change in Breast Thermal Emission on Vitamin E Therapy*

Number improved (>7 points)	12 (43%)
Number unchanged	13 (46%)
Number worsened (>7 points)	3 (11%)

after vitamin E therapy, while a small number of patients (11%) showed a significantly worsening picture (Table 7).

As stress telethermometry is a relatively new technique, there have been a significant number of improvements over the 3 years of use. Computers get "smarter" as more information is added to their data bases. Table 8 shows the improvement in both specificity (i.e., fewer false-positive results) and in sensitivity (fewer false-negative results). Patient No. 5 (Table 5), originally scored as low risk, now has a test score in the high-risk category after rescoring on the newest algorithm. Further evidence of improvement comes from evaluation of the study by Snyder et al. (1979), wherein 5% of biopsy-proved cancers had low-risk scores. Rescored on the newest algorithm, only 2% of cancers fall into the low-risk category. While such cases represent false negative results, there is some evidence that thermally inactive or "cold" tumors have more favorable prognoses. Gautherie and Gros (1980) state that there is an unequivocal relationship between tumor growth rate and metabolic heat production and that lymphatic involvement is very well correlated with decreased tumor doubling time. Hobbins and King (1980) agree, calling contact thermography the most significant marker for malignant grade of the tumor.

The major criticism of stress telethermometry is that there have been too few patients reported. Table 9 summarizes the studies reported to date, including the present one. All of these reports, with data covering a total of over 3,000 well-followed patients and over 200 biopsy-proved cancers, conclude that stress telethermometry is extremely useful as a risk indicator that successfully separates asymptomatic patients into risk categories. It is particularly useful in helping physicians to decide whether to order x-ray mammography for patients under age 50.

There is no question that early detection of breast cancer improves survival. There is no doubt that, to reach all women, breast screening must be the responsibility of the primary care physician. Our data and those of others clearly show stress

Table 8. *Improvements in Data Analysis and Computer Programming*

	Benign (%)				Malignant (%)				
		Class				Class			Sensitivity +
Algorithm	1	2	3	Specificity	1	2	3	Sensitivity	Specificity
13.3	33	41	26	74	7	28	65	65	139
13.4	40	46	14	86	6	37	57	57	143
14.0	37	46	17	83	2	27	71	71	154

Table 9. *Summary of Stress Telethermometry Data**

Reported studies:	No. patients	No. cancers
Snyder	315	162
Jurist	721	19
Dorsey	294	6
Morese	753	9
Brooks	1,030	6
TOTALS	3,113	202

*Central data base: 21,500 tests.

telethermometry to be an effective office screening method for the early detection of breast disease and a most useful tool for monitoring the metabolic functions of the breast.

REFERENCES

Brooks, P. G., S. Gart, A. J. Heldfond, M. L. Margolin, and A. S. Allen. 1981. Measuring the effect of caffeine restriction on fibrocystic breast disease. J. Reprod. Med. 26:279.

Brooks, P. G., S. Gart, and A. J. Heldfond. 1983. Breast screening in the primary care office: A plea for early detection. J. Reprod. Med. 27:685.

Brooks, P. G., A. J. Heldfond, M. L. Margolin, A. S. Allen, and S. Gart. 1980. Graphic Stress Telethermometry: An ideal office screening device for the detection of breast disease. J. Reprod. Med. 25:1–4.

Dorsey, J. H., A. C. W. Montague, and G. L. Stonesifer. 1981. Graphic stress telethermometry, *in* Diagnosis and Treatment of Breast Cancer, E. F. Lewison and A. C. W. Montague, eds. William and Wilkins, Baltimore, pp. 61–64.

Gautherie, M., and C. M. Gros. 1980. Breast thermography and cancer risk prediction. Cancer 45:51–56.

Hicks, M. J., J. R. Davis, J. M. Layton, and A. I. Present. 1979. Sensitivity of mammography and physical examination of the breast for detecting breast cancer. JAMA 242:2080–2083.

Hobbins, W. B., and B. J. King. 1980. Report of thermographic breast biopsy correlation. ACTA Thermographica 5:43–45.

Jurist, J. M., and D. B. Myers. 1981. Stress thermography in breast cancer. Biomed. Sci. Instrum. 17:1–4.

London, R. S., D. M. Solomon, E. D. London, D. Strummer, J. Bankoski, and P. P. Nair. 1978. Mammary dysplasia: Clinical response and urinary excretion of 11-deoxy-17 ketosteroids and pregnandiol following alpha-tocopherol therapy. Breast 4(2):19.

Minton, J. P., M. K. Foecking, D. J. T. Webster, and R. H. Matthews. 1979. Caffeine, cyclic nucleotides, and breast disease. Surgery 86:105.

Shaber, G. S. 1980. Breast cancer screening: Thermography's role, *in* Breast Disease, Diagnosis and Treatment, G. F. Schwartz and D. Marchant, eds. Elsevier/North Holland, New York, pp. 153–172.

Shapiro, S., P. Strax, and L. Venet. 1972. Changes in 5-year breast cancer mortality in a breast cancer screening program, *in* Proceedings of the Seventh National Cancer Conference. American Cancer Society and National Cancer Institute, New York, pp. 663–687.

Snyder, R., R. C. Watson, and N. Cruz. 1979. Graphic stress telethermometry: A possible supplement to physical examination in screening for abnormalities in the female breast. Am. J. Diag. Gynecol. Obstet. 1:197.

Current Controversies in Breast Cancer, edited
by F. C. Ames, G. R. Blumenschein, and E. D. Montague.
University of Texas Press, Austin © 1984.

Efficacy of Breast Self-Examination in the Discovery of Breast Cancer

James L. Hoehn, M.D.,* Willard (Pat) Pierce, Ph.D.,† and
Thomas G. Olsen, M.D.‡

*Departments of *Surgery and ‡Radiology, Marshfield Clinic, and †Marshfield Medical
Foundation, Marshfield, Wisconsin*

Breast self-examination has become a popular health topic and has had the enthusiastic support of many lay groups. The scientific literature has several conflicting reports as to its efficacy: Foster et al. (1978), Grenwald et al. (1978), Feldman et al. (1981), and Huguley and Brown (1981) report earlier detection through breast self-examination, whereas Thiessen (1971), Smith et al. (1980), and Senie et al. (1981) show no particular benefit through self-examination. Also several editorialists (Moore 1978 and Cole and Austin 1981) have criticized the studies in favor of self-examination for not specifically mentioning whether or not the patient was practicing breast self-examination at the moment of discovery of the breast cancer. They cautioned against the widespread endorsement of breast self-examination until benefit can be demonstrated scientifically. Additionally, the size of breast and density of breast as well as the location of the tumor within the breast were not discussed in these papers. Many reports come from breast cancer detection centers with large heterogeneous populations, and many investigators were involved in the retrospective review and extraction of data. We have attempted to look at breast self-examination efficacy by specifically addressing some of the above criticisms.

METHODS

Within a 24-month period (August 1978 through July 1980), 100 consecutive breast cancers in 97 patients were seen and treated by a single surgeon. For subsequent discussion of data, each cancer has been treated as a single patient. At the time of initial evaluation of the patient, a common historical data base was obtained (Table 1). Specifically, the patient was asked if she was practicing self-examination at the time of discovery of the abnormality. The frequency of breast self-examination was grouped into the following categories: Regular (from daily to once every 2 months), occasional (every 2 months to once a year), and never (less frequent than once a year).

Table 1. *Clinical Parameters*

Menopausal status
How abnormality was found
Practice of breast self-examination
Clinical stage
Pathologic size
Pathologic nodal status
Histologic type

Table 2. *Radiographic Parameters*

Volume of breast
Density of breast
Location of cancer
Depth of cancer

Retrospectively, a single radiologist reviewed all the available mammograms. The radiographic parameters are listed in Table 2. The volume of the breast is approximated in cubic centimeters as determined by the formula $V = 2/3 \pi$ ([width + Height]/3)^3 in which width is determined by measurement from the cephalocaudad view of the mammogram and height is determined by measuring the perpendicular through the nipple to the chest wall on the medial to lateral projection. The breast density was classified $N_1 P_1 P_2 D_Y$ as per Wolfe (1976). The location of the tumor within the breast was categorized into medial, lateral, and central locations and not seen. Depth was classified relative to the point midway between the nipple and the chest wall on both views. The classification of exact location depended on which side of the line the bulk of the tumor lay. Only 82 preoperative mammograms were available for analysis. Six patients had obvious advanced local disease and were not subjected to mammography preoperatively. Three patients were 30 years of age or younger and did not receive mammograms. Five patients had biopsies performed elsewhere, and so tumors were no longer present within the breast. Two patients had mammograms taken elsewhere and these were not recalled for this study. The preoperative mammograms on the remaining two patients were not ordered.

RESULTS

Of the entire group of 100 breast cancers, 23 occurred in premenopausal, 72 in postmenopausal, and 5 in perimenopausal women. For subsequent discussion, the postmenopausal and perimenopausal women are grouped together. Fifty-eight percent had pathologically negative nodes, 41% had positive nodes, and one patient's lymph nodes were not sampled.

Pathologic Staging

Clinical staging was evaluated and was not pertinent for further consideration. A T_1 lesion is defined as 2 cm or less, T_2, 2.1 to 5.0 cm; and T_3, 5.1 to 10.0 cm. To facilitate discussion, the microscopic lesions are grouped with the T_1 lesions. When evaluating the pathologic status seven tumors were either not measured, or the multiple fragments were such that they could not be reliably added together. In the remaining 93 patients with adequate data, 54.8% were T_1, 38.7% T_2, and 6.5% T_3. The breakdown varied between the pre- and postmenopausal groups. In the premenopausal group, 38.1% were T_1, 57.1% T_2, and 4.8% T_3. In the postmenopausal group, 59.7% were T_1, 33.3% T_2, and 6.9% T_3 ($P = > 0.15$).

Histology

The tumor histologies of the entire group were not unlike those reported in other series. Sixty-three percent of the tumors were infiltrating duct carcinoma, 14% infiltrating lobular carcinoma, 8% intraductal carcinoma, 4% tubular carcinoma, 3% mucinous carcinoma, 2% lobular carcinoma in situ, and 6% others.

Frequency of Breast Self-Exam

The frequency of breast self-examination is known for 90 cancers and varies with menopausal status. In the premenopausal women, 42% claimed regular practice of breast self-examination, 32% practiced it occasionally, and 26% never practiced. For the postmenopausal group, 21% claimed regular practice, 32% occasional, and 47% never. The differences between the regular and never in the pre- and postmenopausal groups is statistically significant $P = < 0.05$.

Method of Detection

For the entire group of 100 cancers, 54% were discovered by accident, 18% by self-examination, 14% by routine physical examination, and 13% by x-ray. One cancer was found at the time of a prophylactic contralateral mastectomy. In the premenopausal group, 47.8% were found by accident, 34.8% by breast self-examination, 13% by physical examination, and 4.4% by x-ray. In the postmenopausal group, 55.8% were found by accident, 13.0% by breast self-examination, 14.3% by physical examination, 15.6% by x-ray, and 1.3% by others. For those tumors found by breast self-examination, the differences between the pre- and postmenopausal group is statistically significant in that $P = < 0.05$.

Influence of Method of Discovery on Tumor and Nodal Status

The method of discovery was correlated with pathologic tumor size as well as nodal status. Of the T_1 carcinomas, 47% were found by accident, 65% by breast self-examination, 37% by physical examination, and 85% by x-ray. More T_1 carcinomas were found by x-ray than any other method. However, more T_1 lesions were found by breast self-examination than by physical examination or by accident. When lymph node status was also evaluated, the advantage of the smaller tumor size was lost. In those patients with tumors found by accident, 41% had lymph node disease; by breast self-examination, 44%; by physical examination, 50%; and by x-ray, 31%.

Tumor Size Relative to Practice of Breast Self-Exam, Not Method of Discovery

Of the entire group, 23% claimed regular breast self-examination, 29% occasional, 38% never, and 10% unknown. Corresponding nodal disease status was 39%, 28%, 50%, and 60%, respectively. Of the 54 patients who found the tumor by accident, five reported regular breast self-examination, 17 occasional, 27 never, and five unknown. Their nodal disease status increased with decreased frequency of breast self-examination with 20%, 35%, 52%, and 40% having positive nodes, respectively. Additionally, the tumor size increased with decreased frequency of breast self-examination. Of the five patients who regularly performed breast self-examination, 80% had T_1 lesions; of those performing occasional examination 57% had T_1 lesions; of those never performing examination, 33% had T_1 disease; and of those with unknown self-exams, 20% had T_1 lesions. Therefore, it seems that regular breast self-examination is beneficial in detecting changes in breast substance, even though it may not be the actual mechanism of discovery of a breast cancer.

Radiologic Parameters

Density and Volume

Upon review of the 82 mammograms available, the carcinoma was not seen in 15 (18.3%). Ten of these obscured carcinomas lay in D_Y breasts. In categorizing the entire group, 19.5% had N_1 breasts, 32.9% P_1, 24.4% P_2, and 23.2% D_Y. In evaluating the premenopausal group, 7.7% had N_1 breasts, 17.6% P_1, 11.7% P_2, and 58.9% D_Y. For the postmenopausal group, 21.5% had N_1 breasts, 36.9% P_1, 27.7% P_2, and 13.9% D_Y ($P = < 0.005$). With increasing breast volume, there was an increasing frequency of N_1 patterns and decreasing frequency of D_Y patterns (Figure 1). Although the pathologic tumor size did not vary with breast density, nodal involvement was directly related to density in that 25% of patients with N_1 breasts had nodal disease, 30% of those with P_1, 40% with P_2, and 58% with D_Y ($P = < 0.1 > 0.05$). Additionally, with increasing breast volume there was no change in pathologic tumor size, but there was an inverse correlation between breast volume and nodal involvement (Table 3). Breast self-examination was more efficient in discovering carcinomas in small breasts and x-ray in larger breasts (Figure 2). When density is considered, 42% of tumors in D_Y breasts were found by breast

Table 3. *Breast Size Relative to Tumor Size and Nodal Disease*

Size	Nodal Positivity		Lesions T_1	
	No. Pts.	%	No. Pts.	%
<700	5/10	50	8/10	80
701–1400	10/24	42	10/24	42
1401–2400	6/16	38	7/16	44
2401–3100	5/15	33	6/15	40
>3100	4/17	24	10/17	54

Density and Volume of Breast

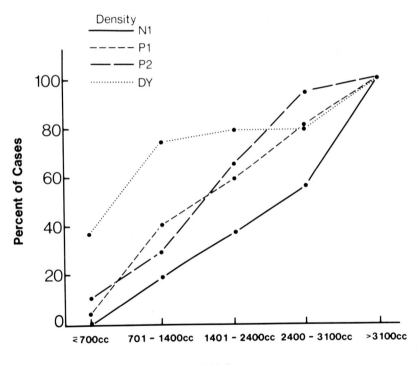

FIG. 1. This figure relates breast density and volume illustrating that there are more D_Y breasts in the smaller breast size and more N_1 breasts with the larger volumes. Breast density is classified as N_1, P_1, P_2, D_Y, as per Wolfe (1976).

How Tumor Was Found By Volume of Breast

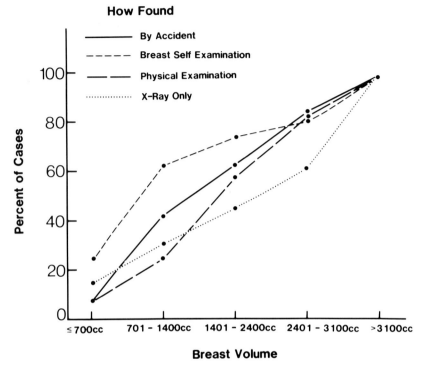

FIG. 2. This figure illustrates method of discovery by volume of breast; x-ray is most efficient in finding lesions in the larger breasts and self-examination in the smaller denser breast.

self-examination, and only 16% were found by x-ray. In N_1 breasts, however, x-ray found 31%, and breast self-examination only 6%.

Location And Depth of Tumor

Analysis showed no relationship between mechanism of discovery and location of the tumor within the breast when categorized by medial, central, and lateral locations. As for depth of tumor, there were actually smaller tumor sizes for the deep lesions when compared to the superficial ones (T_1, 60% versus 37.5%, respectively). In the 15 carcinomas not seen by x-ray, 73.3% were T_1 lesions. There was no difference in nodal involvement between the superficial and deep tumors; 37.5% of the superficial tumors and 31.4% of the deep lesions were associated with nodal disease.

DISCUSSION

The number of patients performing breast self-examination on a regular basis has been reported in the literature ranging from 18% (Foster et al. 1978) to 34% (Huguley et al. 1981). In our series, 23% practiced breast self-examination regularly, but in only 18 patients was breast self-examination practiced at the time of discovery of the breast cancer. When tabulating tumor size relative to mechanism discovery, x-ray was the most efficient in finding small tumors. Eighty-five percent of T_1 lesions were found by x-ray, and 61% by self-examination. However, tumor size is not as good a predictor of future outcome as nodal involvement. Breast self-examination was not different than other methods of discovery when its use was correlated with frequency of nodal disease.

Feldman et al. 1981 found no difference between monthly and episodic breast self-examination, indicating that prior knowledge of breast architecture was important. When evaluating tumor and nodal status relationship to use of breast self-examination, not mechanism of discovery, we have shown that breast self-examination is efficacious in finding more T_1 lesions and is effective in finding lesions in patients with less lymph node involvement.

Size and density of the breast are related. Although tumor size does not vary with either, nodal disease does. Perhaps this is because the tumor is obscured in the small, dense breasts. Most likely it is because the D_Y pattern is most often seen in the premenopausal woman, and increased nodal disease reflects a different biologic aggressiveness of the tumor. The most efficient mechanism for finding smaller tumors was x-ray, particularly in large, fatty breasts, but x-ray was less effective than breast self-examination in the small, dense breasts. Patients with small, dense breasts may be candidates for more intensive educational efforts on breast examination coupled with a more formalized program of physical examination and mammography. Educational efforts might also be applied to the postmenopausal group; forty-seven percent of these women never performed breast self-examination in this study.

Breast self-examination, the patient's part in total health care, must be integrated with a routine physical examination of the breast and mammography. Even though breast self-examination is effective in finding smaller lesions, there is still room for improvement in detecting early breast cancers; between 28% and 39% of our patients who practiced some form of breast self-examination had positive lymph nodes. This group is still at high risk for future failure.

ACKNOWLEDGMENTS

The authors gratefully acknowledge the computer skills of William R. Carl and the patient secretarial help of Loretta Keding.

BIBLIOGRAPHY

Cole, P., and H. Austin. 1981. Breast self-examination: An adjunct to early cancer detection. Am. J. Public Health 71:572–574.

Feldman, J. G., A. C. Carter, A. D. Nicastri, and S. T. Hosat. 1981. Breast self-examination, relationship to stage of breast cancer at diagnosis. Cancer 47:2740–2745.

Foster, R. S., S. P. Lang, M. C. Costanza, J. K. Worden, C. R. Haines, and J. W. Yates. 1978. Breast self-examination practices and breast-cancer stage. N. Engl. J. Med. 299:265–270.

Grenwald, P., P. C. Nasca, C. E. Lawrence, J. Horton, R. P. McGarrah, T. Gabriele, and K. Carlton. 1978. Estimated effect of breast self-examination and routine physician examinations on breast cancer mortality. N. Engl. J. Med. 299:271–273.

Huguley, C. M., and R. L. Brown. 1981. The value of breast self-examination. Cancer 47:989–995.

Moore, F. D. Breast self-examination. 1978. N. Engl. J. Med. 299:304–305.

Senie, R. T., P. P. Rosen, M. L. Lesser, and D. W. Kinne. 1981. Breast self-examination and medical examination related to breast cancer stage. Am. J. Public Health 71:583–590.

Smith, E. M., A. M. Francis, and L. Polissar. 1980. The effect of breast self-exam practices and physician examinations in extent of disease at diagnosis. Prev. Med. 9:409–417.

Thiessen, E. U. 1971. Breast self-examination in proper perspective. Cancer 28:1537–1545.

Wolfe, J. N. 1976. Risk for breast cancer development determined by mammographic parenchymal pattern. Cancer 37:2486–2492.

Current Controversies in Breast Cancer, edited
by F. C. Ames, G. R. Blumenschein, and E. D. Montague.
University of Texas Press, Austin © 1984.

Epidemiology of Male Breast Cancer

Wick R. Williams, Ph.D., Michael D. Badzioch, M.S., and
David E. Anderson, Ph.D.

*Department of Genetics, The University of Texas M. D. Anderson Hospital and Tumor
Institute at Houston, Houston, Texas*

The breast is the leading site of cancer in women, accounting for 26% of the incidence of all female cancer, with 91,000 cases diagnosed in 1979 in the United States. In contrast, breast cancer in men is rare, accounting for approximately 1% of all male cancer, with only 700 diagnosed cases in the United States in 1979. The rarity of the condition in men has precluded our having as complete an understanding of the disease as we have in women.

Recently, we have initiated a study of male breast cancer involving patients seen at The University of Texas M. D. Anderson Hospital and Tumor Institute at Houston. Of particular interest in our study was the examination of family histories and determination of the extent to which male breast cancer results from an inherited liability.

Interest in a family study was motivated by two reasons: first, by the observation that men with breast cancer have been reported in families that also include affected women. In the monograph by Jacobsen (1946), for instance, three out of 200 randomly selected breast cancer patients were men. A positive family history of breast cancer was observed for two of the three men. In addition, three men with breast cancer were observed among relatives of the 197 women patients. Families with more than one affected man with breast cancer have also been reported (Marger et al. 1975, Everson et al. 1976, Teasdale et al. 1976, Schwartz et al. 1980). However, other than isolated case reports, which undoubtedly represent a biased sample, our understanding of the familial nature of male breast cancer and its relationship to female breast cancer remains obscure.

The second reason has a more theoretical basis. If breast cancer in men is part of the same disease process as familial breast cancer in women, then, in accordance with some genetic models of disease transmission (i.e. a multifactorial model) relatives of affected men would be expected to inherit a higher mean liability than relatives of affected women and, consequently, would have a greater frequency of the disease. Thus, selection of families through affected men may be a useful strategy for obtaining some insight into the underlying cause of the observed familial nature of the disease, i.e., whether the consequence of major loci, polygenes, or environmental determinants. Identification of such high-risk families is of concern from the standpoint of prevention and therapy, as well as providing a resource for further study aimed at understanding the cause of breast cancer and for identifying biological markers that have an association with the disease.

In the following article, we describe our study population, review selected clinical and epidemiologic features of the disease in men, and present preliminary results of our family study involving relatives of men patients. This study represents the first major attempt at investigating the familial aspects of male breast cancer. As noted by Lynch (1981), "There is a paucity of knowledge about the genetic aspects of breast cancer in males . . . knowledge of the epidemiology in men could contribute to a better comprehension of its cause in both men and women."

STUDY POPULATION

The study population consists of all men with histologic diagnoses of breast cancer seen at U.T. M. D. Anderson Hospital. Patients were identified by a search of the data base of the Department of Patient Studies (Epidemiology). Initially, only patients admitted after 1970 were considered, resulting in 65 patients. The sampling frame was subsequently extended to include those admitted after January 1, 1960, to increase the size of the study population. The study is a continuing research project; however, for purposes of this report, August 31,1982, was used as a cutoff point, and our results apply only to patients admitted prior to this date. The resulting sample consists of 93 men.

Information on the clinical features of the disease was abstracted from the medical records of the patients. For purposes of this study, we have abstracted information that may be relevant to understanding the cause and familial nature of the disease, particularly those features also associated with a positive family history in relatives of women who have breast cancer, such as age at diagnosis, laterality, histological type of cancer, presence of second primary tumors, medical history (exposure to radiation, previous estrogen therapy), and history of cancer in relatives of the proband.

Questionnaires were sent to the patients or, if deceased, to their spouses or near relatives (siblings) requesting demographic, medical, and family information on the proband and his relatives. The questionnaires were followed by telephone calls to encourage cooperation. This information is being verified by sending identical questionnaires to more than one person in each pedigree. The primary goal was to extend information on the proband to include his first-degree relatives, i.e., parents, siblings, and children, and some second-degree relatives, i.e., grandparents, uncles, and aunts. The sampling scheme is similar to that employed by Jacobsen (1946). Information on more distant relatives was not considered, as it is usually less complete and prone to selection bias.

EPIDEMIOLOGIC AND CLINICAL FEATURES

We reviewed the racial composition, age at diagnosis, laterality, and presence of second primary tumors in our study population. The results are summarized in

Table 1. *Racial Composition and Clinical Features of Study Population*

Race	Number	Mean Age at Diagnosis	Laterality L/R
White	71	56.4	0.9
Black	13	67.2	2.0
Hispanic	9	61.9	3.5
Total	93	58.4	1.15

Table 1. Other studies at U.T. M. D. Anderson Hospital, based upon male breast cancer review selected prognostic factors and the natural history of the disease (Yap et al. 1979), results of chemotherapy (Yap et al. 1980), and results of different treatment regimens (Robison and Montague, 1982).

Racial Composition

Seventy-one patients (76%) were white; 68 were residing in the continental United States at the time of diagnosis. Of these, 62% were from Texas, 15% from contiguous states, and the remaining 23% from more distant states. The second largest racial group was blacks, which was represented by 13 (14%) men. All were reported to be living in Texas. Nine (10%) men were of Hispanic descent; the majority (6) were from Mexico, one was from Guatemala, and one was from Texas.

Age at Diagnosis

The age distribution of patients in our sample is presented in Figure 1. The overall mean age at diagnosis was 58.4 years. The youngest patient was 26 years old and the oldest patient was 87. The overall mean age at onset did not differ significantly from the 59.6 years reported by Crichlow (1972) in a summary of 1,888 men who had breast cancer. Within racial categories, whites were the youngest, having a mean age of 56.4, Hispanics were next, with a mean age of 61.9 years, followed by blacks, with a mean age of 67.2 years.

Laterality

Information on laterality was available on 90 patients. Forty-seven developed breast cancer in the left breast, and 41 developed it in the right breast. The corresponding ratio of left to right was 1.15, which is in agreement with 1.07 reported by Crichlow (1972) in a summary of 1,158 men patients. He also reported a bilateral rate of 1.4%. In our sample, there were two documented instances of bilaterality, for a frequency of 2.2%, in close agreement with Crichlow's finding.

The observation that breast cancer occurs more frequently in the left than the

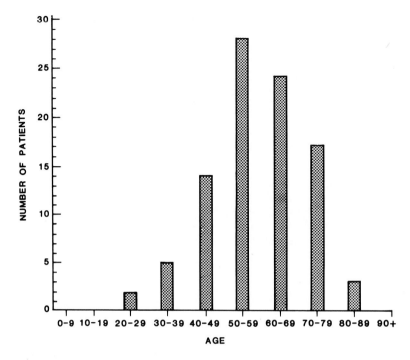

FIG. 1. The distribution of age at diagnosis in our study population.

right breast in men is concordant with the situation in women; the frequency of bi-laterality among men patients is not markedly different from the 3.3% reported among unselected women patients seen at U.T. M. D. Anderson Hospital (Anderson, personal communication).

Other Primary Tumors

We attempted to ascertain whether male patients were more or less susceptible to second malignancies either before or after the diagnosis of breast cancer. Of the 93 patients, the presence of second primary cancers was observed in 17 patients, or 18% of all cases. The 18% is somewhat higher than the 9.2% reported by Crichlow (1972) or the 12.5% reported by Langlands et al. (1976). The type of second primary tumors observed and their frequencies are shown in Table 2. The second malignancies were prostate cancers, three squamous cell carcinomas, and two malignant melanomas. No other malignancy was represented more than once. Slightly more than half of the second primary lesions were diagnosed after the breast cancer was detected. The average interval between the diagnosis of breast cancer and the appearance of the second primary tumor (exclusive of breast cancer) was 4.1 years.

Table 2. *Second Primary Tumors in the Study Population*

Secondary Primary	Number
Cutaneous:	
squamous cell carcinoma	3
malignant melanoma	2
basal cell carcinoma	1
Prostatic carcinoma	4
Colonic carcinoma	2
Thyroid carcinoma	2
Pharyngeal carcinoma	1
Bladder carcinoma	1
Lymphoma	1

FAMILY HISTORY

Preliminary findings of the survey of breast cancer in relatives of the men patients are presented below. The results pertain only to pedigrees of our white patients residing in the United States at the time of diagnosis. There are presently two reasons for limiting the results to this subset of families: The first is that family information on patients from foreign countries has been difficult to obtain and verify, and therefore is still incomplete; the second reason is that limiting the study to whites eliminates potential heterogeneity due to cultural and genetic differences among the three races. It is our intent to continue adding patients to our study. When a reasonable sample of black and Hispanic patients has been accumulated, we will then be able to test for such heterogeneity and determine whether any differences exist with regard to the familial nature of male breast cancer among the three racial groups.

A positive family history of breast cancer was observed in 22 of the 66 patients, resulting in an observed familial incidence of 33%. In 17 of the 22 families with positive histories, the disease occurred in at least one first-degree relative (mother, sister, or daughter). Four of the 17 had more than one first-degree relative with breast cancer. In three families there were two affected sisters of the proband, and in the fourth family a mother and sister of the proband were affected.

For a deleterious trait such as breast cancer, the incidence in women is so high that it would not be unlikely to observe families with more than one affected member solely by chance. To test whether the observed frequency of breast cancer in relatives of men patients is compatible with a chance occurrence, we calculated the number of cases that would be expected in each of six different types of first-degree relatives of our patients. The observed distribution of first-degree relatives is shown in Table 3. Men and women have been grouped into three age categories. For each cell, the expected number of cases was calculated by multiplying the number of observations (affecteds and normals) by the probability a person in the particular age group would be affected, as determined from incidence rates published by the National Cancer Institute (Young et al. 1981). The observed and expected numbers

Table 3. *Distribution of Breast Cancer in First-Degree Relatives of Men Patients*

Age of Proband		Mother's Age			Father's Age			Sister's Age			Brother's Age			Daughter's Age			Son's Age		
		0–49	50–69	70+	0–49	50–69	70+	0–49	50–69	70+	0–49	50–69	70+	0–49	50–69	70+	0–49	50–69	70+
0–49	Affected	0	0	1	0	0	0	0	1	0	0	0	0	0			0	0	
	Normal	1	4	11	0	9	8	11	8	2	7	19	4	16	0	0	26	6	
50–69	Affected	1	1	3	0	0	0	2	6	1	0	0	0	0	0	0	0		
	Normal	0	7	28	2	18	20	3	32	20	11	47	21	32	8	0	33		
70+	Affected		0	1		0	0	0	0	1	0	0	0	0	1	1	0		
	Normal		1	7		4	5	0	1	7	0	4	12	6	4	8	3		
Total	Affected	1	1	5	0	0	0	2	7	2	0	0	0	0	1	1	0	0	
	Normal	1	12	46	2	31	33	14	41	29	18	70	37	54	12	8	62	6	

Table 4. *Observed and Expected Frequencies of Breast Cancer in Mothers and Sisters of Male Probands, Assuming No Familiality**

	Mothers		Sisters	
	Observed	Expected	Observed	Expected
Affected	7	5.7	11	5.3
Normal	59	60.3	84	89.7
Total	66		95	

*χ^2 2 d.f. = 6.41; $P < .05$.

for most cells are small; therefore these numbers were pooled for each type of relative. Results are presented in Table 4.

The observed numbers of affected mothers and affected sisters are greater than those expected by chance; in particular, the observed number of affected sisters is more than twice the expected frequency. The younger ages of daughters and the low incidence in men precluded their having roles in the detection of familiality. On the basis of the observed and expected frequencies in mothers and sisters of men patients (chi-square test), the null hypothesis that breast cancer in men does not have an underlying familial relationship with breast cancer in women must be ruled out.

The heritability of liability (H) measures the extent to which common familial factors contribute to the development of a disease (Falconer 1965). The range of H is from 0–1, reflecting the two extreme situations of no familial aggregation of the trait (H = 0) versus a high degree of familial aggregation (H = 1). For traits with a heritability greater than zero, no distinction is made regarding the cause of the observed familial aggregation, it may be genetic or environmental.

The heritability of liability to breast cancer was calculated from the observed frequency of the disease in first-degree relatives of men patients. The estimate of H is .37 (S.E. = .084), a moderate figure, although significantly greater than zero (χ^2 1 d.f. = 4.4, $P < .05$). Using this estimate of the heritability and assuming a multifactorial disease process, the expected frequency of affected relatives was calculated. As seen in Table 5, allowing for a correlation among relatives, the discrepancy between the observed and expected frequencies of disease is no longer significant.

Table 5. *Observed and Expected Frequencies of Breast Cancer in Mothers and Sisters of Male Probands, Assuming Multifactorial Disease Process (H = .37)**

	Mothers		Sisters	
	Observed	Expected	Observed	Expected
Affected	7	9.9	11	9.6
Normal	59	56.1	84	85.4
Total	66		95	

*χ^2 1 d.f. = 1.25; $P > .05$.

CLINICAL FEATURES AND FAMILY HISTORY

Studies of families of women who have breast cancer have revealed that a positive history is more likely to occur among patients diagnosed at an early age, generally premenopausally (Anderson 1977). It has also been observed that bilaterality in women is associated with a positive family history of breast cancer (Anderson 1977). Bilaterality in conjunction with premenopausal onset has an even more pronounced association with the degree of familiality (Anderson 1972). The relationship between age at diagnosis, laterality, and presence of second tumors to a family history of breast cancer in relatives of men who have breast cancer is presented below.

Age and Family History

To test whether an early age at diagnosis was associated with a family history of breast cancer, patients in our series were partitioned into four classes according to age at diagnosis. Results are presented in Table 6.

A trend toward increasing familiality with decreasing age at diagnosis was not observed in our sample of men patients. That men in our series do not conform to the findings in women, whereby a positive family history is associated with early age at diagnosis, may well be related to hormonal differences in the two sexes, i.e., in women it may not necessarily be early age at diagnosis but premenopausal hormone levels that are associated with a family history of breast cancer.

Laterality and Family History

The number of men with bilateral cancers in our sample, two, was too small to test whether bilaterality in men is associated with a family history of the disease; however, it is interesting to note that bilateral breast cancer and cancer of the vagina were observed in a sister and mother of one of the two men.

Table 6. *Association of Age at Diagnosis with a Family History of Breast Cancer (White Sample)**

| Family | Age of Onset | | | | |
History	0–49	50–59	60–69	70+	All Ages
Positive	4	9	6	3	22
	(22.2%)	(40.9%)	(33.3%)	(37.5%)	(29.0%)
Negative	14	13	12	5	44
	(77.8%)	(59.1%)	(66.7%)	(62.5%)	(71.0%)
Total	18	23	18	8	66

*χ^2 3 d.f. = 1.63; $P > .05$.

Table 7. *Association of Second Primary Tumors with a Family History of Breast Cancer (White Sample of Families)* *

| Family History | Second Primaries | |
	Yes	No
Positive	4	18
	(28.6%)	(34.6%)
Negative	10	34
	(71.4%)	(65.4%)
Total	14	52

*χ^2 1 d.f. = .21; $P > .05$.

Other Primary Tumors and Family History

Finally, it was of interest to test whether relatives of men with second primary tumors and, hence, a possibly enhanced genetic predisposition to cancer, have a higher risk of breast cancer. As seen in Table 7, a second cancer occurring in the proband does not affect the observed frequency of breast cancer.

DISCUSSION

Breast cancer is etiologically heterogeneous, involving both genetic and environmental factors. From a clinical standpoint, it is important to try to identify the cause in each affected person, since this information may have a role in the subsequent clinical course of the disease as well as in determining the appropriate therapeutic approach. Knowledge of whether the cause is genetic or environmental is also of concern to relatives of patients, whose future medical needs and decisions will depend, to some extent, on their levels of risk.

In addition to abstracting information from family histories of our patients, we also collected information about possible environmental risk factors in an attempt to determine to what extent breast cancer in men may have been environmentally induced. Environmental causes we were concerned with include exogenous estrogens and ionizing radiation.

A history of exposure to exogenous estrogens was reported by two patients. One who developed breast cancer reported taking exogenous estrogens and undergoing orchiectomy as treatment for prostate cancer. A second patient, a 74-year-old man, received a male hormone for general well-being. After taking about 50 such tablets, he noticed swelling in both breasts, which subsided after he stopped taking medication. This was followed by tiny cysts, bloody discharge from the left nipple, and 3 years later a diagnosis of breast cancer.

Ionizing radiation is suspected of being responsible for breast cancer in some men treated for other cancers, eczema, gynecomastia, cystic acne, etc. Among men in our study, x-ray therapy was reported by three patients, one of whom had received treatment for "breast-swelling" at age 14, another who received treatment for cystic acne of the chest, and one who reported receiving 6–8 x-ray treatments per year for 10–12 years after having had severe pneumonia as a teenager. Two other patients reported working around x-ray equipment.

Trauma has been suggested as a risk factor for male breast cancer, and although physical injury was reported by some patients in our study prior to evidence of malignancy, it is probable that such injuries are merely coincident with breast cancer. A causative relationship would be difficult to establish.

Information on possible environmentally induced cases of breast cancer among men in our study is very incomplete. Nevertheless, we suspect that some of the cases mentioned above may have been environmentally induced. None of the patients reporting histories of x-ray treatment had family histories of breast cancer. One of the men receiving hormones had a daughter who also had breast cancer.

Other risk factors for breast cancer in men include gynecomastia, chromosome abnormalities, and a family history of breast cancer. Gynecomastia has been cited as a risk factor for breast cancer in men. It may be induced by drugs, but also occurs without known cause. During the course of our investigation, information was gathered on a man in whom breast cancer was suspected. The resulting diagnosis was bilateral gynecomastia without evidence of malignancy; therefore, he was not included as part of our study population. Of interest, however, was the mention of breast cancer in both the father and paternal grandfather of the patient. Clinical gynecomastia has been observed in 0% to 20% of men with breast cancer (Meyskens et al. 1976); however, microscopic gynecomastia has been reported in 26% (Scheike and Visfeldt 1973) and 40% (Heller et al. 1978) of men with breast cancer. The frequency of gynecomastia in the general population is not negligible. Gynecomastia develops in 60% to 70% of adolescent boys during puberty (Nydick et al. 1961), while the frequency among adult men has been reported to be between 30% and 40% (Carlson 1980). When compared with the frequency of gynecomastia in normal men, the frequency of gynecomastia in men with breast cancer does not appear to be excessive. The role of genetic and environmental factors in the development of gynecomastia and its relationship to breast cancer in men and familial breast cancer requires further scientific investigation.

Breast cancer has been observed in males with chromosome abnormalties. In males with Klinefelter's syndrome, an XXY karyotype, the incidence of breast cancer has been reported to be approximately 13 to 66 times as great as in men with normal karyotypes (Jackson et al. 1965, Harnden et al. 1971, Langlands et al. 1976). Breast cancer has also been reported in phenotypic men with XX karyotypes (Giammarini et al. 1980). Patients with these chromosome abnormalities have altered hormonal profiles, including decreased testosterone and a high frequency of gynecomastia. None of the men in our series were known to have chromosome abnormalities; however, karyotyping was not performed.

Family History

The preliminary finding of our study, a positive history of breast cancer in 33% of the families of men who have breast cancer, is higher than the reported incidence of 15.5% in families of women who have breast cancer seen at U.T. M. D. Anderson Hospital (Anderson, personal communication). This latter figure, abstracted from medical records, is incomplete; breast cancers in relatives were not documented, and the rate is nonspecific with regard to the type of relative and frequency of occurrence, and therefore is not a good comparison.

The results of other surveys are summarized in Table 8. There are a number of differences between the studies so that direct comparisons are not strictly valid. For instance, studies based upon death certificates underestimate frequencies of occurrence by exclusion of persons who were successfully treated. The salient feature is recognizable without reviewing the details of each study: the observed frequencies of occurrence in both mothers and sisters in our study, 10.6% and 11.6%, respectively, are higher than those reported for mothers and sisters in these other studies in which relatives were selected through women with breast cancer or through a random series of patients with breast cancer (predominantly women).

An estimate of the heritability of liability to breast cancer is only available from one other study, the pedigrees collected by Jacobsen (1946). The estimate is .28 (Williams 1983, submitted for publication), lower than the estimate derived from our sample of families (.37), corroborating the above finding that selection through an affected man identifies a genetically high-risk group.

When information on second-degree relatives is complete, it is our intention to fit more complicated models of family resemblance to the pedigree data and to evaluate which of these are compatible with the observed segregation patterns of breast cancer in relatives of affected men.

Table 8. *A Summary of Breast Cancer in Mothers and Sisters from Other Studies*

Study	Source of Information	Mothers		Sisters	
		Number	Frequency of Affection	Number	Frequency of Affection
Jacobsen 1946	interview	200	10.5	381	3.4
Penrose et al. 1948	death certificate	408	6.2	307	7.5
Smithers et al. 1952	death certificate	556	5.2	460	3.5
Bucalossi et al. 1954	interview	222	2.7	432	2.8
Woolf 1955	death certificate	200	2.0	561	1.4
Anderson et al. 1958	death certificate & interview	440	2.0	1108	4.3
Macklin 1959	death certificate	205	5.2	498	2.8
Murphy and Abbey 1959	death certificate & interview	199	3.5	372	0.5
Papadrianos et al. 1967	interview	1802	9.0		

A survey of breast cancer among relatives of men patients compiled through a state-wide tumor registry should be initiated to verify the results of our study.

ACKNOWLEDGMENTS

We are grateful to Dr. D. C. Rao, Head, Division of Biostatistics, Washington University Medical School, St. Louis, Missouri, for provision of computer time used in the analysis of the data. The calculation of the heritability was performed using the program ATRIBUTE, developed by D. C. Rao and R. Lew (Morton et al. 1983). Partial support of the Harris 125 S computer (Dr. Rao's laboratory) was provided by grant NIGMS GM 28719. Support for W. R. Williams was provided by training grant CA 09299 from the National Institutes of Health.

REFERENCES

Anderson, D. E. 1972. A genetic study of human breast cancer. JNCI 48:1029–1034.

Anderson, D. E. 1977. Breast cancer in families. Cancer 40:1855–1860.

Anderson, V. E., H. O. Goodman, and S. C. Reed. 1958. Variables Related to Human Breast Cancer. University of Minnesota Press, Minneapolis, pp. 1–172.

Bucalossi, P., U. Veronesi, and A. Pandolfi. 1954. Il problema dell'erdeditarieta nell' uomo. II. Il cancro della mammella. Tumori 40:365–402.

Carlson, H. E. 1980. Gynecomastia. N. Engl. J. Med. 303:795–799.

Crichlow, R. W. 1972. Carcinoma of the male breast. Surg. Gynecol. Obstet. 134:1011–1018.

Everson, R. B., F. P. Li, J.-F. Fraumeni, J. Fishman, R. E. Wilson, D. Stout, and H. J. Norris. 1976. Familial male breast cancer. Lancet 1:9–12.

Falconer, D. S. 1965. The inheritance of liability to certain diseases estimated from the incidence among relatives. Ann. Hum. Genet. 29:51–76.

Giammarini, A., M. Rocchi, W. Zennaro, and G. Filippi. 1980. XX male with breast cancer. Clin. Genet. 18:103–108.

Harnden, D. G., N. MacLean, and A. O. Langlands. 1971. Carcinoma of the breast and Klinefelter's syndrome. J. Med. Genet. 8:460–461.

Heller, K. S., P. P. Rosen, D. Schottenfeld, R. Ashikari, and D. W. Kinne. 1978. Male breast cancer: A clinicopathologic study of 97 cases. Ann. Surg. 188:60–65.

Jackson, A. W., S. Muldol, C. H. Ockey, and P. J. O'Connor. 1965. Carcinoma of the male breast in association with Klinefelter syndrome. Br. Med. J. 23:223–225.

Jacobsen, O. 1946. Heredity in breast cancer. A genetic and clinical study of two hundred probands. H. K. Lewis, London, pp. 1–306.

Langlands, A. O., N. MacLean, and C. K. Kerr. 1976. Carcinoma of the male breast: Report of a series of 88 cases. Clin. Radiol. 27:21–25.

Lynch, H. T. 1981. Genetic heterogeneity and breast cancer: Variable tumor specta, *in* Genetics and Breast Cancer, H. T. Lynch, ed. VanNostrand Reinhold Company, New York, p. 168.

Macklin, M. T. 1959. Comparison of the number of breast cancer deaths observed in relatives of breast-cancer patients and the number expected on the basis of mortality rates. JNCI 22:927–951.

Marger, D., N. Urdaneta, and J. J. Fischer. 1975. Breast cancer in brothers. Case reports and a review of 30 cases of male breast cancer. Cancer 36:458–461.

Meyskens, F. L., D. C. Tormey, and J. P. Neifeld. 1976. Male breast cancer: A review. Cancer Treat. Rev. 3:83–89.

Morton, N. E., D. C. Rao, and J. M. Lalouel. 1983. Methods in genetic epidemiology. S. Karger Press, New York (in press).

Murphy, D. P., and H. Abbey. 1959. Cancer in Families. Harvard Univ. Press, Cambridge, pp. 1–76.

Nydick, M., J. Bustos, J. H. Dale, and R. W. Rawson. 1961. Gynecomastia in adolescent boys. JAMA 178:449–454.

Papadrianos, E., C. D. Haagensen, and E. Cooley. 1967. Cancer of the breast as a familial disease. Ann. Surg. 165:10–19.

Penrose, L. S., H. J. Mackenzie, and M. N. Karn. 1948. A genetical study of human mammary cancer. Ann. Eugen. Lond. 14:234–266.

Robison, R., and E. D. Montague. 1982. Treatment results in males with breast cancer. Cancer 49:403–406.

Scheike, O., and J. Visfeldt. 1973. Male breast cancer. Gynecomastia in patients with breast cancer. Acta. Pathol. Microbiol. Scand. 81:A359.

Schwarz, R. M., R. B. Newell, J. F. Hauch, and W. H. Fairweather. 1980. A study of familial male breast carcinoma and a second report. Cancer 46:2697–2701.

Smithers, D. W., P. Rigby-Jones, D. A. G. Galton, and P. N. Payne. 1952. Cancer of the breast. Br. J. Radiol. Suppl. No. 4:1–89.

Teasdale, C., J. F. Forbes, and M. Baum. 1976. Familial male breast cancer. Lancet 1:360–361.

Woolf, C. M. 1955. Investigations on genetic aspects of carcinoma of the stomach and breast. Univ. Calif. Pub. Public Health 2:265–350.

Yap, H. Y., C. K. Tashima, G. R. Blumenschein, and N. E. Eckles. 1979. Male breast cancer: A natural history study. Cancer 44:748–754.

Yap, H. Y., C. K. Tashima, G. R. Blumenschein, G. N. Hortobagyi, and N. Eckles. 1980. Chemotherapy for advanced male breast cancer. JAMA 243:1739–1741.

Young, J. L., C. L. Percy, and A. J. Asire. 1981. Surveillance, epidemiology, and end results: Incidence and mortality data, 1973–1977. Natl. Cancer Inst. Monogr. 57:98–101.

Current Controversies in Breast Cancer, edited
by F. C. Ames, G. R. Blumenschein, and E. D. Montague.
University of Texas Press, Austin © 1984.

Predominance of Estrophilin-Negative and Poorly Differentiated Breast Cancer in Black Patients

Suresh Mohla, Ph.D.,*§ Calvin C. Sampson, M.D.,† John P. Enterline,
M.S.,* Walter M. Griffin, M.S.,* Tariq Khan, M.D.,‡ Lasalle D.
Leffall, Jr., M.D., F.A.C.S.,‡ and Jack E. White, M.D., F.A.C.S.*†

*Departments of *Oncology, †Pathology, ‡Surgery, and §Pharmacology, College of
Medicine, Howard University Cancer Center, Washington, D.C.*

Breast cancer is the cancer of highest incidence and causes the most deaths among American women; one out of 11 women will develop breast cancer during her lifetime (Cancer Facts and Figures 1982). While breast cancer occurs more frequently in white than in black women, mortality rates in the two groups are comparable (Cutler and Young 1975, White and Enterline 1980). This is due to a poorer survival rate from breast cancer among blacks than among whites. Recent reports clearly indicate that breast cancer in blacks is not only detected in a relatively more advanced stage than in whites but also shows a consistently lower rate of survival within stages of the disease (Myers and Hankey 1980, Nemota et al. 1980). Thus, a question arises as to whether biological differences (independent of socioeconomic status) may account for the survival differential within stages between blacks and whites.

Estrogen receptors (estrophilin, ER) and progesterone receptors (PR) in breast cancer have been shown to play an important role in predicting a patient's response to endocrine therapy and overall prognosis (Allegra et al. 1979, Bloom et al. 1980, DeSombre and Jensen 1976, Horwitz et al. 1975, Jensen et al. 1975, Knight et al. 1977, Maynard et al. 1978, McGuire 1978, McGuire et al. 1975, 1977a, b, Rich et al. 1978, Walt et al. 1976, Witliff et al. 1976).

It has been observed that 60% to 70% of breast cancer patients contain ER and that nearly two-thirds of ER-positive patients respond favorably to endocrine therapy; less than 10% of ER-negative patients have a favorable response to endocrine therapy. To further identify probable responders to endocrine therapy, it has been suggested that PR should be measured in addition to ER in tumor specimens from patients with breast cancer (Horwitz et al. 1975). The rationale for this suggestion is based on the fact that in estrogen target tissues, the synthesis of PR is regulated by estrogens (Friefeld et al. 1974, Koenders et al. 1977, McGuire et al. 1977b, Milgrom et al. 1973, Mohla et al. 1981a, Rao and Weist 1972, Toft and O'Malley 1972). Thus, the presence of PR indicates a biologically active ER.

Earlier reports have shown a significant association between the growth fraction of a breast cancer (as measured by the thymidine labeling index, TLI) and ER. A low TLI was associated with ER positivity and a high TLI with ER negativity; thus, dedifferentiation in breast cancer is associated with high TLI and absence of ER (Meyer et al. 1977, Rao and Meyer 1977). A significant association between tumor grade and ER has previously been documented. It has been osberved that while well- and moderately well-differentiated tumors usually contain ER, poorly differentiated tumors are devoid of ER in the majority of cases (Fisher et al. 1981, Lesser et al. 1981, Maynard et al. 1978, Mohla et al. 1980, 1981b, c, 1982a, b, Parl and Wagner 1980, Rich et al. 1978). Recent observations have also indicated a relationship between the disease-free interval, ER receptors,and tumor differentiation; ER-positive tumors had a longer disease-free interval compared to ER-negative tumors (Knight et al. 1977, Rich et al. 1978). While the disease-free interval is independent of ER in both well- and moderately well-differentiated tumors, a shorter disease-free interval in poorly differentiated ER-negative and a longer disease-free interval in poorly differentiated ER-positive tumors has been observed (Maynard et al. 1978).

Earlier studies from Japan (Matsumoto and Sugano 1978, Ochi et al. 1978) on the distribution of ER and PR revealed significant ethnic differences in the incidence of ER-positive tumors in postmenopausal Japanese patients: "The incidence in Japanese patients was similar for premenopausal and postmenopausal patients, whereas in Western patients the incidence was higher in postmenopausal patients." Further, recent data (Collings et al. 1980, Lesser et al. 1981, Savage et al. 1981) have demonstrated significant differences in the distribution of ER between black and white patients.

Thus, we investigated whether an unknown biological difference may play a role in explaining the poorer survival rate in black patients with breast cancer. This study was conducted to investigate whether the distribution of ER and PR in black American women with breast cancer at the Howard University Hospital differs from the national norm. Preliminary data on 146 black breast cancer patients have been published (Mohla et al. 1980, 1981b, c, 1982a, b).

MATERIALS AND METHODS

Patient Population

All tissue samples were derived from Howard University Hospital between June 1977 and April 1982. There was no apparent bias in patient selection. The data reported here are from 228 women patients (ages 28–97 years). An additional 48 patients with breast cancer underwent surgery during this period. Their tissue samples were not received for receptor determinations. The histopathologic examinations of their slides did not reveal anything different that could change the results of this study.

Tissue Collection, Pathology, and Preparation

Fresh tumor specimens were received from the operating room in an ice bath immediately following excision. All histologic preparations were examined and graded (Bloom and Richardson 1957). Based on the criteria, each case was placed into one of three categories: (1) well differentiated (WD); (2) moderately well differentiated (MWD); or (3) poorly differentiated (PD).

Tissue homogenization, cytosol preparation, and incubation of cytosols for ER and PR assays, which were analyzed using the sucrose density gradient method, have been previously described (Mohla et al. 1981a, 1982b). The results were expressed as fmoles of receptor per mg of cytosol protein (Lowry et al. 1951). For ER, a value of > 10 fmoles/mg protein was classified as ER positive $(+)$; a value between $3-10$ fmoles/mg was classified as borderline $(\pm)$; and a value of < 3 fmoles/mg was classified as ER negative $(-)$. Tumor specimens with > 10 fmoles/mg of 8S + 4S PR or > 3 fmoles/mg of 8S-complex were classified as PR+. Tritiated estradiol [estradiol $(2,4,6,7\text{-}^3H(N)]$ and ^3H-R5020 [promegestone $(17\alpha\text{-Methyl-}^3H)$] were used as ligands for ER and PR, respectively. Each sample was assayed in the absence or presence of 200-fold excess nonradioactive competitor.

Chi-square or Mantel-Haenszel analyses were used in testing differences between various parameters.

RESULTS

The distribution of ER and PR in 228 specimens from patients with breast cancer revealed 45% (98/228) ER+, 15%$\pm$ (35/228), and 42% ER$-$ (95/228). A typical sucrose gradient profile of ER+ cytosol in breast cancer is shown in Figure 1. The median age $(\pm \text{SEM})$ of ER+, ER $\pm$, and ER$-$ patients was 59.89 $\pm$ 1.38, 56.94 $\pm$ 2.13, and 53.49 $\pm$ 1.55 years, respectively. Thirty-nine percent of ER+ patients (34/88) were also PR+ compared to 13% (4/32) and 3% (3/88) PR+ in ER$\pm$ and ER$-$ patients, respectively. The distribution of PR+ in ER+, ER$\pm$, and ER$-$ patients was statistically significant (chi-square analysis, $X^2 = 35.7$, df $= 2$, $P < .001$). Postmenopausal patients showed a higher percentage (49%) of ER+ and a slightly lower percentage (36%) of ER$-$ compared to premenopausal patients, where 29% and 55% showed ER+ and ER$-$ results, respectively (Table 1). The distribution of ER and menopausal status was statistically significant ($P < .02$) whether the ER$\pm$ patients were grouped separately or combined with the ER$-$ group (Table 1).

The majority of patients (197/228; 86%) exhibited tumor histopathologic evidence of infiltrating ductal carcinoma (IDCA). Estrogen receptor-positive samples were observed in 88/197 (45%) of all IDCAs; 27 (14%) and 82 (42%) of the IDCAs were ER $\pm$ and ER$-$, respectively.

Only 4% (10/228) of the tumors showed well-differentiated (WD) tumors, 33% (76/228) were moderately well differentiated (MWD), and 62% (142/228) were

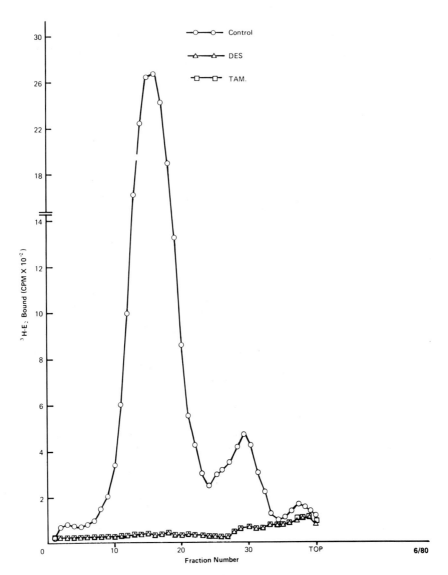

FIG. 1. Sucrose density gradient profile of estrogen receptors in breast cancer. Cytosol (in 10 mM Tris buffer, pH 7.4, containing 0.5 mM dithiothreitol, 0.1 mM EDTA, and 10% glycerol) was incubated with 10 mM ^{3}H-estradiol in the presence (triangles) or absence (circles) of 200-fold excess diethylstilbestrol (DES) or in the presence of 500-fold excess tamoxifen (TAM) (squares). After 4 hours at 0°C, the samples were treated with dextran-coated charcoal, and 0.2 ml of the sample was layered over a 10% to 30% sucrose gradient. The samples were centrifuged at 485,000 x g for 16 hours in a Beckman SW-60 rotor. One-tenth-milliliter fractions were collected and counted for radioactivity. Specific binding was observed in both the 8S (peak-fraction #17) and 4S (peak-fraction #29) complexes in this specimen. Gamma globulin (7.7S) and bovine serum albumin (4.6S) were used as standard marker proteins and sedimented in fractions 20 and 28, respectively (data not shown). Tamoxifen was a gift from Stuart Pharmaceuticals, Division of ICI Americas Inc., Wilmington, Delaware. (Reproduced from Mohla et al. 1982b, with permission of J. B. Lippincott Company).

Table 1. *Distribution of Estrogen Receptors in Breast Cancer: Relationship to Menopausal Status*

Menopausal Status	Estrogen Receptors*			Significance[†]
	>10	3−10	< 3	
				$\chi^2 = 8.10$
Premenopausal	19	10	36	df[†] = 2
Postmenopausal	79	25	59	$P < .02$
	>10	<10		
				$\chi^2 = 6.25$
Premenopausal	19	46		df = 1
Postmenopausal	79	84		$P < .02$

*fmoles/mg protein.
[†]Abbreviations are as follows: χ^2 = chi square; df = degrees of freedom; P = probability.

poorly differentiated (PD). Tumor differentiation of 48 patients whose tissue samples were not received for receptor determination showed a similar distribution of tumor grade (4% WD, 65% PD, and 31% MWD). There was a significant correlation between tumor grade and ER+ whether the small number of WD tumors were pooled along with MWD or analyzed as separate groups (Table 2). Thus, about 70% of all ER− tumors (90/130) were PD. Similarly, PR+ was also significantly correlated with tumor differentiation (Table 3). Conversely, tumor grade was not correlated with menopausal status, whether WD tumors were combined with the MWD group or assessed as separate groups (Table 4). However, ER+ was correlated with tumor grade even when adjusted for menopausal status (Table 5). Forty percent of WD and MWD tumors in premenopausal and 59% in postmenopausal patients were ER+. In contrast, 23% and 42% of PD tumors were ER+ in premenopausal and postmenopausal patients, respectively (Table 5). The relationship between tumor

Table 2. *Relationship Between Estrogen Receptor And Tumor Grade In Breast Cancer*

Tumor Grade*	Estrogen Receptors		Chi-Square Analysis[‡]
	>10[†]	<10	
WD	7	3	$\chi^2 = 7.48$
MWD	39	37	df = 2
PD	52	90	$P = .024$
WD + MWD	46	40	$\chi^2 = 5.55$
			df = 1
PD	52	90	$P = .0185$

* Abbreviations are as follows: WD = well differentiated; MWD = moderately well differentiated; PD = poorly differentiated.
[†]fmoles/mg protein.
[‡]Abbreviations are as follows: χ^2 = chi square; df = degrees of freedom; P = probability.

Table 3. *Relationship Between Progesterone Receptors (PR) And Tumor Grade*

PR*	Tumor Grade[†]			Chi-Square Test[‡]
	WD	MWD	PD	
>10	4	18	19	$\chi^2 = 6.11$
				df = 2
<10	6	52	109	P < .05
	WD + MWD		PD	
>10	22		19	$\chi^2 = 4.22$
				df = 1
<10	58		109	P < .05

*fmoles/mg protein.
[†]Abbreviations are as follows: WD = well differentiated; MWD = moderately well differentiated, and PD = poorly differentiated.
[‡]Abbreviations are as follows: χ^2 = chi square; df = degrees of freedom; P = probability.

Table 4. *Relationship Between Tumor Grade And Menopausal Status In Breast Cancer*

Menopausal Status	Tumor Grade*			Chi-Square Analysis[†]
	WD	MWD	PD	
Premenopausal	1	24	40	$\chi^2 = 2.04$
				df = 2
Postmenopausal	9	52	102	P = .36
	WD + MWD		PD	
Premenopausal	25		40	$\chi^2 = .00003$
				df = 1
Postmenopausal	61		102	P = .9862

*Abbreviations are as follows: WD = well differentiated; MWD = moderately well differentiated; PD = poorly differentiated.
[†]Abbreviations are as follows: χ^2 = chi square; df = degrees of freedom; P = probability.

Table 5. *Relationship Between Estrogen Receptor (ER) And Tumor Grade Adjusted For Menopausal Status**

Menopausal Status		WD[†] + MWD	PD
Premenopausal	ER[‡] > 10	10	9
	ER < 10	15	31
Postmenopausal	ER > 10	36	43
	ER < 10	25	59

*Mantel-Haenszel analysis; chi square = 5.80; degree of freedom = 1; probability = 0.0160.
[†]WD = well differentiated; MWD = moderately well differentiated; PD = poorly differentiated.
[‡]fm/mg protein.

Table 6. *Relationship Between Tumor Grade And Histopathology In Patients With Breast Cancer*

Tumor Histopathology	No. Patients	(%)	Tumor Grade* WD	MWD	PD
IDCA[†]	197	(86)	6	65	126
Intraductal	4	(1.8)	1	0	3
Tubular	1	(0.4)	1	0	0
Mucoid	10	(4.4)	1	8	1
Medullary	7	(3)	0	2	5
Pappillary	2	(0.9)	1	0	1
Lobular	6	(2.6)	0	0	6
Adenoidcystic	1	(0.4)	0	1	0
Total	228		10 (4.4%)	76 (33.3%)	142 (62.3%)

*WD = well differentiated; MWD = moderately well differentiated; PD = poorly differentiated.
[†]Infiltrating ductal carcinoma.

grade and histology is shown in Table 6. Tumor grade was independent of histology when the small members of WD tumors were grouped with MWD tumors (Table 7). If WD tumors were kept as a separate group, then the data were statistically significant. Whether this significance is due to the small number of WD tumors in the IDCA group or some other factor(s) is difficult to assess.

The data indicate a relatively lower incidence of ER+ tumors in the patient population at Howard University Hospital than published reports indicate exists in other institutions. The data in Table 8 indicate that whether a value of ER > 3, > 7, or > 10 fmoles/mg protein was considered as ER+, statistically significant differences were observed when the results in our study were compared with published data from other institutions. When the present findings were compared with those noted in earlier reports of Jensen et al. (1975) the distribution of ER in our patient population was found to be significantly different ($P < .001$). In these data

Table 7. *Relationship Between Tumor Grade And Histopathology*

Histology	Tumor Grade* WD	MWD	PD	Chi-square analysis[§]
IDCA[†]	6	65	126	$\chi^2 = 6.64$ df = 2 $P = 0.036$
Other[‡]	4	11	16	
	WD + MWD		PD	
IDCA	71		126	$\chi^2 = 1.25$ df = 1 P = ns
Other	15		16	

*WD = well differentiated; MWD = moderately well differentiated; PD = poorly differentiated.
[†]IDCA = infiltrating ductal carcinoma.
[‡]Mucoid 10; medullary 7; lobular 6; intraductal 4; papillary 2; tubular 1; adenoidcystic 1.
[§]χ^2 = chi square; df = degrees of freedom; P = probability; ns = not significant.

Table 8. *Estrogen Receptors In Breast Cancer: Data Comparison Of Present Findings With Other Institutions*[*]

ER[†]	Other Studies (%)		Present Study (%)	Chi-square analysis
>3	392/521[‡]	(75)	133/228 (58)	$\chi^2 = 20.83$ df = 1 $P < .001$
>7	225/328[§]	(69)	108/228 (47)	$\chi^2 = 24.36$ df = 1 $P < .001$
>10	1100/1983[‡]	(55.5)	98/228 (43)	$\chi^2 = 12.35$ df = 1 $P < .001$
>10	102/140[∥]	(73)	98/228 (43)	$\chi^2 = 30.00$ df = 1 $P < .001$
ER (fmoles/gm tumor) >1000 pre or >2500 post	46[#]	(34)	25 (11)	
500–1000 pre or 1000–2500 post	10	(9)	18 (8)	$\chi^2 = 28.38$ df = 2 $P < .001$
<500 pre or <1000 post	77	(57)	171 (81)	

[*] Abbreviations are as follows: ER = estrogen receptor; χ^2 = chi square; df = degrees of freedom; P = probability; pre = premenopausal; post = postmenopausal.
[†] fmoles/mg protein.
[‡] McGuire 1978.
[§] Bloom et al. 1980.
[∥] Parl and Wagner 1980.
[#] Jensen et al. 1975.

(Jensen's and the current findings) ER values of > 1000 fmoles/gm tissue for premenopausal and > 2500 fmoles/gm for postmenopausal patients were designated as ER+; ER values of 500–999 fmoles/gm for premenopausal and 1000–2499 fmoles/gm for postmenopausal women were designated as ER±, and ER values of < 500 and < 1000 fmoles/gm tissue for premenopausal and postmenopausal patients, respectively, were defined as ER−.

A further observation that was significantly different from what has been previously reported was a higher incidence of PD tumors in our patient population. The distribution of PD, MWD, and WD tumors (62%, 33%, and 4%, respectively) was significantly different from published data from other institutions (Table 9). Thus, it appears that our patient population displayed a higher frequency of PD and a lower frequency of WD tumors at the time of diagnosis.

Table 9. *Breast Cancer and Tumor Differentiation: Data Comparison Of Present Findings With Other Institutions*

	Present Study (%)	Maynard[*] (%)	Rich[†] (%)	Parl[‡] (%)	Heuson[§] (%)	Matsumoto[‖] (%)	Boyd[#] (%)
N[¶]	228	220	140	116	85	102	698
Tumor grade[**]							
WD	10 (4)	41 (19)	26 (19)	20 (17)	18 (21)	10 (10)	111 (16)
MWD	76 (33)	82 (37)	86 (61)	57 (49)	38 (45)	57 (56)	377 (54)
PD	142 (62)	97 (44)	28 (20)	39 (34)	29 (34)	35 (34)	210 (30)
Chi-square analysis[††]		$\chi^2 = 27.41$	$\chi^2 = 66.46$	$\chi^2 = 31.53$	$\chi^2 = 30.70$	$\chi^2 = 22.58$	$\chi^2 = 79.33$
		df = 2	df = 2	df = 2	df = 2	df = 2	df = 2
		$P < .001$	$P < .001$	$P < .001$	$P < .001$	$P < .001$	$P < .001$

[*]Maynard et al. 1978.
[†]Rich et al. 1978.
[‡]Parl and Wagner 1980.
[§]Heuson et al. 1975.
[‖]Matsumoto and Sugano 1978.
[#]Boyd et al. 1981.
[**]WD = well differentiated; MWD = moderately well differentiated; PD = poorly differentiated.
[††]χ^2 = chi square; df = degrees of freedom; P = probability.

DISCUSSION

Our data indicate a lower incidence of ER+ and a higher incidence of ER− tumors compared with published data from other institutions. These data are consistent with recent reports on the differences in ER distribution between black and white breast cancer patients (Collings et al. 1980, Lesser et al. 1981, Savage et al. 1981). These results also confirm earlier data on 146 black patients published from this institution (Mohla et al. 1980, 1982a, b).

The results also showed several similarities in ER distribution: postmenopausal patients showed higher ER incidence than premenopausal patients and a higher incidence of PgR in ER+ than in ER− patients. Earlier data from this institution also showed a higher incidence of ER positivity in tumor specimens taken from the primary than from the metastatic tumor site (Mohla et al. 1982a, b). These data are in agreement with earlier findings from several laboratories (McGuire et al. 1975, 1977b).

A further observation that was significantly different from what has been previously reported was a higher incidence of PD tumors in our patient population. However, the incidence of ER positivity in WD, MWD, and PD tumors was similar to what has been reported (Fisher et al. 1981, Lesser et al. 1981, Maynard et al. 1978, Mohla et al. 1982a, b, Parl and Wagner 1980, Rich et al. 1978); ER positivity was lower in PD tumors compared to WD or MWD tumors. Further, this relationship between ER and tumor grade is independent of menopausal status.

Several factors have been implicated to influence ER status of a tumor specimen. These include menopausal status and seasonal variation (Hughes et al. 1976, McGuire et al. 1975), rate of cell replication (Meyer et al. 1977, Rao and Meyer 1977), local lymphocytic reaction and tissue cellularity (Meyer et al. 1977, Rao and Meyer 1977, and tumor grade (Fisher et al. 1981, Lesser et al. 1981, Maynard et al. 1978, and Mohla et al. 1981b, Mohla et al. 1982a, b, Parl and Wagner 1980, Rich et al. 1978). Although the rate of cell proliferation, tissue cellularity, and local lymphocytic reaction were not studied in this investigation, our data clearly indicate that the high frequency of ER− and low frequency of ER+ tumors may, among other reasons, be due to the higher incidence of PD tumors in our patient population.

As previously mentioned, even though breast cancer occurs more frequently in white than in black women (Cutler and Young 1975), the breast cancer mortality rates for these two groups are comparable (White and Enterline 1980). This is due to the fact that black women with breast cancer have a notably poorer survival rate than their white counterparts (Myers and Hankey 1980). While certain risk factors (family history, benign breast disease, early onset of menarche, late menopause, delayed age at first pregnancy, nulliparity, failure of ovulation, obesity, high intake of fats in diet, socioeconomic status, body weight) have been implicated in the incidence of breast cancer (Blot et al. 1977, Cole and Cramer 1977, Lesser et al. 1981, MacMahon et al. 1973, Mohla and Criss 1981b, Vorherr 1980), relatively little is known about such risk factors relating to survival. One reason for this survival difference is that breast cancer in blacks is detected at a more advanced stage than in whites (Mohla et al. 1982a, b, Myers and Hankey 1980). However, black women also have poorer survival within each stage of the disease compared to whites (Nemoto et al. 1980). Thus, the biological differences observed in our study, i.e., a high incidence of PD and ER− tumors, may provide at least a partial explanation for within-stage survival differences between blacks and whites. It has been shown that loss of differentiation results in loss of ER, which in turn has been associated with an increase in tumor growth fraction (Meyer et al. 1977, Rao and Meyer 1977). Furthermore, data from other studies suggest both a longer disease-free interval in ER+ patients compared to ER− patients and a longer disease-free interval in PD ER+ patients compared to PD ER− patients (Knight et al. 1977; Maynard et al. 1978; Rich et al. 1978). A determination of whether these findings help to explain poor within-stage survival among blacks will require further study. However, earlier studies (Walt et al. 1976) have shown that "estrogen receptor negative patients have a shorter lifespan after discovery of the tumors and are more likely to develop dominant visceral metastases," known to be associated with very poor prognoses. In contrast, the dominant metastatic sites in ER+ patients were soft tissues and bone; this distribution of metastatic sites between ER+ and ER− patients was highly significant ($P < .0005$; Walt et al. 1976). Further, "life expectancy from the time breast lump was noted until death demonstrated increased longevity in the estrogen receptor positive group," which was independent of stage or delay in seeking medical treatment (Walt et al. 1976). "It is possible that ER positive patients are likely to live longer due at least in part to their greater responsiveness to hormonal therapy but also possibly to the less immediately lethal distribution of their metastases" (Walt et al. 1976).

The clinical significance of the results we report here to the management of breast cancer patients lies in the observations that ER− and PD tumors indicate both histopathological and biochemical evidence of dedifferentiation and, hence, may also indicate aggressive disease. These results may provide a partial explanation of the overall poorer survival of black breast cancer patients compared to whites. Whether these results are due to ethnic differences or environmental factors, or both, remains to be elucidated.

ACKNOWLEDGMENTS

This investigation was supported by Grant Numbers NCI 5P30-CA-14718 and NCI 2R18-CA-18510-06, awarded by the National Cancer Institute, U.S. Department of Health and Human Services.

REFERENCES

Allegra, J. C., M. E. Lippman, E. B. Thompson, R. Simon, A. Barlock, L. Green, K. Huff, M. T. Hoan, and S. C. Aitken. 1979. Distribution, frequency, and quantitative analysis of estrogen, progesterone, androgen, and glucocorticoid receptors in human breast cancer. Cancer Res. 39:1447–1454.

Bloom, H. J. G., and W. W. Richardson. 1957. Histological grading and prognosis in breast cancer. Br. J. Cancer 11:359–369.

Bloom, N.D., E. H. Tobin, B. Schreibman, and G. A. Degenshein. 1980. The role of progesterone receptors in the management of advanced breast cancer. Cancer 45:2992–2997.

Blot, W. J., J. F. Fraumeni, and B. J. Stone. 1977. Geographic patterns of breast cancer in the United States. JNCI 59:1407–1411.

Boyd, N. F., J. W. Meakin, J. L. Hayward, and T. C. Brown. 1981. Clinical estimation of the growth rate of breast cancer. Cancer 48:1037–1042.

Cancer Facts and Figures. 1982. American Cancer Society, New York, pp. 15.

Cole, P., and D. Cramer. 1977. Diet and cancer of endocrine target organs. Cancer 40:434–437.

Collins, J. R., J. Levin, and N. Savage. 1980. Racial Differences in oestrogen receptor and peroxide status of human breast cancer tissue. S. Afr. Med. J. 57:444–446.

Cutler, J. J., and J. L. Young. 1975. Third national cancer survey: Incidence data. U.S. Department of Health, Education, and Welfare publication No. (NIH) 75-787, pp. 122, 134.

DeSombre, E. R., and E. V. Jensen. 1976. Steroid receptors in breast cancer, *in* Control Mechanisms in Cancer, W. E. Criss, J. Ono, and J. R. Sabine, eds. Raven Press, New York, pp. 67–82.

Fisher, E. R., C. K. Osborne, W. L. McGuire, C. Redmond, W. A. Knight, B. Fisher, G. Bannayon, A. Walder, E. J. Gregory, A. Jacobsen, D. M. Queen, D. E. Bennet, and H. C. Ford. 1981. Correlation of primary breast cancer histopathology and estrogen content. Breast Cancer Res. & Treat. 1:37–41.

Friefeld, M. L., P. D. Feil, and C. W. Bardin. 1974. The in vitro regulation of progesterone receptors in guinea pigs: Dependence on estrogen and progesterone. Steroids 23:93–103.

Funderburk, W. W., E. Rosero, and L. D. Leffall. 1972. Breast lesions in blacks. Surg. Gynecol. Obstet. 135:58–60.

Heuson, J. C., G. Leclercq, E. Longeval, C. Deboel, W. H. Mattheiem, and R. Heimann. 1975. Estrogen receptors: prognostic significance in breast cancer, *in* Estrogen Receptors in Human Breast Cancer, W. L. McGuire, P. P. Carbone, and E. P. Vollmer, eds. Raven Press, New York, pp. 57–72.

Horwitz, K. B., W. L. McGuire, O. H. Pearson, and A. Segaloff. 1975. Predicting response to endocrine therapy in human breast cancer: A hypothesis. Science 189:726–727.

Hughes, A., H. I. Jacobsen, R. K. Wagner, and P. W. Jungblut. 1976. Ovarian independent fluctuations of estradiol receptor levels in mammalian tissues. Mol. Cell Endocrinol. 5:379–388.

Jensen, E. V., S. Smith, E. M. Moran, E. R. DeSombre. 1975. Estrogen receptors and hormone dependency in human breast cancer, *in* Hormones and Breast Cancer, M. Namer, and C. M. Lelannes, eds. Inserm, Paris, pp. 29–37.

Knight, W. A., R. B. Livingston, E. J. Gregory, and W. L. McGuire. 1977. Estrogen receptor as an independent prognostic factor for early recurrence in breast cancer. Cancer Res. 37:4669–4671.

Koenders, A. J. M., A. G. Moespot, S. J. Zolingen, and J. J. Bernard. 1977. Progesterone and estradiol receptors in DMBA-induced mammary tumors before and after ovariectomy and after subsequent estradiol administration, *in* Progesterone Receptors in Normal and Neoplastic Tissues, W. L. McGuire, J. P. Raynaud, and E. E. Baulieu, eds. Raven Press, New York, pp. 71–101.

Leclercq, G., J. C. Heuson, M. C. Deboel, N. Legros, E. Longeval, and W. H. Mattheiem. 1977. Estrogen and progesterone receptors in human breast cancer, *in* Progesterone Receptors in Normal and Neoplastic Tissues, W. L. McGuire, J. P. Raynaud, and E. E. Baulieu, eds. Raven Press, New York, pp. 141–153.

Lesser, M. L., P. P. Rosen, R. T. Senie, K. Duthie, C. Menendez-Botet, and M. K. Schwartz. 1981. Estrogen and progesterone receptors in breast carcinoma: Correlations with epidemiology and pathology. Cancer 48:299–309.

Lowry, O. H., N. J. Rosenbrough, A. L. Farr, and R. J. Randall. 1951. Protein measurement with the folin phenol reagent. J. Biol. Chem. 193:265–275.

MacMahon, B., P. Cole, and J. Brown. 1973. Etiology of human breast cancer: A review. JNCI 50:21–42.

Matsumoto, K., and H. Sugano. 1978. Human breast cancer and hormone receptors, *in* Endocrine Control in Neoplasia, R. K. Sharma, and W. E. Criss, eds. Raven Press, New York, pp. 191–208.

Maynard, P. V., R. W. Blamey, C. W. Elston, J. L. Haybittle, and K. Griffiths. 1978. Estrogen receptor assay in primary breast cancer and early recurrence of the disease. Cancer Res. 38:4292–4295.

McGuire, W. L. 1978. Hormone receptors: Their role in predicting prognosis and response to endocrine therapy. Semin. Oncol. 5:428–433.

McGuire, W. L., P. P. Carbone, and E. P. Vollmer. 1975. Estrogen Receptors in Human Breast Cancer. Raven Press, New York.

McGuire, W. L., K. B. Horwitz, O. H. Pearson, and A. Segaloff. 1977a. Current status of estrogen and progesterone receptors in breast cancer. Cancer 39:2934–2947.

McGuire, W. L., J. P. Raynaud, and E. E. Baulieu. 1977b. Progesterone Receptors in Normal and Neoplastic Tissues. Raven Press, New York.

Meyer, J. S., B. R. Rao, S. C. Stevens, and W. L. White. 1977. Low incidence of estrogen receptor in breast carcinomas with rapid rates of cellular replication. Cancer 40:2290–2298.

Myers, M. H., and B. F. Hankey. 1980. Cancer patient survival experience. US Dept. of Health, Education and Welfare publication No. (NIH) 80-2148, pp. 1–15.

Milgrom, E. L., T. M. Atger, and E. E. Baulieu. 1973. Mechanisms regulating the concentration and conformation of progesterone receptor(s) in the uterus. J. Biol. Chem. 248:6366–6374.

Mohla, S., N. Clem-Jackson, and J. B. Hunter. 1981a. Estrogen receptors and estrogen-induced gene expression in the rat mammary glands and uteri during pregnancy and lactation: Changes in progesterone receptor and RNA polymerase activity. J. Steroid Biochem. 14:501–508.

Mohla, S., and W. E. Criss. 1981b. The relationship of diet to cancer and hormones, *in* Nutrition and Cancer: Etiology and Treatment, G. R. Newell and N. M. Ellison, eds. Raven Press, New York, pp. 93–110.

Mohla, S., J. P. Enterline, C. C. Sampson, T. Khan, L. Leffall, Jr., and J. E. White. 1982a. A predominance of poorly differentiated tumors among black breast cancer patients: Management and screening implications. Prog. Clin. Biol. Res. 83:249–258.

Mohla, S., C. C. Sampson, J. P. Enterline, and J. E. White. 1981c. Predominance of poorly differentiating tumors in black breast cancer patients: Correlation with estrogen (ER) and progesterone (PgR) receptors. (Abstract) J. Cell. Biol. 91:208a.

Mohla, S., C. C. Sampson, T. Khan, J. P. Enterline, L. Leffall, Jr., and J. E. White. 1982b. Estrogen and progesterone receptors in breast cancer in black Americans: Correlations of receptor data with tumor differentiation. Cancer 50:552–559.

Mohla, S., C. C. Sampson, T. Khan, L. Leffall, Jr., and J. E. White. 1980. Estrogen and progesterone receptors in human breast cancer in black Americans. (Abstract) Eighth Annual Meeting of the South Eastern Cancer Research Association, Atlanta, Georgia, p. 11.

Mohla, S., C. C. Sampson, T. Khan, L. Leffall, Jr., and J. E. White. 1981d. Estrogen and progesterone receptors in human breast cancer in black Americans. (Abstract) J. Medical and Ped. Oncol. 9:95.

Nemoto, T., J. Vana, R. N. Bedwani, H. W. Bakder, F. H. McGregor, and G. P. Murphy. 1980. Management and survival of female breast cancer: Results of a national survey by the American College of Surgeons. Cancer 45:2917–2924.

Ochi, H., T. Hayashi, K. Nakao, E. Yayoi, T. Kawahara, and K. Matsumoto. 1978. Estrogen, progesterone and androgen receptors in breast cancer in the Japanese: Brief communication. JNCI 60:291–293.

Parl, F. F., and R. K. Wagner. 1980. The histopathological evaluation of human breast cancers in correlation with estrogen receptor values. Cancer 47:362–367.

Rao, B. R., and J. S. Meyers. 1977. Estrogen and progestin receptors in normal and cancer tissues, *in* Progesterone Receptors in Normal and Neoplastic Tissues, W. L. McGuire, J. P. Raynaud, and E. E. Baulieu, eds. Raven Press, New York, pp. 155–169.

Rao, B. R., and W. G. Weist. 1972. Progesterone receptor in rabbit uterus. I. Characterization and estradiol-17 B augmentation. Endocrinology 92:1229–1240.

Rich, M. A., P. Furmanski, S. C. Brooks, and the Breast Cancer Prognostic Study Surgery and Pathology Associates. 1978. Prognostic value of estrogen receptor determinations in patients with breast cancer. Cancer Res. 38:4296–4298.

Rosen, P. P., C. J. Menendez-Botet, J. S. Nisselbaum, J. A. Urban, V. Mike, A. Fracchia, and M. K. Schwartz. 1975. Pathological review of breast lesion analyzed for estrogen receptor protein. Cancer Res. 35:3187–3194.

Savage, N., J. Levin, N. G. DeMoor, and M. Lange. 1981. Cytosolic oestrogen receptor content of breast cancer tissue in blacks and whites. S. Afr. Med. J. 58:623–624.

Toft, D. O., and B. W. O'Malley. 1972. Target tissue receptors for progesterone: The influence of estrogen treatment. Endocrinology 90:1041–1045.

Vorherr, H. 1980. Breast Cancer: Epidemiology, Endocrinology, Biochemistry and Pathobiology. Urban and Schwarzenberg, Baltimore, pp. 25–80.

Walt, J. A., A. Singhakowinta, S. C. Brooks, and A. Cortez. 1976. The surgical implications of estrophile protein estimations in carcinoma of the breast. Cancer 80:506–512.

White, J. E., and J. P. Enterline. 1980. Cancer in non-white Americans. Current Probl. Cancer 4:1–34.

Witliff, J. L., B. W. Beatty, E. D. Savlov, W. B. Patterson, and R. A. Cooper, Jr. 1976. Estrogen receptors and hormone dependency in human breast cancer, *in* Recent Results in Cancer Research, G. St. Arneult and L. Israel, eds. Springer-Verlag, Heidelberg, pp. 59–77.

Current Controversies in Breast Cancer, edited
by F. C. Ames, G. R. Blumenschein, and E. D. Montague.
University of Texas Press, Austin © 1984.

Epidemiology of Breast Cancer in Hispanics Compared to Anglos

Paul K. Mills M.S., M.P.H., and Guy R. Newell, M.D.

Department of Cancer Prevention, The University of Texas M. D. Anderson Hospital and Tumor Institute at Houston, Houston, Texas

This study was conducted to examine differences in breast cancer incidence between Anglo and Hispanic populations and to suggest possible mechanisms that may explain why these two ethnic groups experience differences in risk of developing this common cancer.

The study has compared breast cancer incidence rates among Hispanics with those among Anglos (nonHispanic whites) from selected areas, both in this country and abroad. Large differences in incidence of breast cancer between these two ethnic groups were found. In an attempt to explain these variations, particular attention was focused on nutrition, fertility, socioeconomic status, urban or rural living patterns, and other possible factors.

MATERIALS AND METHODS

Sources of Data

All statistics used in this report were obtained from incidence rates published by selected population-based tumor registries in this country and abroad. Age-adjusted incidence rates per 100,000 population were adjusted to the 1970 U.S. census using rates for men or women when appropriate. The areas compared in this report appear in Figure 1. Summary information on the selected registries is given in Table 1.

For this report, data for the years 1968 to 1972 were examined from the Cali, Colombia, tumor registry, which was initiated in 1962. This registry canvasses a current population of 762,000, principally comprised of mestizos (persons of Spanish and Indian ancestry) and a small minority of blacks. Data came from Waterhouse et al. (1976).

Incidence of data was also obtained from Puerto Rico, which is populated by whites (mostly of Spanish descent), blacks, and mulattos. Since the aboriginal Indian population has few survivors, there is currently less Indian admixture among Puerto Ricans than is found among Hispanics on the mainland. There was also a large importation of Africans to Puerto Rico, especially in the early colonial period.

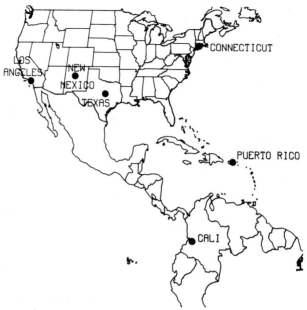

FIG. 1: Study areas.

Table 1. *Sources of Incidence Data*

Registry	Years Covered	Population	Population Characteristics
Cali, Colombia	1968–1972	762,000	Mestizos (Spanish and Indian ancestry)
Puerto Rico	1968–1972	2.7 million	Spanish decent white (80%) and blacks (20%)
Texas	1962–1966	4.0 million	Anglos (53%) Spanish surnamed (32%) Nonwhite (10%)
New Mexico	1969–1976	1.0 million	Spanish or Mexican American (38%) American Indians (7%) Black (2%) Anglo (52%)
Los Angeles County	1972–1976	7.5 million	Spanish ancestry, blacks, and Anglos
Connecticut	1973–1977	3.0 million	Anglo (93%)

The tumor registry in Puerto Rico began in 1950 and includes a population of 2.7-million persons comprised of 80% whites of Spanish descent and 20% blacks. Puerto Rican incidence rates also include the years 1968 to 1972 and are reported in Waterhouse et al.

Incidence data for six urban areas of Texas (including Houston, Laredo, Harlingen, San Antonio, Corpus Christi, and El Paso) were collected from the tumor registry set up by Eleanor Macdonald at the University of Texas M. D. Anderson Hospital and Tumor Institute at Houston beginning in 1951 and covering the years 1944 to 1966. As of 1966, the registry included a population of approximately 4-million people living in those six Texas cities with a distribution of 53% Anglo, 32% Spanish-surnamed, and 10% nonwhite persons. In this comparison, the data from Texas included the years 1962 to 1966. Spanish surnames were determined from a list of 6,000 Spanish surnames prepared by the U.S. Immigration and Naturalization Service. Data from this registry were reported in Macdonald and Heinz (1978).

The New Mexico tumor registry was established in 1969 and covers a population of approximately one million people, one-third of whom live in the state capital of Albuquerque. Thirty-eight percent of New Mexicans have Spanish or Mexican-American heritage, 7% are American Indians, 2% are black, and the remaining 52% are termed Anglo (of European descent, primarily from the British Isles). Surnames were divided into Spanish and nonSpanish categories using information from hospital charts and the detailed Spanish surname list from the 1970 U.S. census, in addition to a list of names developed specifically for New Mexico. New Mexico tumor registry data presented here include the years 1969 to 1976.

The Los Angeles County University of Southern California Cancer Surveillance Program is a rapid reporting system that collects from hospital pathology records all reported incidences of cancer in Los Angeles County (Hisserich et al. 1975). Surnames were divided into Spanish and nonSpanish categories using the detailed Spanish-surname list from the 1970 U.S. census. The Los Angeles data include the years 1972 to 1976.

The Connecticut tumor registry is the oldest population-based cancer registry in the country and currently canvasses a population of over three million persons, 93% of whom are white. Data presented in this report cover the years 1973 to 1977 and were obtained from the recent Surveillance, Epidemiology, and End Results SEER Publication (Young et al. 1981).

Limitations

There are several limitations inherent in using data from such different sources for comparative purposes. First, the definition of "Hispanic" or "Spanish-surnamed" or "Latin" is not always consistent, either in numerator or denominator data. This problem has been addressed by other investigators (Hernandez et al. 1975). The most probable net effect of misclassifying persons into the wrong ethnic group (in the Texas, New Mexico, and Los Angeles areas) would be to underestimate the differences truly present between ethnic groups and, hence, to create a dampening effect on the real differences. If, however, large numbers of Anglo women married Hispanics and were counted as Hispanics, this would inflate, for example, the rates of breast cancer reported for Hispanic women and deflate Anglo rates. Alvirez has reported that the proportion of Hispanic persons marrying non-Hispanics in Albuquerque in 1971 was 24% (Alvirez and Bean 1976). Figures from the 1970 U.S. census show that 18% of Spanish-origin couples in the U.S. were married to persons not of Spanish origin (U.S. Department of Commerce 1972).

Recent data from the National Center for Health Statistics show that in 19 reporting states approximately 12% of live births were to couples in which the mother was of Hispanic origin and the father was of nonHispanic origin. Similarly, 15% of live births in those states were to couples including a nonHispanic mother and an Hispanic father.

In addition, even though rates are standardized to the same population, temporal changes in cancer incidence in different areas may explain some of the observed variation. For example, incidence data from the six cities in Texas include the period 1962–1966, while the Los Angeles data cover the period 1972 to 1976. Hence, the effect of period of reporting on incidence of certain sites may be worthy of attention.

RESULTS

Breast cancer incidence is consistently higher in Anglo women than in Hispanic women in three geographic areas in which both ethnic groups reside (Texas, New Mexico, and Los Angeles). In addition, there is a smooth gradient among these three areas for both ethnic groups, the lowest incidence occurring in Texas, followed by New Mexico, and the highest in Los Angeles. In the two geographic areas studied with only Hispanic women, Colombia and Puerto Rico, the breast cancer rates are slightly lower than the low rates seen for Hispanic women in Texas. These are depicted in Figure 2.

Age-specific incidence rates for breast cancer for three SEER populations are shown in Figure 3. Anglo females in both New Mexico and Connecticut have similar rates that are higher than those for Hispanics in New Mexico. These higher rates in New Mexico and Connecticut women are most evident in the postmenopausal period.

Age-specific incidence rates for breast cancer in Hispanics and Anglos in New Mexico are shown in Figure 4. Rates for Hispanics in Los Angeles are also shown and are intermediate between the two New Mexico ethnic groups, although they more closely resemble the New Mexico Hispanics in both magnitude and shape.

DISCUSSION

Characteristics of Whites and Persons of Spanish Origin

The terms "Mexican-American," "Spanish-surnamed American," and "Hispanic" refer to a distinct minority of the U.S. population descended from Spaniards who migrated to the New World in the 16th century and subsequently intermarried with the native Indian population. Some selected demographic and socioeconomic characteristics of whites and persons of Spanish origin are given in Table 2 (Thomas 1979). In 1970, Mexican Americans had a median age of 20.8 years as compared to 27.5 years for other whites. Indicators of socioeconomic status showed Mexican Americans in 1976 to have lower incomes, less education, and predominantly blue-

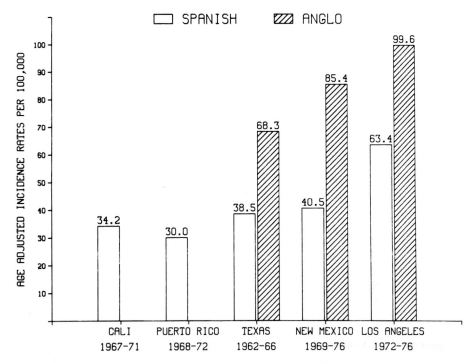

FIG. 2: Breast cancer incidence rates in Spanish and Anglo populations.

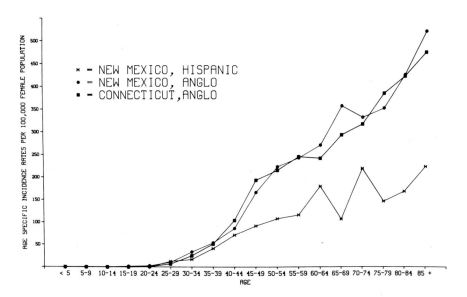

FIG. 3: Breast cancer age-specific incidence rates in three Surveillance, Epidemiology, and End Results (SEER) populations 1973–1977.

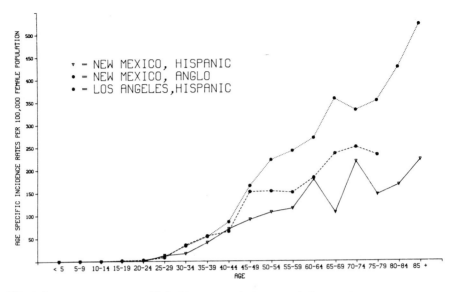

FIG. 4: Breast cancer age-specific incidence rates in three populations 1973–1977.

Table 2. *Selected Demographic and Socioeconomic Characteristics of Whites and Persons of Spanish Origin**

Variable	White	Spanish Origin
Median age, yr.	27.5	20.8
Percent native born	95.1	84.4
No. children/1000 15 to 24 yr.-old married women	933	1,264
Median yr. school completed	12.1	9.6
Mean family size	3.51	4.28
Mean 1969 family income ($)	11,348	8,550
Median family income ($)	9,957	7,533
% families under poverty level	8.6	20.4

*Adapted from Thomas 1979.

collar occupations as compared to the total U.S. population (U.S. Department of Commerce 1976). No other ethnic group identified by the U.S. Census has as high a fertility level as the Mexican Americans (Uhlenberg 1973), and the overall high rate of fertility among Mexican-American women under the age of 20, combined with the typical large family size, suggests a high risk for poorer maternal health in this ethnic group (Schrieber 1981).

Finally, the intermingling of Spanish and Indian cultures mentioned above is noteworthy in that most of the Indian cultures of the New World were based on the

Table 3. *Risk Factors for Breast Cancer*

Predisposing Factor	Increased Risk
Menarche before age 12	1.5
Menopause after age 55	2
Weight > 155 lb	1.5
Age at first birth > 30	1.5
Family history of breast cancer (premenopause)	
mother	3.5
mother and grandmother	5
two close relatives with premenopausal bilateral breast cancer	9

cultivation of corn, and the subsequent protein source for the Hispanic is thought to be based on corn and bean intake. Using a "24-hour recall" methodology, the Ten State Nutrition Survey, conducted between 1968 and 1970, concluded that almost one-third of low-income Hispanics reported no meat consumption but had the highest legume and milk consumption of all groups studied (U.S. Department of Health, Education and Welfare 1972). In contrast, low-income Anglos reported the highest cereal and pastry consumption).

Additionally, Hispanics demonstrate a higher prevalence towards obesity than other socioeconomic groups. This may reflect a reported cultural preference among rural Hispanics in New Mexico and Colorado for the obese body type, which is not characteristic of other segments of the U.S. population (Schulman and Smith 1963).

The known risk factors for breast cancer are shown in Table 3. This discussion will focus on differences in patterns of exposure to these risk factors in Anglos and Hispanics.

Fertility, Reproductive Habits, and Age at First Birth

The high rate of fertility and reproductive habits of the Hispanic female, including marital status, pregnancy, menstruation, and lactation, may well protect her from the excess breast cancer risk experienced by her Anglo counterpart. In particular, there is a consistent pattern of protection conferred by early age of first pregnancy and multiple pregnancies. This relationship, first recognized in 1926 (Petrakis 1982), has been replicated in many studies, including a multinational study that demonstrated an inverse linear relation between timing of first pregnancy and risk of breast cancer until age 30. Women with first full-term pregnancies before age 20 had a relative risk of breast cancer one-third that of women whose first childbirth occurred after age 35 (MacMahon et al. 1970). Of special interest was the fact that this relationship persisted after controlling for parity, which is strongly related to age at first childbirth.

The possibility that the relationship between timing of first birth and breast cancer risk could be due to either the direct protective effect of an early pregnancy or to another factor that both reduces fertility, thus delaying pregnancy, and increases the risk of breast cancer has been investigated (Lilienfeld et al. 1975). The results of this inquiry suggest that it is an early first birth per se that confers protection against breast cancer. This contention is further strengthened by the observation that only full-term pregnancies are associated with an altered risk level (MacMahon et al. 1973).

Menopausal Status

The age-specific incidence rates for breast cancer for three SEER populations, Anglo females in Connecticut and New Mexico and Hispanic females in New Mexico (Figure 3), indicate two interesting trends. First, as expected, the Anglo females in both New Mexico and Connecticut experience higher risks than the New Mexico Hispanics. This is in agreement with international trends demonstrated in Figure 2. Second and most interesting, the difference in rates between the Anglo and Hispanic females is most evident and dramatic in the postmenopausal period. Indeed, before age 45 the rates in the Hispanic females, though not as high as the Anglo rates, follow the same gradually rising trend that is observed in the Anglos. It is only after menopause that the departure in rates is observed, suggesting that ethnicity may explain differences in the postmenopausal type of breast cancer but is not related to the premenopausal type. The etiologic forces involved in the occurrence of premenopausal breast cancer seem to operate equally in both ethnic groups. Breast cancer risk in one study (Stavraky and Emmons 1974) increased with increasing age at first pregnancy among postmenopausal women only. This would agree with the generally later age at first pregnancy experienced by Anglo females. In the same study among the premenopausal women, increased breast cancer was associated with what is currently known about the geographic distribution of breast cancer with breast cancer mortality rates for urban areas being consistently higher than rural areas (Blot et al. 1977).

Demographic, Geographic, Socioeconomic, and Migration Factors

An examination of breast cancer incidence (Figure 2) reveals this is not only a disease afflicting Anglo women more than their Hispanic counterparts but also is a distinctly urban disease even within the Hispanic population. This is in agreement with what is currently known about the geographic distribution of breast cancer with breast cancer mortality rates for urban areas being consistently higher than rural areas (Blot et al. 1977).

More important, studies from various areas of the world have demonstrated a major increase in the urban breast cancer rate for the postmenopausal period (de-Waard 1978). The fact that inhabitants of New Mexico (a predominantly rural population) experience higher rates of breast cancer than their Texas (more urbanized) counterparts may reflect the time period of reporting, since breast cancer incidence in Texas has been increasing over time in both Anglos and Hispanics. The Texas data were collected between 1962 and 1966, while the New Mexico data were collected between 1972 and 1976.

Demographic differences in ethnic groups are recognized, however, and within the Hispanic population in this country there is diversity in urban/rural residential patterns, socioeconomic levels, and other indicators of demographic status. The age-specific incidence curve for New Mexican Hispanics, a predominantly rural, lower-socioeconomic population differs from that of Hispanics in Los Angeles (Figure 4). The rates of Hispanics in Los Angeles are shown to more closely approximate the rates observed in white females in both Connecticut and New Mexico. This may well reflect the more affluent, urbanized lifestyle experienced by Hispanic females in Los Angeles.

If Mexican Americans are dichotomized by place of birth and Standardized Incidence Ratios are examined (Table 4), it becomes evident that Mexican Americans experience lower overall risk for cancer but extremely elevated risk for cancer of the stomach (Menck et al. 1975). American born Mexican-American females, at least in Los Angeles, experience a higher risk for breast cancer than their immigrant counterparts although they are still at lower risk than other white women. This is in agreement with migrant studies that indicate that for Chinese, Japanese, and Latin Americans breast cancer rates are lowest for women in their native countries; in addition, rates in migrants are intermediate in magnitude between those for women in their native countries and white women in the United States. These Standardized Incidence Ratios suggest that rates for the descendants of Mexican migrants are higher than rates for their predecessors who migrated. This is consistent with the suggestion that exposure to western culture at an early age increases the risk for breast cancer more than exposure later in life.

The admixture of American Indian blood into the genome of the Hispanic population of this country is reflected in the cancer incidence and mortality rates presented in Table 5. Like Hispanics, American Indians experience overall lower risk for cancer incidence than do white Americans. Similarly, the common genetic component in American Indian and Hispanic blood places both groups at excess risk for gall-

Table 4.* SIR† (100 For Other Whites) For Mexican Americans, by Sex, Nativity, and Site, Los Angeles County, 1972–1973

Site	Male				Female			
	Immigrant		Indigenous		Immigrant		Indigenous	
	No.	SIR	No.	SIR	No.	SIR	No.	SIR
Cancer, all sites	449	62	893	78	559	69	1,252	86
Stomach	50	214	53	159	23	148	39	192
Breast	–	–	–	–	96	40	372	83

* Adapted from Menck 1975.
† Standardized Incidence Ratios.

Stavraky, K., and S. Emmons. 1974. Breast cancer in premenopausal and postmenopausal women. JNCI 53:647–654.

Tanner, J. M. 1973. Trends toward earlier menarche in London, Oslo, Copenhagen, The Netherlands and Hungary. Nature 243:95–96.

Thomas, D. B. 1979. Epidemiologic Studies of Cancer in Minority Groups in the Western United States. Natl. Cancer Inst. Monog. 53:103–113.

Uhlenberg, P. 1973. Fertility patterns within the Mexican-American population. Soc. Biol. 20: 30–39.

U.S. Department of Commerce. Bureau of the Census. 1976. Persons of Spanish origin in the United States: March, 1975. Current Population Report, ser. P-20, no. 290. Washington, D.C.

U.S. Department of Health, Education, and Welfare. Centers for Disease Control. 1972. Ten-State Nutrition Survey, 1968–1970 (V-Dietary), (HSM) 73-13011. Washington, D.C.

U.S. Department of Commerce. Bureau of the Census. 1972. Marital status. 1970 Census of populations, subject report PC(2)-4C. Washington, D.C.

Ventura, S. J. 1982. Births of Hispanic Parentage, 1979, *in* Monthly Vital Statistics Report, National Center for Health Statistics, vol. 31, no. 2, Public Health Service, Hyattsville, Maryland, pp. 129–160.

Waterhouse, J. C., Muir, P. Correa, and J. Powell. 1976. Cancer Incidence in Five Continents, vol. III. I.A.R.C. Springer-Verlag, Berlin.

Wynder, E. L. 1979. Dietary habits and cancer epidemiology. Cancer 43:1955–1961.

Young, J. L., C. L. Percy, and A. J. Asire. 1981. Surveillance, Epidemiology and End Results. Incidence and Mortality Data: 1973–77. Natl. Cancer Inst. Monog. 57.

THE JEFFREY A. GOTTLIEB MEMORIAL LECTURE

Current Controversies in Breast Cancer, edited
by F. C. Ames, G. R. Blumenschein, and E. D. Montague.
University of Texas Press, Austin © 1984.

Operable Breast Cancer: The Challenge of Adjuvant Chemotherapy

Gianni Bonadonna, M.D.

*Division of Medical Oncology, Istituto Nazionale per lo Studio e la Cura dei Tumori,
Milan, Italy*

I am highly honored and greatly flattered to be invited by the Program Committee to deliver the Jeffrey A. Gottlieb Memorial Lecture this year. I have always admired Jeff Gottlieb, both as a man and research physician. He was among the first medical oncologists who dedicated his professional life to the systematic design and evaluation of drug therapies for solid tumors, a poorly defined area of medical treatment in the early seventies. His human figure stood up as an example for patients and colleagues when the cause he was fighting for suddenly became his own cause. Without sparing himself all psychological and physical discomforts involved in the chemotherapy of cancer, Jeff continued to effectively play the role of research physician with courage and dignity. The message he leaves to all of us is not only that of intellectual and professional integrity but of human tolerance before the inevitable outcome.

I have selected the topic "The Challenge of Adjuvant Chemotherapy" because I believe that investigation of the multimodality approach for cancer in general and for mammary carcinoma in particular is a major task for the medical oncologists of my generation. Actually, the initial, and often successful, efforts to integrate systemic treatment with local-regional modalities have considerably helped to consecrate the importance of medical oncology in the primary treatment of patients with neoplastic diseases. Chemotherapy, once conceived and utilized almost exclusively in the management of clinically disseminated or primary inoperable neoplasms is now emerging as a necessary tool to improve the cure rate of given tumors or patient subsets.

REASONS FOR THE LIMITS OF CURRENT CHEMOTHERAPY REGIMENS IN CLINICALLY ADVANCED BREAST CANCER

After more than a decade of clinical research efforts involving thousands of patients, we can conclude, as summarized in Table 1, that: (a) the incidence of complete remission (CR) remains very low, for even under the most favorable clinical presentations, i.e. limited disease in the soft tissues, the incidence of CR rarely ex-

Table 1. *Expected Average Results with Various Drug Combinations in Clinically Metastatic Breast Cancer*

1. Complete plus partial remission	45–75%
2. Complete remission	5–20%
3. Median duration of response	7–13 months
4. Median survival of responders	12–33 months
5. Treatment results are not affected by increasing the number of drugs.	
6. The response rate is not affected by estrogen-receptor status.	
7. Second-line chemotherapy has limited efficacy.	

ceeds 20% and, most important, is not durable; (b) regardless of menopausal and estrogen receptor (ER) status, median duration of response and survival are not statistically improved by the addition of one or more drugs, either in concomitant, sequential, or alternating fashion, to a known effective cytotoxic combination; (c) present results would negate a clear therapeutic advantage of combined chemohormonal therapy over chemotherapy alone, although the value of such combined approach remains to be unquestionably confirmed in the subgroup of patients having ER-positive tumors; (d) salvage chemotherapy in women previously treated with cytotoxic drugs has very limited efficacy in terms of response rate, duration of response, and survival.

Thus, in advanced breast cancer given appropriate dose levels of effective drugs, the varying effects of these drugs reported in the literature appear to be more attributable to patient selection, i.e. varying mixes of known and unknown prognostic variables such as performance status, disease extent, and tumor aggressiveness, than to the effect of different forms of drug combination (Bonadonna and Valagussa 1983). In malignant neoplasms, including breast cancer, the single most important variable affecting the results of current treatments is the tumor mass. In fact, as pointed out by De Vita in the 1982 James Ewing Lecture, "tumor mass negatively influences the outcome of surgery and radiotherapy by its influence on invasiveness and the propensity to metastasize before local treatment is applied. Tumor mass negatively affects the outcome of cancer chemotherapy in a manner quite different from the way in which it does surgery or radiotherapy. Cancer chemotherapy fails because cells develop resistance to anticancer drugs."

In recent years, the mathematical model of Goldie and Coldman (1979, 1982), who have adapted to cancer treatment the 40-year-old mutation theory of Luria and Delbruck (1943) developed for bacterial cells, has lent considerable support to the cornerstone principle of cancer chemotherapy concerning the "inverse relationship between neoplastic cell burden and the curability with drugs." The assumptions of Goldie and Coldman can be summarized as follows: a) growing neoplastic cells are genetically unstable and develop somatic mutations that lead to phenotypic resistance to drugs they have never been exposed to; b) large fluctuation in the proportion and absolute number of drug-resistant tumor cells probably exists in compara-

Table 2. *Dominant Variables Affecting Cure Rates in Cancer Patients**

A. For surgery or radiotherapy
   1. Degree of regional invasion
   2. Presence and extent of metastatic disease
B. For chemotherapy
   1. Total neoplastic cell burden and the mix of drug-sensitive and drug-resistant tumor cells
   2. Mutation rates to a state of permanent resistance to the drugs employed
   3. Growth and regrowth rates
   4. Dose levels employed
   5. Treatment schedule (intervals, duration, methods of delivery of non-cross-resistant drugs).
C. For surgery or radiotherapy and chemotherapy
   1. The residual tumor cell burden and mix left after local-regional modality
   2. All of the variables listed under B. above

*Adapted from Skipper 1982c.

bly staged individuals with tumors of the same histologic subtype; c) as tumor size increases, the probability of resistant clones increases. Thus, for reasons quite independent of growth kinetics, in clinically advanced cancer, including breast cancer, we should expect that neoplastic cell populations are double-drug or multidrug resistant since the total tumor cell burden in most instances ranges from 10^{11} to 10^{12}. Conceptually, there are two types of resistance, both of which are related to tumor mass: 1) temporary resistance due to low growth fraction or pharmacologic sanctuaries; and 2) permanent resistance, which is related to mutant lines developing specific and permanent resistance to one or more anticancer drugs (De Vita 1982). As pointed out by Skipper (1982a), clinical resistance is observed when 10% to 50% of the surviving neoplastic cells are resistant to the drug(s) being used; in addition, multidrug-resistant neoplastic cells will markedly reduce the effectiveness of 3-, 4-, or 5-drug combinations. Therefore, the most effective means for preventing the emergence of multidrug-resistant phenotypes is to treat cancer patients with combination chemotherapy at an earlier stage, i.e. in its micrometastatic phase. By eradicating the single-drug-resistant cells we can lower the probability of the emergence of double-drug- or multidrug-resistant populations. Table 2 lists the dominant variables that affect the cure rates in animals, and most probably in humans, with cancer.

EVOLUTION IN THE TREATMENT OF MICROMETASTASES

For many years the rationale for surgery plus chemotherapy in the treatment of breast cancer patients with histologically positive axillary nodes has been apparent to many research physicians. The results of the earliest surgery-chemotherapy trials, carried out in particular by the National Surgical Adjuvant Breast Project

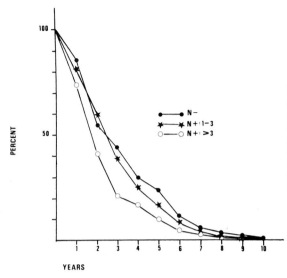

FIG. 1. Relapse-free survival by nodal status in breast cancer patients treated with radical mastectomy alone (excluding 10-year survivors). (N−) negative nodes; (N+:1−3) one to three positive nodes; (N+: > 3) more than three positive nodes. Data of the Milan Cancer Institute.

(NSABP) and the Scandinavian groups, seemed to suggest an advantage in this approach but were not highly encouraging for biological and pharmacological reasons that now are easy to explain: the dosages of triethylenethiophosphoramide (Thio-TEPA) and cyclophosphamide were not administered long enough.

There can be little doubt that optimal local-regional modalities (i.e. surgery or radiotherapy or both) are the best means for curing breast cancer that is not already widespread. However, until about 12–15 years ago, many clinicians thought that a considerable fraction of surgical failures was the result of the release of viable tumor cells during surgery. Although some of the metastases may be indeed secondary to surgery, their ubiquitous patterns leave little doubt that the vast majority of treatment failures are due to widespread micrometastases that occur prior to local-regional therapy. This modern concept is exemplified by the findings illustrated in Figure 1. In a consecutive case series of 716 women treated in Milan with radical mastectomy alone (Valagussa et al. 1978), the median relapse-free survival (RFS) was very similar among the three nodal groups examined. The slope of the curves was, however, slightly steeper for women with more than three axillary nodes involved. A median RFS of 20 to 30 months and the similar shape of the curves cannot be easily explained, except with the assumption that the disease was already widespread microscopically at the time of surgery. As pointed out by Fisher et al. (1981b), the probability of developing distant metastases or dying of cancer is not related to the extent of local treatment. This finding and the known fact that about 25% of women with histologically negative axillary nodes manifest distant treatment failure provide additional evidence that "positive regional nodes are indicators of a host-tumor relationship that permits the development of metastases and that they are not important instigators of distant disease." There is consistent evidence,

Table 3. *Influence of Nodal Status* on The Percentage of Breast Cancer Patients Suffering Relapse in Varying Intervals After Surgery[†]*

| | % Relapsing in Intervals (Years) | | | |
	0−1.5	0−3	0−5	5−10
N−	8.8	15.0	21.0	6.9
N+	30.4	51.7	63.6	11.9
N+ 1−3	19.1	39.4	53.9	12.6
N+ >3	42.6	65.0	74.3	9.3
Total	18.9	34.7	44.5	9.0

*(N−) negative nodes, (N+) positive nodes, (N+ 1−3) one to three positive nodes, (N+ >3) more than three positive nodes.
[†]Data of Milan Cancer Institute.

Table 4. *Influence of Nodal Status* on the Percent of Patients Relapsing in 10 Years Who Relapsed in the Intervals Indicated[†]*

| | % Relapsing in Intervals (Years) | | |
	0−1.5	0−3	0−5
N−	29.7	54.9	76.9
N+	41.6	70.3	86.4
N+ 1−3	28.9	60.5	82.2
N+ >3	53.5	77.8	89.6
Total	38.6	66.7	84.1

*(N−) negative nodes, (N+) positive nodes, (N+ 1−3) one to three positive nodes, (N+ >3) more than three positive nodes.
[†]Data of Milan Cancer Institute.

with almost superimposable results in case series subjected to prospective controlled trials (Fisher et al. 1975b, Valagussa et al. 1978), that the total 10-year RFS is affected by the histologic status of axillary nodes (for patients with negative nodes about 75%, with positive nodes about 25%).

Furthermore, the number of involved regional nodes represents a simple and reliable prognostic factor. From the findings reported in Tables 3 and 4, which are also derived from our previous surgical series (Valagussa et al. 1978), one can appreciate the relationship between nodal status and percent of patients relapsing at various intervals: The higher the number of histologically positive nodes, the higher the fraction of patients showing early relapse, i.e. within the first 18 months following radical mastectomy. Thus, tumor cell burden in the axilla may indirectly reflect not only the risk of developing distant micrometastatic disease but also the tumor cell burden of micrometastases. However, since the residual tumor stem cell burden in surgical failures ranges from $< 10^1$ to $\geq 10^9$ (Skipper 1982b), it would be of practical importance to clearly establish in individual patients the actual tumor cell burden of micrometastases, or at least to estimate with sufficient accuracy its median value in given subgroups. The incidence and the prognostic importance of blood

Table 5. *Importance of Estrogen Receptor (ER) Status in Resectable Breast Cancer*[*]

Author	Stage	No. Pts.	Years of Analysis		% RFS ER+	ER−	P
Knight[†]	I–II	145	1.6		86	66	0.01
Rich	I–II	285	1.6		93	73	not reported
Allegra	I–II	292	2		91	62	0.001
Cooke	I–II	144	3		85	35	0.001
				N+	55	30	0.05
				N−	75	32	0.01
Maynard[‡]	I–II	232	3		71	63	0.05
Valagussa	T_{1-3a}, N−	464	5		82	45	0.0005
Crowe	I	510	5		78	67	0.0341

[*]Adapted from Bonadonna and Valagussa 1983.
[†]Some patients received adjuvant treatment.
[‡]Minor local recurrences excluded from analysis.

vessel invasion was recently re-emphasized by Weigand et al. (1982). In 175 breast cancer patients, the incidence was 35%, and the association of poor prognosis with blood vessel invasion (70% recurrence by 2 years) was independent of clinical tumor size and menopausal and nodal status.

In recent years, ER status has also been consistently identified as an important prognostic parameter in patients treated with local-regional modality alone. Table 5 reports the RFS related to ER status in seven representative case series in which patients were treated with surgery alone. As can be seen, inspite of nonuniform patient selection and timing of analysis, the RFS was invariably and significantly superior in women with ER-positive tumors compared to women with ER-negative tumors. In particular, two research groups have shown that patients with operable disease confined to the breast (with negative nodes) and with ER-negative tumors fall into a significantly poorer prognostic group compared to patients with ER-positive tumors. The apparent discrepancy in the RFS of pre- vs postmenopausal women reported by Valagussa et al. (1981) and Crowe et al. (1982) may be due to the different median follow-up times (36 vs 60 months, respectively); the American group has noted that within the premenopausal group ER-positive women have a recurrent rate identical to ER-negative women, and this finding became apparent only after prolonged follow-up.

The true prognostic importance of the labeling index (Meyer and Hixon 1979, Bertuzzi et al. 1981) remains to be confirmed by the long-term analysis of a large series including consecutive patients.

The First Modern Adjuvant Trials

The concept of widespread micrometastases and the advent of cyclical chemotherapy to control systemic disease provided a background for modern adjuvant trials. The initial series, which have provided considerable support to the scientific

Table 6. *First CMF Adjuvant Trial Carried Out in Milan: Summary of 7-Year Results in Pre- and Postmenopausal Pts. with Positive Nodes (N+)*

	Control (%)	CMF* (%)	P
Relapse-Free Survival			
Total	35.8	49.2	<0.002
N+ 1–3	42.3	60.4	0.003
N+ >3	22.2	28.4	0.18
Premenopause	35.4	56.1	<0.001
N+ 1–3	46.7	72.5	0.0007
N+ >3	19.2	25.5	0.09
Postmenopause	37.3	43.3	0.43
N+ 1–3	40.0	48.8	0.42
N+ >3	28.2	32.9	0.79
Survival			
Total	56.3	66.6	0.12
Premenopause	55.3	70.6	0.03
Postmenopause	59.6	62.7	0.79

*CMF = cyclophosphamide, methotrexate, 5-fluorouracil.

hypothesis that effective and prolonged chemotherapy should improve the RFS over surgery alone, were those designed by the NSABP group (Fisher et al. 1975a) and by the Milan group (Bonadonna et al. 1976). To adequately test the validity of the new combined treatment, the correct methodology required the use of a concomitant control group with surgery alone. Of the five research teams utilizing such a concomitant control group (NSABP, Milan Cancer Institute, Ostschweizerische Arreitsgemeinschaft Für Klinische Onkologie [OSAKO], Guy's-Manchester Group, and Multicenter Breast Cancer Chemotherapy Group [MBCCG]), four have demonstrated that systemic treatment started within 2 to 4 weeks from conventional surgery resulted in a significantly improved RFS (Bonadonna and Valagussa 1983). Table 6 summarizes the 7-year results of the first cyclophosphamide, methotrexate, and 5-fluorouracil (CMF) adjuvant study performed in Milan. It is important to emphasize that the difference in RFS between the control and the CMF group has remained proportionately about the same from the third year from surgery (Bonadonna and Valagussa 1983). Subsequent prospective studies that have not utilized a concomitant control group have reported comparable treatment results.

Reproducibility of Trial Results

Although interstudy comparisons raise many controversial problems concerning patient sample, drug combinations, doses and schedules, average time on study, and reporting techniques, Table 7 indicates that the overall reported results are remarkably similar, although there are percent differences among various subsets (Bonadonna and Valagussa 1983). The findings strongly suggest that when breast cancer has been treated with surgery alone the RFS has not significantly changed over

Table 7.* *Reproducibility of 5-Year Adjuvant Results[t]*

Primary Therapy	RFS	Institutions
Surgery alone	45%	NSABP, Milan, UT M. D. Anderson Hospital
Surgery + CMF	59–64%	Milan, Memorial, Guy's— Manchester
Surgery + PAM	53–55%	NSABP, SWOG, COG, Guy's—Manchester Group.

*Adapted from Bonadonna and Valagussa 1983.
[t]Abbreviations are as follows: RFS = relapse-free survival; NSABP = National Surgical Adjuvant Breast Project; CMF = cyclophosphamide, methotrexate, 5-fluorouracil; PAM = phenylalanine mustard; SWOG = Southwest Oncology Group; COG = Central Oncology Group.

the past 20 years, a conclusion also supported by the Natural History Data Base (Moon et al. 1981). As far as adjuvant chemotherapy is concerned, the comparability of total RFS within the various groups utilizing either CMF or phenylalanine mustard (PAM) chemotherapy was indeed very good. The results differ in pre- vs postmenopausal patients but, inspite of percent differences, RFS was always inversely related to the number of involved axillary nodes. Table 8 shows the comparative 5-year results from the Milan CMF adjuvant trials. The details of the two successive studies were reported in previous publications (Bonadonna and Valagussa 1983, Tancini et al. 1983). All three CMF groups received drug therapy following the same dose regimen, including the dose attenuation schedule. The comparative RFS and total survival failed to show significant differences. The trend in the RFS favoring CMF given for only six cycles, particularly in women with more than three positive nodes (49.3%) and in postmenopausal women (63.1%), is

Table 8. *Comparative 5-Year Results in Breast Cancer Pts. with Positive Nodes (N+) Treated in Milan in Two Successive Trials with CMF**

	Control	vs	CMF 12 cycles	CMF 12 cycles	vs	CMF 6 cycles
	%		%	%		%
RFS[t]						
Total	44.6		59.5	59.0		65.5
N+ 1–3	48.1		69.4	72.3		76.1
N+ >3	33.0		40.5	37.4		49.3
Premenopausal	43.4		65.9	59.3		66.5
Postmenopausal	49.3		55.7	57.6		63.1
Survival	66.2		78.4	72.7		76.9

*CMF = cyclophosphamide, methotrexate, 5-fluorouracil.
[t]RFS = relapse-free survival.

difficult to explain at this point of the actuarial analysis. Relapse-free survival was directly related to the dose levels administered, and in all three CMF groups there was no increased incidence of second neoplasms compared to the control group.

Are the Most Desirable Trials Being Tested?

A successful trial is one that yields the correct answer to the specific question posed. With the evidence that adjuvant chemotherapy could significantly affect the growth of distant micrometastases, a number of randomized trials were mounted in the attempt to elucidate whether (a) drug combinations were superior to single-agent chemotherapy; (b) the addition of endocrine therapy or immunotherapy to chemotherapy could improve the results over chemotherapy alone; (c) treatment duration could be safely reduced; (d) the delivery of sequential or alternating non-cross-resistant regimens could yield results superior to a single-drug combination. Table 9 presents representative examples of such trials, most of which are still in a very early phase. Available results would indicate that adjuvant combination chemotherapy, regardless of drugs and dose schedules utilized, appears significantly superior to single-agent chemotherapy, at least when PAM is utilized. At the present moment, the most convincing results are those reported by the Southwest Oncology Group (SWOG), which randomly tested CMF plus vincristine and prednisone

Table 9. *Trials Being Tested**

Trials	Examples
Single-drug vs multidrug chemotherapy	PAM vs CMF(VP) or CFP
	PAM vs PAM + F
	F vs CMF
	CTx vs CMF
Optimal duration of treatment	CMF: 12 vs 6 cycles
	ChMF: 6 vs 18 cycles
	CA: 6 vs 10 cycles
Chemotherapy plus hormones	CMF ± Tx
	PAM + F ± Tx
Chemotherapy plus immunotherapy	CMF ± levamisole
	CMF ± BCG
	CMF(VP) ± MER
	FAC ± BCG
Chemotherapy in N− patients	surgery ± CMF[†]
Sequential chemotherapy	CMFP → AV
	CMF → A
	A → CMF
Alternating chemotherapy	CMF/A

* Abbreviations are as follows: PAM = 1-phenylalanine mustard; C = cyclophosphamide; M = methotrexate; P = prednisone; F = fluorouracil; CH = chlorambucil; A = Adriamycin; V = vincristine; Tx = tamoxifen; BCG = bacillus Calmette-Guerin; MER = methanol extraction residue (of BCG); (N−) = negative nodes.
[†] Limited to ER negative patients.

(CMFVP) vs PAM and found that multidrug therapy was superior to monochemotherapy in all classic prognostic subgroups (Rivkin 1982).

Although some investigators believed that chemotherapy could exert its beneficial effect on premenopausal women through suppression of the ovarian function, to my knowledge there is no single ongoing randomized trial testing adjuvant castration alone vs adjuvant chemotherapy. The value of combined chemohormonal therapy relies at present on the studies at Case Western University (Hubay 1981) (low dose CMF ± tamoxifen (Tx)) and NSABP (PAM plus 5-fluorouracil (5-FU) ± Tx) groups. Both research groups have observed a significant improvement of RFS of patients receiving Tx (at 4 years: CMF 58% vs CMF + Tx 62%; at 2 years: PAM + 5-FU 61% vs PAM + 5-FU + Tx 78%). Though promising, the results are still premature for general conclusions to be drawn, particularly those of the NSABP group (Fisher et al. 1981a). It is also important to recall that the best results reported by the Case Western Reserve group with CMF plus Tx (Hubay et al. 1981) were indeed similar to the results achieved with CMF alone in Milan. This was most probably due to the low-dose regimen of CMF utilized by the American investigators.

The addition of immunotherapy with bacillus Calmette-Guérin (BCG) or levamisole failed in three randomized studies (Bonadonna and Valagussa 1983) to affect the RFS. The only apparent positive study with adjuvant immunotherapy was published in 1980 by a French group. Lacour et al. (1980) claimed an improved 3-year RFS following administration of polyadenylic-polyuridylic acid (PolyA-PolyU) in patients with axillary node involvement. However, when the analysis was broken down into subsets (menopausal and nodal groups) no significant difference was detected.

Finally, the role of adjuvant radiotherapy in combination with chemotherapy has been investigated. Current results would negate that the addition of postoperative irradiation to an effective adjuvant chemotherapy regimen could reduce, in patients subjected to Halsted or modified radical mastectomy, the recurrence rate from 3 to 5 years after surgery (Bonadonna et al. 1983). Thus, unless a woman has been subjected to a surgical breast-saving procedure (i.e. excisional biopsy, lumpectomy, segmental resection, or quadrantectomy), radiotherapy does not appear to play an important therapeutic role either with or without concomitant or sequential chemotherapy, as recently confirmed by the NSABP findings (Fisher et al. 1981b).

Optimal Treatment Duration and Number of Drugs

The optimal duration of adjuvant treatment remains, at present, unknown. The comparability of the RFS and survival results between 6 and 12 cycles of CMF (Table 8) is both of theoretical and practical importance. Also considering that the 5-year RFS for the entire group of patients with positive nodes receiving 6 CMF cycles (59%) is superimposable on the RFS reported by Memorial Hospital investigators (Hakes et al. 1982) who have administered 24 CMF cycles (59%), one can conclude that the maximal tumor cell kill is achieved, at least with CMF, within the first 6 months of adjuvant therapy. Two other randomized studies utilizing cyclophosphamide and Adriamycin (CA) administered for 15 versus 30 weeks (Henderson et al. 1982) and chlorambucil, methotrexate, and 5-FU (chMF) for 6 versus 18 cycles (Jungi et al. 1981), respectively, have shown in the 3-year analysis, that RFS was comparable between short-term and long-term chemotherapy. Also, present findings are in keeping with the basic tenet of the mutation theory and re-emphasize the need to properly test alternating non-cross-resistant regimens to prevent or limit the emergence of phenotypes that are resistant to a single effective combination.

The effect of timing of initiation of chemotherapy on RFS was first reported by Nissen-Meyer (1979) who noticed a marked decrease in the efficacy of adjuvant cyclophosphamide when the drug was not started immediately after surgery. A recent publication of a group at The University of Texas M. D. Anderson Hospital and Tumor Institute at Houston (Buzdar et al. 1982) indicated that there is no relation between RFS and length of delays in initiation of a combination of 5-FU, Adriamycin, and cyclophosphamide (FAC). Also, this information would correspond to the concept of primary cell resistance. In fact, considering the relatively long median doubling time of breast cancer cells as well as the fraction of cells in the G_o phase of the cell cycle, it is conceivable that a treatment delay of 2 to 4 months will not appreciably affect the likelihood of killing sensitive tumor cells while the recurrence rate is related to the growing fraction of resistant cell population.

How many drugs are required to achieve optimal results? As shown in Table 10, many women will have a high (i.e. $\geq 10^9$) tumor cell burden after surgery and, as a consequence, micrometastases will be doubly or multidrug resistant. Therefore, more than one combination, given in sequential or alternating fashion, could theoretically provide better results than current single combinations. Only in the rare, presently not identifiable, situations in which the total residual tumor cell burden will be low (i.e. $\leq 10^3$) adjuvant treatment utilizing a lesser number of drugs could be sufficient to achieve cure or long-term control of micrometastases. Some of the reported positive results in subsets treated with PAM could indeed be explained by the hypothesis of a direct relationship between tumor cell burden and phenotypic heterogeneity.

CONCLUSION

In the recent history of local-regional treatment of breast cancer, we have learned from our successes and failures; in particular, failures have forced changes in both theory and practice. Now that adjuvant chemotherapy is becoming a reality, for some positive clinical findings have been consistently achieved all over the world, it is time to learn from our successes and failures in the area of systematic therapy. Can we better identify some of the reasons for failures during and after the best current treatments for clinically and microscopically disseminated breast cancer? If this could be done, it might influence future planning and the rate of future progress.

The direct relationship between total neoplastic cell burden and the probability of the presence (or emergence) of single-, double-, or multidrug-resistant tumor cells

Table 10. *Minimum Number of Drugs that may be Required in an Adjuvant Situation Following Mastectomy or Primary Radiotherapy**

Subgroups with the Same Nodal and Menopausal Status	Total Residual Burden or Tumor Stem Cells After Surgery		Expected Number of Drug-Resistant Cells in the Residual Burden[†]		Minimum Number of Drugs Necessary to Achieve Cure
			Single-Drug Resistant	Double-Drug Resistant	
I	low	$(\leqslant 10^3)$	0	0	1
II	medium	(10^6)	10^2	0	2
III	high	$(\geqslant 10^9)$	$\geqslant .10^5$	some	$\geqslant 3$

* Adapted from Skipper 1982c.
[†] Based on common mutation rates and the direct relationship between tumor cell burden and phenotypic heterogeneity.

currently appears to be not only a fascinating hypothesis but also an important bio-logical concept upon which new treatment strategies can be planned. Drug-resistant neoplastic cells may arise as a result of mutations of drug-sensitive cells before ini-tiation of chemotherapy, and double-drug-resistant cancer cells usually arise from single-drug-resistant cells, not directly (i.e. in a single step) from the drug-sensitive phenotypes. Thus clinical resistance is not an instantaneous nor an all-or-none phe-nomenon. Rather, "it is a step-by-step process that may not be clinically apparent until selection has proceeded to the point in which 10% to 50% of the surviving tumor cells are drug-resistant" (Skipper 1982b). Depending on the tumor size and the mutation rate, there is a possibility that no cells are resistant to a given drug at the initiation of treatment (Table 11). We also must expect the proportion and abso-lute numbers of drug-resistant tumor cells of a specific type to fluctuate consider-ably in tumors of the same size and type. This predictable fluctuation helps to explain the quite different degrees and duration of response to chemotherapy fre-quently observed in similarly staged and treated individuals (Skipper 1982a).

As stressed by Skipper (1982c), "future progress in the area of cancer chemo-therapy may depend on paying closer attention to the heterogeneity of tumor stem cell populations and the continually changing burden and mix that occurs during treatment. Such changes necessitate strategies that will (a) maximize the proba-bility of eradicating both the drug-sensitive and drug-resistant tumor stem cells present at the initiation of chemotherapy and (b) minimize the probability of the emergence of double-drug- or multi-drug-resistant cells during treatment." The likelihood of eradicating single- and double-drug-resistant cells and preventing emergence of new drug-resistant cells during treatment, might be increased by the optimum delivery of 3, 4, or more drugs versus delivery of 2 drugs. Considering the recent results achieved in Hodgkin's disease with the MOPP/ABVD program (Bo-nadonna 1982), the alternating delivery of two non-cross-resistant combinations at maximum tolerated doses could provide significant improvement of end results over those achieved to date. Goldie et al. (1982) have listed the situations in which treat-ment alternation might not prove to be the optimal strategy: 1) When in a given tumor one resistant fraction is considerably larger than the other, even if the values for their mutation rates are identical; 2) When two resistant cell compartments will

Table 11. *Approximate Average Numbers of Expected*[*]
Single-Drug-Resistant Tumor Cells[†]

Mutation Rate	Total Tumor Cell Burden[‡]			
	10^4	10^6	10^8	10^{10}
10^{-4}	10^1	10^3	10^5	10^7
10^{-6}	0	10^1	10^3	10^5
10^{-8}	0	0	10^1	10^3

[*]Considerable fluctuation must be expected.
[†]Adapted from Skipper 1982c.
[‡]Encircled values: possible or probable presence of some double-drug-resistant phenotypes.

not exhibit the same kinetic behavior. Thus, alternating sequence therapies that do not incorporate stringent requirements may fail to show therapeutic advantage. Theoretically, less substantial deviations from this symmetry are most likely to occur in the treatment of patients with micrometastases, and, therefore, alternating chemotherapy may constitute the optimal therapeutic approach in an adjuvant situation. In the treatment of experimental animals with tumors, often the dose schedule and the methods of delivering drug combinations have a greater effect on end results than the number of drugs in a combination. Therefore, retrospective and prospective simulations, if used with prudence, will help to provide conceptual guidance toward the use of an optimal number of non-cross-resistant drugs and optimum delivery (Goldie et al. 1982, Skipper 1982a, c).

How should practicing physicians approach the problem of adjuvant chemotherapy for breast cancer? In my opinion, a few practical rules should be kept in mind. First of all, clinicians should avoid premature arbitrary conclusions such as: Surgery plus chemotherapy is of no value in postmenopausal women or in patients with more than three positive nodes; or, surgery plus one drug is as effective as surgery plus two or more non-cross-resistant drugs. As previously outlined, the biological and the clinical problems are indeed much more complex than the all-or-none phenomenon. Second, a cautious attitude should be maintained in patient selection and treatment delivery. Adjuvant chemotherapy is indicated today only in conventionally high-risk groups, namely those with positive axillary nodes or with blood vessel invasion. At present, the high-risk subgroup of patients with negative regional nodes remains to be more clearly defined, in spite of the initial evidence for poor prognosis in a subset of these women—those with ER-negative tumors.

The Milan observation showing that the 5-year results are similar following 6 or 12 cycles of CMF indicates that, apparently, there is no need to prolong adjuvant chemotherapy beyond the sixth month, at least when only one combination is utilized. The interpretation of the above-mentioned findings suggests that the breast cancer cell populations that survive 6 cycles of CMF often are CMF-resistant, i.e. resistant to one, two, or all of the drugs in CMF. The observation that the first few cycles of adjuvant CMF select resistant neoplastic cells may well be applicable to other known drug combinations, and, therefore, has implications with respect to the design of future adjuvant regimens (i.e. alternating chemotherapy), especially for women with more than three positive nodes. The administration of a single adjuvant combination for a relatively short period of time, as well as its delivery in an alternating fashion with a non-cross-resistant regimen, will probably minimize the risk of long-term complications such as carcinogenesis and organ damage (e.g. sterility, cardiomyopathy, and liver fibrosis) associated with high cumulative doses of alkylating agents, Adriamycin, and methotrexate.

Since all tested two- to five-drug combinations appear to yield comparable results, a third recommendation is to focus in clinical practice on the correct application of an established regimen, in which too many changes, particularly in the dose levels, should be avoided.

In conclusion, the initial adjuvant trials have achieved limited, but consistent, results, particularly in women with minimal axillary node involvement. Also, because of limited follow-up, present findings cannot indicate that the cure rate has been increased in given subsets. Since no other therapeutic means have been able in decades to consistently and significantly decrease the failure rate following local-regional therapy, I see no major obstacles to the general use of known chemotherapeutic regimens by qualified medical oncologists for high-risk groups. We should not, however, be content with present achievements; research should vigorously continue in the attempt to identify more effective and less toxic treatments. Therefore, future goals must include the achievement of higher RFS for different groups and subgroups and the reduction of toxicity, but not at the expense of a long-term RFS.

ACKNOWLEDGMENTS

This work was partially supported by Contract No. N01-CM-07338, Division of Cancer Treatment, National Cancer Institute, U.S. Department of Health and Human Services.

REFERENCES

Bertuzzi, A., M. G. Daidone, G. Di Fronzo, and R. Silvestrini. 1981. Relationship among estrogen receptors, proliferative activity and menopausal status in breast cancer. Breast Cancer Res. Treat. 1:253–262.

Bonadonna, G. 1982. Chemotherapy strategies to improve the control of Hodgkin's disease. The Richard and Hinda Rosenthal Foundation Memorial Lecture. Cancer Res. (in press).

Bonadonna, G., E. Brusamolino, P. Valagussa, A. Rossi, L.Brugnatelli, C. Brambilla, M. De Lena, G. Tancini, E. Bajetta, R. Musumeci, and U. Veronesi. 1976. Combination chemotherapy as an adjuvant treatment in operable breast cancer. N. Engl. J. Med. 294:405–410.

Bonadonna, G., and P. Valagussa. 1983. Chemotherapy of breast cancer. Current views and results. Int. J. Radiat. Oncol. Biol. Phys. (in press).

Bonadonna, G., P. Valagussa, R. Zucali, M. Del Vecchio, and U. Veronesi. 1982. Feasibility of adjuvant chemotherapy plus radiotherapy in operable breast cancer, *in* Alternatives to Mastectomy, S. Hellman, J. R. Harris, eds. J. B. Lippincott, Philadelphia (in press).

Buzdar, A. U., T. L. Smith, K. C. Powell, G. R. Blumenschein, and E. A. Gehan. 1982. Effect of timing of initiation of adjuvant chemotherapy on disease-free survival in breast cancer. Breast Cancer Res. Treat. 2:163–169.

Crowe, J. P., C. A. Hubay, O. H. Pearson, J. S. Marshall, J. Rosenblatt, E. G. Mansour, R. E. Herman, J. C. Jones, W. J. Flynn, W. L. McGuire, and participating investigators. 1982. Estrogen receptor status as a prognostic indicator for stage I breast cancer patients. Breast Cancer Res. Treat. 2:171–176.

Fisher, B., P. Carbone, S. G. Economou, R. Frelick, A. Glass, H. Lerner, C. Redmond, M. Zelen, D. L. Katrých, N. Wolmark, E. R. Fisher, and cooperating NSABP investigators. 1975a. L-phenylalanine mustard (L-PAM) in the management of primary breast cancer: a report of early findings. N. Engl. J. Med. 292:117–122.

Fisher, B., C. Redmond, A. Brown, N. Wolmark, J. Wittliff, E. R. Fisher, D. Plotkin, D. Bowman, S. Sacks, J. Wolter, R. Frelick, R. Desser, N. LiCalzi, P. Geggie, G. E. Elias, D. Prager, P. Koontz, H. Wolk, N. Dimitrov, B. Gardner, H. Lerner, H. Shibata, and other NSABP investigators. 1981a. Treatment of primary breast cancer with chemotherapy and tamoxifen. N. Engl. J. Med. 305:1–6.

Fisher, B., N. Slack, D. Katrych, and N. Wolmark. 1975b. Ten year follow-up results of patients with carcinoma of the breast in a cooperative clinical trial evaluating surgical adjuvant chemotherapy. Surg. Gynecol. Obstet. 140:528–534.

Fisher, B., N. Wolmark, C. Redmond, M. Deutsch, E. R. Fisher, and Participating NSABP Investigators. 1981b. Findings from NSABP Protocol No. B-04: Comparison of radical mastectomy with alternative treatments. II. The clinical and biologic significance of medial-central breast cancers. Cancer 48:1863–1872.

Goldie, J. H., and A. J. Coldman. 1979. A mathematical model for relating the drug sensitivity of tumors to their spontaneous mutation rate. Cancer Treat. Rep. 63:1727–1733.

Goldie, J. H., A. J. Coldman, and G. A. Gudauskas. 1982. Rationale for the use of alternating non-cross resistant chemotherapy. Cancer Treat. Rep. 66:439–449.

Hakes, T. B., V. E. Currie, R. J. Kaufman, D. Kinne, H. Oettgen, and C. Pinsky. 1982. CMF ± levamisole breast adjuvant chemotherapy: 5-year analysis. (Abstract) Proc. Amer. Soc. Clin. Oncol. 1:83.

Henderson, I. C., R. Gelman, L. M. Parker, A. T. Skarin, R. J. Mayer, M. B. Garnick, and G. P. Canellos. 1982. 15 vs 30 weeks of adjuvant chemotherapy for breast cancer patients with a high risk of recurrence: A randomized trial. (Abstract) Proc. Amer. Soc. Clin. Oncol. 1:75.

Hubay, C. A., O. H. Pearson, J. S. Marshall, T. A. Stellato, R . S. Rhodes, S. M. Debanne, J. Rosenblatt, E. G. Mansour, R. E. Hermann, J. C. Jones, W. J. Flynn, C. Eckert, W. L. McGuire, and 27 participating investigators. 1981. Adjuvant therapy of stage II breast cancer. 48-month follow-up of a prospective randomized clinical trial. Breast Cancer Res. Treat. 1:77–82.

Jungi, W. F., P. Alberto, F. W. Brunner, F. Cavalli, L. Barrelet, and H. S. Senn. 1981. Short or long-term adjuvant chemotherapy for breast cancer, *in* Adjuvant Therapy of Cancer III, S. E. Salmon and S. E. Jones, eds. Grune & Stratton, New York, pp. 395–402.

Lacour, J., F. Lacour, A. Spira, M. Michelson, J. Y. Petit, G. Delage, D. Sarrazin, G. Contesso, and J. Viguier. 1980. Adjuvant treatment with poly adenylic-poly uridylic acid (Poly A-Poly U) in operable breast cancer. Lancet 2:161–164.

Luria, S. E., and M. Delbruck. 1943. Mutations of bacteria from virus sensitivity to virus resistance. Genetics 28:491–511.

Meyer, J. S., and B. Hixon. 1979. Advanced stage and early relapse of breast carcinomas associated with high thymidine labeling indices. Cancer Res. 39:4042–4047.

Moon, T., S. E. Jones, S. L. Davis, G. Bonadonna, P. Valagussa, U. Veronesi, and T. J. Powles. 1981. Development of a Natural History Data Base for breast cancer, *in* Adjuvant Therapy of Cancer III, S. E. Salmon, and S. E. Jones, eds. Grune & Stratton, New York, pp. 471–481.

Nissen-Meyer, R. 1979. One short chemotherapy course in primary breast cancer: 12-year follow-up in series 1 of the Scandinavian adjuvant chemotherapy study group, *in* Adjuvant Therapy of Cancer II, S. E. Jones, and S. E. Salmon, eds. Grune & Stratton, New York, pp. 207–213.

Rivkin, S., H. Glucksberg, and M. Foulkes. 1982. Adjuvant chemotherapy for operable breast cancer with positive axillary nodes. (Abstract) Proc. Amer. Soc. Clin. Oncol. 1:74.

Skipper, H. E. 1982a. Some additional observations, views, concepts, and theories that seem applicable in the practice of cancer treatment. (Booklet 3) Southern Research Institute, Birmingham, Alabama.

Skipper, H. E. 1982b. On the origin of singly and doubly-drug resistant neoplastic cells: cross-resistance, lack of cross-resistance, and occasional collateral sensitivity and some implications. (Booklet 8) Southern Research Institute, Birmingham, Alabama.

Skipper, H. E. 1982c. Human cancers: shapes and slopes of remission and survival curves and variables that affect them. Part III. Breast Cancer. (Booklet 17) Southern Research Institute, Birmingham, Alabama.

Tancini, G., G. Bonadonna, P. Valagussa, S. Marchini, and U. Veronesi. 1983. Adjuvant CMF in breast cancer: comparative 5-year results of 12 versus 6 cycles. J. Clin. Oncol. 1:1–10.

Valagussa, P., G. Bonadonna, and U. Veronesi. 1978. Pattern of relapse and survival following radical mastectomy. Analysis of 716 consecutive patients. Cancer 41:1171–1178.

Valagussa, P., G. Di Fronzo, P. Bignami, R. Buzzoni, G. Bonadonna, and U. Veronesi. 1981. Prognostic importance of estrogen receptors to select node negative patients for adjuvant chemotherapy, *in* Adjuvant Therapy of Cancer III, S. E. Salmon and S. E. Jones, eds. Grune & Stratton, New York, pp. 329–333.

Weigand, R. A., W. M. Isenberg, J. Russo, M. J. Brennan, M. A. Rick and Breast Cancer Prognostic Study Associates. 1982. Blood vessel invasion and axillary lymph node involvement as prognostic indicators for human breast cancer. Cancer 50:962–969.

Index

N